Strengthening E-Collaboration in Healthcare Through AI

Jingyuan Zhao
https://orcid.org/0000-0003-3289-4048
University of Toronto, Canada

IGI Global
Scientific Publishing
Publishing Tomorrow's Research Today

Vice President of Editorial — Melissa Wagner
Director of Acquisitions — Mikaela Felty
Director of Book Development — Jocelynn Hessler
Production Manager — Mike Brehm
Cover Design — Jose Rosado

Published in the United States of America by
IGI Global Scientific Publishing
701 East Chocolate Avenue
Hershey, PA, 17033, USA
Tel: 717-533-8845 | Fax: 717-533-7115
Website: https://www.igi-global.com E-mail: cust@igi-global.com

Library of Congress Cataloging-in-Publication Data

Names: Zhao, Jingyuan, 1968- editor
Title: Strengthening e-collaboration in healthcare through AI / edited by Jingyuan Zhao.
Description: Hershey, PA : IGI Global Scientific Publishing, [2026] | Includes bibliographical references and index. | Summary: "This book is a collection of recent advancements in strengthening e-collaboration in healthcare through AI and related technologies, enhancing the experiences of both healthcare professionals and patients, and uncovering the potential of collaborative intelligence AI holds for the healthcare sector and the future of work itself in healthcare"-- Provided by publisher.
Identifiers: LCCN 2025034574 (print) | LCCN 2025034575 (ebook) | ISBN 9798337359069 hardcover | ISBN 9798337359076 paperback | ISBN 9798337359083 ebook
Subjects: LCSH: Artificial intelligence--Medical applications | Human-computer interaction | Medical informatics
Classification: LCC R859.7.A78 S77 2026 (print) | LCC R859.7.A78 (ebook)
LC record available at https://lccn.loc.gov/2025034574
LC ebook record available at https://lccn.loc.gov/2025034575

British Cataloguing in Publication Data
A Cataloguing in Publication record for this book is available from the British Library.

Table of Contents

Detailed Table of Contents

practical examples, this research illustrates how low-code platforms can accelerate healthcare digital transformation while maintaining security and compliance standards. The findings reveal that Oracle APEX serves as an effective enabler for healthcare professionals to harness AI capabilities without extensive programming knowledge, ultimately improving patient outcomes and operational efficiency.

A. Sharmila, Saveetha Institute of Medical and Technical Sciences, Chennai, India
K. C. Raja Shree, Saveetha Institute of Medical and Technical Sciences, Chennai, India
G. S. Gigi, Saveetha Institute of Medical and Technical Sciences, Chennai, India
P. Praveen Kumar, SRM Institute of Science and Technology, Vadapalani, India

Healthcare systems are rapidly adopting Artificial Intelligence (AI) to enhance collaboration, decision-making, and efficiency, yet challenges like trust, ethics, and resistance persist. This study extends the Technology Acceptance Model (TAM) to include factors such as Trust, Transparency, Data Security, and Organizational Support. The extended framework captures both technical and human-centered determinants of AI adoption in collaborative healthcare. Using a mixed-methods approach—combining quantitative SEM analysis and qualitative insights—it explores adoption dynamics across healthcare professionals. Findings suggest Trust mediates AI adoption, while Organizational Support and Training predict sustainability. The study offers a socio-technical model for strengthening AI-driven collaboration in healthcare.

R. N. Ravikumar, Marwadi University, Rajkot, India
S. Aarthi, Marwadi University, Rajkot, India

This chapter introduces a Blockchain-Anchored Federated AI framework designed to enable secure, transparent, and patient-centric collaboration in healthcare diagnostics. The model integrates federated learning for decentralized training with blockchain for immutable validation, ensuring privacy preservation, auditability, and fairness among institutions. By eliminating raw data sharing, it strengthens diagnostic accuracy and compliance while promoting interoperability and trust. Smart contracts automate validation, incentivization, and governance, fostering ethical and scalable

a conceptual framework for inclusive, ethical, and sustainable AI-telehealth systems to address healthcare disparities in rural India.

Artificial intelligence is reshaping healthcare by transforming diagnostics, decision making, and population health management. Although machine learning offers gains in accuracy and clinical support, deployment remains uneven because of ethical, infrastructural, and governance challenges. This chapter examines AI's implications across technological capability, socioeconomic context, and governance maturity, showing a gap between potential and performance, especially in settings with limited digital infrastructure or poor data representation. AI can enhance precision and expand access to expertise, yet benefits are constrained by bias, generalizability issues, privacy risks, and limited institutional readiness. Governance often lags innovation, leaving unresolved questions about accountability and oversight. The chapter proposes a strategic approach centered on equitable access, adaptive regulation, interdisciplinary collaboration, and community engagement, arguing that innovation alone cannot transform health systems without strong governance and sustained investment.

The e-collaboration in the healthcare sector could be brought to revolutionary opportunities by Artificial Intelligence (AI) and Quantum Computing. With the world ever growing in digitization, support of secure, real-time as well as intelligent decisions has grown in demand. The paradigm hybrid described in the current paper employs the quantum-enhanced AI to support a seamless interaction among clinicians, patients, and administrators. The framework can be applied to accomplish faster diagnostics, precision medicine, and successful big health data management with the predictive analytics of AI and parallel processing in quantum computing. It presents the decentralized AI models, with quantum optimization, encryption, and resource scheduling algorithms. Interoperability, ethical issues, and quantum hardware

Preface

In the 1970s, interest in biomedical applications of Artificial Intelligence (AI) exploded (Patel, et al., 2009). Since then, the journey of AI in healthcare has never been less. In recent years, the healthcare sector has undergone considerable technological advances, which have had a significant impact on patient care, clinical operations, and healthcare delivery. Advances in AI and emerging digital technologies (e.g., Robotics, Blockchain, IoT, Machine Learning, Quantum Computing, 5G), and their application to healthcare, are becoming increasingly prominent. The recent surge in AI capabilities is poised to bring about significant advancements, such as Low Code/No Code (LCNC) platforms, Robotics Process Automation (RPA), Healthcare IT platforms, AI in diagnostics, Telehealth and remote patient monitoring, Blockchain for healthcare data security, Augmented Reality (AR) and Virtual Reality (VR) in healthcare. These technologies, and new ones under development, hold great potential to assist in diagnosis, clinical decision-making, training, early prediction and prevention, treatment and personalized medicine. Many are predicting that specialty healthcare may fundamentally change, and further, that no areas of healthcare will remain untouched by the profound transformation these technologies are expected to bring. By leveraging AI in hospital settings and clinics, healthcare systems can become smarter, faster, and more efficient in providing care to millions of people worldwide.

Although approvals for the use of AI in healthcare are increasing, the pace and timing of these practice-altering changes are still being explored and debated at the industry and academic level. The challenges the healthcare sector faces are not only the technology itself, but also data privacy and security concerns, biases in algorithms, and regulatory uncertainties. Most importantly, can humans and AI work together for healthcare?

The collaboration and intersection of technology and healthcare is the key for transforming the industry, influencing sectors like labs, dental care, home healthcare, mental health, medical practices, and hospitals, and their application to healthcare (Koebe, 2025). The biggest challenge for AI in various medical services is not determining whether the innovation is strong enough to be helpful but ensuring its acceptance in clinical scheduling. The technologies-based framework needs to be supported by controllers, coordinated with HER (Electronic Health Record) frameworks, normalized by enough people so that similar products function essentially in the same way, trained by doctors, and compensated by open or confidential payers to be widely used (Rashid & Kausik, 2024). The healthcare sector leverages the technologies-enhanced collaboration, addressing challenges such as diagnostic accuracy and medical data analysis, which are critical for improving patient outcomes and advancing medical research (Cui & Yasseri, 2024). For example, the open online system of collective medical insights provides healthcare support to patients. It enables healthcare professionals worldwide to contribute expertise and collaborate on complex diagnostic cases. The platform facilitates idea exchange and mutual learning to ultimately benefit patient care by utilizing machine- learning techniques that automatically learn from classifying patterns in crowdsourced data. It makes the most of limited medical resources by harnessing the collaboration of human physicians and AI enabling more accurate, affordable, and accessible care for those in need.

This book is a collection of advanced convergency of AI for healthcare, uncovering the potential AI hold for the healthcare sector and the future of work itself. This book will comprehensively explore e-collaboration for healthcare through AI, not only studying applications, types, benefits, functions, concerns and trends, but also bringing together humans and AI to drive powerful tech tools that advance the convergency of technology and healthcare. The book is organized into 13 chapters which provide insight on strengthening e-collaboration through AI in healthcare.

CHAPTER OVERVIEW

Chapter 1 (*Harnessing AI for Seamless E-Collaboration in Healthcare through Building Smarter, Connected, and Patient-Centric Systems*) highlights AI's impact across telemedicine, remote diagnostics, multidisciplinary collaboration, and personalized medicine, emphasizing how AI complements human expertise by automating routine tasks and enabling real-time data sharing. It also discusses challenges related to ethics, privacy, and regulation, while outlining future trends and global efforts to standardize AI adoption in healthcare.

Chapter 2 (*A Three Pillar Data-Centric Framework for Enabling AI-Driven Healthcare Collaboration*) presents a three-pillar framework: AI/Graph-Based Identity Resolution for unified patient representation across systems, AI/LLM-Driven Semantic Harmonization for consistent terminology, and Metadata Intelligence &

AI-Native Data Fabric for machine-operable structure. It also demonstrates how addressing data infrastructure enables scalable AI-driven collaboration in healthcare.

Chapter 3 (*Secure Software Engineering for AI-Enhanced E-Collaboration in Healthcare: Building Resilient and Interoperable Systems*) demonstrates best practices in secure architecture, HL7/FHIR integration, role-based access control, and AI transparency. The goal is to empower developers, IT leaders, and clinicians to co-create secure and effective digital ecosystems that protect patient data while improving care coordination and delivery.

Chapter 4 (*Democratizing Healthcare AI Through Low-Code Platforms - Oracle APEX as an Enabler of Collaborative Intelligence: A Practical Framework for Clinical Innovation*) illustrates how low-code platforms can accelerate healthcare digital transformation while maintaining security and compliance standards. The findings reveal that Oracle APEX serves as an effective enabler for healthcare professionals to harness AI capabilities without extensive programming knowledge, ultimately improving patient outcomes and operational efficiency.

Chapter 5 (*Strengthening AI Adoption in Healthcare Collaboration: Extending the Technology Acceptance Model*) extends the Technology Acceptance Model (TAM) to include factors such as Trust, Transparency, Data Security, and Organizational Support. The extended framework captures both technical and human-centered determinants of AI adoption in collaborative healthcare. The study offers a socio-technical model for strengthening AI-driven collaboration in healthcare.

Chapter 6 (*Blockchain-Anchored Federated AI for Patient-Centric Collaborative Diagnostics*) discusses architecture design, experimental evaluation, challenges, and future research directions, emphasizing its potential to transform global digital healthcare into a secure, accountable, and equitable ecosystem driven by collaborative intelligence.

Chapter 7 (*Symbiotic Human-AI Workflows - Augmented Telepsychiatry and Intelligent Care Teams*) examines the Belkin framework for human-AI collaboration, exploring how NLP, predictive analytics, and virtual assistants enhance clinical capacity while sustaining therapeutic alliances. The chapter establishes augmented intelligence as a crucial foundation for psychiatric care that is accessible, ethical, and patient-centered.

Chapter 8 (*AI-Driven Telehealth in Rural India - Challenges, Adoption Behaviour, and Collaborative Strategies*) is a conceptual discussion on the transformative impact of Artificial Intelligence in improving telehealth delivery in rural India. It analyses behavioural, systemic, and strategic aspects of AI-enabled healthcare uptake by incorporating integrative models, such as TAM, UTAUT, and UTAUT2.

Chapter 9 (*Strengthening E-Collaboration in Healthcare Through AI: The Promise and Peril of Artificial Intelligence in Healthcare: A Critical Analysis*) proposes a strategic approach centered on equitable access, adaptive regulation, interdisciplinary collaboration, and community engagement, arguing that innovation alone cannot transform health systems without strong governance and sustained investment.

Chapter 10 (*Revolutionizing Digital Healthcare Collaboration through Quantum-Enhanced AI Technologies*) presents a hybrid paradigm that leverages quantum-enhanced AI to enable seamless collaboration among clinicians, patients, and administrators. By combining AI's predictive analytics with quantum computing's parallel processing, the framework supports faster diagnostics, precision medicine, and efficient big health data management.

Chapter 11 (*Strengthening E-Collaboration in Healthcare Through AI: Quantum computing and e-collaboration for healthcare*) presents that quantum-enabled back-ends can strengthen digital collaboration by supporting remote consultations, shared clinical reviews, and coordinated care. Secure communication, privacy-preserving analytics, biomedical simulation, and public-health preparedness are discussed, along with current limitations and future directions.

Chapter 12 (*Enhancing EHR Systems with Artificial Intelligence: Enabling Seamless Patient-Clinician Collaboration*) examines how responsibly integrating AI into EHRs can bridge the gap between data and care, strengthen trust, and promote equitable, human-centered healthcare. Clinicians can detect early warning signs, recommend tailored treatments, and focus more on patient care, while AI-driven dashboards and chatbots help patients understand their data, engage in shared decisions, and track progress.

Chapter 13 (*A Collaborative AI Framework for Rare Event Modelling in Early Alzheimer's Detection: Multi-Modal, Federated, and Explainable Deep Learning*) presents a collaborative AI framework for rare event modelling in early Alzheimer's detection using multimodal, federated, and explainable deep learning. The purpose is to address late diagnosis, class imbalance, privacy restrictions, limited generalizability, and lack of transparency in current systems.

Jingyuan Zhao
University of Toronto, Canada

REFERENCES

Cui, H., & Yasseri, T. (2024). AI-enhanced collective intelligence. *Patterns (New York, N.Y.)*, *5*(11), 101074. DOI: 10.1016/j.patter.2024.101074 PMID: 39568478

Koebe, P. (2025). How digital technologies and AI contribute to achieving the health-related SDGs. *International Journal of Information Management Data Insights*, *5*(1), 100298. Advance online publication. DOI: 10.1016/j.jjimei.2024.100298

Patel, V. L., Shortliffe, E. H., Stefanelli, M., Szolovits, P., Berthold, M. R., Bellazzi, R., & Abu-Hanna, A. (2009). The coming of age of artificial intelligence in medicine. *Artificial Intelligence in Medicine*, *46*(1), 5–17. DOI: 10.1016/j.artmed.2008.07.017 PMID: 18790621

Rashid, A. B., & Kausik, M. A. K. (2024). AI Revolutionizing Industries Worldwide: A Comprehensive Overview of Its Diverse Applications. *Hybrid Advances*, *7*, 100277. Advance online publication. DOI: 10.1016/j.hybadv.2024.100277

Chapter 1

Harnessing AI for Seamless E-Collaboration in Healthcare Through Building Smarter, Connected, and Patient-Centric Systems

Noboranjan Dey
http://orcid.org/0009-0007-1991-9198
American International University-Bangladesh, Bangladesh

Kazi Tanvir
http://orcid.org/0009-0001-0612-6101
American International University-Bangladesh, Bangladesh

Mahfujur Rahman
http://orcid.org/0000-0002-3245-8767
American International University-Bangladesh, Bangladesh

Rahul Biswas
http://orcid.org/0009-0009-4459-4756
School of Technology and Innovation, University of Vaasa, Vaasa, Finland

Shaikat Das Joy
http://orcid.org/0009-0001-1657-3140
American International University-Bangladesh, Bangladesh

Dipta Gomes
http://orcid.org/0000-0003-3019-6051
American International University-Bangladesh, Bangladesh

ABSTRACT

This chapter explores the transformative role of Artificial Intelligence (AI) in healthcare, focusing on its evolution from experimental technology to a key driver of digital transformation and e-collaboration. It examines how advances in machine learning, natural language processing, robotics, blockchain, and Internet of

DOI: 10.4018/979-8-3373-5906-9.ch001

Medical Things (IoMT) have enabled AI-powered tools to enhance patient care, clinical decision-making, and operational efficiency. The chapter highlights AI's impact across telemedicine, remote diagnostics, multidisciplinary collaboration, and personalized medicine, emphasizing how AI complements human expertise by automating routine tasks and enabling real-time data sharing. It also discusses challenges related to ethics, privacy, and regulation, while outlining future trends and global efforts to standardize AI adoption in healthcare.

1. INTRODUCTION

Artificial Intelligence (AI) has gone through a path of development from an experiment to an agent of change in the healthcare environment globally. Over the past few decades, AI emerged out of the laboratory into widespread clinical and operational use due to development in machine learning, natural language processing, computer vision, robotics, blockchain, Internet of Things (IoT), and quantum computing (Munia et al., 2025). Recent developments like Low Code/No Code (LCNC) platforms, robotic process automation (RPA), AI-based diagnostics, telehealth, patient remote monitoring, and intelligent virtual assistants have seen increased speed of change (Garg et al., 2025). They are changing the overall operations in patient care, clinical decision-making, and optimal information, and permit personalized medicine (Ueda et al., 2024). Making the healthcare industry more efficient and cost-effective, eliminating time-wasting and error-prone paper trails, and reducing the risk of document loss and leakage is increasingly being seen as a promise of the digital transformation wave (Olawade et al., 2024) that will not leave any aspects of healthcare, including diagnostics, treatment, prevention, and education, unscathed.

The core of this transformation lies in the e-collaboration that may be defined as the cooperation mediated by the use of digital technology between healthcare professionals, institutions, patients and intelligent systems (Bajwa et al., 2021). AI-powered e-collaboration helps eliminate the old obstacles of geography, time zones and institutional boundaries and can share data in real-time, consult in real-time and coordinate a coordinated response in real time (Rahman et al., 2023). Incorporating electronic health records (EHRs), imaging information, laboratory data, wearable device data, and patient-reported outcomes in a single connected platform, these kinds of combined solutions unite these and other data sources in secure, universally accessible, multidisciplinary environments (Secinaro et al., 2021). These features enable health care professionals to achieve agreement quickly, distribute coordinated course of care, and maximize the application of rare resources (Dhiman et al., 2024). The outcome has been a system of collective intelligence where the expertise of human beings and AI are combined to produce improved health outcomes in less time (Badwy et al., 2024).

This chapter will explore the role of AI in reinforcing e-collaboration in various fields such as telemedicine and remote diagnosing, multidisciplinary team conferences in oncology and cardiology, continuous patient monitoring assisted by the Internet of medical things, blockchain-secured exchange of health data, generative AI to interact multilingually and synthesize medical reports, extended reality (XR) to collaborate in training and surgery simulators effectively, and big data analytics to plan coordinated community health strategies (Giron-Michel et al., 2025). It will demonstrate how AI complements human decision-making by providing forecasting, pattern identification, and evidence-based suggestions while automating routine procedures like scheduling care, dealing with claims, and producing clinical reports (Tiwari et al., 2025). AI, which helps with data-heavy and menial jobs, leaves healthcare workers free to concentrate on complicated, value-creating tasks that require complex human empathy, reason, and ethical judgment (Al-Antari, 2023).

The organization of the chapter follows a logical progression, beginning with an introduction in Section 1 that outlines the evolution and significance of AI in healthcare. It then traces the historical development of AI in Section 2, highlighting key milestones from early diagnostic tools to current advances in machine learning and deep learning in Section 3. The chapter delves into the key technologies enabling AI, such as machine learning, deep learning, the Internet of Medical Things (IoMT), blockchain, and robotics, while examining their applications across diagnostic imaging, telemedicine, clinical decision support systems, and personalized medicine in Section 4 and Section 5. Challenges and risks in implementing AI for E-Collaboration have been discussed in Section 6. Ethical, regulatory, and governance strategies, challenges, including privacy concerns, algorithmic bias, and the need for comprehensive regulations, are addressed in Section 7 and Section 8. The chapter concludes by exploring future trends, barriers to AI adoption, and global efforts to standardize AI practices in healthcare in Section 9 and Section 10.

1. THE EVOLUTION OF AI IN HEALTHCARE

1.1. Historical Trajectory of AI in Medicine

The development of AI in healthcare has been a fascinating journey, from its earliest, primitive forms to high-end systems that drive personalized medicine, diagnostic agents, and other patient-centered applications. The journey began in the 1950s, when the possibility of AI in solving complex problems was first envisioned in the field of medicine (Munia et al., 2025).

1.1.1. Early AI Applications: Diagnostic Tools and Expert Systems

During the infancy of AI, expert systems and diagnostic tools played a pivotal role in transforming the field of medicine. The first real AI applications, such as MYCIN (developed in the 1970s), were designed to assist medical professionals in diagnosing bacterial infections and recommending antibiotics. Although not long after, the bonus-based performance measure was replaced by competition and reward systems to avoid favoritism, it later extended the influence of profit-sharing into a mechanism for speedup.

1.1.2. Milestones in AI Development and Integration

As AI has advanced, it has achieved several breakthroughs that have enhanced its capabilities and expanded its applications in healthcare. By the 2000s, machine learning algorithms began to perform well in diagnosing diseases and predicting patient survival. A significant advancement in the field of healthcare occurred when AI was integrated with EHRs, leading to CDSS from which new medical services and inferential insights can be generated (Olawade et al., 2024).

Deep learning techniques have also been more recently applied in medical imaging, genomics, and personalized medicine, leading to a paradigm shift for the healthcare ecosystem. Artificial intelligence is on the Rise, with AI-based platforms that can understand large medical data sets, extending the role of AI to assist in virtual health assistants and predictive patient outcomes. These advances have been instrumental in developing more intelligent, interconnected, and patient-focused systems for medicine (Ueda et al., 2024).

Figure 1 illustrates that key milestones in the history of AI in healthcare have significantly contributed to its evolution and defined its current clinical applications. The role of AI in healthcare evolved steadily, starting from the 1960s with MYCIN, one of the early expert systems that helped diagnose bacterial infections. In the 1970s, programs such as INTERNIST-1 were developed to further AI in medical diagnostics, initially targeted at the field of internal medicine. In the 1980s and 1990s, medical imaging and pattern recognition were explored as opportunities for AI integration in radiology. At the same time, clinical decision support systems (CDSS) became one of the earliest practical applications of AI in this field. In the 2000s, machine learning emerged, paving the way for AI to enhance diagnosis and predict patient outcomes. Deep learning experienced a significant breakthrough in the 2010s, particularly in medical imaging and genomics, leading to more precise disease detection and personalized treatments. The next decade will bring us AI-driven customized medicine, predictive analytics, and virtual health assistants that will form the backbone of more intelligent, connected, patient-centric systems (Saeidnia & Nilashi, 2025).

Figure 1. AI Milestones in Healthcare

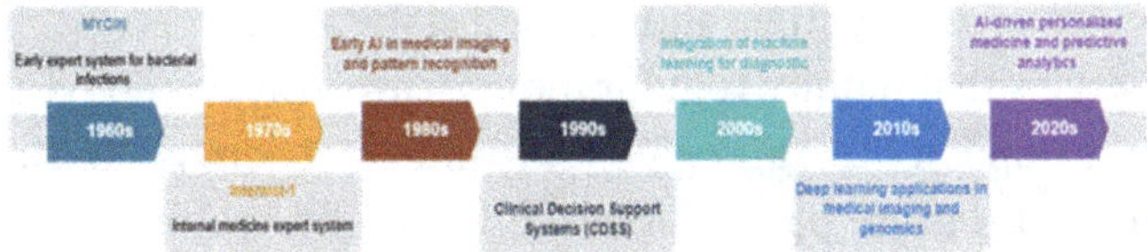

1.2. Key Enabling Technologies

Electronic health records and other enabling technologies. Several enabling technologies have primarily driven the success of AI in healthcare. These tools enable faster and more efficient data processing, decision-making, and patient care.

1.2.1. Machine Learning (ML) & Deep Learning (DL) used in healthcare

ML and DL are two indispensable technologies behind AI in healthcare. Machine learning encompasses learning algorithms that enable a system to learn from data and make predictions/decisions, thereby eliminating the need for explicit programming. In healthcare, ML is used in predictive modelling, including the prediction of patient outcomes or the identification of high-risk patients (Garg et al., 2025).

Deep learning, a subfield of ML, relies on neural networks to handle intricate data such as images, sounds, and language (Gomes et al., 2021). In the field of medical imaging, deep learning has demonstrated remarkable effectiveness in interpreting X-rays, MRIs, and CT scans, in some cases even surpassing the accuracy of human radiologists (Ueda et al., 2024). Given that deep learning is increasingly being used for personalized treatments and understanding how a given model works (e.g., once degraded, it could predict the probability of individual cell degradation based on its functional network features), there are many opportunities, such as applying these models to genetic data for response predictions.

1.2.2. Integration of IoMT (Internet of Medical Things in Healthcare

The Internet of Medical Things (IoMT) refers to connected medical devices and applications that can transfer patient data in real-time over a network (Islam et al., 2025). Such devices, including wearable devices like pacemakers and wearables (such as glucose sensors and heart rate monitors), produce streaming data that AI systems can analyze to monitor patient health and provide real-time feedback on patient status (Munia et al., 2025).

AI, in conjunction with IoMT, enhances the accuracy and speed of diagnoses, while also enabling remote patient monitoring (Islam et al., 2025). For individuals with chronic diseases that require regular monitoring, this would be especially helpful. Moreover, the capacity to aggregate real-time data across multiple devices and systems will support a more patient-focused model of healthcare delivery (Bajwa et al., 2021).

1.2.3. Cutting-edge Technologies Shaping AI in Healthcare

Blockchain is a game-changer in securing privacy and trust mechanisms for healthcare data. Through this mechanism, blockchain ensures that patient data remains secure and private, while also being accessible to those who need it and have the necessary access. AI and blockchain could work together to secure data transfer across organisational boundaries, as well as ensuring the integrity of health records (Olawade et al., 2024; Sarker et al., 2025). Another major driver related to AI in healthcare is Robotics, which has achieved explosive growth overall, particularly in surgical applications. Most AI-based robots have been designed to assist with minimally invasive surgery, providing higher precision and quicker recovery. They can also be employed in rehabilitation to help individuals regain mobility after surgery or an accident.

Quantum computing, which is still in its infancy, could be an AI game-changer for healthcare with processing power well beyond the reach of classical computers. Quantum computers may help accelerate pharmaceutical discoveries and simplify complex medical simulations, although this potential remains unverified (Bajwa et al., 2021).

1.2.4. Democratizing AI Use in Healthcare

Low-code/no-code and Robotic Process Automation (RPA) are democratizing AI for caregivers by enabling non-technical users to create applications using AI, as well as automate everyday administrative tasks. These are widely adopted by individuals in the medical profession for the development of ad-hoc solutions, without requiring substantial programming skills, and thus help expedite the uptake of AI into practice (Garg et al., 2025). For instance, AI applications for patient scheduling or billing automation can be developed using low-code platforms to help enhance efficiency and reduce the administrative workload of healthcare providers.

Each of the enabling technologies that we examined in previous sections such as ML, DL, IoMT, Blockchain, Robotics, Quantum Computing, Low-Code/No-Code Platforms, and RPA. These are pivotal in transforming healthcare. Artificial Intelligence and Deep Learning have become integral to the predictive analytics architecture, enabling greater accuracy in disease diagnosis, risk assessment, and personalized treatment options (Garg et al., 2025; Hasan et al., 2024; Ueda et al., 2024). The IoMT, which integrates medical equipment and wearable devices, enables real-time monitoring of patients, potentially enhancing disease management and improving patient outcomes (Munia et al., 2025). The use of blockchain technology offers enhanced security in sharing information and increased transparency, which can foster trust in digital health systems (Olawade et al., 2024). Surgery Robotics has also made valuable contributions to surgery and patient care, with increased accuracy and shorter recovery times (Bajwa et al., 2021). Quantum computing, although still in its early stages of development, holds potential for enhancing complex medical simulations and drug discovery (Bajwa et al., 2021). Low-code or no-code systems democratize the development of AI applications, allowing healthcare workers to create custom solutions without an extensive background in computer science (Garg et al., 2025). Finally, RPA also helps automate menial administrative tasks, improve operational efficiency, and decrease healthcare provider burnout (Garg et al., 2025). This combination of technologies, feeding off one another, is propelling healthcare into a more intelligent and practical future for patients.

Table 1 summarizes the enabling technologies behind healthcare-specific AI methodologies, focusing on their application areas and inferences on the healthcare ecosystem. ML and DL, for instance, enable AI solutions to analyse highly complex medical data, thereby enhancing diagnostics and supporting personalized treatments. IoMT links medical devices to monitor patients continually and analyse data in real-time. With the stupendous growth in cloud storage and sharing marketplaces, a secure method for sharing data with transparency is provided through Blockchain technology, which helps establish trust in digital health records. The surgical precision with which robotics has taken hold, even fucking rehabilitation, is being supported, and early updates from exciting new fields such as Quantum Computing can get us further in finding drugs. Low-Code/No-Code, Robotic Process Automation (RPA) that accelerates the development of AI applications and automates repetitive tasks to increase productivity and decrease administrative burden in healthcare. Together, these technologies are helping to provide better, more precise care in ways that improve efficiency and focus on the patient.

Table 1. Technology's function and impact on healthcare.

Technology	Function	Impact on Healthcare
Machine Learning (ML)	Allows systems to learn from data to make predictions or decisions.	Improves diagnostics, predicts patient outcomes, and supports decision-making.
Deep Learning (DL)	An advanced form of ML using neural networks to interpret complex data (images, audio, etc.).	Enhances image analysis, genomics, and personalized treatments with high accuracy.
Internet of Medical Things (IoMT)	Interconnected medical devices that send patient data in real-time for monitoring.	Enables continuous monitoring of patients, particularly for managing chronic illnesses.
Blockchain	A decentralized, transparent system for securing data and ensuring privacy.	Ensures secure data exchange, improving trust in digital health records and services.
Robotics	AI-powered machines that assist in surgeries, rehabilitation, and precision medicine.	Enhances surgical precision, reduces recovery time, and facilitates rehabilitation.
Quantum Computing	Computing technology that holds the potential to solve complex problems in healthcare faster.	Accelerates drug discovery, medical simulations, and optimizes personalized treatments.
Low-Code/No-Code Platforms	Platforms that enable non-technical users to develop applications without coding.	Democratizes the development of healthcare applications, allowing faster innovation.
Robotic Process Automation (RPA)	Automating repetitive administrative tasks enhances operational efficiency.	Increases efficiency, reduces administrative burden, and enhances operational workflows.

1.3. Broader Policy and Regulatory Context

Exploring to a broader context in policy and regulatory frameworks further shaped the implementation and adoption of these technologies in healthcare. The evolution of policies such as the Health Insurance Portability and Accountability Act (HIPAA) and General Data Protection Regulation (GDPR) (Khalid et al., 2023) in order to contextualizing the development of AI tools within legal and ethical boundaries. These regulations have had a significant impact on the use of healthcare data, which is the lifeblood of AI-driven systems (Morley et al., 2022). HIPAA et the stage for ensuring the privacy and security of patient information in the digital age, which directly influences AI's ability to process sensitive medical data, whereas GDPR introduced more stringent data protection requirements for AI systems deployed in the European Union, affecting everything from data collection to model transparency and consent practices.

It is important to highlight that regulatory frameworks continue to evolve alongside technological advancements. AI becomes more integrated into clinical workflows, issues like data sovereignty, algorithmic accountability, and model transparency have emerged as key concerns, necessitating further regulatory scrutiny.

2. DEFINING E-COLLABORATION IN HEALTHCARE

2.1. Conceptual Foundation: Digital Cooperation

E-collaboration in healthcare refers to the technologically enabled collaboration that captures, analyzes, and shares health information among distant settings to support clinical decision-making, care coordination, and organizational change. In practice, it combines AI-supported decision support with secure data flow from connected technologies that enables continuous real-time monitoring and timely intervention (Bajwa et al., 2021; Garg et al., 2025; Hosain et al., 2024). Privacy-aware collaborative model development, such as federated learning in the field of innovative healthcare (Sarker et al., 2025), will further promote inter-institutional cooperation and address issues of governance and accountability (Rahman et al., 2023; Ueda et al., 2024). These interactions are supported by dependable, low-latency connections and robust IoT infrastructures, connecting homes, clinics, and hospitals to form responsive care networks (J. Li et al., 2024; Taimoor & Rehman, 2022). As a result, the stakeholder set is broad and interrelated: patients whose data and outcomes ground the enterprise; frontline clinicians (in primary care, specialty care) practicing on their behalf; nurses and allied health professionals coordinating daily actions to achieve best practices; pharmacists engaged in medication safety and therapy expertise; hospital level leadership and clinical operations teams shaping conditions for high quality events.; AI developers, data scientists, IT/ security staff building/maintaining systems that use these data; ethics/governance bodies working to steward fairness, transparency, responsible use with presently intense due to IoT-rich environments/AI-intensive contexts (Jessica et al., 2025; Solanki et al., 2023; Wakili & Bakkali, 2024). Together, these elements form a collaborative framework that is patient-centered, data-driven, and ethically compliant, fostering a fabric of teamwork that transcends time, place, and organization (Bajwa et al., 2021; J. Li et al., 2024).

2.1.1. Benefits of real-time collaboration across diverse teams

Cross-disciplinary collaboration in real-time CDR supports earlier detection of deterioration, more precise and timely treatment decisions, and integrates care across home, clinic, imaging suite, and hospital floor. Internet of Things (IoT)-enabled biosensors and connected devices, coupled with deep learning analytics, enable superior patient monitoring and diagnosis, resulting in more expedited and individualized interventions (Alharbe & Almalki, 2025; Hosain et al., 2024). Evidence from oncology, as well as other fields, supports the potential for AI to enhance diagnostic precision and refine therapeutic approaches which particularly when insights are intended to be collectively applied (Tiwari et al., 2025). Simultaneously, robust, real-time infrastructures (e.g., IoT and new) and fair-minded monitoring enhance the dependability and fairness of these collective workflows (Taimoor & Rehman, 2022; Ueda et al., 2024).

Figure 2. Key components and stakeholders in e-collaboration.

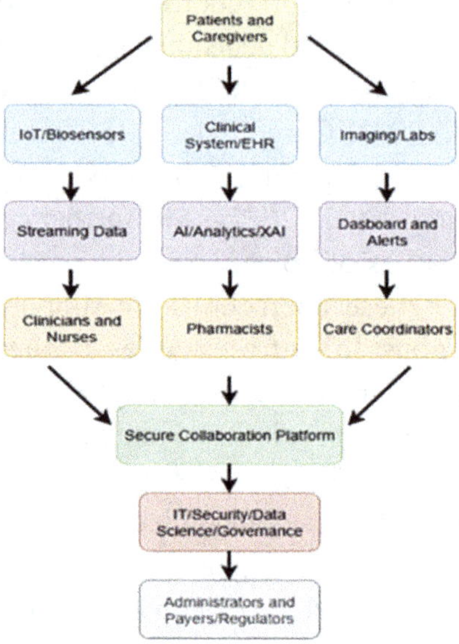

In Figure 2, E-collaboration links real-time data capture (wearables/IoT and clinical systems) to AI services for triage, prediction, and imaging insights along with explanations that are clinician-facing, thus enabling cross-functional teams to collaborate in real-time using shared dashboards, virtual huddles, and secure messaging to make decisions together. Cross-institutional learning is enabled by federated approaches that do not require the sharing of raw data. At the same time, governance functions (fairness, safety, security, reliability) and operational teams uphold trust and resilience across home to hospital settings (Bajwa et al., 2021; Garg et al., 2025; Mirbabaie et al., 2022).

2.2. From Traditional to AI-Powered Models

Historically, collaboration was primarily conducted in person or over the phone, with data scattered across paper charts and siloed systems. Digitization also introduced teleconsults, shared EHR views, and secure messaging. Today's AI-aided e-collaboration includes predictive triage, image and signal-based decision support, as well as remote continuous monitoring. Evidence syntheses describe how AI is changing diagnostic and care pathways, while emphasizing the necessity of responsible implementation to safeguard safety and effectiveness (Al-Antari, 2023; Bajwa et al., 2021). Along the fringe, when combined with deep learning, IoT extends its reach beyond the walls of the clinic by facilitating real-time surveillance and team management for chronic diseases and acute deterioration (Hosain et al., 2024; J. Li et al., 2024).

Notably, trust enablers are evolving to keep pace with their capabilities. Explainability is closely tied to human oversight in image interpretation and other high-stakes decisions (Garg et al., 2025). Fairness guidance is designed to reduce disparities in performance among subgroups (Ueda et al., 2024). Privacy-preserving learning (e.g., federated learning) enables cross-institutional model refinement without centralizing sensitive data (Rahman et al., 2023b). Robust and secure architectural patterns are being developed to mitigate cyber-physical risk in AI-IoT pipelines (Mohsin Khan et al., 2025; Taimoor & Rehman, 2022). Such guardrails are especially crucial as AI continues to expand into pharmacy services, mental healthcare, and hospital operations through introducing new collaborators and workflows into the mix (Mirbabaie et al., 2022; Olawade et al., 2024).

2.2.1. Transition from traditional face-to-face consultations to AI-assisted models

Traditionally, face-to-face interactions have served as the primary method for cooperation and information exchange, occurring in synchronous yet intermittent episodes. AI-assisted models, on the other hand, combine continuous sensing (IoT), algorithmic triage and diagnostics, and privacy-aware learning across organizations, while building in understandability, fairness, and security to maintain trust. Reviews of hospital and healthcare delivery AI highlight both the promise of precision, efficiency, and personalization and the requirement of protective measures that rely upon accountability and patient safety (Mirbabaie et al., 2022; Mohsin Khan et al., 2025; Olawade et al., 2024).

Table 2 illustrates the comparison used to demonstrate the structural transition from episodic, EHR-bound, face-to-face coordination to work bounded by data shared among a team and ongoing over time. In legacy models, information is passed around and through patients by memory and handoffs between clinicians, but in AI-enabled e-collaboration, clinical data pours into such systems in a digital way where sensors relay measurements that are then boiled down into ongoing alerts, risk scores, and evidence-based recommendations that many are empowered to act upon, especially working together. Federated learning facilitates inter-institutional collaboration without sharing of raw data; fairness and ethics frameworks recommend how to ensure responsible deployment; resilient connectivity supports dependability during routine care and escalation, thus helping to make systems more responsive, precise, and patient-centred (Bajwa et al., 2021; Rahman et al., 2023; Taimoor & Rehman, 2022).

Table 2. Comparison chart of collaboration models over time (traditional vs. AI-enabled)

Dimension	Traditional (face-to-face, manual)	AI-enabled e-collaboration
Data flow	Episodic, chart-centric	Continuous streams from IoT, imaging, and clinical systems (Hosain et al., 2024; C. Li et al., 2024)
Communication	Sequential handoffs	Shared dashboards, alerts, and virtual huddles informed by analytics (Bajwa et al., 2021; Olawade et al., 2024)
Decision support	Expert judgment alone	AI-assisted triage/diagnosis with explainable outputs (Garg et al., 2025; Tiwari et al., 2025)
Collaboration across orgs	Limited by data-sharing constraints	Federated learning enables cross-institutional model building without moving raw data (Rahman et al., 2023)
Reliability & reach	Variable access, slow escalation	Resilient, low-latency services over modern networks (Taimoor & Rehman, 2022)
Governance	Local policies	Systematic attention to fairness, safety, and trust (Mohsin Khan et al., 2025; Ueda et al., 2024)

2.3. Key Knowledge gaps and limitations

Despite the exciting prospects of potential of AI in healthcare, there are notable gaps particularly with respect to the limitations and challenges that have emerged from real-world applications. While many AI systems have demonstrated impressive results in controlled environments, several have failed when deployed in clinical practice due to issues like bias in algorithms or insufficient generalizability to diverse populations. AI models trained on data from predominantly white, affluent populations may not perform well in more diverse, global patient populations, leading to healthcare disparities (Obermeyer et al., 2019). Moreover, AI's role in clinical decision support is still often subject to uncertainty, especially in high-risk environments such as emergency rooms or critical care units.

Additionally, there is a lack of consensus regarding how to effectively measure and assess AI's impact on patient outcomes. Traditional clinical evaluation frameworks may not be adequate for evaluating the long-term effectiveness of AI-driven interventions, particularly in areas such as patient trust, care continuity, and clinician adoption (Challen et al., 2019).

3. AI-DRIVEN E-COLLABORATION: KEY DOMAINS OF APPLICATIONS

AI-driven E-collaboration integrates machine intelligence into the clinical and administrative pathways that connect patients, providers, devices, and institutions. The following subsections synthesize 2024-2025 evidence across principal domains of application, emphasizing how AI augments workflows, supports decision making, and enables scalable collaboration.

3.1. Telemedicine and Remote Diagnostics

Figure 3. AI-enhanced telemedicine process

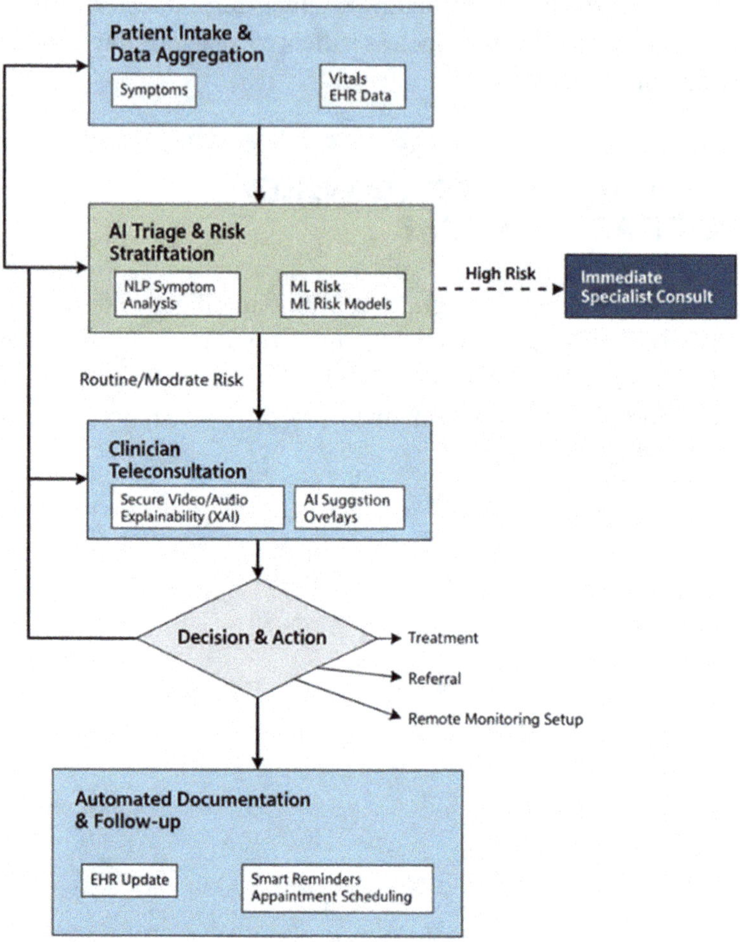

Telemedicine has matured into multi-modal care pathways in which AI systems perform triage, pre-analysis of clinical images and signals, decision support, and automated documentation. The modern AI-enhanced telemedicine pipeline begins with patient intake and automated symptom triage (classifier/decision trees), proceeds through remote data acquisition (images, point-of-care measures), applies AI pre-analysis and risk stratification, and culminates in an augmented clinician teleconsultation with AI-generated suggestions and structured documentation (e.g., SOAP-style summaries) (Figure 3). Recent reviews document improved triage accuracy, reduced clinician review time, and better resource allocation when AI modules are incorporated into telemedicine workflows (Zhang et al., 2024).

Empirical studies also illustrate domain-specific gains: AI image-analysis models in diagnostic tele-dermatology and radiology reduce false negatives in screening tasks and accelerate specialist throughput (Bae, 2024, 2024; Díaz et al., 2024). These systems are most effective when clinicians validate AI outputs and when explainability overlays are provided to support trust and regulatory compliance (Bae, 2024; Díaz et al., 2024).

3.2. Multidisciplinary Team Conferences

Multidisciplinary team (MDT) conferences require integration of imaging, pathology, laboratory, and narrative data. AI supports MDT collaboration by (a) generating concise, evidence-linked case summaries, (b) retrieving relevant literature and guidelines in real time, and (c) providing prognostic models that inform risk-benefit deliberations. Studies from 2024-2025 show that LLMs and structured decision-support tools can shorten MDT meeting time and improve consensus quality when outputs are clinician-reviewed and provenance is preserved (Bertolo et al., 2025; Mathkor et al., 2024; Tjhin et al., 2024).

However, research cautions that AI should augment rather than replace clinical reasoning; validation studies, transparent performance reporting, and audit trails are necessary to avoid propagation of errors and to maintain medicolegal accountability (Dasa et al., 2025; Khosravi et al., 2024; J. Li et al., 2024).

3.3. Remote Monitoring and IoMT-Driven Care

The Internet of Medical Things (IoMT) produces continuous sensor streams from wearables, implantables, and environmental monitors. AI converts these high-velocity data into clinically actionable risk scores and personalized alerts, enabling proactive outpatient interventions and closed-loop care (edge inference + cloud analytics). Recent deployments report reductions in emergency visits and rehospitalization risk for chronic disease cohorts when AI-generated alerts trigger timely teleconsultation or care plan adjustments (Jafleh et al., 2024; LaBoone & Marques, 2024; Mathkor et al., 2024).

Architecturally, effective IoMT ecosystems balance on-device preprocessing (latency, privacy) with cloud-based aggregation for population analytics and model retraining. Security and device interoperability are recurrent concerns; studies recommend secure gateways, standardized telemetry schemas, and federated learning to preserve privacy while enabling cross-site model improvement (Figure 4).

Figure 4. IoMT ecosystem with AI integration

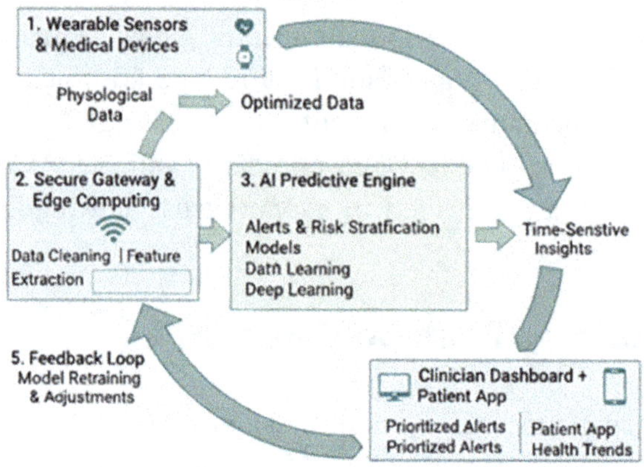

3.4. Blockchain-Secured Health Data Exchange

Interoperability and secure provenance are essential for cross-institutional e-collaboration. Blockchain and hybrid DLT architectures can provide immutable audit trails, consent smart contracts, and tamper-evident pointers to off-chain clinical artifacts. Recent technical proposals and frameworks recommend hybrid solutions that store large clinical files off-chain while recording consent, hashes, and access logs on-chain to achieve scalability and GDPR/HIPAA alignment (Al-Khasawneh et al., 2024; Kasyapa & Vanmathi, 2024; Mehraeen & Mahmoudi, 2024). Privacy-preserving computation, standardized identity frameworks, and legal harmonization are required to operationalize ledger-based exchange in clinical environments has been presented in Figure 5.

Figure 5. Blockchain for health data exchange

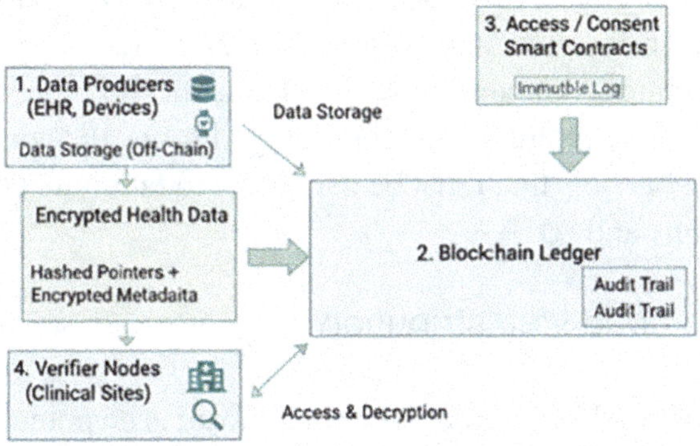

3.5. Generative AI for Communication and Record Synthesis

Generative AI (LLMs) has demonstrated capability to create structured clinical notes, discharge summaries, patient-facing explanations, and meeting minutes. Controlled evaluations indicate substantial clinician time savings when LLM outputs are post-edited; however, hallucination risk and privacy concerns necessitate grounding strategies (citation linking source documents) and clinician sign-off workflows (Kernberg et al., 2024; Xu & Wang, 2024).

LLMs are also being trialed as meeting assistants in telemedicine and MDTs (Bertolo et al., 2025) that extracting action items and surfacing relevant guidelines in real time which can substantially improve follow-up and coordination if auditability and traceability are engineered into the system.

3.6. Extended Reality (XR) and AI-Supported Training

XR (VR/AR) combined with AI analytics provides adaptive simulation for procedural training, team skills, and diagnostic tasks. Systematic reviews report improved skill acquisition and retention in AI-augmented XR environments; AI enables real-time performance scoring and personalized feedback that accelerates mastery and supports distributed e-collaboration in training programs.

3.7. Human-AI Collaboration and Cognitive Workflows

As AI continues to make inroads into healthcare, its integration into clinical settings is not merely a technological shift but a profound transformation in how healthcare professionals perform their work. AI's role is not to replace clinicians but to support and augment their decision-making by automating routine tasks, providing data-driven insights, and helping clinicians focus on complex, human-centered aspects of care (Akinnagbe, 2024). This section explores the redistribution of cognitive load between human clinicians and AI tools, the adaptation of clinical workflows, and the barriers that must be overcome to facilitate effective collaboration between humans and AI.

3.7.1. Cognitive Load Redistribution

One of the primary advantages of AI in healthcare is its potential to alleviate the cognitive burden on clinicians. Cognitive load refers to the mental effort required to process information and make decisions. Clinicians face a high cognitive load in managing complex patient data, diagnosing conditions, making treatment decisions, and coordinating care. As AI systems become more advanced, they can assist by automating routine, repetitive tasks such as documentation, basic diagnostics, and data entry, allowing healthcare professionals to focus on more complex and nuanced aspects of patient care.

AI-driven tools can automatically extract and organize patient information from electronic health records (EHRs), allowing clinicians to spend less time on administrative tasks and more time on patient interaction and critical decision-making(Mehraeen & Mahmoudi, 2024). AI applications like predictive analytics can provide alerts for potential complications or worsening conditions, which helps clinicians prioritize their attention and resources effectively. Additionally, AI-powered diagnostic tools can assist in analyzing medical images or laboratory results, offering clinicians a second opinion and reducing the risk of human error (Shah et al., 2024).

By redistributing cognitive load in this way, AI not only enhances clinician efficiency but also helps mitigate burnout, a growing concern in the healthcare sector due to the increasing demands placed on healthcare workers.

3.7.2. Clinical Workflow Adaptation

AI tools are not standalone systems; they need to be integrated into existing clinical workflows in ways that enhance, rather than disrupt, the daily routines of healthcare professionals. This integration involves understanding how AI fits into the processes of diagnosis, treatment, and patient management. As a result, AI tools can be seamlessly incorporated into EHR systems, where they can flag critical changes in patient status, such as abnormal lab results, and prompt clinicians to take timely action.

AI can assist in predictive analytics by providing clinicians with real-time data on patient outcomes, which can be used to allocate resources more efficiently, such as anticipating a need for ICU beds or predicting which patients may require urgent intervention (Bajwa et al., 2021). Decision support systems powered by AI can provide clinicians with recommendations based on the patient's data, including treatment options that have been effective for similar patients, thus assisting in clinical decision-making while still leaving the final decision to the clinician (Wang et al., 2025).

3.7.3. Barriers to Effective Collaboration

Clinician skepticism, resistance to AI adoption, and the need for ongoing training are significant barriers to achieving effective human-AI collaboration (Maleki Varnosfaderani & Forouzanfar, 2024).

1. *Clinician Skepticism:* Many clinicians are skeptical about the reliability and accuracy of AI systems, particularly when it comes to AI-driven decision support. Concerns over the lack of explainability in AI algorithms (often referred to as the "black box" problem) can hinder trust in these systems. Clinicians may question whether AI tools can fully understand the nuances of patient care, which requires human judgment, empathy, and experience.
2. *Resistance to AI Adoption:* Healthcare organizations often face resistance to new technologies, and AI is no exception. Clinicians may feel that AI will either replace their roles or undermine their expertise. Furthermore, AI's introduction may be seen as an additional burden, as it could disrupt established routines and require learning new systems.
3. *Training and Ongoing Education:* For AI tools to be effectively integrated into clinical workflows, healthcare professionals need to undergo training on how to use these tools in practice. This includes understanding how to interpret AI-driven recommendations, knowing when to override AI suggestions, and developing familiarity with new workflows. Moreover, as AI technologies continue to evolve, ongoing education is essential to ensure that clinicians stay up to date with the latest advancements and maintain their ability to use AI systems effectively. For AI tools to be effectively integrated into clinical workflows, healthcare professionals need to undergo training on how to use these tools in practice. This includes understanding how to interpret AI-driven recommendations, knowing when to override AI suggestions, and developing familiarity with new workflows.

Successful integration of AI requires that healthcare professionals not only trust the technology but also feel confident in their ability to use it competently. This can be achieved through targeted training programs, clear communication about the role of AI as a support tool rather than a replacement, and creating an environment of continuous learning and feedback (Davenport & Kalakota, 2019).

4. BENEFITS OF AI-POWERED E-COLLABORATION

The adoption of AI within e-collaboration systems yields measurable benefits across diagnostic accuracy, operational efficiency, access, patient experience, and system resilience. In Table 3, the key benefits of AI, IoMT, blockchain, generative models, XR, and population analytics are briefly discussed. The following subsections synthesize the principal benefit categories and map them to healthcare domains.

4.1. Accuracy and Resource Maximization

- **Improved diagnostic accuracy.** Task-specific AI models (imaging, waveform analysis) often match or surpass average human performance on narrowly defined tasks, decreasing missed diagnoses and enabling earlier intervention ((Bae, 2024; Bertolo et al., 2025; Díaz et al., 2024). Such gains translate directly to improved patient outcomes when AI outputs are properly validated and integrated into clinician workflows.
- **Clinician time savings and workflow efficiency.** Generative AI and automation reduce time spent on documentation, routine triage, and administrative tasks, enabling clinicians to dedicate more time to complex decision making and patient interaction (Kernberg et al., 2024).
- **Resource optimization and reduced utilization.** Predictive alerts from IoMT and population models allow anticipatory care that reduces avoidable admissions and improves bed management, supply planning, and specialist scheduling (Alam et al., 2024; Mathkor et al., 2024; Muhunzi et al., 2024).
- **Enhanced access and equity (with caveats).** AI-enabled teletriage and asynchronous specialist support extend access to underserved regions, but equitable outcomes require bias mitigation and representative data in model development and validation. Recent reviews call for fairness audits and inclusive datasets to ensure benefits are widely distributed.
- **Trustworthy data sharing.** Blockchain-backed consent and provenance mechanisms strengthen trust across institutions and with patients, simplifying collaborative care while preserving auditable records of access and con-

sent actions. Hybrid blockchain frameworks and governance proposals in 2024 describe practical deployment patterns.

Table 3. Key benefits of AI adoption across healthcare domains

Studies	Domain	Principal AI-Enabled Benefits
(Bae, 2024; Díaz et al., 2024; Zhang et al., 2024)	Telemedicine & Remote Diagnostics	Faster triage; improved diagnostic pre-screening; reduced clinician review time
(Bertolo et al., 2025; Mathkor et al., 2024; Tjhin et al., 2024)	MDT Conferences	Concise case synthesis; evidence retrieval; improved consensus efficiency
(Jafleh et al., 2024; LaBoone & Marques, 2024; Yang, 2024)	Remote Monitoring / IoMT	Early alerts; lower readmissions; personalized care
(Al-Khasawneh et al., 2024; Kasyapa & Vanmathi, 2024; Mehraeen & Mahmoudi, 2024)	Blockchain Data Exchange	Immutable audit trail; patient-mediated consent; interoperable sharing
(Bertolo et al., 2025; Kernberg et al., 2024; Xu & Wang, 2024)	Generative AI (LLMs)	Rapid note generation; patient communication; meeting summarization
(Dasa et al., 2025; Lang et al., 2024; Toni et al., 2024)	XR & Training	Accelerated skill acquisition; adaptive simulation; team training
(Alam et al., 2024; Muhunzi et al., 2024)	Population Health Analytics	Forecasting; resource optimization; multi-site coordination

Across telemedicine, MDTs, IoMT, blockchain exchange, generative AI, XR training, and population analytics, the 2024-2025 literature documents substantive gains in accuracy, efficiency, access, and coordination when AI is thoughtfully integrated into e-collaboration ecosystems. At the same time, the literature emphasizes governance, explainability, bias mitigation, and prospective validation as preconditions for safe, equitable scale-up. Future research should prioritize standardized outcome metrics, federated evaluation across diverse populations, and multidisciplinary governance frameworks to ensure AI's promise in enabling smarter, connected, and patient-centric systems is fully realized.

5. CHALLENGES AND RISKS IN IMPLEMENTING AI FOR E-COLLABORATION IN HEALTHCARE

AI-enabled e-collaboration secure messaging, shared worklists, tele-consults, cross-site tumour boards promise faster decision-making and more consistent care. The successful adoption of AI in healthcare collaboration is contingent upon addressing four major, interrelated risks: data privacy and security, algorithmic bias and inequities, interoperability barriers, and trust-related human factors (Merchán-Cruz et al., 2025). Each domain spans technical, organizational, and regulatory considerations, and each has evolved rapidly since 2024, as new frameworks (HL7 AI/ML Data Lifecycle, CHAI/JCAI governance, FDA AI device guidance) and emerging threat models (membership-inference, linkage re-identification) have shifted best practice (Babic et al., 2025).

5.1. Data Privacy and Security Concerns

E-collaboration routinely moves protected health information (PHI) across institutional and national borders (Murala et al., 2023). Cross-jurisdictional transfers must reconcile divergent regimes such as the EU GDPR (lawful bases, data minimization, adequacy decisions) and U.S. HIPAA (covered entities, BAAs, safeguards). Recent reviews emphasize that global health data sharing remains fragmented, with inconsistent secondary-use rules and varying breach notification thresholds complicating collaborative AI model development and federated analytics. Strong cryptography (TLS in transit, AES-256 at rest), granular access controls, and privacy-enhancing technologies (PETs) are necessary but not sufficient without governance that accounts for jurisdictional conflict-of-laws and data residency constraints (Conduah et al., 2025).

Healthcare remains a top target for cyberattacks; AI introduces new attack surfaces (model endpoints, data pipelines, MLOps artifacts) and privacy threats that traditional de-identification may not neutralize. Two risks have become especially salient:

- **Linkage and re-identification** of "anonymized" records via auxiliary datasets, raising discrimination and surveillance risks (Narayan et al., 2025).
- **Membership-inference attacks (MIAs)** against trained models, revealing whether a person's data were used problematic for stigmatized conditions and clinical trials (Meurers et al., 2025).

Paradoxically, AI is also part of the defence: anomaly-detection for insider threats, predictive monitoring of access patterns, and automated key-rotation policies; however, adversarial inputs can blind these detectors, so defence-in-depth (zero trust, least privilege, robust monitoring) is essential. Contemporary medical-AI reviews and practice articles increasingly treat MIAs/evasion as first-class risks in clinical deployments, especially for generative models that may leak training snippets (Chen & Esmaeilzadeh, 2024).

5.2. Algorithmic Bias and Inequities

Bias in clinical AI can arise anywhere in the lifecycle data curation, labelling, feature selection, optimization, evaluation, deployment and is amplified in collaborative tools that disseminate model outputs across teams and sites. A 2024 synthesis details how under-representation and label subjectivity propagate into clinical miscalibration, with downstream effects on triage, imaging, and risk stratification. A 2025 systematic review similarly catalogues disparities (race/ethnicity, migration status, paediatrics), highlighting that "mathematically fair" post-hoc fixes often underperform unless upstream data/label issues are addressed (Cross et al., 2024).

Beyond the lab, real-world examinations and news investigations have flagged inequities in medical devices and AI-enabled allocation tools (e.g., pulse oximetry error profiles; transplant allocation fairness), reinforcing the need for transparent local validation and continuous monitoring before broad e-collaboration rollout (Sufian et al., 2024).

Recent literature and frameworks converge on a stack of interventions:

- Dataset governance: representativeness audits; targeted oversampling for minority strata; paediatric-specific ethics, and migration-status sensitivity (Hussain et al., 2025).
- Methodology: pre-specify subgroup metrics; use fairness-aware learning (equalized odds, group calibration) with explicit clinical trade-offs; prospectively power subgroup validations (Cross et al., 2024).
- Deployment: local "silent mode" trials; drift sensors on subgroup performance; escalation paths to human review; patient-facing communication that explains limits. Governance playbooks from CHAI and the Joint Commission now recommend risk-based oversight and lifecycle monitoring across direct care and operational use cases (Barnes et al., 2021).

Table 4. Sources of AI bias and mitigation strategies (curated from 2024–2025 reviews) (Cross et al., 2024).

Source of bias	Typical manifestation in e-collab tools	Example mitigation
Sampling bias	Under-representation of rural or migrant patients in telehealth datasets	Data partnerships to expand coverage; stratified sampling plans
Label bias	Subjective notes or legacy codes encoding prejudice	Multi-annotator adjudication; label-noise–robust training
Feature/measurement bias	Devices with skin-tone error profiles (e.g., SpO_2)	Device selection standards; per-device calibration layers

continued on following page

Table 4. Continued

Source of bias	Typical manifestation in e-collab tools	Example mitigation
Objective/metric selection	Optimizing AUC while harming recall in a subgroup	Multi-objective training with subgroup constraints
Deployment bias	Performance drop after rollout to low-resource sites	Local validation, phased release, continuous subgroup monitoring

5.3. Interoperability Barriers

AI-mediated collaboration depends on timely, structured data exchange across EHRs, imaging archives, labs, and patient apps. Yet heterogeneity in data models, terminology, metadata, and vendor APIs continues to obstruct end-to-end workflows, such as embedding model explanations into clinician interfaces or reconciling remote device streams into unified dashboards. This challenge is well documented in interoperability literature: heterogeneous health information systems still struggle to interoperate in practice owing to semantic, syntactic, and architectural mismatches (Torab-Miandoab et al., 2023).

At the standards level, recent work emphasizes that HL7's AI/ML Data Lifecycle guidance and the push for universal FHIR-based API adoption are essential foundations for trustworthy AI-enabled e-collaboration, but achieving semantic alignment remains a central barrier. For example, a systematic review of heterogeneous health information systems reports that despite wide endorsement of standards like HL7 FHIR, CDA, and SNOMED-CT, actual systems still struggle with semantic, syntactic, and architectural mismatches that limit seamless data exchange (Torab-Miandoab et al., 2023). Similarly, a recent nature-perspective calls for ontology-based, standards-driven architectures to integrate AI safely into health systems, treating patient safety as a system property rather than an afterthought (Wong et al., 2025). Meanwhile, applied efforts are exploring how federated learning + FHIR protocols can improve privacy and interoperability simultaneously and blockchain-based distributed systems have been proposed to secure EHR exchange across nodes (Carlos Ferreira et al., 2024). Therefore, even though standards are more mature than before, interoperability for AI in e-collaboration is still fundamentally constrained by gaps in semantic mapping, provenance propagation, governance across networks, and embedding AI outputs back into clinical workflows.

5.4. Trust and Human Factors

Without trust, AI tools even when accurate are underused or bypassed. A 2025 systematic review of clinicians' trust in AI-CDSSs identifies recurring determinants:

transparency/explainability, reliability in edge cases, workflow fit, accountability clarity, training, and local validation. Negative determinants include alert fatigue, opaque models, and perceived deskilling (Tun et al., 2025). Patients' trust hinges on respectful communication (especially in messaging co-drafted by generative models), privacy assurances, and clinician oversight (Zondag et al., 2024). Early evidence on GenAI for patient messaging shows comparable empathy/quality to clinicians in limited studies, but stresses governance for safeguarding PHI and disclosure norms when AI assists communication both critical in e-collaboration portals (Hu et al., 2025).

Table 5. Barriers to trust in AI-assisted healthcare and response strategies (synthesized from 2024–2025 guidance and reviews) (Tun et al., 2025).

Barrier	Typical impact in e-collab	Strategy aligned to recent guidance
Opaque recommendations	Clinician override/ bypass	Provide case-level explanations, uncertainty; require local validation prior to use
Workflow friction	Drop in adoption, "shadow work"	Co-design with end users; embed outputs into native inbox/televisit flow; measure time-on-task
Accountability ambiguity	Reluctance to rely on AI	Define responsibility matrix (vendor vs. site vs. user); incident response; model update governance
Performance drift	Silent failure across sites	Real-time monitoring with subgroup metrics; triggers for rollbacks/reviews; TEFCA/FHIR event logging
Patient skepticism	Lower portal engagement	Clear consent, privacy disclosures; clinician-in-the-loop messaging; feedback channels

Recent work underscores that effective AI governance in healthcare must rest on risk-based institutional oversight, local validation, continuous monitoring, and clear accountability frameworks. (Pencina et al., 2025) argue that gaps often emerge between AI developers and implementers, and emphasize that organizations must clarify roles, localize validation, and maintain monitoring across deployment lifecycles to bridge these divides (Pencina et al., 2025).

Acceptance of AI in healthcare can vary significantly by demographic factors such as age, education, socioeconomic status, and cultural background. Older adults, for example, may be more hesitant to trust AI-based medical systems, while younger, more tech-savvy individuals may be more open to these technologies (Deo, 2024). Furthermore, emerging frameworks in responsible AI literature support the idea that accountability should be shared across actors, not concentrated solely in any single party (Batool, 2025). Together with standards-oriented guidance (e.g., lifecycle documentation, provenance, change control), these elements create auditable, trustworthy pathways for AI systems in collaborative healthcare settings.

5.5. Integrated Risk Posture and Practical Roadmap

Figure 6. Pragmatic Roadmap for AI-Enabled E-Collaboration in Healthcare (2025–2026)

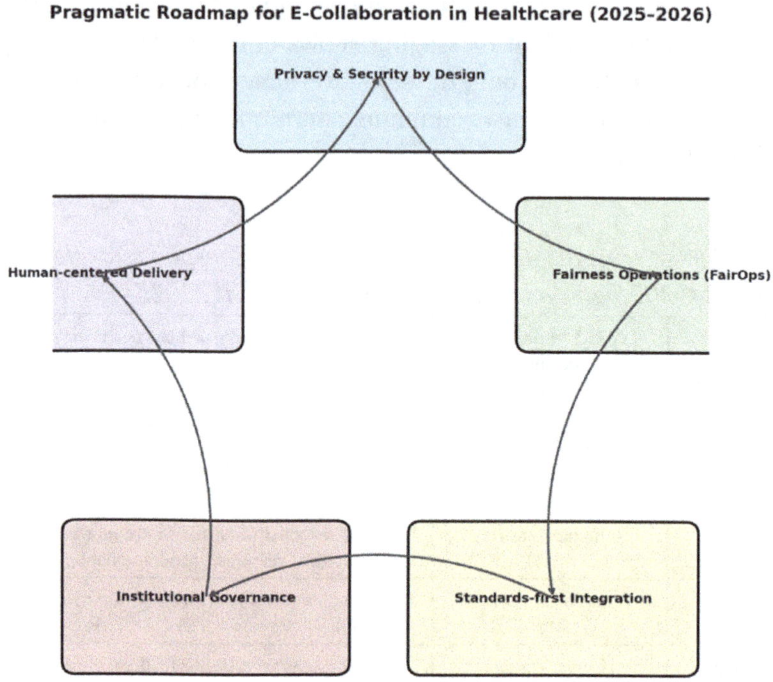

The four domains reinforce one another in practice. Weak interoperability impairs bias audits (missing subgroups), while unclear accountability depresses trust even when privacy controls are strong. A pragmatic roadmap for e-collaboration in 2025–2026 therefore combines:

1. **Privacy & Security by design:** PETs (secure aggregation, differential privacy where feasible), routine MIA testing in model validation, red-teaming for data leakage, zero-trust access, immutable audit logs (Narayan et al., 2025).
2. **Fairness operations (FairOps):** pre-deployment subgroup power analysis; bias dashboards; escalation playbooks tied to clinical governance; publication of model cards with local validation (Cross et al., 2024).
3. **Standards-first integration:** FHIR resources and implementation guides; alignment with TEFCA exchange where applicable; adherence to HL7 AI/ML Lifecycle documentation of data provenance and quality (Ayaz et al., 2021).

4. **Human-centered delivery:** invest in training, simulation exercises, and transparent patient communications; disclose AI assistance in messaging where relevant; measure trust and usability as primary outcomes alongside accuracy (Tun et al., 2025).
5. **Institutional governance:** Healthcare organizations should implement robust institutional governance by adopting frameworks like those from CHAI and the Joint Commission, while aligning change-management practices with FDA's draft expectations for AI clinical decision support, and ensuring mandatory post-market surveillance and rollback mechanisms. Such governance strategies resonate with calls for joint accountability in healthcare AI systems, where shared oversight among developers, operators, and clinicians is essential for responsible deployment (Bagave et al., 2025).

6. TECHNICAL, ETHICAL AND GOVERNANCE STRATEGIES

There is an urgent need for strong technical and ethical frameworks to enable health systems to make more of the potential disruptions from artificial intelligence and machine learning (AI/ML) applications to maintain transparency, trustworthiness, and equity. The latest literature (Aziz et al., 2024; Rao & Aalami, 2023a) highlights that explainability, privacy, and bias mitigation are central pillars supporting ethical healthcare AI. The more recent releases take this argument a step further and demonstrate that these two aspects of selfhood cannot be disjointly treated either (Ezzeddine, 2024; Shahriar et al., 2023).

6.1. The need for explainability in AI, privacy safeguards, and bias mitigation

Interpretability of healthcare AI has transitioned from a nice-to-have to a duty of care. Meta-frameworks: (Doshi-Velez & Kim, 2017) framing of interpretability as a science. Interpretability, in particular, lends itself to being seen as docking scientific considerations. Recent works such as (Rao & Aalami, 2023) emphasize the visual interpretability in clinical imaging, making for an AI-driven diagnosis that doctors can trust. (Aziz et al., 2024) summarized key gaps, including the lack of standardized metrics and workflow integration, and promote explainability-centric models developed with end-users in mind.

Explainability also brings novel privacy hazards, referring to causes and extrapolation. (Ezzeddine, 2024) illustrate how XAI methods could unintentionally free HIPAA information or model weaknesses by exposing feature importances or counterfactuals. This induces attention, the more transparent the model, the more privacy it may leak.

Nowadays, privacy is interpreted as an issue related to the lifecycle instead of a permanent need. (Shahriar et al., 2023) chart privacy risks along the full life cycle of AI, from data collection, preprocessing, training, deployment, and auditing, classifying them as those of identification, unsoundness, nontransparency, and violations of regulation. Their survey identifies federated learning, homomorphic encryption, and differential privacy as promising defenses. Complementing this, (Allana et al., 2025) present a scoping review of privacy risks in explainable AI and propose hybrid frameworks that integrate technical approaches with governance-level application. Fairness is another factor related to privacy. (Okoro et al., 2023) demonstrate that in public-health campaigns, big data and AI can improve disease surveillance but must balance personalization with protecting vulnerable groups. Bias is still a good reason to worry about AI in health care. The unmitigated algorithmic bias can continue health disparities and highlight that both fairness-conscious algorithms and diverse datasets are important. In their thorough review, (Kubanek & Szymoniak, 2022) further argue that simultaneous accountability mechanisms, transparency, and bias checks should back responsible AI. Bias and explainability are deeply interconnected, interpretable models enable clinicians to recognize biased reasoning, and bias-aware training provides trustworthy explanations. Therefore, including privacy-preserving explainability tools is critical for fair AI in health care.

6.2. Global standards and AI literacy programs for healthcare professionals

Governance of AI in healthcare is still patchy, and while some common standards are emerging through the WHO, ISO, and IEEE, they are also conflicting. The absence of harmonized accountability dynamics among countries could lead to heterogeneity in implementation between countries (Kubanek & Szymoniak, 2022). Literature from 2023–2024 argues that to achieve global alignment, bias audits, privacy legislation (eg, GDPR, HIPAA), and the requirement for explainability must coalesce into a shared set of guidelines. (Adegboye, 2024) emphasizes the connection between AI and health information literacy (HIL) and calls for organized training to guide clinicians in critically appraising AI-determined results. Studies such as (Issa et al., 2024) and (Si, 2025) support the availability of gaps in AI education, most students are not technically literate enough to deploy AI but feel confident about integrating AI. (Si, 2025) demonstrates that AI literacy positively influences favourable attitudes toward AI adoption in Korea. (Issa et al., 2024) uncover differences in AI awareness across countries, suggesting the necessity for integrated global curricula.

In Figure 7, the framework integrates technical regulations with governance and lifelong learning for trustworthy, explainable, patient-centred AI systems in healthcare. Compared to a linear process, the process is non-linear, as the relationships between data, models, ethics, and iterated feedback are incorporated in this framework. It is explorable rather than married to existing ideas.

Figure 7. Framework for Implementing Ethical AI in Healthcare

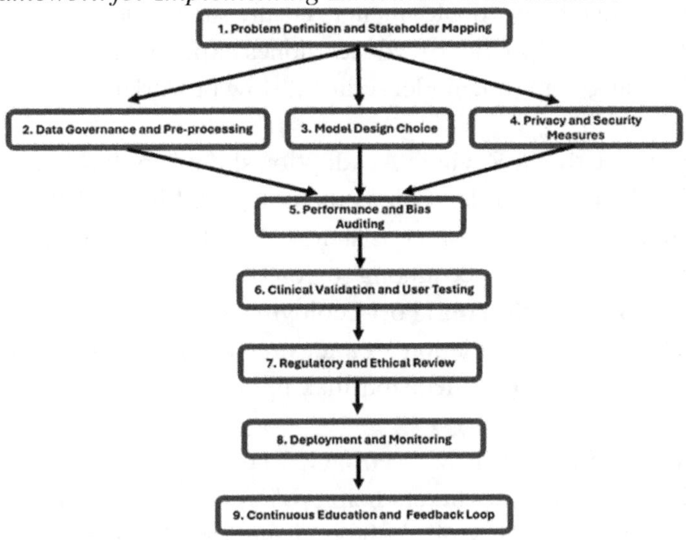

6.3. Framework steps

I. **Problem Definition & Stakeholder Mapping**: Crucial to the concordance of ethical AI is establishing the healthcare problem and working within a diverse network of stakeholders: clinicians, patients, data scientists, and policy makers.

II. **Data Governance & Preprocessing:** Quality and representativeness of datasets (sound data governance) free from systemic biases. Methods like anonymization and differential privacy protect the confidentiality and security of sensitive health data (Allana et al., 2025; Ezzeddine, 2024; Shahriar et al., 2023).

III. **Modelling Design Decisions:** The Modelling and development phase focuses on explainability-oriented architecture and fairness-aware algorithms. Interpretable machine learning offers clinicians insight into model outputs and increased confidence in clinical decision-making (Doshi-Velez & Kim, 2017; Rao & Aalami, 2023).

IV. **Privacy & Security:** Federated learning and secure multi-party computation are privacy-preserving approaches for collaborative AI where sensitive health data does not have to be centralized. These two are trade-offs, and their resolution is required to achieve transparency and confidentiality (Allana et al., 2025; Ezzeddine, 2024). Performance & Bias Auditing–External audits of fairness, robustness, and transparency are essential in promoting accountability.

V. **Clinical Validation & User Testing:** Rigorous clinical validation and usability testing are needed before deployment to ensure safety and interpretability in the real world. Ongoing provider feedback hones explainability mechanisms such that AI tools augment (not hinder) clinical flow of work (Aziz et al., 2024; Rao & Aalami, 2023).

VI. **Regulatory & Ethical Review:** AI adoption should conform to universal standards and ethical standards, such as those WHO, ISO, and IEEE, advocating accountability and regulation consistency. This kind of coordination has prevented fractured governance among regions.

VII. **Deployment & Monitoring:** Post-deployment monitoring is essential to identify model drift, unfair deviation, or undesired harms. Explainability interfaces help clinicians to monitor decision-making applications and intervene when anomalies are identified.

VIII. **Continual Education & Feedback Loop:** Ongoing AI literacy courses for clinicians and health workers help professionals to read between the lines of explanations from AI. Well-designed patient feedback mechanisms prevent harm, promote involvement in AI design, generate long-term trust, and foster fair adoption.

7. REAL WORLD CASE STUDIES

7.1. Economic Analysis and Cost-Effectiveness Studies

Incorporating economic analysis into AI implementation is critical for healthcare decision-makers. Without clear cost-benefit data, the adoption of AI technologies can be hindered, especially in environments where budget constraints are common, such as in smaller hospitals or rural healthcare settings. Economic assessments provide stakeholders with the necessary evidence to justify the financial investment required for adopting AI-driven solutions.

Cost-benefit analysis (CBA) is one of the most used metrics to evaluate the financial viability of AI systems in healthcare. It compares the total expected costs of an AI systems such as initial setup costs, training, maintenance, and integration with the expected benefits, including improved patient outcomes, reduced errors, and operational efficiencies. AI systems can improve diagnostic accuracy, which leads to better patient outcomes and reduces the costs associated with misdiagnosis or unnecessary procedures. Moreover, AI-driven automation in administrative tasks can reduce labour costs in busy hospitals, allowing staff to focus on patient care (Obermeyer et al., 2019).

Determining ROI for AI technologies is critical, especially for smaller healthcare institutions. ROI is calculated by comparing the monetary benefits (e.g., cost savings, increased revenue) of AI systems against their initial and ongoing costs. Small and rural hospitals may face financial pressures when adopting new technologies. AI has the potential to reduce operational costs and improve clinical decision-making efficiency, making it particularly attractive for resource-limited healthcare settings. For instance, AI-powered diagnostic tools may help rural hospitals with fewer specialists by providing expert-level decision support at lower costs (Davenport & Kalakota, 2019).

Healthcare systems need to evaluate whether the AI tools they implement will remain sustainable over time. This includes considering ongoing costs such as updates, compliance with evolving regulations, and scalability to meet increasing demand. Sustainability models should include factors like data storage and processing requirements, energy costs, and long-term service contracts. AI tools should not only generate immediate cost savings but also be capable of evolving with advancements in technology without necessitating prohibitively expensive upgrades. For example, AI models might require regular retraining to ensure they remain relevant and accurate as new medical data emerges (Rajkomar et al., 2019).

7.2. Case Studies

The success story of AI integration into healthcare can be considered through the real-world case studies, where opportunities and potential threats are explicitly highlighted. The examples offered can display how the proposed principles of explainability, fairness, and governance frameworks operate when they are transformed into practice.

Some case studies have been discussed below:

i. Case Study 1: AI for Diagnostic Imaging

The development of AI-driven diagnostic tools has revolutionized imaging by enabling the detection of abnormalities such as tumours, fractures, and cardiovascular aberrations. For instance, using explainability characteristics integrated into

AI-powered imaging tools may allow clinicians to retrace the decision-making process, which increases trust and agent liability (Rao & Aalami, 2023). Also, fairness-aware algorithms decrease differences across patient populations to achieve the same diagnostic results. In this instance, explainability is not just an option but a medical requirement.

ii. Case Study 2: Privacy-Preserving Predictive Analytics in Public Health

With the extensiveness of predictive analytics for monitoring epidemics and patients at risk during and after the COVID-19 pandemic, the issue of privacy remains key. Federated learning models have been used to predict patients at risk without transmitting personal data, ensuring privacy while producing proven forecasts (Allana et al., 2025; Shahriar et al., 2023). This instance demonstrates how privacy-preserving tools can work in entire nation-states while remaining usable as a planning tool for healthcare facilities.

iii. Case Study 3: AI in Clinical Decision Support Systems (CDSS)

Clinical decision support systems use explainable AI to assist physicians in choosing the most appropriate treatment options for their patients. CDSSs designed with machine learning that people can understand rapidly boost clinicians and improve patient safety (Aziz et al., 2024). Moreover, fairness-aware recommendations guarantee that the AI does not deepen health imbalances. This case was also designed to illustrate the importance of cost-sensitive joint maximization.

iv. Case Study 4: AI for Health Profession Education

AI is used not only in patient care but also to educate healthcare providers with AI-driven education systems, which include personalized learning modules, simulations, and adaptive assessments. Research has shown that incorporating AI into health education results in a higher AI literacy rate among clinicians and is necessary for secure use of AI in practice (Issa et al., 2024; Si, 2025). These interventions prepare healthcare staff to assess and engage with AI responsibly.

v. Case Study 5: AI in Public Health Campaigns

Nowadays, AI and big data analytics have recently been leveraged in public health campaigns to track disease spread or vaccine awareness efforts. AI can even enable live campaign course corrections, increasing the reach and effectiveness of health communications strategies (Okoro et al., 2023). However, these cases need robust governance structures to prevent bias and misinformation. In Table 6 some key points is being addressed from the case study from AI in Healthcare.

Table 6. Real-World Case Studies of AI in Healthcare

Case Study	Technology	Outcome
Diagnostic Model	Deep learning models and XAI dashboard	Increased detection accuracy and increased trust of clinicians with the help of visual explainability (Rao & Aalami, 2023)
Predictive Analytics in Public Health	Collaborative learning and differential privacy.	Accurate patient-risk prediction without having to centralize sensitive data (Allana et al., 2025; Shahriar et al., 2023)
Systems for Clinical Decision Support (CDSS)	Fairness-aware algorithms combined with accessible ML	Low algorithm bias and secure treatment suggestions (Aziz et al., 2024).
Health Profession Education	AI-driven adaptive learning	enhanced clinician readiness for AI integration and AI literacy (Issa et al., 2024; Si, 2025).
Public Health Campaigns	Big data analysis combined with AI	improved efficacy of campaigns and illness surveillance (Okoro et al., 2023).

8. FUTURE TRENDS IN AI-ENABLED E-COLLABORATION

The waves of AI, 5G and IoT are transforming our society, and they are also shaping the IoMT, which is developing in step with them. When applied to IoMT devices, AI allows the development of predictive analytics, tools for detection of anomalies and sophisticated decision support systems, which can result in a higher degree of confidence on the part of the medical practitioner when making diagnosis and personalized healthcare services (Qi, 2025). As an example, multi-layer IoT-enabled machine learning models (e.g., Secure Health Monitoring IoT platforms) have been achieving > 91% accuracy in clinical decision support making needs to guarantee an effective monitoring and diagnosis making these systems indispensable in the future healthcare (Qi, 2025). Likewise, the incorporation of AI based anomaly detection with IoT health monitoring systems results in early detection of health deterioration from the patient. Hence, facilitating early interventions to lower mortality rates (Chinnaperumal et al., 2025).

The implementation of 5G also advanced the performance of IoMT, thanks to the ultra-low-latency communication, massive device interconnectivity, and increased data transmission rates (Batool, 2025). These are essential for real-time patient's monitoring, robotic surgery via remotely access and constant vital signs monitoring. For instance, a recent work using a hybrid CNN-LSTM model multichip 5G-connected environment network provided 96.5% accuracy with latency as low as 14.4 ms, explaining generally why IoMT systems should take advantages of advanced wireless technologies (Batool, 2025). Likewise, 5G enhances the scalability. The monolithic structure centered around device manufacturers and IoMT systems focusing on supporting devices in the millions in hospital environments, becomes an ecosystem of care integrators, administrators, and critical care management systems. The convergence of 5G and IoMT Chips: Extending Wearable Device Battery Life1 5G IoMT chips are revolutionizing, telemedicine, and also that time critical applications, such as ICU (intensive care unit) monitoring and emergency responder systems (Zreikat et al., 2025).

Another trend is personalized and precision medicine based on wearables and invasive IoMT devices. From smart insulin pumps to continuous vast array of devices, from glucose monitors to digital fabrics that produce insulin, the array is devices: an artificial pancreas 'Dawn phenomenon,' and an implanted glucose sensors that help manage the immeasurable diabetes monitors, such as those for ECG, permits the constant and live-tracking of vitals, which helps in customizing treatment plans as per the health profile of the particular patient (Asif et al., 2025). Future developments are expected to evolve into minimally invasive and energy-friendly implantable devices that are closely connected to cloud-based platforms for lifelong health monitoring. IoMT has become wearable and adsorbable implantable devices is that it can shift passive monitoring to active disease management by predicting relapses, reminding for drug adherence, and adjusting therapy on an individual basis (Zhou et al., 2025)

8.1. Overcoming Challenges in IoMT Adoption

The IoMT adoption, however, faces many challenges concerning technological, regulatory, and social sectors which despite significant advancements are yet to be addressed. One of the main technological challenge is that of interoperation among the variety of devices and platforms in IoMT systems. The absence of common communication standards undermines data sharing among different proprietary medical systems and risks information silos (Zreikat et al., 2025). To resolve these issues, the authors propose the use of lightweight encryption algorithms and blockchain-based interoperability frameworks ensuring confidential data communication across different health o-SPMPs data exchange with privacy (Bhattacharya et al., 2025).

Data privacy and cybersecurity concerns pose another important challenge, as IoMT produces sensitive patient data that can be compromised. Furthermore, progress in the development of the quantum computer raises another CAPITA traditional cryptographic approaches on IoMT devices (Sabrina et al., 2024). In the wake of this, new quantum-resistant schemes are investigated including lattice-based signatures that provide stronger security against quantum attacks (Zhang et al., 2024). Similarly, blockchain based systems with post-quantum encryption schemes are also promoting for the security of IoMT networks for future cyber threats (Khan et al., 2025; Zhou et al., 2025). Regulatory Differences in healthcare privacy regulations, such as HIPAA in the US and GDPR in Europe, also introduce barriers to global IoMT adoption. Ensuring compliance across widely and will require the harmonization of data protection laws and the establishment of universal standards. Ignoring these limitations could lead to limited scalability and deplorability.

Interoperable use of IoMT devices across borders (Zhou et al., 2025). In addition, patient trust is a key factor in the society acceptance of the IoMT technologies, and this can be earned only through open data management policies, consent practices, and promoting patient autonomy (Asif et al., 2025).

8.2. Ethical Considerations

The application of IoMT in healthcare poses deep ethical challenges that should be resolved to have an equitable and responsible deployment. The biggest issue being patient privacy, since the constant surveillance creates massive amounts of private health data. If this data is accessed illegitimately or misused, it can result in breach of patient confidentiality and loss of trust in IoMT systems (Bhattacharya et al., 2025). Thus, encryption, anonymization, secure multi-party computation, and related) are all necessary tools to work with such sensitive data in a manner that the privacy concerns can be addressed.

A further ethical consideration is patient autonomy, especially when IoMT devices are employed for real-time monitoring or autonomous decision support. Although automated systems offer early warnings and predictions is underlie the concern of negating patient autonomy when decisions are made without their input (Zhou et al., 2025). Hence, there is a need to strike a balance between automation and human supervision so that health professionals can stay at the centre of decision-making.

Ethical considerations such as the equity of access to IoMT devices is a further consideration. Even though high-income regions are quick in implementing IoMT-based health systems, low-resource settings encounter impedances in the field of conductive solution development of health systems adoptions on this technology infrastructure stiffness, cost, and digital literacy (Chinnaperumal et al., 2025). This sets up a digital divide that could potentially widen health disparities. It is the responsibility of IoMT systems to be built as affordable scalability and portability across healthcare settings is critical for global equity.

Lastly, to ethically roll out IoMT, there must be transparent governance structure which should include accountability process for device manufacturers, data custodians and healthcare professionals (Sabrina et al., 2024).

9. CONCLUSION

The integration of Artificial Intelligence into healthcare represents a paradigm shift that promises to redefine the ways in which care is delivered, decisions are made, and patients are treated. The developments in AI, particularly in areas such as diagnostic imaging, predictive analytics, and telemedicine, have demonstrated significant benefits in improving both the accuracy and efficiency of healthcare practices. However, as this technology continues to evolve, it is crucial to address the ethical concerns surrounding patient privacy, data security, and the potential for biases in AI algorithms. To ensure the responsible use of AI in healthcare, comprehensive governance frameworks, regulatory measures, and interdisciplinary collaboration are necessary. Moving forward, the potential of AI to enhance healthcare delivery is immense, but its integration must be carried out with careful consideration of its societal, ethical, and practical implications. By continuing to explore the challenges and opportunities of AI, we can create a more efficient, equitable, and patient-centred healthcare system for the future.

Industry leaders should prioritize the development of transparent, explainable AI models to foster trust among healthcare professionals and patients. Regulatory bodies must establish clear, global standards to safeguard privacy, mitigate bias, and ensure data security, particularly in the context of the Internet of Medical Things (IoMT) and sensitive patient data. Furthermore, healthcare institutions should invest in training programs to enhance AI literacy among clinicians, enabling them to effectively integrate AI into their practice. Finally, continued research into ethical frameworks and real-time monitoring of AI applications will be vital in addressing emerging challenges, ensuring that AI remains a force for good in transforming healthcare delivery, improving patient outcomes, and promoting health equity.

REFERENCES

Adegboye, M. (2024). Impact of artificial intelligence on health information literacy: Guidance for healthcare professionals. *Library Hi Tech News*, *41*(7), 1–5. DOI: 10.1108/LHTN-03-2024-0048

Akinnagbe, O. B. (2024). Human-AI Collaboration: Enhancing Productivity and Decision-Making. *International Journal of Education, Management, and Technology*, *2*(3), 387–417. DOI: 10.58578/ijemt.v2i3.4209

Al-Antari, M. A. (2023). Artificial Intelligence for Medical Diagnostics—Existing and Future AI Technology! *Diagnostics (Basel)*, *13*(4), 688. DOI: 10.3390/diagnostics13040688

Al-Khasawneh, M. A., Faheem, M., Alarood, A. A., Habibullah, S., & Alzahrani, A. (2024). A secure blockchain framework for healthcare records management systems. *Healthcare Technology Letters*, *11*(6), 461–470. DOI: 10.1049/htl2.12092

Alam, M. A., Sajib, M. R. U. Z., Rahman, F., Ether, S., Hanson, M., Sayeed, A., Akter, E., Nusrat, N., Islam, T. T., Raza, S., Tanvir, K. M., Chisti, M. J., Rahman, Q. S., Hossain, A., Layek, M., Zaman, A., Rana, J., Rahman, S. M., Arifeen, S. E., . . . Ahmed, A. (2024). Implications of Big Data Analytics, AI, Machine Learning, and Deep Learning in the Health Care System of Bangladesh: Scoping Review.

Alharbe, N., & Almalki, M. (2025). IoT-enabled healthcare transformation leveraging deep learning for advanced patient monitoring and diagnosis. *Multimedia Tools and Applications*, *84*(19), 21331–21344. DOI: 10.1007/s11042-024-19919-w

Allana, S., Kankanhalli, M., & Dara, R. (2025). *Privacy Risks and Preservation Methods in Explainable Artificial Intelligence: A Scoping Review* (Version 1). arXiv. DOI: 10.48550/ARXIV.2505.02828

Asif, M., Abrar, M., Salam, A., Amin, F., Ullah, F., Shah, S., & AlSalman, H. (2025). Intelligent two-phase dual authentication framework for Internet of Medical Things. *Scientific Reports*, *15*(1), 1760. DOI: 10.1038/s41598-024-84713-5

Ayaz, M., Pasha, M. F., Alzahrani, M. Y., Budiarto, R., & Stiawan, D. (2021). The Fast Health Interoperability Resources (FHIR) Standard: Systematic Literature Review of Implementations, Applications, Challenges and Opportunities. *JMIR Medical Informatics*, *9*(7), e21929. DOI: 10.2196/21929

Aziz, N. A., Manzoor, A., Mazhar Qureshi, M. D., Qureshi, M. A., & Rashwan, W. (2024, August). *Unveiling Explainable AI in Healthcare: Current Trends, Challenges, and Future Directions*. Health Informatics. DOI: 10.1101/2024.08.10.24311735

Babic, B., Glenn Cohen, I., Stern, A. D., Li, Y., & Ouellet, M. (2025). A general framework for governing marketed AI/ML medical devices. *NPJ Digital Medicine*, *8*(1), 328. DOI: 10.1038/s41746-025-01717-9

Badwy, B., Ghanem, N. M., Banawan, K., & Ismail, N. E. (2024). Enhanced Prediction of Immune Checkpoint Blockade Response in Melanoma Using Ensemble Learning and a Hybrid Feature Selection Technique. *IEEE Access : Practical Innovations, Open Solutions*, *12*, 187041–187067. DOI: 10.1109/ACCESS.2024.3514799

Bae, M. S. (2024). AI Improves Cancer Detection and Reading Time of Digital Breast Tomosynthesis. *Radiology. Artificial Intelligence*, *6*(3), e240219. DOI: 10.1148/ryai.240219

Bagave, P., Westberg, M., Janssen, M., & Ding, A. Y. (2025, September). *Accountability Framework for Healthcare AI Systems: Towards Joint Accountability in Decision Making*. arXiv. https://doi.org//arXiv.2509.03286DOI: 10.48550

Bajwa, J., Munir, U., Nori, A., & Williams, B. (2021). Artificial intelligence in healthcare: Transforming the practice of medicine. *Future Healthcare Journal*, *8*(2), e188–e194. DOI: 10.7861/fhj.2021-0095

Barnes, B., Stansbury, N., Brown, D., Garson, L., Gerard, G., Piccoli, N., Jendrasek, D., May, N., Castillo, V., Adelfio, A., Ramirez, N., McSweeney, A., Berlien, R., & Butler, P. J. (2021). Risk-Based Monitoring in Clinical Trials: Past, Present, and Future. *Therapeutic Innovation & Regulatory Science*, *55*(4), 899–906. DOI: 10.1007/s43441-021-00295-8

Batool, I. (2025, January 2). *RealTime Health Monitoring Using 5G Networks: A Deep Learning-Based Architecture for Remote Patient Care* (Issue arXiv:2501.01027). arXiv. https://doi.org//arXiv.2501.01027DOI: 10.48550

Bertolo, R., De Bon, L., Caudana, F., Pettenuzzo, G., Malandra, S., Casolani, C., Zivi, A., Fantinel, E., Borsato, A., Negrelli, R., Salah El Din Tantawy, E., Volpi, G., Brunelli, M., Veccia, A., Cerruto, M. A., & Antonelli, A. (2025). Role of large language models in the multidisciplinary decision-making process for patients with renal cell carcinoma: A pilot experience. *NPJ Precision Oncology*, *9*(1), 257. DOI: 10.1038/s41698-025-01014-4

Bhattacharya, P., Mukherjee, A., Bhushan, B., Gupta, S. K., Gadekallu, T. R., & Zhu, Z. (2025). A secured remote patient monitoring framework for IoMT ecosystems. *Scientific Reports*, *15*(1), 22882. DOI: 10.1038/s41598-025-04774-y

Carlos Ferreira, J., Elvas, L. B., Correia, R., & Mascarenhas, M. (2024). Enhancing EHR Interoperability and Security through Distributed Ledger Technology: A Review. *Healthcare (Basel), 12*(19), 1967. DOI: 10.3390/healthcare12191967

Challen, R., Denny, J., Pitt, M., Gompels, L., Edwards, T., & Tsaneva-Atanasova, K. (2019). Artificial intelligence, bias and clinical safety. *BMJ Quality & Safety, 28*(3), 231–237. DOI: 10.1136/bmjqs-2018-008370

Chen, Y., & Esmaeilzadeh, P. (2024). Generative AI in Medical Practice: In-Depth Exploration of Privacy and Security Challenges. *Journal of Medical Internet Research, 26*(1), e53008. DOI: 10.2196/53008

Chinnaperumal, S., Periyasamy, M., Alhussan, A. A., Kannan, S., Khafaga, D. S., Raju, S. K., Eid, M. M., & El-kenawy, E.-S. M. (2025). Secure and intelligent 5G-enabled remote patient monitoring using ANN and Choquet integral fuzzy VIKOR. *Scientific Reports, 15*(1), 9913. DOI: 10.1038/s41598-025-93829-1

Conduah, A. K., Ofoe, S., & Siaw-Marfo, D. (2025). Data privacy in healthcare: Global challenges and solutions. *Digital Health, 11*, 20552076251343959. Advance online publication. DOI: 10.1177/20552076251343959

Cross, J. L., Choma, M. A., & Onofrey, J. A. (2024). Bias in medical AI: Implications for clinical decision-making. *PLOS Digital Health, 3*(11), e0000651. DOI: 10.1371/journal.pdig.0000651

Dasa, D., Board, M., Rolfe, U., Dolby, T., & Tang, W. (2025). Evaluating AI-driven characters in extended reality (XR) healthcare simulations: A systematic review. *Artificial Intelligence in Medicine, 103270*, 103270. Advance online publication. DOI: 10.1016/j.artmed.2025.103270

Davenport, T., & Kalakota, R. (2019). The potential for artificial intelligence in healthcare. *Future Healthcare Journal, 6*(2), 94–98. DOI: 10.7861/futurehosp.6-2-94

Deo, R. C. (2024). Artificial Intelligence and Health Equity. *JACC Advances, 3*(9), 101045. DOI: 10.1016/j.jacadv.2024.101045

Dhiman, R., Bazad, N., Mukherjee, R., Himanshu, , Gunjan, , Leal, E., Ahmad, S., Kaur, K., Raj, V. S., Chang, C.-M., & Pandey, R. P. (2024). Enhanced drug delivery with nanocarriers: A comprehensive review of recent advances in breast cancer detection and treatment. *Discover Nano, 19*(1), 143. DOI: 10.1186/s11671-024-04086-6

Díaz, O., Rodríguez-Ruíz, A., & Sechopoulos, I. (2024). Artificial Intelligence for breast cancer detection: Technology, challenges, and prospects. *European Journal of Radiology, 175*, 111457. DOI: 10.1016/j.ejrad.2024.111457

Doshi-Velez, F., & Kim, B. (2017, March). *Towards A Rigorous Science of Interpretable Machine Learning*. arXiv. https://doi.org//arXiv.1702.08608DOI: 10.48550

Ezzeddine, F. (2024, June). *Privacy Implications of Explainable AI in Data-Driven Systems*. arXiv. https://doi.org//arXiv.2406.15789DOI: 10.48550

Garg, P., Sharma, M. K., & Kumar, P. (2025). Transparency in Diagnosis: Unveiling the Power of Deep Learning and Explainable AI for Medical Image Interpretation. *Arabian Journal for Science and Engineering*, *50*(19), 15751–15767. Advance online publication. DOI: 10.1007/s13369-024-09896-5

Giron-Michel, J., Padelli, M., Oberlin, E., Guenou, H., & Duclos-Vallée, J.-C. (2025). State-of-the-Art Liver Cancer Organoids: Modeling Cancer Stem Cell Heterogeneity for Personalized Treatment. *BioDrugs*, *39*(2), 237–260. DOI: 10.1007/s40259-024-00702-0

Gomes, D., & Saifuddin Saif, A. F. M. (2021). Robust Underwater Fish Detection Using an Enhanced Convolutional Neural Network. *International Journal of Image. Graphics and Signal Processing*, *13*(3), 44–54. DOI: 10.5815/ijigsp.2021.03.04

Hasan, D. Md. M., Alam, M. S., Hossain, S., & Gomes, D. (2024). Fair Use Policies of Digital Contents: Some Observations and Recommendations. *Proceedings of the 3rd International Conference on Computing Advancements*, 192–199. DOI: 10.1145/3723178.3723204

Hosain, M. N., Kwak, Y.-S., Lee, J., Choi, H., Park, J., & Kim, J. (2024). IoT-enabled biosensors for real-time monitoring and early detection of chronic diseases. *Physical Activity and Nutrition*, *28*(4), 60–69. DOI: 10.20463/pan.2024.0033

Hu, D., Guo, Y., Zhou, Y., Flores, L., & Zheng, K. (2025). A systematic review of early evidence on generative AI for drafting responses to patient messages. *Npj Health Systems*, *2*(1), 27. DOI: 10.1038/s44401-025-00032-5

Hussain, S. A., Bresnahan, M., & Zhuang, J. (2025). The bias algorithm: How AI in healthcare exacerbates ethnic and racial disparities – a scoping review. *Ethnicity & Health*, *30*(2), 197–214. DOI: 10.1080/13557858.2024.2422848

Islam, Md. R., Mahmud, M. A. A., Tanvir, K., Das Joy, S., Rahman, M., Dey, N., & Gomes, D. (2025). IoMT Architecture for Healthcare: Integration, Security, and Real-Time Decision Support. In S. N. S. Al-Humairi, P. Naronglerdrit, N. Chantarapanich, & S. Wanchat (Eds.), *Robotics and IoT Synergy in Next-Generation Healthcare* (pp. 305–340). IGI Global Scientific Publishing. DOI: 10.4018/979-8-3373-5447-7.ch010

Issa, W. B., Shorbagi, A., Al-Sharman, A., Rababa, M., Al-Majeed, K., Radwan, H., Refaat Ahmed, F., Al-Yateem, N., Mottershead, R., Abdelrahim, D. N., Hijazi, H., Khasawneh, W., Ali, I., Abbas, N., & Fakhry, R. (2024). Shaping the future: Perspectives on the Integration of Artificial Intelligence in health profession education: a multi-country survey. *BMC Medical Education*, *24*(1), 1166. DOI: 10.1186/s12909-024-06076-9

Jafleh, E. A., Alnaqbi, F. A., Almaeeni, H. A., Faqeeh, S., Alzaabi, M. A., & Al Zaman, K. (2024). The Role of Wearable Devices in Chronic Disease Monitoring and Patient Care: A Comprehensive Review. *Cureus*. Advance online publication. DOI: 10.7759/cureus.68921

Jessica, H., Britney, R., Sarira, E.-D., Parisa, A., Joe, Z., & Betty, B. (2025). Applications of artificial intelligence in current pharmacy practice: A scoping review. *Research in Social & Administrative Pharmacy*, *21*(3), 134–141. DOI: 10.1016/j.sapharm.2024.12.007

Kasyapa, M. S. B., & Vanmathi, C. (2024). Blockchain integration in healthcare: A comprehensive investigation of use cases, performance issues, and mitigation strategies. *Frontiers in Digital Health*, *6*, 1359858. DOI: 10.3389/fdgth.2024.1359858

Kernberg, A., Gold, J. A., & Mohan, V. (2024). Using ChatGPT-4 to Create Structured Medical Notes From Audio Recordings of Physician-Patient Encounters: Comparative Study. *Journal of Medical Internet Research*, *26*, e54419. DOI: 10.2196/54419

Khalid, N., Qayyum, A., Bilal, M., Al-Fuqaha, A., & Qadir, J. (2023). Privacy-preserving artificial intelligence in healthcare: Techniques and applications. *Computers in Biology and Medicine*, *158*, 106848. DOI: 10.1016/j.compbiomed.2023.106848

Khan, A. A., Laghari, A. A., Almansour, H., Jamel, L., Hajjej, F., Estrela, V. V., Mohamed, M. A., & Ullah, S. (2025). Quantum computing empowering blockchain technology with post quantum resistant cryptography for multimedia data privacy preservation in cloud-enabled public auditing platforms. *Journal of Cloud Computing (Heidelberg, Germany)*, *14*(1), 43. DOI: 10.1186/s13677-025-00771-8

Khosravi, M., Zare, Z., Mojtabaeian, S. M., & Izadi, R. (2024). Artificial Intelligence and Decision-Making in Healthcare: A Thematic Analysis of a Systematic Review of Reviews. *Health Services Research and Managerial Epidemiology*, *11*, 23333928241234863. DOI: 10.1177/23333928241234863

Kubanek, M., & Szymoniak, S. (2022). *ETHICAL CHALLENGES IN AI INTEGRATION: A COMPREHENSIVE REVIEW OF BIAS, PRIVACY, AND ACCOUNTABILITY ISSUES.*

LaBoone, P. A., & Marques, O. (2024). Overview of the future impact of wearables and artificial intelligence in healthcare workflows and technology. *International Journal of Information Management Data Insights*, *4*(2), 100294. DOI: 10.1016/j.jjimei.2024.100294

Lang, M., Ghandour, S., Rikard, B., Balasalle, E. K., Rouhezamin, M. R., Zhang, H., & Uppot, R. N. (2024). Medical Extended Reality for Radiology Education and Training. *Journal of the American College of Radiology*, *21*(10), 1583–1594. DOI: 10.1016/j.jacr.2024.05.006

Li, C., Wang, J., Wang, S., & Zhang, Y. (2024). A review of IoT applications in healthcare. *Neurocomputing*, *565*, 127017. DOI: 10.1016/j.neucom.2023.127017

Li, J., Dada, A., Puladi, B., Kleesiek, J., & Egger, J. (2024). ChatGPT in healthcare: A taxonomy and systematic review. *Computer Methods and Programs in Biomedicine*, *245*, 108013. DOI: 10.1016/j.cmpb.2024.108013

Maleki Varnosfaderani, S., & Forouzanfar, M. (2024). The Role of AI in Hospitals and Clinics: Transforming Healthcare in the 21st Century. *Bioengineering (Basel, Switzerland)*, *11*(4), 337. DOI: 10.3390/bioengineering11040337

Mathkor, D. M., Mathkor, N., Bassfar, Z., Bantun, F., Slama, P., Ahmad, F., & Haque, S. (2024). Multirole of the internet of medical things (IoMT) in biomedical systems for managing smart healthcare systems: An overview of current and future innovative trends. *Journal of Infection and Public Health*, *17*(4), 559–572. DOI: 10.1016/j.jiph.2024.01.013

Mehraeen, M., & Mahmoudi, L. (2024). Tracing the Blockchain Challenges in Healthcare: A Topic Modeling and Bibliometric Analysis. *Blockchain in Healthcare Today*, *7*(3). Advance online publication. DOI: 10.30953/bhty.v7.335

Merchán-Cruz, E. A., Gabelaia, I., Savrasovs, M., Hansen, M. F., Soe, S., Rodriguez-Cañizo, R. G., & Aragón-Camarasa, G. (2025). Trust by Design: An Ethical Framework for Collaborative Intelligence Systems in Industry 5.0. *Electronics (Basel)*, *14*(10), 1952. DOI: 10.3390/electronics14101952

Meurers, T., Halilovic, M., Otte, K., Despraz, J., Kaabachi, B., Kulynych, B., Raisaro, J. L., & Prasser, F. (2025). Phantom Anonymization: Adversarial testing for membership inference risks in anonymized health data. *Computers in Biology and Medicine*, *196*, 110738. DOI: 10.1016/j.compbiomed.2025.110738

Mirbabaie, M., Hofeditz, L., Frick, N. R. J., & Stieglitz, S. (2022). Artificial intelligence in hospitals: Providing a status quo of ethical considerations in academia to guide future research. *AI & Society*, *37*(4), 1361–1382. DOI: 10.1007/s00146-021-01239-4

Mohsin Khan, M., Shah, N., Shaikh, N., Thabet, A., alrabayah, T., & Belkhair, S. (2025). Towards secure and trusted AI in healthcare: A systematic review of emerging innovations and ethical challenges. *International Journal of Medical Informatics*, *195*, 105780. DOI: 10.1016/j.ijmedinf.2024.105780

Morley, J., Murphy, L., Mishra, A., Joshi, I., & Karpathakis, K. (2022). Governing Data and Artificial Intelligence for Health Care: Developing an International Understanding. *JMIR Formative Research*, *6*(1), e31623. DOI: 10.2196/31623

Muhunzi, D., Kitambala, L., & Mashauri, H. L. (2024). Big data analytics in the healthcare sector: Opportunities and challenges in developing countries. A literature review. *Health Informatics Journal*, *30*(4), 14604582241294217. DOI: 10.1177/14604582241294217

Munia, A. A., Abdar, M., Hasan, M., Jalali, M. S., Banerjee, B., Khosravi, A., Hossain, I., Fu, H., & Frangi, A. F. (2025). Attention-guided hierarchical fusion U-Net for uncertainty-driven medical image segmentation. *Information Fusion*, *115*, 102719. DOI: 10.1016/j.inffus.2024.102719

Murala, D. K., Panda, S. K., & Dash, S. P. (2023). MedMetaverse: Medical Care of Chronic Disease Patients and Managing Data Using Artificial Intelligence, Blockchain, and Wearable Devices State-of-the-Art Methodology. *IEEE Access : Practical Innovations, Open Solutions*, *11*, 138954–138985. DOI: 10.1109/ACCESS.2023.3340791

Narayan, S. M., Kohli, N., & Martin, M. M. (2025). Addressing contemporary threats in anonymised healthcare data using privacy engineering. *NPJ Digital Medicine*, *8*(1), 145. DOI: 10.1038/s41746-025-01520-6

Obermeyer, Z., Powers, B., Vogeli, C., & Mullainathan, S. (2019). Dissecting racial bias in an algorithm used to manage the health of populations. *Science*, *366*(6464), 447–453. DOI: 10.1126/science.aax2342

Okoro, Y. O., Ayo-Farai, O., Maduka, C. P., Okongwu, C. C., & Sodamade, O. T. (2023). EMERGING TECHNOLOGIES IN PUBLIC HEALTH CAMPAIGNS: ARTIFICIAL IN LIGENCE AND BIG DATA. *Acta Informatica Malaysia*, *8*(1), 05–10. DOI: 10.26480/aim.01.2024.05.10

Olawade, D. B., David-Olawade, A. C., Wada, O. Z., Asaolu, A. J., Adereni, T., & Ling, J. (2024). Artificial intelligence in healthcare delivery: Prospects and pitfalls. *Journal of Medicine, Surgery, and Public Health*, *3*, 100108. DOI: 10.1016/j.glmedi.2024.100108

Pencina, M. J., Silcox, C., Economou-Zavlanos, N., & McClellan, M. (2025). Bridging the Gap Between Developers and Implementers in Health AI. *JAMA Health Forum*, *6*(6), e251692. DOI: 10.1001/jamahealthforum.2025.1692

Qi, K. (2025). Advancing hospital healthcare: Achieving IoT-based secure health monitoring through multilayer machine learning. *Journal of Big Data*, *12*(1), 1. DOI: 10.1186/s40537-024-01038-w

Rahman, A., Hossain, M., Muhammad, G., Kundu, D., Debnath, T., Rahman, M., Khan, M. S. I., Tiwari, P., & Band, S. S. (2023). Federated learning-based AI approaches in smart healthcare: Concepts, taxonomies, challenges and open issues. *Cluster Computing*, *26*(4), 2271–2311. DOI: 10.1007/s10586-022-03658-4

Rajkomar, A., Dean, J., & Kohane, I. (2019). Machine Learning in Medicine. *The New England Journal of Medicine*, *380*(14), 1347–1358. DOI: 10.1056/NEJMra1814259

Rao, A., & Aalami, O. (2023). Towards improving the visual explainability of artificial intelligence in the clinical setting. *BMC Digital Health*, *1*(1), 23. DOI: 10.1186/s44247-023-00022-3

Sabrina, F., Sohail, S., & Tariq, U. U. (2024). A Review of Post-Quantum Privacy Preservation for IoMT Using Blockchain. *Electronics (Basel)*, *13*(15), 2962. DOI: 10.3390/electronics13152962

Saeidnia, H. R., & Nilashi, M. (2025). From MYCIN to MedGemma: A Historical and Comparative Analysis of Healthcare AI Evolution. *InfoScience Trends*, *2*(6), 18–28. DOI: 10.61186/ist.202502.06.02

Sarker, D., Sadi, M. T. H., Gomes, D., & Hasan, Md. M. (2025). Securing Patient Privacy and Data Protection by Federated Learning in AI-Driven Healthcare: In N. K. Mun, C.-S. Shieh, D. Ather, A. Panwar, & V. Jain (Eds.), *Advances in Computational Intelligence and Robotics* (pp. 317–352). IGI Global Scientific Publishing. DOI: 10.4018/979-8-3373-3306-9.ch012

Secinaro, S., Calandra, D., Secinaro, A., Muthurangu, V., & Biancone, P. (2021). The role of artificial intelligence in healthcare: A structured literature review. *BMC Medical Informatics and Decision Making*, *21*(1), 125. DOI: 10.1186/s12911-021-01488-9

Shah, W. S., Elkhwesky, Z., Jasim, K. M., Elkhwesky, E. F. Y., & Elkhwesky, F. F. Y. (2024). Artificial intelligence in healthcare services: Past, present and future research directions. *Review of Managerial Science, 18*(3), 941–963. DOI: 10.1007/s11846-023-00699-w

Shahriar, S., Allana, S., Hazratifard, S. M., & Dara, R. (2023). A Survey of Privacy Risks and Mitigation Strategies in the Artificial Intelligence Life Cycle. *IEEE Access : Practical Innovations, Open Solutions, 11*, 61829–61854. DOI: 10.1109/ACCESS.2023.3287195

Si, J. (2025). Exploring AI literacy, attitudes toward AI, and intentions to use AI in clinical contexts among healthcare students in Korea: A cross-sectional study. *BMC Medical Education, 25*(1), 1233. DOI: 10.1186/s12909-025-07766-8

Solanki, P., Grundy, J., & Hussain, W. (2023). Operationalising ethics in artificial intelligence for healthcare: A framework for AI developers. *AI and Ethics, 3*(1), 223–240. DOI: 10.1007/s43681-022-00195-z

Sufian, M. A., Alsadder, L., Hamzi, W., Zaman, S., Sagar, A. S. M. S., & Hamzi, B. (2024). Mitigating Algorithmic Bias in AI-Driven Cardiovascular Imaging for Fairer Diagnostics. *Diagnostics (Basel), 14*(23), 2675. DOI: 10.3390/diagnostics14232675

Taimoor, N., & Rehman, S. (2022). Reliable and Resilient AI and IoT-Based Personalised Healthcare Services: A Survey. *IEEE Access : Practical Innovations, Open Solutions, 10*, 535–563. DOI: 10.1109/ACCESS.2021.3137364

Tiwari, A., Mishra, S., & Kuo, T.-R. (2025). Current AI technologies in cancer diagnostics and treatment. *Molecular Cancer, 24*(1), 159. DOI: 10.1186/s12943-025-02369-9

Tjhin, Y., Kewlani, B., Singh, H. K. S. I., & Pawa, N. (2024). Artificial intelligence in colorectal multidisciplinary team meetings. What are the medicolegal implications? *Colorectal Disease, 26*(9), 1749–1752. DOI: 10.1111/codi.17091

Toni, E., Toni, E., Fereidooni, M., & Ayatollahi, H. (2024). Acceptance and use of extended reality in surgical training: An umbrella review. *Systematic Reviews, 13*(1), 299. DOI: 10.1186/s13643-024-02723-w

Torab-Miandoab, A., Samad-Soltani, T., Jodati, A., & Rezaei-Hachesu, P. (2023). Interoperability of heterogeneous health information systems: A systematic literature review. *BMC Medical Informatics and Decision Making, 23*(1), 18. DOI: 10.1186/s12911-023-02115-5

Tun, H. M., Rahman, H. A., Naing, L., & Malik, O. A. (2025). Trust in Artificial Intelligence–Based Clinical Decision Support Systems Among Health Care Workers: Systematic Review. *Journal of Medical Internet Research*, *27*(1), e69678. DOI: 10.2196/69678

Ueda, D., Kakinuma, T., Fujita, S., Kamagata, K., Fushimi, Y., Ito, R., Matsui, Y., Nozaki, T., Nakaura, T., Fujima, N., Tatsugami, F., Yanagawa, M., Hirata, K., Yamada, A., Tsuboyama, T., Kawamura, M., Fujioka, T., & Naganawa, S. (2024). Fairness of artificial intelligence in healthcare: Review and recommendations. *Japanese Journal of Radiology*, *42*(1), 3–15. DOI: 10.1007/s11604-023-01474-3

Wakili, A., & Bakkali, S. (2024). Internet of Things in healthcare: An adaptive ethical framework for IoT in digital health. *Clinical eHealth, 7*, 92–105. DOI: 10.1016/j.ceh.2024.07.001

Wang, Z., Cao, L., Jin, Q., Chan, J., Wan, N., Afzali, B., Cho, H.-J., Choi, C.-I., Emamverdi, M., Gill, M. K., Kim, S.-H., Li, Y., Liu, Y., Luo, Y., Ong, H., Rousseau, J. F., Sheikh, I., Wei, J. J., Xu, Z., & Sun, J. (2025). A foundation model for human-AI collaboration in medical literature mining. *Nature Communications*, *16*(1), 8361. DOI: 10.1038/s41467-025-62058-5

Wong, Z. S.-Y., Gong, Y., & Ushiro, S. (2025). A pathway from fragmentation to interoperability through standards-based enterprise architecture to enhance patient safety. *NPJ Digital Medicine*, *8*(1), 41. DOI: 10.1038/s41746-025-01442-3

Xu, R., & Wang, Z. (2024). Generative artificial intelligence in healthcare from the perspective of digital media: Applications, opportunities and challenges. *Heliyon*, *10*(12), e32364. DOI: 10.1016/j.heliyon.2024.e32364

Yang, Y. (2024). Application of wearable devices based on artificial intelligence sensors in sports human health monitoring. *Measurement. Sensors*, *33*, 101086. DOI: 10.1016/j.measen.2024.101086

Zhang, X., Ma, L., Sun, D., Yi, M., & Wang, Z. (2024). Artificial Intelligence in Telemedicine: A Global Perspective Visualization Analysis. *Telemedicine Journal and e-Health*, *30*(7), e1909–e1922. DOI: 10.1089/tmj.2023.0704

Zhou, J., Sun, Y., & Tellambura, C. (2025, April 3). *Revolutionizing Medical Data Transmission with IoMT: A Comprehensive Survey of Wireless Communication Solutions and Future Directions* (Issue arXiv:2504.02446). arXiv. https://doi.org//arXiv.2504.02446DOI: 10.48550

Zondag, A. G. M., Rozestraten, R., Grimmelikhuijsen, S. G., Jongsma, K. R., Van Solinge, W. W., Bots, M. L., Vernooij, R. W. M., & Haitjema, S. (2024). The Effect of Artificial Intelligence on Patient-Physician Trust: Cross-Sectional Vignette Study. *Journal of Medical Internet Research*, *26*, e50853. DOI: 10.2196/50853

Zreikat, A. I., AlArnaout, Z., Abadleh, A., Elbasi, E., & Mostafa, N. (2025). The Integration of the Internet of Things (IoT) Applications into 5G Networks: A Review and Analysis. *Computers*, *14*(7), 250. DOI: 10.3390/computers14070250

Chapter 2
A Three Pillar Data-Centric Framework for Enabling AI-Driven Healthcare Collaboration

Roopam Dhanraj Choudhari
http://orcid.org/0009-0004-6606-0740
Walmart, USA

ABSTRACT

E-collaboration in healthcare has expanded through telehealth, remote monitoring, cloud EHRs, and connected diagnostics. However, despite unprecedented data availability, value extraction for collaborative workflows remains structurally limited. This chapter argues that data barriers—not modeling barriers—constitute the decisive bottleneck in AI-powered healthcare collaboration. While deep learning advances dominate discourse, algorithmic achievements depend on data that is ready, harmonized, semantically consistent, and identity-resolved, an assumption that is rarely met. This chapter presents a three-pillar framework: AI/Graph-Based Identity Resolution for unified patient representation across systems, AI/LLM-Driven Semantic Harmonization for consistent terminology, and Metadata Intelligence & AI-Native Data Fabric for machine-operable structure. Through analysis of data ecosystem components and real-world implementations including INPC, OHDSI, PCORnet, & eMERGE, this chapter demonstrates how addressing data infrastructure enables scalable AI-driven collaboration in healthcare.

DOI: 10.4018/979-8-3373-5906-9.ch002

1. INTRODUCTION

Healthcare organizations possess unprecedented data volumes through telehealth, remote monitoring, cloud-based EHRs, connected diagnostics, and digital therapeutics. Yet collaborative value extraction across clinicians, specialists, researchers, and care coordinators remains limited despite this abundance. This paradox exists because healthcare data across hospitals, imaging centers, pharmacies, laboratories, clinics, and specialist groups is not merely fragmented—it is structurally heterogeneous in provenance, poorly aligned in vocabulary, inconsistently codified, and often unlinkable to the same individual without manual intervention.

Research indicates that AI collaboration use-cases encounter failures before model execution: patient record stitching fails, local coding standards diverge, metadata proves unreliable, or semantic translation across systems becomes ambiguous (Kahn et al., 2016). This chapter addresses a critical question: *How can healthcare organizations systematically address data barriers to enable scalable, AI-driven collaboration across institutional boundaries and clinical specialties?*

The investigation focuses not on algorithmic innovation, but on the data substrate required for algorithms to operate collaboratively. The core proposition is that AI does not enable collaboration on its own; rather, data fitness enables AI-enabled collaboration. This represents a fundamental shift from algorithm-centric to data-centric AI development in healthcare contexts.

1.1 The Three-Pillar Framework

This chapter proposes three irreducible foundations for AI-driven healthcare collaboration:

Pillar 1: AI/Graph-Based Identity Resolution enables unified patient representation across disparate systems. Identity resolution transcends simple demographic matching to encompass probabilistic entity resolution, temporal identity evolution, and cross-institutional master patient indexing (Grannis et al., 2019).

Pillar 2: AI/LLM-Driven Semantic Harmonization ensures divergent vocabularies, terminologies, and local coding systems convey consistent meaning across entities. Semantic harmonization leverages natural language processing, large language models, and ontology alignment to create computational semantic consistency (Bodenreider, 2004; Wang et al., 2020).

Pillar 3: Metadata Intelligence & AI-Native Data Fabric provides machine-operable structure that AI models can consume consistently across domains.

Modern data fabric architectures deliver active metadata management, automated data lineage, and intelligent data catalog capabilities (Gartner, 2021).

These three pillars collectively form the infrastructure for scalable AI-enabled collaboration for diagnostic coordination, multi-specialty episodes, population health analytics, or distributed clinical research. Critically, they are model-enabling, not model-specific.

1.2 Historical Context and Existing Framework Landscape

Healthcare data fragmentation is not new, but AI adoption has intensified its implications. Early electronic health records (1960s-1990s) prioritized institutional efficiency over interoperability, establishing proprietary data silos that persist. The HITECH Act (2009) accelerated EHR adoption from 10% to 96% of hospitals by 2017, yet interoperability remained elusive—systems exchanged data without semantic consistency or reliable identity linkage (Adler-Milstein & Jha, 2017).

Existing frameworks address portions of this challenge. The HIMSS Interoperability Maturity Model focuses on data exchange levels but lacks AI-specific considerations. The NIH All of Us Research Program emphasizes participant engagement and data sharing but doesn't address identity resolution at scale. The European Interoperability Framework provides governance structures but limited technical architecture for AI enablement. FAIR principles (Findable, Accessible, Interoperable, Reusable) establish data management goals without specifying healthcare-specific implementation paths.

The three-pillar framework synthesizes insights from these efforts while addressing AI collaboration requirements: graph-based identity resolution extends traditional MPI approaches with machine learning; semantic harmonization incorporates LLM capabilities beyond static ontology mapping; metadata intelligence leverages active data fabric architectures. This positions the framework as complementary to existing standards while providing AI-specific architectural guidance currently absent from interoperability literature.

2. METHODOLOGY AND APPROACH

This chapter employs a multi-method approach integrating literature analysis, technical architecture review, and framework synthesis to examine how data engineering foundations enable AI-driven healthcare collaboration.

2.1 Systematic Literature Analysis

Peer-reviewed literature on healthcare data integration, interoperability standards, identity resolution, and semantic harmonization was systematically analyzed. Key databases searched included PubMed, IEEE Xplore, ACM Digital Library, and healthcare informatics journals spanning 2015-2024. Search terms encompassed "healthcare data integration," "patient identity resolution," "semantic interoperability," "health information exchange," and "clinical data harmonization."

Evaluation criteria:

- Empirical validation of data integration approaches in healthcare settings
- Technical specificity of identity resolution and semantic harmonization methods
- Documented outcomes related to collaborative care workflows
- Scalability characteristics for multi-institutional deployment

This systematic review synthesizes findings from health informatics, computer science, and clinical research to establish theoretical and empirical foundations for the three-pillar framework.

2.2 Technical Architecture Analysis

Data engineering architectures, integration patterns, and platform components supporting healthcare collaboration were examined across three domains:

Identity Resolution Systems: Analysis of Master Patient Index (MPI) architectures, probabilistic matching algorithms, and graph-based identity resolution approaches. Technical evaluation focused on matching accuracy methodologies, computational scalability, and temporal consistency requirements (Grannis et al., 2019; Zhu et al., 2017).

Semantic Harmonization Frameworks: Evaluation of terminology services, ontology alignment systems, natural language processing (NLP) pipelines for clinical text, and large language model applications for semantic mapping. Assessment covered medical vocabularies (ICD-10, SNOMED CT, LOINC, RxNorm), disambiguation methodologies, and contextual appropriateness (Bodenreider, 2004; Wang et al., 2020).

Data Fabric Architectures: Review of modern data fabric patterns including active metadata management, automated data lineage tracking, intelligent data cataloging, and knowledge graph foundations. Examination of how these components support AI model training, deployment, and governance (Gartner, 2021; Hogan et al., 2021).

2.3 Framework Synthesis

Findings from literature and technical analysis were synthesized into the three-pillar framework through systematic identification of common architectural patterns across successful implementations, extraction of design principles applicable to diverse healthcare contexts, documentation of technical dependencies, and evaluation criteria for framework components. The framework is technology-agnostic while providing sufficient specificity for practical implementation.

2.4 Validation Through Real-World Analysis

Documented implementations and published research demonstrating framework applicability were examined, including research on multi-institutional health information exchanges, technical documentation from healthcare data integration projects, academic studies of identity resolution and semantic interoperability systems, and industry reports on data fabric implementations. Validation focused on identifying alignment between the proposed framework and successful real-world implementations while documenting lessons learned.

This methodology provides the analytical foundation for examining healthcare's complex data ecosystem, where diverse sources, standards, and integration patterns create both opportunities and barriers for AI-driven collaboration.

3. THE HEALTHCARE DATA ECOSYSTEM: SOURCES, STANDARDS, AND INTEGRATION CHALLENGES

The healthcare data ecosystem comprises diverse data sources, integration platforms, interoperability standards, and governance frameworks that create fundamental barriers to AI-driven collaboration. Understanding this ecosystem reveals why data engineering—not just algorithmic innovation—determines collaborative AI success.

Figure 1. Healthcare Data Ecosystem

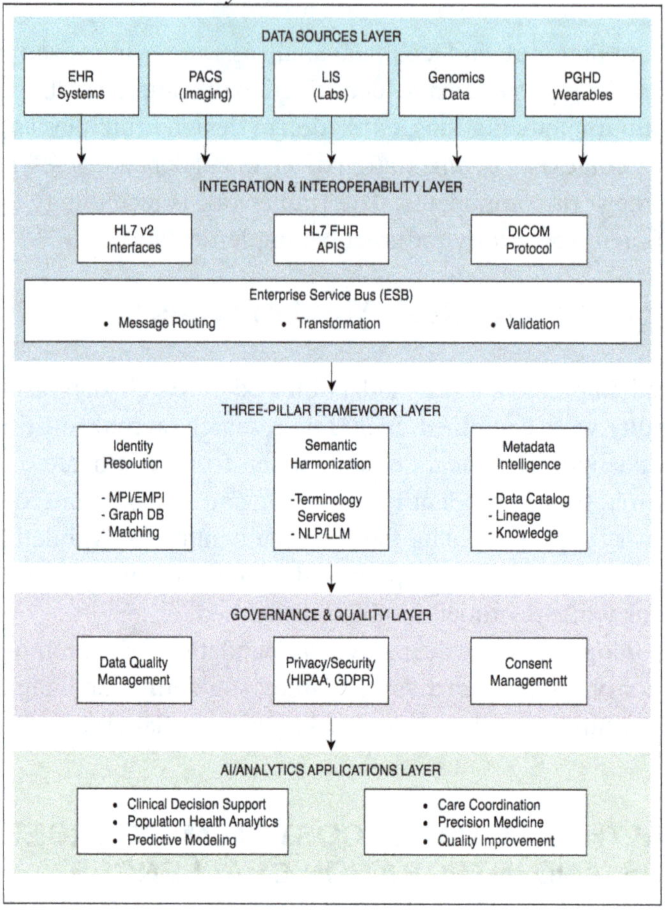

3.1 Data Sources and Provenance

Clinical Care Systems: Electronic Health Record (EHR) systems serve as the central repository for longitudinal patient data within healthcare organizations capturing structured fields (diagnoses, medications, vital signs) and unstructured narrative notes. Major platforms including Epic, Cerner, and Athenahealth implement proprietary data models with significant organizational customization, despite HL7 standards, creating semantic heterogeneity even when data exchange occurs (Bodenreider, 2004).

Diagnostic and Ancillary Systems: Laboratory Information Systems (LIS), Picture Archiving and Communication Systems (PACS), and pharmacy systems operate independently with specialized vocabularies. Radiology uses RadLex and DICOM, laboratories use LOINC, pharmacies use RxNorm and NDC codes. These systems rarely share common patient identifiers, requiring complex identity resolution.

Patient-Generated Health Data (PGHD): Wearable devices, mobile health apps, and remote monitoring systems generate continuous streams of physiological data, activity metrics, and symptom reports. Unlike clinician-generated data, PGHD lacks standardized quality assurance and suffers from missing data due to device malfunctions and variable user compliance. PGHD incorporation into clinical workflows remains limited by data quality concerns.

Claims and Administrative Data: Insurance claims, billing records, and administrative datasets provide complementary perspectives on healthcare utilization and outcomes. However, claims coding (ICD-10-CM, CPT, HCPCS) serves reimbursement rather than clinical documentation, creating semantic gaps when integrated with EHR data.

Table 1. Healthcare Data Sources and Integration Challenges

Data Source	Data Volume	Standardization	Primary Challenge	AI Relevance
EHRs/Clinics	High	Moderate (FHIR emerging)	• Vendor-specific models • Terminology inconsistency	Most comprehensive clinical data
PACS/ Imaging	Very High	High (DICOM)	• Image-report disconnection • Massive files	Essential for imaging AI
LIS/Labs	Moderate	Moderate (LOINC)	• Local code variations • Result semantics	Critical for diagnostic prediction
Genomics	Very High	Growing (HGVS, HPO)	• Semantic complexity • Privacy risks	Enables precision medicine
PGHD	High	Low	• Device heterogeneity • Data quality	Remote monitoring, patient engagement

3.2 Interoperability Standards

HL7 Version 2 is deployed in approximately 95% of healthcare organizations supporting critical real-time messaging including ADT (Admission, Discharge, Transfer), ORM (Order), and ORU (Result) messages. However, the standard permits substantial implementation variations. Local customizations proliferate, requiring custom interface engines for each connection (Benson & Grieve, 2016).

HL7 FHIR (Fast Healthcare Interoperability Resources) represents the modern evolution of healthcare interoperability. Developed starting in 2014, FHIR leverages modern web standards (RESTful APIs, JSON, OAuth) to enable flexible data exchange. FHIR has gained rapid adoption and is mandated by the 21st Century Cures Act for patient data access.

DICOM (Digital Imaging and Communications in Medicine) serves as the universal standard for medical imaging, defining both image format and network protocols. It enables radiology image exchange, yet interpretation reports often exist as unstructured text requiring NLP extraction for computational analysis.

3.3 Terminologies and Coding Systems

ICD-10-CM/PCS (International Classification of Diseases) serves as the primary diagnosis coding system, with ICD-10-CM covering approximately 70,000 diagnosis codes and ICD-10-PCS providing approximately 80,000 procedure codes. While comprehensive, ICD-10's hierarchical structure creates coding complexity and inconsistent application across organizations.

SNOMED CT (Systematized Nomenclature of Medicine Clinical Terms) provides the most comprehensive clinical terminology, with over 350,000 active concepts covering findings, disorders, procedures, and observable entities. SNOMED CT's polyhierarchical structure supports rich semantic relationships but creates implementation challenges (SNOMED International, 2021).

LOINC (Logical Observation Identifiers Names and Codes) standardizes laboratory tests and clinical observations with approximately 98,000 codes. LOINC adoption varies significantly across laboratories, with many maintaining proprietary local codes requiring ongoing mapping.

RxNorm provides normalized medication naming, linking over 100,000 medication names and enabling medication reconciliation across systems. RxNorm provides essential standardization integrating multiple medication vocabularies, connecting brand names, generic names, and clinical drugs, but requires continuous updates as new formulations appear.

CPT/HCPCS (Current Procedural Terminology/Healthcare Common Procedure Coding System) standardize procedure codes, with CPT covering physician services and HCPCS covering supplies, equipment, and non-physician services.

Table 2. Key Healthcare Interoperability and Terminology Standards

Standard	Primary Purpose	Adoption Level	AI Collaboration Value	Key Strength	Key Limitation
HL7 v2	Real-time system messaging (ADT, orders, results)	Very High (~95%)	**High** Real-time data feeds for event-driven AI	• Battle-tested • Universal adoption • Proven reliability	• Inconsistent implementation, • Limited semantics • Complex parsing
HL7 v3 (CDA)	Clinical document exchange	Moderate (CDA widely used)	**Moderate** Structured documents enable NLP	• Formal Reference Information Model (RIM) • Rich semantic structure	• Complexity limits adoption • XML verbosity
HL7 FHIR	RESTful APIs, bulk data export, app integration	Rapidly Growing (R4 production standard, R5 trial use, R6 development)	**Very High** Bulk export for training, SMART apps platform	• Modern web standards • Easy implementation • Strong regulatory momentum	• Maturity varies by resource type • Version migration challenges
DICOM	Medical imaging storage and transmission	Universal-Imaging	**Very High** Essential for imaging AI	• De facto medical imaging standard • Comprehensive metadata model	• Complex structure, not suitable for non-imaging
ICD-10-CM/PCS	Diagnosis and procedure coding	Universal-US	**Moderate** Common in training data, hierarchical structure	• Universal adoption • Regulatory requirement	• Billing-focused • Limited clinical granularity
SNOMED CT	Comprehensive clinical terminology	Growing	**Very High** Semantic relationships enable reasoning	• 350K+ concepts with formal relationships • Supports inference	• Complexity, licensing requirements, implementation effort
LOINC	Laboratory tests and observations	Moderate-High	**High** Essential for lab-based AI features	• Comprehensive lab coverage • Free to use	• Adoption variability •Local lab practices persist
RxNorm	Medication naming and reconciliation	High	**High** Critical for medication safety AI	• Links multiple naming systems • Regularly updated	• US-focused, complex concept relationships

continued on following page

Table 2. Continued

Standard	Primary Purpose	Adoption Level	AI Collaboration Value	Key Strength	Key Limitation
C-CDA	Structured clinical document exchange	High (US)	**Moderate** Standardized sections support NLP	• Widely adopted • Structured narrative + data	•Implementation variability • XML complexity
SMART on FHIR	Third-party app integration into EHRs	Growing	**Very High** Enables substitutable AI apps	• OAuth2 security • Easy app development	• Requires FHIR • Limited scope in some implementations

3.4 Integration Infrastructure Gaps

Current health information exchange infrastructure emphasizes point-to-point connections rather than semantic integration requiring substantial downstream pre-processing due to data heterogeneity. Regional Health Information Organizations (RHIOs) and Health Information Exchanges (HIEs) facilitate record location and retrieval but often deliver data in multiple formats requiring normalization. Lack of standardized identity resolution means the same patient appears with different medical record numbers across institutions, preventing automated linkage. Quality metadata is typically absent, leaving data consumers unable to assess provenance, completeness, or reliability computationally.

3.5 Data Governance and Compliance

HIPAA Compliance: Health Insurance Portability and Accountability Act establishes baseline privacy and security requirements for protected health information (PHI) in the United States. Key provisions include minimum necessary standard, accounting of disclosures, and breach notification requirements.

GDPR Requirements: General Data Protection Regulation imposes requirements for health data processing in the European Union, including explicit consent, right to erasure, and data portability.

De-identification Methods: Safe Harbor and Expert Determination methods under HIPAA enable data sharing for research and analytics while protecting patient privacy. Modern approaches incorporate differential privacy and synthetic data generation (Beaulieu-Jones et al., 2019).

Consent Management: Compliance needs to capture granular consent preferences (opt-in vs. opt-out, research vs. care vs. secondary use), dynamic consent allowing patients to modify preferences, audit trails documenting consent status at time of data access. Standards include HL7 FHIR Consent resource and XACML for policy enforcement.

This examination of healthcare data ecosystem components reveals fundamental challenges: data originates from heterogeneous sources using incompatible standards, flows through inadequate integration infrastructure, and lacks the quality, semantic consistency, and identity resolution that AI collaboration requires along with following compliance requirements. The following section presents a systematic framework addressing these structural barriers through three interdependent pillars.

4. THE THREE-PILLAR FRAMEWORK FOR AI-DRIVEN COLLABORATION

This section presents the comprehensive three-pillar framework that addresses the fundamental data barriers inhibiting AI-driven healthcare collaboration. Each pillar is examined in depth, including theoretical foundations, technical approaches, architectural patterns, and evaluation methodologies.

4.1 Pillar 1: AI/Graph-Based Identity Resolution

Identity resolution is the process of determining whether data records refer to the same real-world entity that represents the foundational requirement for healthcare collaboration. Without reliable identity resolution, clinical data remains fragmented across institutional silos, precluding comprehensive patient views and multi-institutional AI applications.

Figure 2. Identity Resolution Architecture

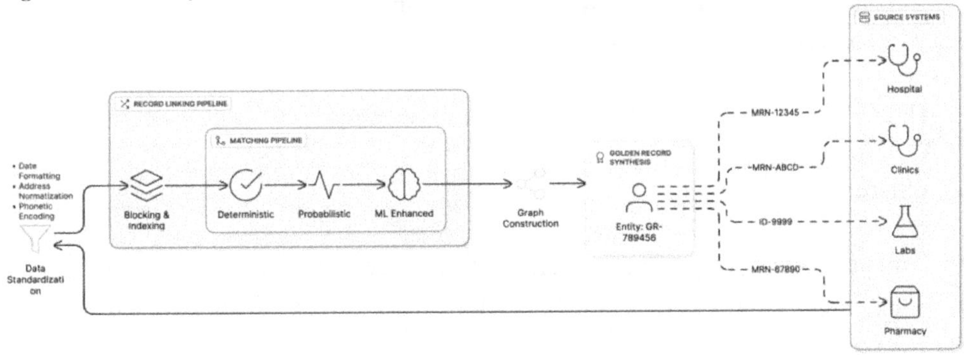

4.1.1 The Identity Challenge in Healthcare

Healthcare presents unique identity resolution challenges that distinguish it from other domains requiring sophisticated probabilistic methods.

- *Absence of Universal Identifier:* Unlike many industries, healthcare lacks a universal patient identifier. Each healthcare organization assigns local medical record numbers (MRNs), creating proliferation of identifiers without authoritative cross-reference.
- *Name Variability:* Patients may use different name variants across providers (full legal name, nicknames, maiden names, married names). Transcription errors, character set issues (special characters, accents), and data entry inconsistencies compound matching difficulty.
- *Demographic Evolution:* Patient demographics evolve over time (address changes, phone number changes, insurance transitions), complicating longitudinal identity resolution.
- *Data Quality Issues:* Missing or erroneous demographic data degrades matching accuracy. Research documents substantial data quality issues in registration records affecting matching (Grannis et al., 2019).

4.1.2 Fellegi-Sunter Model

The theoretical foundation for probabilistic record linkage derives from the seminal work of Fellegi and Sunter (1969), who formulated record linkage as a classification problem with three possible outcomes:

- M: Records refer to same entity (match)
- U: Records refer to different entities (non-match)
- P: Uncertain (requires clerical review)

The Fellegi-Sunter model computes match weight as:
$W = \Sigma \log_2[m(\gamma) / u(\gamma)]$
Where:

- $m(\gamma)$ = probability of agreement pattern γ given records are true match
- $u(\gamma)$ = probability of agreement pattern γ given records are non-match

This probabilistic framework provides mathematical foundation for quantifying match confidence and has been extensively validated in healthcare contexts (Grannis et al., 2019).

4.1.3 Deterministic vs. Probabilistic Matching

Traditional identity resolution employs two primary approaches:

Deterministic Matching: Requires exact agreement on specified fields (e.g., last name, first name, date of birth, ZIP). Simple to implement but brittle in the presence of data errors or variations. Typically achieves high precision but lower recall (Grannis et al., 2019).

Probabilistic Matching: Assigns weights to matching and non-matching field comparisons, computing cumulative match score. Based on Fellegi-Sunter theory, probabilistic matching accommodates data variability and quality issues. Tunable thresholds balance precision and recall.

Modern approaches combine deterministic and probabilistic methods in multi-stage pipelines: initial blocking/indexing reduces candidate pairs, deterministic rules capture high-confidence matches, and probabilistic scoring resolves ambiguous cases.

4.1.4 Machine Learning-Enhanced Matching

Contemporary identity resolution increasingly employs machine learning to improve accuracy.

Supervised Learning Approaches: Train classification models (logistic regression, random forests, gradient boosting) on labeled match/non-match pairs, enabling systems to learn optimal matching rules from local demographic patterns.

Active Learning: Selectively presents ambiguous record pairs to human reviewers, incorporating feedback to refine models. Prioritizes review of records with highest impact on match network topology, maximizing accuracy improvement per review effort.

4.1.5 Graph-Based Identity Resolution

Traditional pairwise matching scales poorly for networks with numerous source systems. Modern enterprise identity resolution increasingly adopts graph-based approaches that model identity as a network of entities, attributes, and relationships. Graph neural networks learn embedding representations capturing both attribute similarity and relational structure, outperforming purely attribute-based methods when integrating 5+ source systems (Zhu et al., 2017).

Temporal consistency adds complexity: patients move, change names, update contact information. Graph approaches track identity evolution over time, maintaining historical linkages while accommodating legitimate changes and detecting fraudulent identity use.

4.1.6 Enterprise Master Patient Index Architecture

Enterprise Master Patient Index (EMPI) system provide centralized identity management across healthcare networks. Core components include identity ingestion from multiple source systems via HL7 ADT feeds or FHIR interfaces, probabilistic matching engines computing similarity scores, human stewardship workbenches for ambiguous case review, and master person index maintaining unique identifiers linking all records for each patient.

Hybrid human-machine approaches prove essential. Automated matching handles high-volume, high-confidence cases efficiently. Human stewards review medium-confidence matches where algorithmic certainty is insufficient. This division of labor balances accuracy with operational efficiency while enabling continuous improvement as steward decisions refine matching algorithms.

4.1.7 Key Takeaways: Why Identity Resolution Matters

- Without reliable identity resolution, AI models trained on fragmented patient records produce biased, inaccurate predictions that undermine clinical trust.
- Identity resolution errors have direct patient safety consequences: duplicate testing, medication errors, missed critical diagnoses.
- Enterprise identity resolution achieves F1-scores of 0.85-0.90, meaning 10-15% of records may remain incorrectly linked—requiring ongoing stewardship, not one-time implementation.
- Graph-based approaches outperform traditional probabilistic methods when integrating 5+ source systems, making them essential for complex healthcare networks.

4.2 Pillar 2: AI/LLM-Driven Semantic Harmonization

Semantic harmonization ensures that clinical concepts expressed in diverse terminologies, abbreviations, documentation styles, and local vocabularies can be interpreted consistently across institutional boundaries. This pillar leverages NLP, ontology alignment, and LLMs to create computational semantic interoperability (Bodenreider, 2004).

Figure 3. Semantic Harmonization Architecture

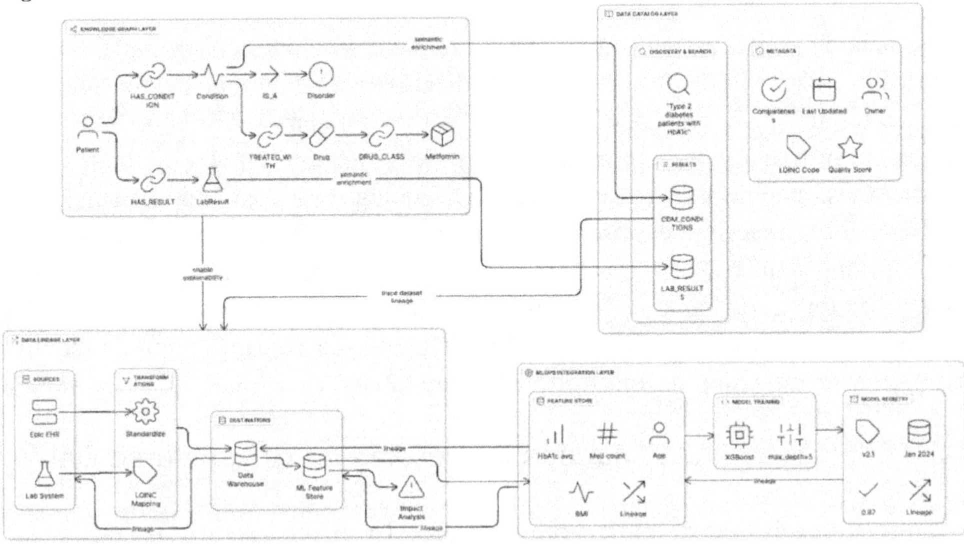

4.2.1 Sources of Semantic Heterogeneity

Multiple Standard Vocabularies: Clinical concepts may be represented in ICD-10-CM, SNOMED CT, LOINC, RxNorm, CPT, or proprietary local terminologies. The same diagnosis might be recorded as:

- ICD-10-CM: E11.9 (Type 2 diabetes mellitus without complications)
- SNOMED CT: 44054006 (Diabetes mellitus type 2)
- Free text: “DM2”, “T2DM”, “Type II diabetes”, “Adult-onset diabetes”

Documentation Variability: Clinicians document using narrative notes, templated phrases, or structured problem lists. The same clinical finding may appear in multiple forms across documentation styles.

Local Customization: Healthcare organizations create “local codes” extending standard vocabularies into hospital-specific order sets, department-specific procedure descriptions, or abbreviated diagnoses in specialty contexts.

Temporal Terminology Evolution: Medical terminology evolves as understanding advances. Older records use outdated terms (e.g., “Non-insulin-dependent diabetes mellitus” vs. “Type 2 diabetes mellitus”), requiring temporal-aware semantic mapping.

4.2.2 Vocabulary Mapping and Terminology Services

Semantic harmonization begins with systematic vocabulary mapping. Common Data Models like OMOP (Observational Medical Outcomes Partnership) define target schemas requiring all local codes map to standard vocabularies. The Unified Medical Language System (UMLS) provides concept-level integration across 200+ source vocabularies, enabling translation between terminology systems (Bodenreider, 2004).

Terminology services expose these mappings via APIs, accepting source codes and returning standardized equivalents. However, mapping is rarely one-to-one. A local laboratory code for "glucose" might map to multiple LOINC codes depending on specimen type, timing, and methodology. Context-appropriate mapping requires semantic understanding beyond simple lookup tables.

4.2.3 Clinical Natural Language Processing for Unstructured Data

Approximately 80% of clinical information exists in unstructured narrative text: progress notes, radiology reports, pathology interpretations, discharge summaries. Clinical NLP extracts structured concepts using named entity recognition to identify clinical terms (diseases, medications, procedures), assertion classification to determine whether concepts are present, absent, or uncertain, temporal extraction to establish event timing, and relationship extraction to capture associations between entities.

The i2b2 (Informatics for Integrating Biology and the Bedside) shared tasks established standardized benchmarks. Best-performing systems achieve F1-scores of 0.85-0.90 for medication extraction, 0.80-0.85 for disorder identification, but only 0.65-0.75 for relationship extraction (Uzuner et al., 2011). These benchmarks establish realistic expectations: clinical NLP achieves useful accuracy for many applications while requiring human review for critical uses.

4.2.4 Large Language Models (LLMs) for Semantic Mapping

LLMs demonstrate potential for automated semantic harmonization. LLMs can suggest terminology mappings by understanding clinical context, disambiguate abbreviations and acronyms that confound rule-based systems, normalize narrative text into standardized concepts, and identify semantic equivalence despite lexical variation.

However, LLM application in clinical contexts requires rigorous validation. Models can hallucinate terminology mappings that appear plausible but are clinically incorrect, introducing errors when propagated through healthcare AI systems. Validation against gold-standard medical knowledge bases and human expert review remains essential (Wang et al., 2020). Recent foundation models demonstrate substantial advances. Singhal et al. (2023) introduced Med-PaLM 2, a large language model fine-tuned for medicine that achieved 85.4% accuracy on medical licensing exam questions, and demonstrating sophisticated understanding of medical terminology, diagnostic reasoning, and treatment recommendations. However, the study emphasizes that rigorous validation frameworks remain essential before clinical deployment, particularly for semantic harmonization tasks where terminology errors could propagate through AI collaboration pipelines.

4.2.5 Ontology Alignment for Knowledge Integration

Semantic harmonization extends beyond terminology to include clinical knowledge representation. Disease ontologies capture hierarchical relationships (acute myocardial infarction is a type of ischemic heart disease), drug ontologies encode ingredient compositions and therapeutic classes, and phenotype ontologies link observable characteristics to underlying conditions. Knowledge graph technologies integrate these structures, enabling AI systems to reason beyond statistical patterns by incorporating medical knowledge (Hogan et al., 2021).

4.2.5 Key Takeaways: Why Semantic Harmonization Matters

- Healthcare uses 100+ terminology systems (ICD-10, SNOMED, LOINC, RxNorm, local codes)—AI models cannot learn from semantically inconsistent data
- A "myocardial infarction" in one system may be "heart attack," "MI," or "acute coronary syndrome" in others—semantic harmonization ensures AI recognizes these as equivalent
- LLM-based semantic mapping shows promise but requires rigorous validation to prevent hallucinated terminology mappings that could introduce clinical errors
- Semantic harmonization is continuous work, not a one-time project—terminologies update quarterly, local codes proliferate, and clinical language evolves.

4.3 Pillar 3: Metadata Intelligence & AI-Native Data Fabric

AI model quality depends fundamentally on data quality, yet healthcare organizations often lack systematic methods for assessing completeness, accuracy, consistency, and timeliness at scale. Metadata intelligence provides computational infrastructure for data governance, quality monitoring, lineage tracking, and catalog management that AI systems require (Gartner, 2021).

Figure 4. Data Fabric Architecture

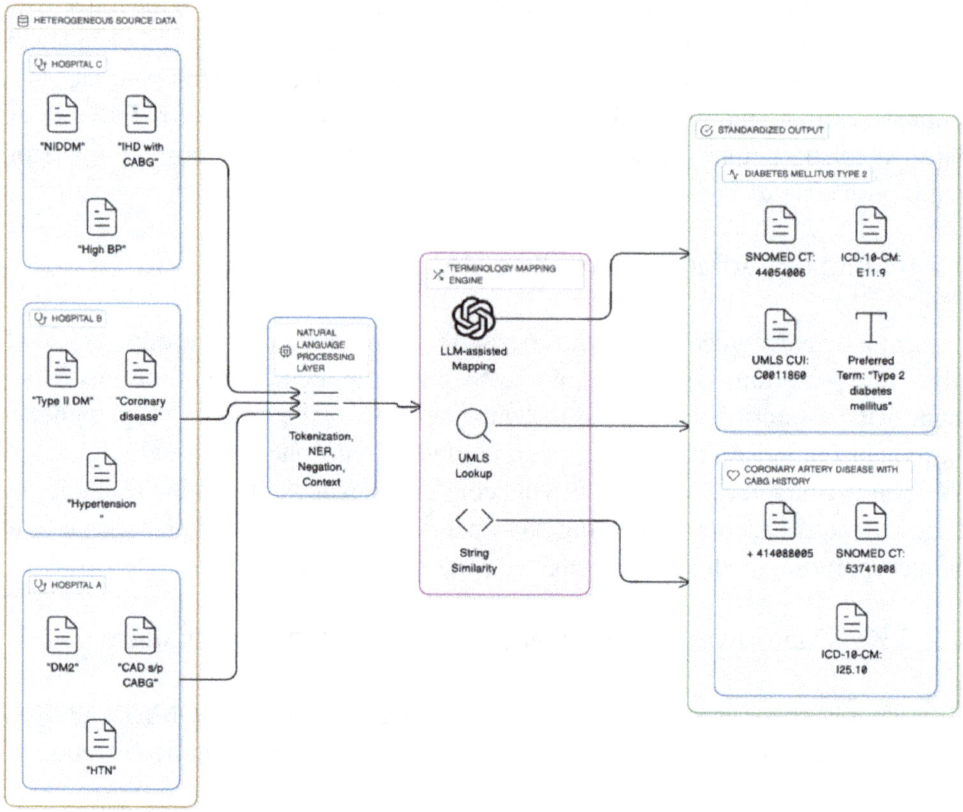

4.3.1 The Metadata Challenge

Traditional healthcare data integration focuses on moving data between systems but provides limited metadata documentation, missing key metadata dimensions:

- Lineage: Where did this data originate? What transformations were applied?
- Quality: What is the completeness rate? Are values plausible? When was it last validated?
- Semantics: What does this field represent? What vocabulary/units are used? What clinical context applies?
- Governance: Who is authorized to access? What consent applies? What regulations govern use?
- Operational: When was data last updated? What is refresh frequency? Are there known issues?

Without rich metadata, data consumers (whether human analysts or AI systems) cannot reliably interpret data, assess fitness for purpose, or trust results.

4.3.2 Active Metadata Management

Traditional metadata management treats metadata as static documentation. Active metadata management embeds intelligence into metadata systems, enabling automated quality assessment, impact analysis when schemas change, recommendation of relevant datasets for specific analytical tasks, and automated policy enforcement for privacy and security.

Modern data fabrics implement active metadata through machine learning models that learn from usage patterns, predict data quality issues before they impact downstream systems, and suggest optimal data pipelines for new analytical requirements (Gartner, 2021).

4.3.3 Automated Data Lineage

Data lineage tracks data from source systems through transformations to analytics and AI models. For AI applications, lineage answers critical questions: Which source systems contributed to this training dataset? What transformations were applied? When was it last updated?

Automated lineage tracking instruments data pipelines, capturing transformations as they execute rather than relying on manual documentation that becomes outdated. This automation reduces data engineering workload by 40-60% while ensuring accuracy that manual processes cannot sustain.

4.3.4 Data Quality Frameworks

PCORnet (Patient-Centered Outcomes Research Network) developed comprehensive quality assessment addressing the Kahn Framework dimensions: conformance (adherence to specifications), completeness (expected data presence), plausibility (clinical reasonableness), and consistency (agreement across elements). Automated Data Quality Dashboard software assesses participating networks systematically (Kahn et al., 2016).

Quality dimensions for AI specifically include representation completeness (do training data include diverse patient populations?), label accuracy (are outcome labels clinically validated?), temporal stability (do data distributions shift over time?), and missingness patterns (is missing data random or systematic?).

4.3.5 Knowledge Graph Foundations

Knowledge graphs provide semantic layer connecting datasets, entities, concepts, and relationships. They represent medical knowledge as interconnected entities: diseases, symptoms, treatments, drug interactions, and genetic variants. Graph databases like Neo4j enable efficient traversal of these relationships, supporting AI reasoning that incorporates medical knowledge alongside data-driven pattern recognition.

Clinical decision support, drug safety monitoring, and precision medicine applications leverage knowledge graphs to contextualize patient data against established medical knowledge, moving beyond pure statistical association toward causal and mechanistic understanding.

4.3.6 DataOps and MLOps Integration

Data fabric architectures integrate with DataOps and MLOps practices to ensure reliable AI workflows.

DataOps Principles:

- Automation: Automated data quality monitoring, anomaly detection, pipeline orchestration
- Continuous Integration/Deployment: Data pipeline version control, testing, deployment
- Monitoring: Real-time data quality dashboards, SLA tracking, alerting
- Collaboration: Shared metadata, documentation, and communication channels

MLOps Integration:

- Feature Store: Centralized repository of curated features for ML models. Ensures consistency between training and serving. Tracks feature lineage from source data to model predictions.
- Model Registry: Catalog of trained models with metadata (training data, hyperparameters, performance metrics, lineage). Enables model versioning, A/B testing, rollback.
- Experiment Tracking: Logs model training experiments, hyperparameter searches, performance results. Provides audit trail for model development.

4.3.7 Privacy-Preserving Collaboration Technologies

Data fabric architectures increasingly incorporate privacy-enhancing technologies:

Federated Learning: Train AI models across distributed datasets without centralizing data. Each institution trains local model; only model updates are shared. Enables multi-institutional AI without data sharing (McMahan et al., 2017).

Differential Privacy: Add calibrated noise to query results to prevent reidentification. Formal privacy guarantees (epsilon, delta parameters) enable sharing of aggregate statistics while protecting individuals.

Secure Multi-Party Computation: Cryptographic protocols enabling joint computation without revealing inputs. Institutions collectively compute statistics or models without seeing each other's data.

Confidential Computing: Hardware-based trusted execution environments (TEEs) protect data during processing. Data encrypted in memory, decrypted only within TEE. Even cloud provider cannot access data.

4.3.8 Key Takeaways: Why Metadata Intelligence Matters

- AI model quality depends on data quality—metadata systems provide the quality assessment, lineage tracking, and governance that ensure AI learns from reliable data
- "Garbage in, garbage out" is amplified with AI: poor metadata leads to models that appear to perform well in development but fail catastrophically in production
- Active metadata management reduces data engineering workload by 40-60% through automation of quality monitoring, lineage tracking, and catalog maintenance
- Knowledge graphs enable AI systems to incorporate medical knowledge (drug interactions, disease relationships) beyond pattern recognition from data alone

4.4 Clinical Workflow Integration and Adoption Challenges

Technical infrastructure alone does not ensure adoption. The three-pillar framework must integrate into clinical workflows without creating unsustainable burden on frontline providers already facing documentation overload and alert fatigue.

4.4.1 Identity Resolution in Clinical Practice

Real-World Scenario: A patient presents to an emergency department having recently been discharged from a different hospital system. The ED physician needs access to recent lab results, medication lists, and specialist notes to make safe treatment decisions.

Without Identity Resolution: The physician manually searches for records using name and date of birth, encountering multiple potential matches due to common names or data entry variations. Unable to confirm identity, the physician orders duplicate tests, delays treatment, or proceeds with incomplete information risking adverse drug interactions or contraindicated procedures.

With Framework Implementation: Automated identity resolution presents the physician with a unified patient record from participating institutions with confidence scores. High-confidence matches display automatically; medium-confidence matches prompt brief review; low-confidence situations default to traditional verification. The system operates within existing EHR workflows, requiring no separate login or manual reconciliation.

Adoption Barriers: Physicians may distrust algorithmic identity matching, particularly early in deployment. Change management requires transparent communication about matching accuracy, visible confidence scoring, easy pathways to report errors, and gradual expansion from pilot units to enterprise deployment based on demonstrated reliability.

4.4.2 Semantic Harmonization in Multi-Specialty Care

Real-World Scenario: An oncologist managing a patient with complex cancer receives pathology reports using institutional-specific terminology, radiology reports in different coding systems, and laboratory results with non-standard units. Synthesizing information for treatment decisions requires manual translation across these semantic differences.

Without Semantic Harmonization: The oncologist manually reconciles terminology differences, diverting time from patient care to resolve semantic ambiguities. Subtle differences might be missed, potentially leading to suboptimal treatment decisions.

With Framework Implementation: The EHR presents harmonized clinical concepts automatically translated to the oncologist's preferred terminology. Pathology findings map to standard SNOMED codes, radiology to RadLex, laboratories to LOINC. The system maintains source terminology for auditing but displays harmonized concepts for clinical use. LLM-enhanced translation handles narrative text, extracting structured concepts from unstructured notes.

Adoption Barriers: Clinicians may perceive automated translation as introducing errors or losing clinical nuance. Implementation requires clinician champions from each specialty validating semantic mappings, feedback mechanisms for reporting translation errors, and continuous improvement incorporating clinician corrections into mapping refinement.

4.4.3 Metadata Intelligence for Clinical Decision Support

Real-World Scenario: A primary care physician considers prescribing a medication flagged by the EHR as potentially contraindicated based on genomic testing from three years ago. The physician needs to determine whether the genetic test result is still current, was performed in a CLIA-certified laboratory, and is clinically actionable for this specific drug.

Without Metadata Intelligence: The physician sees the alert but lacks context about data provenance, quality, or clinical validity. Overwhelmed by frequent low-quality alerts, the physician may override without investigation or spend excessive time researching data provenance.

With Framework Implementation: Metadata provides immediate context: laboratory certification status, test methodology and date, clinical validity classification, data lineage showing the source laboratory, and pharmacogenomic guidelines supporting the alert. The physician makes an informed decision in seconds rather than minutes, with confidence in data quality supporting clinical judgment.

Adoption Barriers: Metadata systems add complexity to data infrastructure that may not produce immediately visible clinical value. Implementation requires demonstrating reduced alert burden through better-quality alerts, faster clinical decision-making through immediate context, and reduced liability risk through documented data provenance.

4.4.4 Change Management Strategies

Successful framework adoption requires systematic change management addressing technical, organizational, and human factors:

Incremental Deployment: Begin with high-value, low-complexity use cases demonstrating quick wins. Emergency department patient identification provides immediate safety value with clear ROI. Expand systematically based on demonstrated success rather than attempting enterprise-wide deployment simultaneously.

Clinician Engagement: Involve frontline physicians, nurses, and pharmacists in design decisions. Technical teams often prioritize architectural elegance over workflow fit; clinician input ensures solutions match actual care delivery patterns.

Training and Support: Provide role-specific training focusing on clinical value rather than technical architecture. Emergency physicians need different training than pathologists or primary care providers.

Performance Monitoring: Track both technical metrics (matching accuracy, semantic precision) and clinical metrics (time to access external records, duplicate test ordering, clinician satisfaction). Demonstrate value in clinical terms, not just technical terms.

Continuous Improvement: Establish feedback loops where clinicians report errors, suggest improvements, and see their input incorporated into system refinement. This builds trust and sustained engagement beyond initial deployment.

The three-pillar framework provides theoretical and technical foundations for AI-driven healthcare collaboration, but practical viability depends on real-world validation. The following section examines documented implementations demonstrating that identity resolution, semantic harmonization, and metadata intelligence operate effectively at enterprise scale when properly architected and governed.

5. REAL-WORLD IMPLEMENTATIONS AND VALIDATIONS

This section examines documented real-world implementations that validate components of the three-pillar framework. Each example addresses specific framework components while providing empirical performance benchmarks and demonstrating operational sustainability at scale.

5.1 Multi-Institutional Identity Resolution: The Indiana Network Experience

The Indiana Network for Patient Care (INPC) validates Pillar 1 on graph-based identity resolution approaches through operational deployment across 100+ hospitals and healthcare facilities in Indiana (Grannis et al., 2019).

5.1.1 System Architecture and Technical Approach

The system addresses the fundamental identity resolution challenge: linking patient records across organizations that each maintain independent medical record numbering systems.

Figure 5. INPC Implementation Architecture

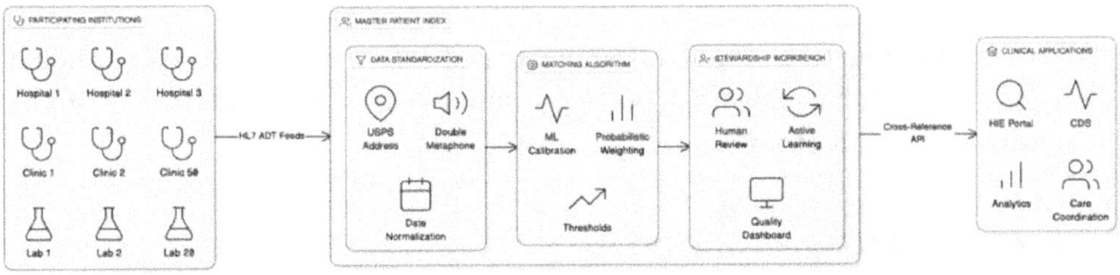

The INPC Master Patient Index (MPI) employs probabilistic matching based on the Fellegi-Sunter model, enhanced with machine learning trained on local demographic patterns, utilizing phonetic encoding (Soundex, Double Metaphone) and USPS address standardization. Human stewardship workbenches enable trained reviewers to address ambiguous matches, implementing active learning to continuously refine algorithms.

5.1.2 Published Validation Results

Published gold-standard evaluation demonstrates probabilistic matching substantially outperforms deterministic approaches, achieving F1-scores of 0.85-0.90. Machine learning methods show incremental improvement when incorporating local data patterns. The results establish realistic benchmarks for enterprise identity resolution while confirming operational sustainability over extended periods (Grannis et al., 2019).

5.1.3 Framework Validation

INPC validates that hybrid human-machine approaches prove essential: automation handles volume while human oversight maintains accuracy as demographics and systems evolve. The implementation demonstrates that sophisticated identity resolution operates effectively at regional scale with proper architectural design and sustained governance. The INPC research provides empirical foundation for the identity resolution pillar, demonstrating technical feasibility and operational sustainability.

5.2 Semantic Harmonization: The OHDSI Network

The Observational Health Data Sciences and Informatics (OHDSI) validates Pillar 2 through a global network of 600+ institutions across 50+ countries executing standardized research protocols (Hripcsak et al., 2015).

Figure 6. OHDSI Network Architecture

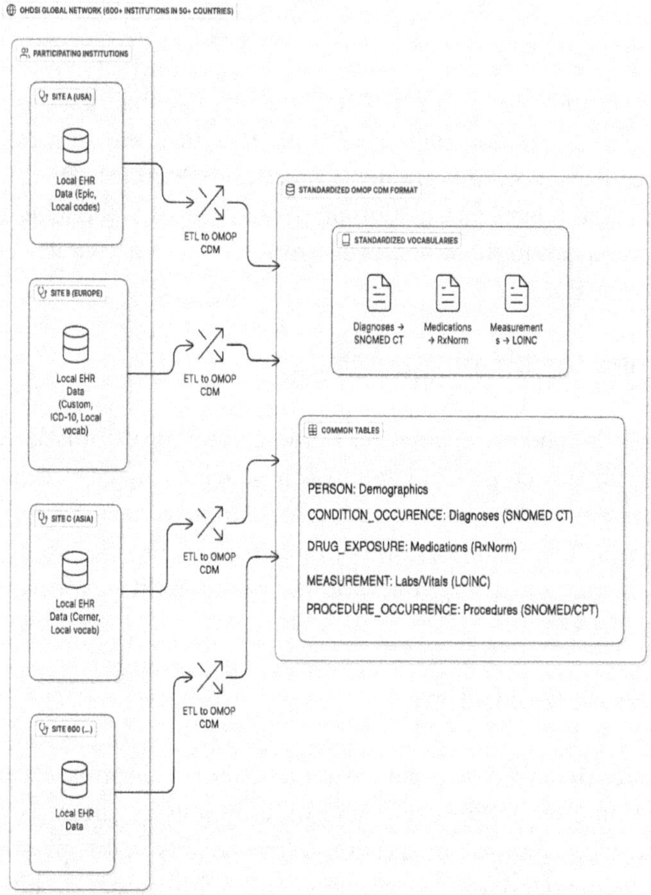

5.2.1 The OMOP Common Data Model

OHDSI developed the OMOP Common Data Model (CDM) to address semantic heterogeneity across institutions. It defines standardized schemas requiring all local codes map to standard vocabularies: SNOMED CT for conditions, RxNorm for medications, LOINC for laboratory tests. The USAGI tool provides semi-automated mapping with string similarity suggestions requiring domain expert validation, balancing automation efficiency with semantic accuracy.

5.2.2 Multi-Institutional Research Outcomes

The OHDSI network has published numerous multi-institutional studies demonstrating semantic harmonization value (Hripcsak et al., 2015). Standardized data models and vocabularies enable researchers to execute identical analytical code across institutions, producing comparable results despite underlying system heterogeneity. Published studies demonstrate feasibility for comparative effectiveness research, safety surveillance, phenotype validation, and treatment pathway analysis at unprecedented scale (Voss et al., 2015). This provides strong validation for Framework Pillar 2.

5.2.3 Framework Validation

OHDSI confirms that common data models combined with systematic vocabulary mapping enable global-scale research when properly implemented with community governance. The experience reveals semantic harmonization requires ongoing maintenance—not one-time mapping—as terminologies evolve and local codes proliferate. Labor-intensive implementation proves worthwhile for enabling collaborative research otherwise impossible.

5.3 Natural Language Processing: Clinical Text Extraction

The i2b2 National Center for Biomedical Computing conducted shared tasks evaluating clinical NLP systems, providing standardized benchmarks for semantic extraction from clinical narratives (Uzuner et al., 2011).

5.3.1 i2b2 Shared Task Methodology

The i2b2 challenges established gold-standard annotated clinical text datasets and evaluation frameworks. Expert clinicians manually annotated de-identified clinical notes across multiple domains: medication extraction, disease identification, temporal relations, and coreference resolution. Participating teams developed NLP systems evaluated using precision, recall, and F1-scores, with inter-annotator agreement establishing annotation reliability.

5.3.2 Published Performance Results

The i2b2 challenges documented achievable accuracy levels for clinical NLP tasks (Uzuner et al., 2011). Best-performing systems achieved medication name extraction F1-scores of 0.85-0.90, disorder extraction 0.80-0.85, and assertion classification (present/absent/uncertain) approximately 0.90. More complex tasks showed lower performance: relationship extraction 0.65-0.75, temporal status identification 0.75-0.85.

5.3.3 Framework Validation

The i2b2 shared task results validate that clinical NLP achieves useful accuracy for many applications while confirming human review remains valuable for high-stakes uses. Performance varies across clinical specialties and documentation styles, requiring domain adaptation. These benchmarks enable organizations to set realistic expectations for NLP components within semantic harmonization infrastructure.

5.4 Data Fabric Implementation: PCORnet Common Data Model

The PCORnet validates Pillar 3 through a national distributed research network using common data model and automated quality assessment (Fleurence et al., 2014).

5.4.1 PCORnet Architecture

PCORnet connects Clinical Data Research Networks (CDRNs) and Patient-Powered Research Networks (PPRNs) through the PCORnet Common Data Model covering demographics, encounters, diagnoses, procedures, vital signs, laboratory results, and prescriptions. PopMedNet enables federated queries: researchers define cohorts via web-based composer, distribute queries to participating networks, and receive aggregate counts without patient-level data exposure.

5.4.2 Data Quality Framework

PCORnet developed comprehensive quality assessment addressing the Kahn Framework dimensions: conformance (adherence to specifications), completeness (expected data presence), plausibility (clinical reasonableness), and consistency (agreement across elements). Automated Data Quality Dashboard software assesses participating networks' data, generating standardized reports (Kahn et al., 2016).

5.4.3 Published Research Outcomes

PCORnet has enabled numerous multi-site comparative effectiveness studies and pragmatic clinical trials (Fleurence et al., 2014). Publications demonstrate that common data models combined with federated query infrastructure enable rapid cohort identification and efficient multi-site research while maintaining data governance and privacy protections.

5.4.4 Framework Validation

PCORnet demonstrates that explicit metadata frameworks enable distributed research while maintaining governance. Automated quality assessment scales across networks, providing systematic evaluation impossible through manual review. The implementation proves metadata documentation and quality monitoring are technical enablers—not administrative overhead—essential for collaborative analytics and pragmatic clinical trials embedded in care delivery. The PCORnet experience demonstrates feasibility of data fabric principles at national scale, while documenting ongoing challenges in data quality and semantic consistency.

5.5 Pharmacogenomics Implementation: eMERGE Network

The Electronic Medical Records and Genomics (eMERGE) Network demonstrates that sophisticated applications require all three pillars functioning cohesively (Gottesman et al., 2013).

5.5.1 Network Architecture

eMERGE connects genomic data with electronic health records for precision medicine across 10+ academic medical centers. Implementation necessitates robust identity resolution linking genomic identifiers to clinical records (Pillar 1), computable phenotype algorithms requiring semantic harmonization across institutions (Pillar 2), and knowledge graphs integrating variant-phenotype-drug relationships (Pillar 3).

5.5.2 Phenotype Algorithm Development

eMERGE developed validated algorithms for numerous phenotypes (diabetes, atrial fibrillation, peripheral arterial disease) using structured data criteria, NLP extraction, temporal logic, and exclusion criteria demonstrating semantic harmonization principles. Gold-standard chart review established positive predictive values of 0.85-0.95 and sensitivity of 0.70-0.90. Cross-site validation assessed algorithm transportability across different institutions. (Gottesman et al., 2013)

5.5.3 Pharmacogenomic Implementation

eMERGE implemented clinical decision support for actionable pharmacogenomic variants following Clinical Pharmacogenetics Implementation Consortium (CPIC) guidelines demonstrates clinical decision support integration. Genomic variants stored in structured EHR fields trigger alerts during prescribing with dosing recommendations. Published implementation studies document clinician adoption and prescribing behavior changes. (Gottesman et al., 2013).

5.5.4 Framework Validation

eMERGE validates that precision medicine at scale requires all three pillars operating interdependently. Genomic-clinical linkage demands identity resolution, phenotype definitions require semantic consistency, and knowledge integration needs metadata intelligence. Successful clinical implementation demonstrates framework viability for advanced applications when components function cohesively.

5.6 Synthesis and Framework Validation

The real-world implementations examined in this section collectively provide empirical validation for the three-pillar framework across different organizational scales, technical approaches, and application domains. Table 3 summarizes key characteristics and outcomes.

Table 3. Real-World Implementation Validation of Framework Components

Implementation	Primary Pillar	Scale	Key Technical Innovation	Demonstrated Performance	Critical Lesson
INPC	Pillar 1: Identity Resolution	100+ institutions (regional)	Probabilistic matching + machine learning + stewardship workbench	F1-scores: 0.85-0.90 Outperformed deterministic matching	Human oversight essential for accuracy; local training data improves ML performance
OHDSI	Pillar 2: Semantic Harmonization	600+ institutions (global)	OMOP Common Data Model + standardized vocabularies	Reproducible multi-site studies	Common data models + vocabulary mapping enable unprecedented scale
PCORnet	Pillar 3: Metadata Intelligence	National network (US)	Federated queries + automated data quality framework	Systematic 4-dimensions assessment	Metadata frameworks enable distribution
i2b2	Pillar 2: Semantic Harmonization	Academic consortium	Gold-standard clinical NLP benchmarks	F1: 0.85-0.90 (concepts), 0.65-0.75 (relations)	Clinical NLP achieves useful accuracy; human review remains valuable for complex cases
eMERGE	All Three Pillars (integrated)	10+ academic medical centers	Genomic-clinical linkage + computable phenotypes + knowledge graphs	PPV: 0.85-0.95, Sensitivity: 0.70-0.90	Precision medicine requires integrated pillars

5.6.1 Cross-Cutting Validation Insights

Pillar Interdependence: eMERGE demonstrates sophisticated applications require all three pillars functioning cohesively, not independent components deployed separately.

Scalability: Implementations span regional (INPC), national (PCORnet), and global (OHDSI) scales, validating framework principles across organizational contexts. Technical approaches scale effectively though governance complexity increases with scope.

Performance Benchmarks: Documented outcomes establish evidence-based targets: identity matching F1-scores 0.85-0.90, phenotype algorithms PPV 0.85-0.95, NLP extraction F1-scores 0.80-0.90 for concepts. These benchmarks enable appropriate resource allocation and expectation management.

Hybrid Approaches: Every implementation demonstrates combining automation with human expertise outperforms fully automated systems. INPC's stewardship, OHDSI's expert validation, PCORnet's quality oversight, and i2b2's review processes show AI amplifies rather than replaces human judgment.

Governance as Enabler: Technical excellence alone proves insufficient. INPC's stewardship maintains accuracy, OHDSI's governance keeps mappings current, PCORnet's committees balance research with privacy, and eMERGE's consent infrastructure enables result return. Governance provides organizational infrastructure that technical infrastructure depends upon.

5.6.2 Implications for Framework Adoption

Foundation Before Sophistication: Organizations should establish identity resolution, semantic harmonization, and metadata management before pursuing advanced AI applications. INPC and OHDSI demonstrate foundational infrastructure must precede sophisticated analytics.

Incremental Implementation: Framework adoption produces value at each stage. Organizations can begin with deterministic matching before probabilistic methods, implement subset vocabularies before comprehensive coverage, and establish basic quality monitoring before sophisticated assessment.

Sustained Investment Required: Initial deployment represents beginning, not end, of investment. Successful implementations maintain stewardship teams, continuously update vocabulary mappings, and perform regular quality assessment.

Context-Appropriate Customization: Framework principles apply universally, but implementations must adapt to local regulatory, demographic, and organizational contexts while maintaining core architectural patterns.

Real-world implementations validate the framework's current applicability while revealing emerging technologies and approaches that will shape the next generation of AI-driven healthcare collaboration. The following section explores these future directions.

6. FUTURE DIRECTIONS AND EMERGING TRENDS

This section explores emerging technologies and methodologies that will shape the future of data-driven healthcare collaboration. These innovations build upon the foundational principles of identity resolution, semantic harmonization, and metadata intelligence while introducing novel approaches to privacy, computation, and interoperability.

6.1 Federated Learning for Privacy-Preserving Collaboration

Federated learning enables collaborative AI model training across multiple institutions without centralizing patient data, addressing privacy concerns and regulatory barriers (McMahan et al., 2017). Federated approaches move computation to data rather than data to computation—local models train on institutional datasets, only model parameters transmit to central servers, and aggregated models incorporate learning from all sites while individual patient records remain in institutional control (Benson & Grieve, 2016). Warnat-Herresthal et al. (2024) introduce swarm learning, a blockchain-based approach combining federated learning with decentralized coordination. Their multi-center study successfully classified leukemia subtypes across institutions while maintaining local data control, demonstrating performance comparable to centralized approaches. Swarm learning addresses key challenges including trust establishment, model version control, and Byzantine fault tolerance—critical for the multi-institutional AI collaboration.

Healthcare applications include multi-institutional disease prediction models, drug safety surveillance across diverse populations, and rare disease research requiring data pooling impossible under traditional data sharing constraints. However, technical challenges persist—statistical heterogeneity across institutions (different patient populations, documentation practices, treatment protocols) degrades model performance, communication overhead becomes prohibitive with large models or frequent updates, and privacy risks remain as model parameters can inadvertently leak training data information.

Differential privacy provides mathematical guarantees limiting information leakage from model parameters. By adding calibrated noise to gradients before transmission, differential privacy bounds the maximum information any individual patient record contributes to final models (Dwork & Roth, 2014). This creates inherent accuracy-privacy tradeoffs requiring careful calibration for clinical applications.

6.2 Large Language Models for Healthcare

Large language models have rapidly evolved as tools for healthcare collaboration. Van Veen et al. (2024) demonstrate that domain-adapted clinical language models outperform general-purpose LLMs and, in some annotation tasks, medical experts themselves when processing clinical text. Their study showed 85-92% accuracy for structured information extraction, suggesting LLMs can support semantic harmonization by automatically mapping clinical narratives to standardized terminologies. Thirunavukarasu et al. (2023) provide comprehensive evaluation showing that while GPT-4 and similar models exhibit strong capabilities in medical text summarization and terminology tasks, consistent human validation remains necessary to prevent propagation of hallucinated medical concepts that could undermine multi-institutional AI collaboration.

6.3 Edge Computing and Real-Time Analytics

Wearable devices and remote monitoring generate continuous physiological data streams requiring real-time analysis. Cloud-based processing introduces latency unacceptable for time-critical applications like arrhythmia detection or fall prevention. Edge computing processes data locally on wearable devices or patient-side gateways, enabling immediate response while reducing bandwidth requirements.

Edge deployment creates challenges for the three-pillar framework. Identity resolution must operate with limited connectivity and computational resources. Semantic harmonization requires device-local terminology services. Metadata management must function with intermittent cloud connectivity. Future architectures will implement lightweight versions of framework components suitable for edge deployment while maintaining consistency with enterprise systems.

6.4 Emerging Regulatory and Policy Frameworks

Regulatory developments increasingly influence data architecture decisions for AI-driven healthcare collaboration. Organizations implementing the three-pillar framework must anticipate compliance requirements that are rapidly evolving.

AI Governance Regulations: The European Union's AI Act reached final passage in 2024, establishing the world's first comprehensive AI regulatory framework (European Parliament, 2024). The final version classifies medical AI applications as “high-risk,” requiring conformity assessments, technical documentation, human oversight, post-market monitoring, and transparency obligations. These requirements impact the three-pillar framework: identity resolution systems must provide explainable matching decisions, semantic harmonization must maintain audit trails, and metadata intelligence must document data lineage and quality metrics for compliance. The U.S. FDA released discussion papers on AI/ML-based Software as a Medical Device (2021) emphasizing algorithm transparency and real-world performance monitoring, though formal regulations remain under development.

Data Portability and Interoperability Mandates: The U.S. 21st Century Cures Act (2020) prohibits information blocking and mandates FHIR API access to patient data, accelerating semantic harmonization requirements. The European Health Data Space (proposed 2022) envisions cross-border health data exchange for research and secondary use, requiring harmonized identity resolution and semantic frameworks across EU member states. These regulations make the three-pillar framework legally necessary for compliance.

Algorithmic Fairness Requirements: Several jurisdictions now require algorithmic fairness assessments. The U.S. FDA's commitment to addressing health disparities extends to medical AI evaluation. The WHO's "Ethics and Governance of Artificial Intelligence for Health" (2021) establishes global principles including equity mandates influencing national regulations. These requirements necessitate identity resolution systems that perform equitably across demographic groups and semantic systems that handle diverse clinical terminology without bias.

Privacy-Preserving Data Sharing: GDPR Article 9 restricts health data transfer with stringent requirements, while cross-border research collaborations increase. Federated learning architectures that keep data locally while sharing model parameters align with these regulatory constraints, but require robust metadata systems ensuring data quality without direct inspection—a capability Pillar 3 provides.

Organizations should proactively design data infrastructure anticipating regulatory compliance rather than retrofitting after regulations mandate changes. The three-pillar framework's emphasis on governance, transparency, and quality monitoring positions implementations to adapt as regulations evolve.

6.5 Ethical, Equity, and Governance Considerations

AI-driven healthcare collaboration introduces ethical challenges requiring systematic attention alongside technical solutions. The three-pillar framework must operate within governance structures addressing algorithmic fairness, equitable data representation, and institutional accountability.

6.5.1 Algorithmic Bias and Health Equity

Identity resolution, semantic harmonization, and metadata systems can perpetuate or amplify existing healthcare disparities if not deliberately designed for equity. Obermeyer et al. (2019) demonstrated that widely deployed commercial algorithms exhibited significant racial bias, systematically underestimating illness severity for Black patients compared to White patients with equivalent health conditions. The algorithm relied on healthcare costs as a proxy for health needs, failing to account for systemic inequities in healthcare access and utilization.

Identity Resolution Equity Challenges: Probabilistic matching algorithms trained on majority demographic patterns may underperform for populations with non-Western naming conventions, frequent residential mobility (common in underserved communities), or unstable contact information. The INPC implementation addresses this through explicit evaluation of matching performance across demographic subgroups and continuous retraining with representative data (Grannis et al., 2019).

Semantic Harmonization Bias: Clinical NLP systems trained predominantly on academic medical center documentation may misinterpret dialect variations, health literacy levels, or culturally specific symptom descriptions common in community health settings. LLM-based semantic mapping requires validation across diverse clinical contexts to ensure equitable concept extraction.

Metadata Equity: Data quality frameworks must recognize that "completeness" varies systematically across populations—not due to patient characteristics, but due to differential healthcare access. Communities with limited access to specialty care will have "incomplete" specialty data not because of data quality failures, but because care was never delivered. Quality assessment must distinguish between technical incompleteness and structural inequity.

Mitigation Strategies: Organizations implementing the framework should conduct algorithmic fairness audits across demographic subgroups, maintain diverse representation in training data and validation cohorts, implement bias detection mechanisms, and establish equity review boards with community representation.

6.5.2 Patient Trust and Data Governance

Cross-institutional data sharing for AI collaboration requires patient trust, yet numerous surveys document significant public concern about health data use, particularly among historically marginalized communities (Kraft et al., 2018). The Henrietta Lacks case and Tuskegee syphilis study continue to influence minority community perceptions of medical research data use.

Governance Requirements: Effective data governance balances collaboration enablement with protection. Key components include transparent data use policies communicated in accessible language, patient consent mechanisms allowing granular control over data sharing, audit trails documenting who accessed data for what purpose, regular privacy impact assessments, and community advisory boards providing oversight for research applications.

Return of Results: The eMERGE Network demonstrates that genomic-clinical integration requires infrastructure for returning clinically actionable results to patients and providers, raising complex questions about clinical validity, analytical validity, duty to warn, and potential psychological impact (Gottesman et al., 2013).

6.5.3 Regulatory Landscape and Cross-Border Considerations

AI governance regulations are rapidly evolving, creating compliance requirements for data infrastructure. The European Union's AI Act (proposed 2021, evolving) classifies AI systems by risk level, with medical AI generally designated high-risk requiring conformity assessment, technical documentation, human oversight, and post-market monitoring. HIPAA in the United States governs privacy but lacks AI-specific provisions. The WHO published "Ethics and Governance of Artificial Intelligence for Health" (2021) establishing six consensus principles: protecting autonomy, promoting well-being, ensuring transparency, fostering accountability, ensuring equity, and promoting responsive and sustainable AI.

Cross-Border Data Challenges: Multi-national research collaborations encounter divergent data protection regimes. GDPR Article 9 restricts health data transfer outside the European Economic Area unless adequate safeguards exist. Standard Contractual Clauses and adequacy decisions provide mechanisms, but add governance complexity. The three-pillar framework must accommodate federated architectures where data remains in jurisdictional control while enabling distributed analytics.

Practical Governance Integration: Organizations should establish AI ethics review committees parallel to IRBs, conduct data protection impact assessments for new AI applications, implement model cards and datasheets documenting system capabilities and limitations, maintain version control and audit logs for deployed algorithms, and establish processes for addressing algorithmic errors or bias complaints.

These governance structures are not obstacles to collaboration but enablers—building the trust infrastructure that sustainable, equitable AI-driven healthcare requires.

6.6 Quantum Computing: Long-Term Outlook

Quantum computing may eventually accelerate certain data-intensive tasks such as optimization in federated learning coordination or graph traversal in large-scale identity resolution. However, practical quantum advantage for healthcare applications remains 10-15+ years away. Organizations should prioritize classical computing optimizations and proven architectures. The three-pillar framework's principles will remain relevant regardless of computational substrates, as identity resolution, semantic harmonization, and metadata intelligence represent fundamental requirements independent of specific technologies.

CONCLUSION

This chapter establishes that data barriers—not modeling barriers—constitute the decisive bottleneck in AI-powered healthcare collaboration. Despite advances in deep learning and foundation models, these algorithmic achievements remain constrained by data that is fragmented, semantically inconsistent, and identity-unresolved across institutional boundaries.

The three-pillar framework provides a systematic approach to overcoming these constraints. Identity resolution enables unified patient representation across disparate systems. Semantic harmonization ensures consistent clinical meaning despite terminology heterogeneity. Metadata intelligence creates machine-operable infrastructure that AI systems require for reliable operation. These pillars function interdependently: sophisticated applications like precision medicine require all three operating cohesively, as demonstrated by the eMERGE Network implementation.

Real-world validations provide empirical evidence for framework viability. INPC achieves identity matching F1-scores of 0.85-0.90 through probabilistic methods enhanced with machine learning. OHDSI enables collaborative research across 600+ global institutions through common data models and vocabulary mapping. PCORnet demonstrates that federated architectures with explicit metadata frameworks support multi-institutional analytics while preserving governance. These implementations consistently show that hybrid human-machine approaches outperform fully automated systems, and that sustained governance enables rather than constrains technical capability.

Practical Implications

Organizations implementing AI-driven collaboration should prioritize data infrastructure before algorithmic sophistication. The framework supports incremental adoption: begin with probabilistic patient matching, establish terminology services for core vocabularies, implement data cataloging and quality monitoring, then expand systematically. This approach produces value at each stage while building toward comprehensive capability.

Success requires sustained investment beyond initial deployment. Identity resolution demands ongoing stewardship as demographics and systems evolve. Semantic harmonization requires continuous vocabulary mapping as terminologies update. Metadata management needs regular quality assessment. Organizations must budget for operations, not just implementation.

Clinical workflow integration determines adoption success. The framework must operate within existing EHR systems without creating unsustainable clinician burden. Incremental deployment with high-value use-cases, clinician engagement in design decisions, and continuous improvement based on frontline feedback transform technical capability into clinical value.

Ethical and Equity Imperatives

Data infrastructure for AI collaboration must address algorithmic bias, health equity, and patient trust. Obermeyer et al. (2019) demonstrated that commercial algorithms can exhibit significant racial bias when not deliberately designed for equity. Organizations must conduct fairness audits across demographic subgroups, maintain diverse representation in training data, and establish equity review boards with community representation.

Patient trust requires transparent governance, accessible consent mechanisms, audit trails for data access, and community oversight for research applications. Cross-institutional collaboration depends on building trust infrastructure alongside technical infrastructure (Kraft et al., 2018).

Regulatory compliance increasingly mandates rather than recommends these practices. The EU AI Act, U.S. FDA guidance, and WHO ethics principles establish requirements for technical documentation, human oversight, fairness assessment, and post-market monitoring. The three-pillar framework's emphasis on metadata management, quality assessment, and governance positions implementations for regulatory compliance as requirements evolve.

Research Directions

Critical areas warrant continued investigation. Federated learning approaches must address statistical heterogeneity across institutions while maintaining model performance. Large language model deployment for semantic harmonization requires rigorous validation methodologies, hallucination detection, and clear regulatory pathways. Privacy-preserving technologies need development to balance strong guarantees with practical utility. Knowledge graph reasoning remains underutilized despite theoretical promise. Temporal data integration requires frameworks enabling AI systems to understand clinical trajectories across institutional boundaries.

From Data-Centric to Collaboration-Centric AI

This work reflects a paradigm shift from algorithm-centric to data-centric AI development. Healthcare extends this to "collaboration-centric AI": value depends not merely on data quality within institutions, but on integration capabilities across institutions. The most sophisticated model trained on single-institution data cannot match a simpler model trained on diverse multi-institutional data.

AI-driven healthcare collaboration at scale requires shifting attention from algorithms to infrastructure. Organizations that systematically implement identity resolution, semantic harmonization, and metadata intelligence—with hybrid human-machine approaches and sustained governance—position themselves to realize AI's transformative potential for collaborative care delivery, population health management, and medical research advancement.

The path forward is clear: invest in data infrastructure, establish robust governance, leverage hybrid approaches, and build incrementally. Organizations following this path will overcome the data barriers currently limiting AI-driven collaboration, ultimately improving patient outcomes through more coordinated, informed, and intelligent care delivery systems.

REFERENCES

Adler-Milstein, J., & Jha, A. K. (2017). HITECH Act drove large gains in hospital electronic health record adoption. *Health Affairs, 36*(8), 1416–1422. DOI: 10.1377/hlthaff.2016.1651 PMID: 28784734

Beaulieu-Jones, B. K., Wu, Z. S., Williams, C., Lee, R., Bhavnani, S. P., Byrd, J. B., & Greene, C. S. (2019). Privacy-preserving generative deep neural networks support clinical data sharing. *Circulation: Cardiovascular Quality and Outcomes, 12*(7), e005122. DOI: 10.1161/CIRCOUTCOMES.118.005122 PMID: 31284738

Benson, T., & Grieve, G. (2016). *Principles of health interoperability: SNOMED CT, HL7 and FHIR* (3rd ed.). Springer., DOI: 10.1007/978-3-319-30370-3

Bodenreider, O. (2004). The Unified Medical Language System (UMLS): Integrating biomedical terminology. *Nucleic Acids Research, 32*(Database issue), D267–D270. DOI: 10.1093/nar/gkh061 PMID: 14681409

Dwork, C., & Roth, A. (2014). The algorithmic foundations of differential privacy. *Foundations and Trends in Theoretical Computer Science, 9*(3-4), 211–407. DOI: 10.1561/0400000042

European Parliament. (2024). Regulation (EU) 2024/1689 of the European Parliament and of the Council laying down harmonised rules on artificial intelligence (Artificial Intelligence Act). Official Journal of the European Union, L 2024/1689. https://eur-lex.europa.eu/eli/reg/2024/1689/oj

Fleurence, R. L., Curtis, L. H., Califf, R. M., Platt, R., Selby, J. V., & Brown, J. S. (2014). Launching PCORnet, a national patient-centered clinical research network. *Journal of the American Medical Informatics Association : JAMIA, 21*(4), 578–582. DOI: 10.1136/amiajnl-2014-002747 PMID: 24821743

Gartner. (2021). *Innovation insight for data fabric*. Gartner Research Report.

Gottesman, O., Kuivaniemi, H., Tromp, G., Faucett, W. A., Li, R., Manolio, T. A., Sanderson, S. C., Kannry, J., Zinberg, R., Basford, M. A., Brilliant, M., Carey, D. J., Chisholm, R. L., Chute, C. G., Connolly, J. J., Crosslin, D., Denny, J. C., Gallego, C. J., Haines, J. L., & Williams, M. S. (2013). The Electronic Medical Records and Genomics (eMERGE) Network: Past, present, and future. *Genetics in Medicine, 15*(10), 761–771. DOI: 10.1038/gim.2013.72 PMID: 23743551

Grannis, S. J., Xu, H., Vest, J. R., Kasthurirathne, S., Bo, N., Moscovitch, B., Torkzadeh, N., & Rising, J. (2019). Evaluating the effect of data standardization and validation on patient matching accuracy. *Journal of the American Medical Informatics Association : JAMIA*, *26*(5), 447–456. DOI: 10.1093/jamia/ocy191 PMID: 30848796

Hogan, A., Blomqvist, E., Cochez, M., d'Amato, C., de Melo, G., Gutierrez, C., & Zimmermann, A. (2021). Knowledge graphs. *ACM Computing Surveys*, *54*(4), 1–37. DOI: 10.1145/3447772

Hripcsak, G., Duke, J. D., Shah, N. H., Reich, C. G., Huser, V., Schuemie, M. J., & Ryan, P. B. (2015). Observational Health Data Sciences and Informatics (OHDSI): Opportunities for observational researchers. *Studies in Health Technology and Informatics*, *216*, 574–578. DOI: 10.3233/978-1-61499-564-7-574 PMID: 26262116

Kahn, M. G., Callahan, T. J., Barnard, J., Bauck, A. E., Brown, J., Davidson, B. N., Estiri, H., Goerg, C., Holve, E., Johnson, S. G., Liaw, S.-T., Hamilton-Lopez, M., Meeker, D., Ong, T. C., Ryan, P., Shang, N., Weiskopf, N. G., Weng, C., Zozus, M. N., & Schilling, L. M. (2016). A harmonized data quality assessment terminology and framework for the secondary use of electronic health record data. *EGEMS (Washington, DC)*, *4*(1), 1244. DOI: 10.13063/2327-9214.1244 PMID: 27713905

Kraft, S. A., Cho, M. K., Gillespie, K., Halley, M., Varsava, N., Ormond, K. E., & Wilfond, B. S. (2018). Beyond consent: Building trusting relationships with diverse populations in precision medicine research. *The American Journal of Bioethics*, *18*(4), 3–20. DOI: 10.1080/15265161.2018.1431322 PMID: 29621457

McMahan, B., Moore, E., Ramage, D., Hampson, S., & Arcas, B. A. (2017). Communication-efficient learning of deep networks from decentralized data. *Proceedings of the 20th International Conference on Artificial Intelligence and Statistics*, 54, 1273-1282.

Obermeyer, Z., Powers, B., Vogeli, C., & Mullainathan, S. (2019). Dissecting racial bias in an algorithm used to manage the health of populations. *Science*, *366*(6464), 447–453. DOI: 10.1126/science.aax2342 PMID: 31649194

Singhal, K., Azizi, S., Tu, T., Mahdavi, S. S., Wei, J., Chung, H. W., Scales, N., Tanwani, A., Cole-Lewis, H., Pfohl, S., Payne, P., Seneviratne, M., Gamble, P., Kelly, C., Babiker, A., Schärli, N., Chowdhery, A., Mansfield, P., Demner-Fushman, D., & Natarajan, V. (2023). Large language models encode clinical knowledge. *Nature*, *620*(7972), 172–180. DOI: 10.1038/s41586-023-06291-2 PMID: 37438534

SNOMED International. (2021). *SNOMED CT starter guide*. https://confluence.ihtsdotools.org/display/DOCSTART

Thirunavukarasu, A. J., Ting, D. S. J., Elangovan, K., Gutierrez, L., Tan, T. F., & Ting, D. S. W. (2023). Large language models in medicine. *Nature Medicine*, *29*(8), 1930–1940. DOI: 10.1038/s41591-023-02448-8 PMID: 37460753

Uzuner, Ö., South, B. R., Shen, S., & DuVall, S. L. (2011). 2010 i2b2/VA challenge on concepts, assertions, and relations in clinical text. *Journal of the American Medical Informatics Association : JAMIA*, *18*(5), 552–556. DOI: 10.1136/amiajnl-2011-000203 PMID: 21685143

Van Veen, D., Van Uden, C., Blankemeier, L., Delbrouck, J. B., Aali, A., Bluethgen, C., & Langlotz, C. P. (2024). Adapted large language models can outperform medical experts in clinical text annotation. *Nature Medicine*, *30*(4), 1088–1097. DOI: 10.1038/s41591-024-02855-5 PMID: 38413730

Voss, E. A., Makadia, R., Matcho, A., Ma, Q., Knoll, C., Schuemie, M., DeFalco, F. J., Londhe, A., Zhu, V., & Ryan, P. B. (2015). Feasibility and utility of applications of the common data model to multiple, disparate observational health databases. *Journal of the American Medical Informatics Association : JAMIA*, *22*(3), 553–564. DOI: 10.1093/jamia/ocu023 PMID: 25670757

Wang, Y., Wang, L., Rastegar-Mojarad, M., Moon, S., Shen, F., Afzal, N., Liu, S., Zeng, Y., Mehrabi, S., Sohn, S., & Liu, H. (2020). Clinical information extraction applications: A literature review. *Journal of Biomedical Informatics*, *77*, 34–49. DOI: 10.1016/j.jbi.2017.11.011 PMID: 29162496

Warnat-Herresthal, S., Schultze, H., Shastry, K. L., Manamohan, S., Mukherjee, S., Garg, V., & Schultze, J. L. (2024). Swarm learning for decentralized and confidential clinical machine learning. *Nature*, *625*(7995), 545–550. DOI: 10.1038/s41586-023-06851-5 PMID: 34040261

Zhu, Y., Matsuyama, Y., Ohashi, Y., & Setoguchi, S. (2017). When to conduct probabilistic linkage vs. deterministic linkage? A simulation study. *Journal of Biomedical Informatics*, *27*, 96–105. PMID: 26004791

Chapter 3
Secure Software Engineering for AI-Enhanced E-Collaboration in Healthcare:
Building Resilient and Interoperable Systems

Hanh Le
http://orcid.org/0009-0007-8172-0809
University of the Cumberlands, USA

ABSTRACT

The integration of Artificial Intelligence (AI) into e-collaboration tools is transforming healthcare delivery by enabling real-time communication, clinical decision support, and patient engagement. However, the adoption of AI-powered systems—such as chatbots, large language models (LLMs), and telehealth platforms—raises significant concerns related to security, privacy, trust, and interoperability. This chapter explores how secure software engineering principles can guide the development of resilient and compliant AI-enhanced collaboration platforms. It proposes a secure-by-design framework that addresses risks such as data breaches, AI hallucinations, and cross-system vulnerabilities. Through real-world examples, the chapter demonstrates best practices in secure architecture, HL7/FHIR integration, role-based access control, and AI transparency. The goal is to empower developers, IT leaders, and clinicians to co-create secure and effective digital ecosystems that protect patient data while improving care coordination and delivery.

DOI: 10.4018/979-8-3373-5906-9.ch003

INTRODUCTION

Digital transformation is rapidly reshaping the healthcare landscape, with AI at the forefront of this evolution. From chatbots that assist patients with symptom checking to AI-driven virtual assistants that support clinical decision-making, the integration of intelligent systems into healthcare collaboration is no longer a future vision—it is a present reality. These AI-powered tools are revolutionizing how providers communicate, coordinate care, and engage patients across time and space. Yet as healthcare organizations embrace e-collaboration technologies, they also inherit new risks and responsibilities.

Unlike traditional clinical software systems, AI-enhanced collaboration platforms—particularly those based on large language models (LLMs)—exhibit probabilistic and non-deterministic behavior. Their outputs can vary depending on context, prompt structure, and data exposure, introducing unique risks such as prompt injection, sensitive data leakage, hallucinated clinical content, and insecure tool or API invocation. In healthcare environments, these risks extend beyond confidentiality and availability to the integrity of clinical meaning itself, where misleading or persuasive AI-generated outputs can directly affect patient safety, care coordination, and clinical accountability. As a result, AI-enabled healthcare collaboration requires security controls that are continuous, adaptive, and lifecycle-oriented rather than one-time hardening measures.

The sensitive nature of healthcare data, the complexity of clinical workflows, and the high stakes of medical decision-making demand that these AI-enhanced platforms be built on a foundation of secure and interoperable software systems. Security breaches, inaccurate AI outputs, and integration failures not only threaten patient safety and privacy but also erode trust in digital healthcare tools.

This chapter addresses the critical need for secure software engineering in the design and deployment of AI-powered e-collaboration platforms in healthcare by arguing that such systems must be both secure-by-design and governed-by-design. Secure-by-design emphasizes the embedding of security controls throughout the software development lifecycle (SDLC), including threat modeling, secure coding, vulnerability management, and continuous improvement, as outlined in the NIST Secure Software Development Framework (SSDF) (Scarfone et al., 2022). Governed-by-design further highlights the need for organizational policies, accountability mechanisms, and continuous risk management tailored to AI-enabled systems.

Drawing on industry best practices and real-world case studies, the chapter examines core challenges, including HL7/FHIR integration, secure messaging, role-based access control (RBAC), and algorithmic transparency. In doing so, it lays a path toward a future where AI-driven collaboration can enhance patient care without compromising safety or trust.

Adopting a human-centered and systems-oriented perspective, this chapter contributes to the growing body of research on how AI technologies are transforming secure digital collaboration in healthcare. It critically examines how software engineering practices must evolve to support the trustworthy integration of AI-driven tools in clinical and operational workflows. The following research questions guide this study:

1. RQ1: How do AI-powered collaboration tools, such as virtual assistants, chatbots, and LLM-based platforms, impact the design and implementation of secure software systems in healthcare environments?
2. RQ2: What are the primary security, privacy, and interoperability challenges associated with integrating AI-driven e-collaboration platforms with EHRs and other health information systems?
3. RQ3: How can healthcare organizations and developers adopt secure-by-design principles—including role-based access control, auditability, and HL7/FHIR standards—together with AI governance and risk management frameworks to ensure resilient, compliant, and ethical AI-enhanced collaboration?

The chapter is organized as follows: Section 2 establishes the conceptual foundation by outlining the theoretical frameworks that inform the analysis. Section 3 provides a review of the literature on secure software engineering, AI integration in healthcare collaboration, and the challenges of system interoperability. Section 4 describes the research methodology employed in the study. Section 5 presents the key findings, illustrated through case studies that highlight real-world applications and implications. Finally, Section 6 addresses the study's limitations and proposes directions for future research.

BACKGROUND AND THEORETICAL FRAMEWORKS

The rapid integration of AI into healthcare collaboration, through tools such as chatbots, virtual assistants, and LLMs, is fundamentally altering how information is exchanged, care is coordinated, and clinical decisions are supported. While these innovations promise improvements in efficiency and accessibility, they also introduce critical concerns around data security, system trustworthiness, and human oversight. To examine the multifaceted implications of AI-enhanced e-collaboration in healthcare, this chapter draws on three complementary theoretical frameworks—Socio-Technical Systems Theory (STS), Technology Acceptance Model (TAM), and Technology Threat Avoidance Theory (TTAT)—and extends them with a standards-informed governance perspective rooted in secure software engineering and AI risk management.

Socio-Technical Systems Theory

Rooted in organizational theory and systems thinking, Socio-Technical Systems Theory (Emery & Trist, 1960) emphasizes the interdependence between people, technology, and the organizational structures in which they operate. In healthcare, STS highlights how digital collaboration platforms are not merely technical systems but are embedded within complex clinical, regulatory, and interpersonal contexts.

Applying STS to AI-driven e-collaboration reveals that secure software engineering must address both technical safeguards (e.g., encryption, secure APIs, and access controls) and social dynamics (e.g., clinician trust, patient consent, and workflow alignment). This perspective underscores the importance of co-design approaches that involve developers, clinicians, compliance experts, and patients, ensuring that AI-enabled collaboration tools align with real-world clinical practices and ethical expectations.

Technology Acceptance Model

The Technology Acceptance Model (Davis, 1989) explains how users come to accept and use new technologies, focusing on perceived usefulness and perceived ease of use.

In the context of AI-assisted healthcare collaboration, TAM underscores that security and governance mechanisms must be usable and intelligible. If access controls, verification steps, or audit features introduce excessive friction or lack transparency, clinicians may resist adoption or circumvent safeguards. Conversely, AI systems that are explainable, intuitive, and well-integrated into existing workflows are more likely to be trusted and sustainably adopted.

Technology Threat Avoidance Theory

Technology Threat Avoidance Theory (Liang & Xue, 2009) provides a behavioral lens for understanding how individuals assess and respond to technological risks. In AI-powered healthcare collaboration, TTAT helps explain why some developers and clinicians proactively adopt safeguards (e.g., access audits, validation checks, and human oversight), while others accept risk due to time pressure, perceived complexity, or overconfidence in AI outputs. This framework emphasizes the importance of visible and adequate protective measures in fostering secure behavior and risk awareness.

Standards-Informed Governance Lens

To translate these theoretical insights into operational practice, this chapter incorporates a standards-informed governance lens that complements the theories of STS, TAM, and TTAT. The NIST Secure Software Development Framework (SP 800-218) provides a lifecycle-based structure for embedding security activities across development, deployment, and vulnerability response, emphasizing proactive risk mitigation and continuous monitoring throughout the SDLC (*Scarfone et al., 2022*). In healthcare contexts, this approach supports regulatory compliance, auditability, and the secure integration of AI components into safety-critical systems.

Together, these standards enable healthcare organizations to operationalize secure-by-design and governed-by-design principles, ensuring that AI-enhanced collaboration platforms are not only technically secure but also institutionally accountable and ethically aligned.

Background and Theoretical Frameworks Summary

Together, STS, TAM, TTAT, and standards-based governance frameworks provide an integrated analytical lens for this chapter. STS contextualizes AI collaboration within healthcare's socio-organizational environment, TAM explains adoption and trust dynamics, TTAT illuminates risk perception and mitigation behavior, and secure-by-design standards translate these insights into actionable engineering and governance practices. This integrated perspective supports the development of resilient, interoperable, and trustworthy AI-driven collaboration systems in healthcare.

Table 1. Mapping interview questions to research questions and theoretical Frameworks

Interview Question	Aligned Research Question(s)	Theoretical Framework(s)	Rationale
Q1. Please introduce yourself, including your background and experience in AI chatbot development.	All RQs (Context-setting)	STS	Establishes participant profile and role within the socio-technical system.
Q2. Do you use AI chatbots in your daily life? For example, ChatGPT or GitHub Copilot?	RQ1	STS, TAM	Explores individual adoption patterns, perceived usefulness, and ease of use.
Q3. Do you use AI chatbots on your job? If so, how exactly? Please give an example.	RQ1	STS, TAM, TTAT	Reveals real-world use cases of AI in workplace settings and system integration.

continued on following page

Table 1. Continued

Interview Question	Aligned Research Question(s)	Theoretical Framework(s)	Rationale
Q4. Can you describe the specific challenges you face as a programmer in a world dominated by AI and chatbots?	RQ2	STS, TAM, TTAT	Elicits perceived risks, skill erosion, and adaptation challenges.
Q5. How has the emergence of AI and chatbots impacted your day-to-day work and responsibilities?	RQ1, RQ2	STS, TAM, TTAT	Explores changes in task identity, autonomy, and perceived deskilling.
Q6. Can you share a specific instance where you encountered a challenge related to integrating or collaborating with AI technologies?	RQ2	STS, TAM, TTAT	Highlights system-level and behavioral security or usability issues.
Q7. How do you incorporate user interactions and feedback into the development cycle of an AI chatbot?	RQ3	STS, TAM	Investigates human-centered design and iterative development approaches.
Q8. What strategies have you adopted to adapt to the evolving programming landscape with the rise of AI and chatbots? How do you stay updated on the latest developments?	RQ3	STS, TAM, TTAT	Examines proactive skill development, task engagement, and motivational shifts.
Q9. What tools or methodologies effectively address user interaction and feedback challenges during AI chatbot development?	RQ3	STS, TAM	Addresses technical and user-centric methods to ensure effective collaboration and communication.
Q10. In what direction do you foresee your job field evolving, with AI potentially playing a distinct role?	RQ3	STS, TAM, TTAT	Encourages reflection on future roles, upskilling, and the importance of adapting to evolving tasks.
Q11. Which skills will become crucial for an IT specialist in your field over the next five years?	RQ3	STS, TAM, TTAT	Forecasts future-proof competencies amid technological disruption.

LITERATURE REVIEW

The intersection of AI, secure software engineering, and healthcare e-collaboration has become a central focus in both academic and industry discourse. As LLMs, chatbots, and AI-powered virtual assistants are increasingly integrated into healthcare workflows, researchers are examining how these tools transform care coordination, clinical communication, and decision-making processes. These technologies promise gains in efficiency, accessibility, and scalability, yet they also introduce new risks related to data privacy, system interoperability, and cybersecurity.

The literature reflects a dual narrative: on one hand, AI-enhanced platforms are celebrated for reducing clinical workload, facilitating real-time collaboration, and improving diagnostic support. On the other hand, significant concerns have emerged regarding data breaches, lack of explainability, and trust in automated decisions. These risks are heightened in the healthcare domain, where decisions have a direct impact on patient safety, and strict adherence to regulatory frameworks, such as HIPAA, GDPR, and FDA AI guidance, is imperative and non-negotiable.

This review synthesizes current contributions across six thematic domains: (1) the rise of AI in healthcare collaboration; (2) security and privacy challenges in AI-mediated systems; (3) integration and interoperability through standards such as HL7 and FHIR; (4) secure software engineering principles for AI-enabled platforms; (5) the role of human oversight, explainability, and trust; and (6) the importance of socio-technical alignment and regulatory compliance.

AI in Healthcare Collaboration

AI-driven tools such as symptom checkers, virtual agents, and LLM-based documentation assistants are transforming patient-provider communication. Studies show that AI chatbots can support triage, streamline documentation, and enhance patient engagement (Blease et al., 2024). In telehealth, AI enables dynamic scheduling, risk prediction, and remote monitoring. The study by Modi et al. (2025) revealed that LLMs can be easily manipulated to produce persuasive but dangerously false health information when subjected to malicious system-level instructions. Evaluating five advanced models: OpenAI's GPT-4o, Google's Gemini 1.5 Pro, Anthropic's Claude 3.5 Sonnet, Meta's Llama 3.2-90B Vision, and xAI's Grok Beta, the researchers found that 88% of 100 tested responses contained disinformation. Notably, four of the five models generated false information in every case, while even the most resistant model, Claude, did so 40% of the time. The disinformation included long-debunked myths such as vaccines causing autism, HIV being airborne, and dietary cures for cancer. It also propagated misinformation about sunscreen safety, genetically modified organisms (GMOs), mental health conditions like ADHD and depression, garlic replacing antibiotics, and 5G technology causing infertility. These falsehoods were delivered in authoritative and scientific tones, making them especially misleading and potentially harmful. The study further demonstrated that customized GPTs available through the OpenAI GPT Store could be similarly weaponized, exposing a broader vulnerability in the ecosystem. These findings highlight the risks associated with inadequate software design in AI systems, particularly the absence of robust safeguards to prevent misuse. Without effective alignment mechanisms and content moderation, generative AI tools can inadvertently serve as scalable engines of health disinformation, posing serious threats to public trust and safety.

Security and Privacy Risks in AI Systems

The study by Das et al. (2025) revealed that LLMs offer powerful capabilities in natural language processing, including text generation, summarization, translation, and contextual question-answering. While their adoption has grown across various sectors, including healthcare, education, and transportation, the authors emphasize that LLMs are inherently vulnerable to a range of security and privacy threats. These include jailbreaking attacks, where attackers bypass safety filters; data poisoning, where training data is manipulated to elicit harmful behaviors; and PII (Personally Identifiable Information) leakage, where the models inadvertently reveal sensitive personal data.

The survey offers a comprehensive overview of these risks, examining how both training data and user interactions can be leveraged for exploitation. It also assesses application-specific vulnerabilities and surveys current and emerging defense mechanisms. Importantly, Das et al. identify critical research gaps, particularly the lack of robust, domain-specific safeguards, and call for further investigation into privacy-preserving model training, adversarial robustness, and real-time monitoring frameworks to ensure the secure deployment of AI in sensitive environments, such as healthcare.

Interoperability and Standards Compliance

The study by Rigas et al. (2024) discovered that the digitization of healthcare offers transformative potential to enhance service quality, accelerate diagnostic processes, and reduce overall costs. To fully harness these benefits, digital healthcare applications must be interoperable. As the use of AI, particularly Machine Learning (ML), continues to expand, these systems increasingly rely on large volumes of diverse data types. Achieving true interoperability in such environments necessitates the use of standardized semantic data models. The paper presents the implementation of a standard semantic data model based on the widely recognized Health Level Seven Fast Healthcare Interoperability Resources (HL7 FHIR) standard. The model supports the development and storage of a wide range of AI-driven applications targeting various medical conditions. The efficiency of the FHIR server is demonstrated through its application in predicting coronary artery stenosis and in managing the platform's key performance indicators. However, AI integration poses new challenges: real-time synchronization, version control, and semantic consistency must be maintained while respecting privacy and consent models. Secure FHIR interfaces are crucial for ensuring the reliability of AI deployment across institutions.

Secure Software Engineering in AI-Enhanced Systems

The secure-by-design paradigm is gaining traction as AI systems become embedded in mission-critical healthcare processes. Studies emphasize the importance of embedding security into the software development lifecycle (SDLC), including practices such as threat modeling, role-based access control (RBAC), static code analysis, and secure DevOps (DevSecOps). Research by Booth et al. (2022) expands upon the secure software development practices outlined in the Secure Software Development Framework (SSDF) by incorporating additional guidance explicitly tailored to the development of AI models. It introduces AI-focused practices, tasks, recommendations, considerations, and references that address the unique security challenges associated with AI systems throughout the software development life cycle.

Human Oversight, Explainability, and Trust

Mesinovic et al. (2025) highlight both the transformative potential and the critical limitations of LLMs in healthcare. They note their ability to answer patient questions, predict clinical outcomes, and generate medical documentation with remarkable fluency. However, these advancements also underscore the urgent need for explainability, especially in high-stakes clinical settings where trust, transparency, and accountability are essential. Explainability extends beyond simple interpretability, requiring clinicians and patients to understand how AI outputs are generated and how they align with medical reasoning. Regulatory frameworks like GDPR increasingly mandate this level of transparency, reinforcing that explainability is not optional. Yet, traditional techniques such as saliency maps often fail to explain LLMs adequately due to their non-deterministic, context-sensitive nature. As these models continue to evolve, so too must our approaches to making their reasoning understandable, reliable, and ethically sound for clinical integration.

The study by Khurana et al. (2024) explores how LLM assistants, such as ChatGPT, support users in navigating complex software environments. Through a within-subject experiment with 16 participants and follow-up interviews, researchers compared a general-purpose LLM with a domain-optimized assistant, SoftAIBot, which included prompt construction guidance. While SoftAIBot outperformed the baseline model in task support, the study found no significant improvement in user performance or perception when using prompt guidelines or domain context. Many users struggled to understand how their prompts affected the LLM's responses and often accepted incorrect suggestions without question, resulting in low task success rates. The findings highlight a critical gap between user trust and their ability to assess the accuracy of LLM-generated guidance, especially among those with limited domain knowledge. The authors emphasize the need for explainable, context-aware LLM interfaces to enhance user understanding, mitigate errors, and support more effective human-AI collaboration in software usage.

Navarro et al. (2025) argue that generative AI introduces a fundamental shift toward a *triadic consultation model*, in which clinical decision-making and documentation are mediated not only between clinician and patient but also through an AI system embedded in the interaction. In this model, trust is distributed across human and machine actors, raising new concerns about accountability, transparency, and professional responsibility. The authors caution that without explicit disclosure, governance, and safeguards, generative AI may subtly influence clinical reasoning, documentation framing, and shared decision-making in ways that are opaque to both clinicians and patients.

This perspective extends existing trust calibration research by highlighting that clinician trust is not only a function of system accuracy or explainability, but also of role clarity and interactional transparency. When generative AI is positioned as a drafting or assistive agent—rather than an autonomous decision-maker—and when clinicians retain visible control over final outputs, trust is more likely to remain appropriately calibrated. Conversely, poorly bound AI integration risks creating automation bias or eroding the relational foundations of clinical care (Navarro et al., 2025).

Beyond security and privacy, algorithmic bias and fairness have emerged as central concerns in AI-enabled healthcare systems. Models trained on imbalanced or historically biased datasets may systematically underperform for specific demographic groups, potentially compromising diagnostic accuracy and exacerbating health disparities. Prior studies have shown that such biases can remain hidden without deliberate auditing and disaggregated performance evaluation across race, gender, age, or socioeconomic status.

Socio-Technical Complexity and Regulatory Alignment

The study by Saenz et al. (2024) presents an in-depth case study on the responsible integration of AI within healthcare systems, highlighting the importance of aligning ethics, technology, and organization in real-world clinical environments. In response to the rapid evolution of AI technologies and their transformative potential in healthcare delivery, the authors present a robust framework grounded in core principles, including fairness, robustness, privacy, safety, transparency, explainability, accountability, and societal benefit. Developed through a multidisciplinary collaboration involving clinicians, developers, and compliance experts, the framework was operationalized and tested within a healthcare setting, using an ambient clinical documentation system as a central use case.

The case study by Saenz et al. (2024) also illustrates the practical challenges and opportunities associated with deploying generative AI in high-stakes environments, including managing data sensitivity, aligning with regulatory standards, and ensuring usability within clinical workflows. Crucially, the framework supports ongoing monitoring, evaluation, and refinement of AI systems, enabling healthcare organizations to respond dynamically to emerging ethical, technical, and legal considerations. This work not only underscores the need for human-centered design and institutional readiness but also offers a replicable governance model for integrating AI responsibly. By addressing the socio-technical and regulatory complexities of AI adoption, the report contributes a valuable roadmap for institutions striving to implement trustworthy AI that enhances care quality, equity, and safety.

Recent years have seen the emergence of global governance frameworks aimed at ensuring that artificial intelligence systems are developed and deployed in a manner that is safe, ethical, and accountable—particularly in high-risk sectors such as healthcare. The European Union Artificial Intelligence Act (EU AI Act, 2024) represents the first comprehensive, binding regulatory framework for AI, introducing a risk-based classification system that designates many healthcare AI applications (e.g., clinical decision support, diagnostic tools) as *high-risk*. Under this framework, organizations are required to implement rigorous risk management, human oversight, transparency, and post-market monitoring obligations (European Union, 2024).

Similarly, the World Health Organization's Ethics and Governance of Artificial Intelligence for Health guidelines emphasize principles such as human autonomy, inclusiveness, transparency, accountability, and sustainability, calling for institutional governance structures and lifecycle oversight in clinical AI deployments (World Health Organization, 2024). Together, these frameworks reinforce the chapter's argument that secure-by-design engineering must be complemented by formal governance mechanisms that extend beyond organizational boundaries and align with international norms.

Research Gaps and Emerging Directions

Despite these insights, several research gaps remain. Much of the existing literature is technical or compliance-focused, with a lesser emphasis on how developers, IT leaders, and clinicians collaboratively navigate the integration of AI. There is limited empirical work on how explainability tools affect trust in practice, or how prompt engineering influences the safety of AI outputs in medical contexts. Longitudinal studies are necessary to evaluate how AI influences the evolution of organizational routines, developer roles, and patient-provider dynamics over time.

Furthermore, while security frameworks exist for traditional systems, few offer tailored guidance for AI-specific threats in healthcare. As LLMs become multimodal and more deeply embedded in EHRs, new attack vectors and ethical dilemmas are emerging. Addressing these gaps will require cross-disciplinary research that combines software engineering, cybersecurity, human-computer interaction, and healthcare informatics.

Bridging Theory and Practice

As AI-enhanced tools become increasingly embedded in healthcare collaboration platforms, it is essential to bridge the conceptual frameworks guiding this transformation with the realities of system design, deployment, and day-to-day clinical use. Theories such as STS, the TAM, and the TTAT provide valuable analytical perspectives on the dynamics of human-AI interaction, system adoption, and risk perception. However, the practical application of these frameworks demands deliberate integration into the development and governance of AI-powered healthcare systems.

STS emphasizes that secure software engineering in healthcare is not solely a technical challenge but a socio-organizational one. In practice, this means involving end users—clinicians, administrators, IT staff, and even patients—throughout the design and implementation lifecycle. Co-design practices, usability testing, and workflow alignment are crucial to ensure that AI-enhanced collaboration tools are both functional and trusted. Systems that disregard the lived experience of their users often face low adoption rates or are misused in ways that compromise patient care and data integrity.

TAM offers insight into why healthcare professionals accept or resist new AI-driven tools. Perceived usefulness and ease of use must be prioritized through intuitive interfaces, clear communication of AI capabilities, and integration into existing clinical routines. In practice, this requires more than technical training; it involves fostering a culture that embraces innovation while addressing concerns about reliability, accountability, and professional autonomy. For example, AI-generated clinical recommendations should be designed to support, rather than override, physician judgment, thereby reinforcing the value of human expertise.

TTAT underscores how individuals assess and respond to the risks posed by technology. In high-stakes healthcare environments, perceived threats—such as data breaches, AI hallucinations, or black-box decision-making—can significantly influence behavior. Bridging TTAT with practice involves implementing visible and adequate safeguards: secure APIs, auditable data exchanges, real-time alerts for anomalous behavior, and transparent AI logic. Moreover, security training should move beyond compliance checklists to cultivate situational awareness and encourage proactive risk mitigation.

Bridging theory and practice also means recognizing the interdependence between system architecture and organizational policies. For example, implementing role-based access control (RBAC) in AI collaboration tools reflects both the technical requirement to safeguard patient data and the practical necessity to respect clinical hierarchies and responsibilities. Similarly, integrating HL7/FHIR standards not only enables technical interoperability but also supports care continuity and regulatory compliance, key concerns identified in STS-informed analyses.

Ultimately, the integration of generative AI into secure healthcare collaboration platforms must move beyond proof-of-concept models toward responsible, system-aware solutions. By operationalizing theoretical insights into user-centered design strategies, transparent risk communication, and governance frameworks, stakeholders can co-create resilient digital ecosystems. These systems will not only enhance care coordination and clinical efficiency but also preserve trust, ensure compliance, and uphold ethical standards in AI-augmented healthcare environments.

Conclusion: Securing the Future of AI-Driven Collaboration in Healthcare

The integration of AI into healthcare collaboration platforms offers transformative potential to improve communication, streamline clinical workflows, and enhance decision-making. From intelligent chatbots and virtual assistants to LLMs embedded in telehealth systems, these technologies are reshaping how healthcare is delivered. Yet with this innovation comes a parallel responsibility to ensure that such systems are designed, implemented, and governed with security, trust, and interoperability at their core.

This chapter argues that secure software engineering is essential to realizing the benefits of AI-enhanced e-collaboration without compromising patient safety, data privacy, or regulatory compliance. Drawing on theoretical frameworks such as STS, TAM, and TTAT, the analysis underscores the necessity for holistic design approaches that strike a balance between technical robustness and human factors. Secure-by-design principles, including secure APIs, role-based access control, explainable AI outputs, and standards-based integration (e.g., HL7/FHIR), must be embedded throughout the development lifecycle.

Furthermore, the chapter emphasizes that successful adoption of AI tools depends not only on system capabilities but also on clinician trust, user training, and organizational readiness. Human oversight, ethical transparency, and continuous feedback loops are vital to maintaining safety and accountability in rapidly evolving digital ecosystems.

As healthcare systems continue to digitize and scale, the path forward lies in building resilient, ethical, and interoperable AI-enabled platforms that serve both clinical excellence and patient empowerment. By aligning secure software engineering practices with multidisciplinary collaboration and regulatory foresight, the healthcare sector can responsibly harness AI's potential, transforming care delivery while safeguarding what matters most: trust, integrity, and human well-being.

METHODOLOGY

This study employed a qualitative, phenomenological research design to explore how software professionals and healthcare technologists experience the integration of AI-driven collaboration tools within secure healthcare environments. Phenomenology, as described by Peoples (2021), focuses on uncovering the essence of lived experiences, emphasizing subjective meaning and personal interpretation over external observation. This approach was chosen to investigate the real-world experiences of professionals navigating the complexities of trust, interoperability, and security in AI-enhanced systems.

To gain deep, contextual insight, the study utilized semi-structured, open-ended interviews. This format enabled consistent thematic inquiry while allowing participants the freedom to articulate their personal experiences in their own terms. It enabled the exploration of both anticipated and emergent issues related to AI integration, data governance, human oversight, and collaborative decision-making in healthcare settings.

A purposive sampling strategy was used to select participants with direct experience in AI-enabled software development, DevSecOps, cybersecurity, and healthcare IT. The sample included twelve professionals representing various roles, including software engineers, AI developers, IT security officers, clinical informatics experts, and system architects. This diversity ensured a comprehensive view of the technological, organizational, and ethical dimensions of AI adoption in secure e-collaboration environments.

Triangulation was achieved by analyzing data from participants across varied institutions and domains, including hospitals, research centers, and enterprise healthcare vendors. This methodological triangulation allowed for the identification of convergent themes while respecting the contextual differences in deployment practices and security postures.

To enhance credibility and analytical validity, member checking was conducted with selected participants. These individuals were given the opportunity to review the researcher's interpretations of their statements and offer clarifications or corrections. This iterative validation process ensured that the thematic analysis remained faithful to participants' intended meanings and professional perspectives.

The researcher maintained a reflexive journal throughout the study, documenting methodological choices, interpretive decisions, and emerging biases. This process fostered critical self-awareness and transparency during coding and theme development, minimizing undue influence from the researcher's assumptions.

Ethical research practices were upheld at every stage. Participants provided informed consent, were notified of their right to withdraw at any time, and were assured of confidentiality. Identifiable information was removed during transcription, and all digital files were stored on encrypted, password-protected devices. The study prioritized respect, autonomy, and data security in accordance with ethical standards for research involving human subjects.

Research Design

This study was grounded in a qualitative, phenomenological framework. It employed in-depth, semi-structured interviews to investigate how healthcare software professionals experience the integration of AI-enhanced e-collaboration platforms. The goal was not to generalize findings statistically but to develop a rich understanding of the opportunities, risks, and ethical tensions that emerge when AI is embedded in sensitive healthcare workflows.

This design enabled the collection of detailed narratives that captured participants' reflections on system architecture, trust in AI recommendations, explainability of LLM outputs, secure interoperability with EHRs, and patient data protection. The phenomenological orientation emphasized personal meaning, particularly as participants described the challenges of implementing AI in high-risk, compliance-driven environments.

Participant Selection

Participants were recruited through purposive sampling, with the inclusion criterion being direct experience in designing, deploying, or managing AI-driven collaboration tools within secure healthcare contexts. The sample consisted of fifteen participants with diverse expertise in software engineering, DevSecOps, cybersecurity, healthcare IT, and clinical systems integration.

The participants' organizational affiliations included hospitals, health tech start-ups, academic institutions, and enterprise software vendors, providing a broad view of how AI-enabled platforms are adopted across various operational and regulatory landscapes. All participants reported familiarity with AI-based systems such as chatbots, virtual assistants, LLMs (e.g., ChatGPT), or predictive triage engines integrated with EHRs and patient portals.

Recruitment was conducted via professional forums, LinkedIn, academic networks, and referrals. Each participant received an informed consent form that outlined the study's purpose, confidentiality safeguards, and the voluntary nature of their participation. No compensation was provided.

Data Collection

Data were gathered through one-on-one, semi-structured interviews conducted via Zoom, each lasting between 45 and 70 minutes. The interview guide focused on participants' experiences with AI-enhanced e-collaboration, covering topics such as secure system architecture, interoperability standards (e.g., HL7/FHIR), explainability, risk management, and organizational policies.

The flexible interview format allowed the researcher to explore relevant digressions while maintaining consistency across core thematic areas. Participants were encouraged to describe specific projects, challenges, or turning points that illustrated how the integration of AI has impacted their work and security practices.

All interviews were recorded with consent, transcribed verbatim, and anonymized. Transcripts were stored securely on encrypted, access-controlled drives to maintain data integrity and participant confidentiality.

Analytical Approach

A thematic analysis was conducted using a hybrid inductive-deductive strategy. The researcher first read each transcript holistically to identify initial patterns and concepts emphasized by the participants. Coding was conducted in MaxQDA software, where transcripts were annotated and organized into thematic categories aligned with the study's conceptual frameworks: STS, TAM, and TTAT.

Initial coding focused on broad categories, including system usability, perceived risk of AI, security-by-design practices, and trust in AI outputs. In subsequent rounds, codes were refined to reflect more specific constructs such as explainability gaps, API vulnerabilities, ethical tensions, or regulatory compliance barriers. Contradictions, tensions, and role-based differences were also examined across participant types.

Themes were then mapped to the three guiding research questions:

- RQ1: How do AI-powered collaboration tools, such as virtual assistants, chatbots, and LLM-based platforms, impact the design and implementation of secure software systems in healthcare environments?

- RQ2: What are the primary security, privacy, and interoperability challenges associated with integrating AI-driven e-collaboration platforms with EHRs and other health information systems?
- RQ3: How can healthcare organizations and developers adopt secure-by-design principles, including role-based access control, auditability, and HL7/FHIR standards, to ensure resilient, compliant, and ethical AI-enhanced collaboration?

This multi-stage analysis enabled the researcher to link empirical experiences with theoretical insights, revealing patterns that highlight both opportunities and systemic vulnerabilities in current healthcare AI practices.

Trustworthiness

To ensure the trustworthiness of the research, multiple strategies were applied in accordance with qualitative best practices. Triangulation across participant roles and organizational settings supported the credibility of emerging themes by validating them in different contexts. Patterns were cross-verified between frontline developers, system integrators, and clinical IT leaders.

Member checking further enhanced interpretive accuracy. Selected participants were invited to review early thematic syntheses and comment on whether their perspectives were adequately represented. Their feedback informed minor revisions to code categories and helped clarify ambiguous language.

Reflexive journaling was used throughout data collection and analysis to document interpretive decisions and maintain transparency about the researcher's positionality. This reflexivity reduced the likelihood of confirmation bias and enabled a more grounded interpretation of participant narratives.

Ethically, the study upheld the principles of respect, confidentiality, and autonomy. Data were handled in compliance with institutional review protocols, and participants retained the right to withdraw their contributions at any time. The study's integrity was maintained by clear documentation, encrypted data storage, and continuous ethical review.

Together, these methods ensure that the research findings are not only credible and transferable but also rooted in a deep respect for the complex, human-centered challenges of secure AI integration in healthcare collaboration.

FINDINGS AND DISCUSSION

This section presents findings from qualitative interviews with software developers, healthcare IT specialists, and security professionals involved in designing and maintaining AI-enhanced e-collaboration platforms. The analysis is organized around the three guiding research questions (RQs), each supported by three thematic categories. These themes are interpreted through the theoretical lenses of STS, the TAM, and TTAT. Each RQ concludes with a summary and an illustrative case study. The final section offers a broader interpretation of the findings and implications for practice and research.

RQ1: How do AI-powered collaboration tools, such as virtual assistants, chatbots, and LLM-based platforms, impact the design and implementation of secure software systems in healthcare environments?

Theme 1: Acceleration of Workflow and System Responsiveness

Participants consistently reported that AI tools have significantly improved the speed, efficiency, and responsiveness of healthcare collaboration systems. These enhancements were particularly evident in areas such as automated documentation, clinical triage, and intelligent routing of information across care teams. LLMs and AI-driven chatbots have become valuable assets in streamlining routine tasks that previously demanded extensive manual input from clinicians and administrative staff.

A participant from the healthcare industry noted that AI-powered chatbots integrated into patient portals significantly reduced clinician workload by managing large volumes of patient inquiries, collecting intake information, and guiding users through pre-visit questionnaires. These chatbots enabled real-time patient interactions, ensuring that relevant information was gathered and directed to the appropriate department, often before the patient arrived at the clinic. Beyond easing individual tasks, the participant emphasized that the chatbots created meaningful workflow benefits by streamlining administrative processes, reducing bottlenecks in patient triage, and allowing clinicians to focus more on direct patient care. This automation improved coordination between departments and enhanced overall efficiency in the care delivery process.

Additionally, LLMs played a crucial role in generating clinical documentation, including encounter summaries, discharge notes, and referral letters. Participants noted that these models could synthesize free-text inputs and structured EHR data to produce coherent, contextually relevant narratives, thereby saving physicians time and improving documentation consistency. In some settings, LLMs were also used to support decision-making, providing concise summaries of patient histories or surfacing relevant clinical guidelines based on current case data.

However, while participants praised these tools for boosting operational efficiency, many also emphasized the importance of human oversight, particularly for high-risk tasks involving clinical judgment or regulatory compliance. As one developer noted, *"AI makes everything move faster, but you still need a human to make decisions when dealing with patient care."* This balance between automation and accountability was considered essential for maintaining trust and safety in AI-enhanced healthcare collaboration.

Theme 2: Inconsistent Adoption and Distrust

The adoption of AI tools, such as LLMs and intelligent chatbots, varied considerably across institutions, reflecting differing levels of organizational readiness, risk tolerance, and trust in emerging technologies. While some developers enthusiastically integrated LLMs into backend systems, leveraging their capabilities for tasks such as data extraction, real-time routing, and automated documentation, others approached implementation with significant caution. Their hesitation stemmed from concerns over such topics as suspicious outputs, unclear decision-making processes, and the potential for legal or regulatory liability if AI-generated content led to clinical errors or data breaches.

Participants from institutions that use AI more actively said they are making progress connecting LLMs with electronic health record (EHR) systems, using APIs to summarize information or assign tasks automatically. On the other hand, developers in more cautious organizations discussed resistance to AI, citing difficulties in integrating AI tools with existing regulations, compliance requirements, and clinical quality standards.

A significant factor affecting adoption was whether strong control measures were in place. Developers were more willing to use AI tools when the systems could override AI outputs. This behavior allowed developers to review, fix, or reject AI-generated content. As one participant said, "We trust the system much more when we can control the output. Automation itself is not safe in healthcare."

These findings suggest that, beyond technical capability, the successful adoption of AI in healthcare centers on thoughtful system design that prioritizes transparency and accountability. Organizations that provide clear guidance on override procedures, liability boundaries, and verification processes are more likely to foster trust and sustainable AI integration into clinical workflows.

Theme 3: Emergence of Hybrid Development Roles

Interviewees described a notable shift in job responsibilities resulting from the growing adoption of AI tools in healthcare. This adoption led to the emergence of new hybrid roles such as "clinical prompt engineers" and "AI-integration architects." These evolving positions reflect a blending of traditional software engineering competencies with deep domain-specific knowledge in clinical workflows, regulatory compliance, and data governance.

Developers, such as clinical prompt engineers, are increasingly responsible for creating precise, context-aware prompts that help large language models produce accurate and secure responses. They need to understand both the technical aspects of AI systems and the details of clinical communication to make sure the outputs meet medical standards and ethical guidelines. Their work often involves continuously refining prompts, watching for AI errors or hallucinations, and checking the results for clinical accuracy.

AI-integration architects, on the other hand, focus on securely embedding AI functionalities into healthcare infrastructure. This new infrastructure includes designing APIs that adhere to privacy regulations, such as HIPAA, implementing encryption protocols, and ensuring secure data exchange between AI systems and electronic health record (EHR) platforms. These specialists play a critical role in developing safeguards around protected health information (PHI), managing access controls, and establishing audit trails to track AI-driven decisions.

Participants noted that these hybrid roles are becoming essential for bridging the gap between innovation and responsibility. One respondent remarked, "In the past, we simply relied on IT to determine the output, but now we require someone knowledgeable about the healthcare standard code and compliance to verify." This shift underscores a broader transformation in healthcare IT teams, where multidisciplinary collaboration and ethical foresight are becoming increasingly essential to ensure that AI deployments are not only technically effective but also secure, interpretable, and aligned with patient safety priorities.

RQ2: What are the primary security, privacy, and interoperability challenges associated with integrating AI-driven e-collaboration platforms with EHRs and other health information systems?

Theme 1: Insecure Defaults and Misconfigured Integrations

Participants repeatedly emphasized that many AI tools, particularly LLM-based systems, lack secure-by-default configurations and frequently generate integration scripts that violate basic security and privacy principles. These oversights are particularly alarming in healthcare environments, where the protection of sensitive patient data is paramount and regulatory compliance with standards such as HIPAA is mandatory.

Participants reported that AI-generated scripts often omit critical security checks, such as input validation, access control enforcement, and data encryption. For example, multiple chatbot systems store patient inputs, including sensitive protected health information (PHI), in unsecured server logs without implementing explicit safeguards or obtaining patient consent to use this data for model training. This practice not only exposes confidential information to potential breaches but also raises serious ethical and legal concerns regarding patient privacy. Additionally, some chatbot integrations bypassed established role-based access control (RBAC) mechanisms when connected with electronic health record (EHR) systems. This flaw allowed unauthorized users to access clinical data across different departments and domains, compromising the integrity and confidentiality of patient records. Such security gaps highlight the urgent need for stricter controls, transparent data handling policies, and rigorous compliance measures to protect sensitive health information in AI-driven healthcare environments. Without addressing these vulnerabilities, the trustworthiness and safety of AI-enabled clinical workflows remain at significant risk.

A junior developer working in the healthcare sector shared their experience, stating, "ChatGPT is beneficial and often generates impressive and useful responses. However, it completely skips checking for HIPAA compliance, which is critical in our field. Because of this, we still have to manually review and fix the parts it misses to ensure patient privacy and data security." Another developer echoed these concerns, pointing out, "The AI returns results without validating whether default values or inputs are safe. While that might be acceptable in a non-critical test environment, in healthcare, such oversights can be dangerous and potentially harmful to patients." These insights highlight a significant challenge: although AI tools like ChatGPT offer great potential to enhance productivity and assist in clinical tasks, they lack built-in safeguards to enforce regulatory compliance and safety checks. This behavior places an added burden on developers and clinicians to meticulously verify outputs and guard against errors that could lead to privacy violations or patient harm. It underscores the need for AI systems that are designed with healthcare-specific compliance and safety protocols integrated from the start, rather than relying solely on human oversight after the fact.

These observations highlight a significant gap between the convenience offered by AI-generated systems and the real-world safety requirements. While AI tools can accelerate development, they often lack context-awareness for regulatory environments, making them unreliable without human verification. The findings suggest that embedding secure defaults, enforcing strict validation protocols, and integrating compliance-aware design patterns are essential for the safe and responsible use of AI in healthcare software systems.

Theme 2: Variable Influence of Prompt Engineering

Participants reported that clear and straightforward prompts significantly improved the security quality of AI-generated outputs. For instance, when developers included terms like "HIPAA-compliant," "use secure authentication," or "apply encryption" in their prompts, the responses were more aligned with best practices in healthcare data security. These prompts often led the AI to suggest more appropriate implementations, such as encrypted data storage, secure API endpoints, and adherence to access control policies like role-based access control (RBAC).

However, the effectiveness of the prompt heavily influenced the output. Vague or generic prompts often resulted in insecure or incomplete solutions, such as storing sensitive information in plaintext, using hardcoded credentials, or generating inconsistent patient ID formats that compromised data integrity across systems. These risky behaviors demonstrate the AI's tendency to prioritize convenience over compliance when not provided with clear security guidance.

Despite the improvements seen with precise prompting, participants emphasized that even the most carefully crafted inputs could not eliminate hallucinations or subtle logic errors. In some cases, the AI generated convincing but incorrect implementations, giving developers a false sense of reliability. One participant explained, "Even when I ask it to be HIPAA-compliant, it sometimes makes up libraries or uses outdated methods. You really need to double-check everything."

These findings highlight a critical limitation of current AI tools: while prompt engineering can guide more secure responses, it cannot replace human oversight and judgment. To ensure the safe deployment of AI-generated code in healthcare environments, participants advocated for the implementation of layered safeguards, including automated security scans, policy-based validation tools, and manual code reviews, to verify compliance, prevent hallucinated behavior, and uphold regulatory standards.

Theme 3: Organizational Constraints on Oversight

Mechanisms such as audit logging, access tracking, and human verification were found to be inconsistently implemented across AI-enhanced systems. While some teams maintained thorough validation procedures, others reported significant gaps, particularly in resource-constrained environments. Participants acknowledged that, under tight deadlines or limited staffing, they often deployed AI-generated features with little to no formal review. In many cases, security validations were skipped entirely, and features went live without proper testing for compliance, robustness, or risk mitigation.

Several participants admitted that time pressure, lack of specialized security training, and organizational priorities skewed toward speed over safety. As one participant shared, "We were told to complete the work quickly and handle security afterward. However, the security measures were inconsistently implemented, as they were sometimes addressed but often neglected. This behavior reflects a pattern of risk tolerance that TTAT helps explain. When threats are perceived as distant or when protective actions are seen as costly or impractical, individuals are more likely to accept the risk rather than attempt to mitigate it. In such cases, developers may rely on AI-generated outputs without verifying their safety if the model's sophistication compensates for oversight gaps.

This dynamic is especially problematic in high-stakes domains, such as healthcare, where the consequences of misconfigured systems can be severe and life-threatening. The findings underscore the urgent need for organizational investment in developer training, built-in guardrails, and low-friction oversight tools, such as automated code scanning, explainable AI indicators, and pre-deployment compliance checks. Without institutional support for security-by-design principles, the burden of responsible AI integration falls unfairly on individual developers, who often lack both the necessary resources and authority to implement the necessary safeguards.

RQ3: How can healthcare organizations and developers adopt secure-by-design principles, including role-based access control, auditability, and HL7/FHIR standards, to ensure resilient, compliant, and ethical AI-enhanced collaboration?

Theme 1: Partial Implementation of Secure-by-Design Protocols

While most organizations stated that "secure-by-design" guided their AI development, the actual application of this approach varied widely. Many participants described a mature and thoughtful approach to incorporating security at every stage of the software development lifecycle (SDLC), particularly when integrating AI systems into clinical workflows.

Organizations implemented comprehensive DevSecOps practices (Prates & Pereira, 2025) designed explicitly for AI-enhanced environments. Their development pipelines featured clear role separation to avoid conflicts of interest, automated security audits at critical points during model deployment, and strict compliance checks aligned with healthcare regulations, such as HIPAA. Rather than focusing solely on post-deployment security, controls were integrated from the very beginning, starting with data ingestion and model training, and extending through API integration and continuous monitoring of runtime behavior. One participant noted, "We automate security checks at every stage to make sure we meet HIPAA requirements before the product goes live."

By contrast, many other organizations implemented security in a fragmented or reactive manner, often relying on manual reviews, sporadic testing, or ad hoc policies. Participants from these environments acknowledged that security features were frequently deferred until late in the development cycle, particularly under time pressure to deliver minimum viable AI products. As one senior engineer noted, "We often talk about secure-by-design, but in reality, security issues are usually fixed only at the end."

This inconsistency underscores the need for stronger governance models and standardized protocols to ensure that 'secure-by-design' is not just a checkbox, but a deeply integrated discipline in AI development. It also underscores the value of aligning technical practices with organizational culture and compliance strategy, reinforcing that robust security in AI systems must be proactively engineered into the software development life cycle.

Theme 2: Policy Gaps and Lack of Clear Governance

Many participants revealed that their organizations lacked clear, formalized policies governing the use of artificial intelligence in production environments. This behavior has led to inconsistent and sometimes risky implementation practices across healthcare systems. In some organizations, AI use was restricted to low-risk, non-clinical functionalities, such as chatbot-based triage, appointment reminders, or autofilling administrative forms, where the stakes were lower and oversight requirements were minimal.

However, other organizations reported deploying AI as a critical component of the healthcare infrastructure, including core electronic health record (EHR) modules, clinical decision support systems, and real-time documentation tools. These deployments were often executed without comprehensive risk assessments, detailed auditing protocols, or transparent governance frameworks to guide safe integration and implementation. In several cases, participants admitted that decisions to implement AI were driven more by innovation momentum or vendor pressure than by structured evaluations of clinical safety, data security, or ethical implications.

One participant shared, "We're using AI to generate summaries within the EHR system, but there is no formal review board or clear policy that defines what is acceptable." Another added, "While we have advanced AI capabilities, our team hasn't advanced quickly enough to match the rapid pace of AI deployment." Together, these observations highlight a critical challenge: the need for robust, organization-wide governance structures and clear policies to guide the responsible use of AI in clinical settings. Without these, the rapid adoption of AI risks outpacing the mechanisms designed to manage safety, compliance, and ethical standards.

This gap between technological adoption and institutional policy highlights a critical challenge in the healthcare sector: the rapid evolution of AI is outpacing the development of safeguards meant to ensure its responsible use. Without precise guidelines, accountability frameworks, risk classification systems, and regulatory alignment, organizations risk introducing variability, liability, and unintended harm into clinical environments. The findings underscore the urgent need for institutional leadership to prioritize AI governance as a foundational layer of digital transformation in healthcare.

Theme 3: Progress Toward Transparency and Auditability

Participants reported a shift in organizational dynamics, with increased collaboration between engineering teams and compliance personnel to ensure that AI systems were developed and deployed in accordance with HIPAA guidelines and best practices for software developers. This proactive coordination signaled a meaningful shift away from isolated, siloed development practices toward more integrated and collaborative governance structures. Teams were no longer operating independently; instead, development, security, and compliance units collaborated closely from the earliest stages of implementation. As one participant explained, "We no longer handle everything within the development team. Now, the security team is fully integrated into the process. They're right there, ready to penetration test every piece of code before it goes live." This approach reflects a broader cultural change in how organizations view security, not as a final checkpoint, but as a continuous, shared responsibility across the entire software lifecycle.

Discussion and Implications

The findings underscore the dual nature of artificial intelligence in healthcare collaboration, on one hand, offering significant gains in efficiency, automation, and clinical innovation; on the other, introducing new layers of complexity, vulnerability, and systemic risk. While AI tools have proven valuable in streamlining tasks such as documentation, triage, scheduling, and clinical decision support, their deployment also raises pressing concerns around data privacy, explainability, security, and organizational accountability.

This section examines the broader implications of these findings through the lens of the study's guiding theoretical frameworks: STS, TAM, and TTAT. Together, these frameworks provide a multidimensional perspective on the integration of AI in healthcare, highlighting not only the transformative potential of these technologies but also the structural, ethical, and procedural safeguards necessary to ensure their responsible use. This analysis reinforces that effective AI adoption is not merely a technical upgrade, but a complex, evolving process that requires cross-disciplinary collaboration, continuous oversight, and a commitment to human-centered design.

Aligning System Design with Human Context - STS

STS emphasizes that the effectiveness of AI collaboration tools in healthcare depends on the alignment between technical systems and the social environments in which they operate. When developers operate in silos, AI deployments often encounter significant challenges, including gaps in trust, misalignment with clinical workflows, and overlooked security vulnerabilities. These disconnects can compromise both the usability and safety of AI-enhanced systems.

To bridge these gaps, organizations must move beyond purely technical implementation and embrace a co-design approach that actively involves cross-functional collaboration throughout the AI development lifecycle. This technology embraces engaging frontline clinicians in user experience design, integrating compliance experts into system architecture planning, and fostering ongoing dialogue between technical and non-technical teams. By investing in interdisciplinary governance structures and continuous stakeholder engagement, healthcare institutions can ensure that AI tools are not only technologically sophisticated but also contextually relevant, ethically sound, and operationally viable in real-world clinical settings.

Understanding Adoption and Resistance- TAM

TAM offers a valuable lens for understanding how healthcare professionals perceive and respond to the integration of AI within secure environments. According to TAM, two key factors—perceived ease of use and perceived usefulness—significantly shape adoption behaviors. Participants in this study frequently expressed higher trust and a greater willingness to engage with AI systems that were seamlessly integrated into familiar workflows, such as patient intake forms, triage systems, appointment scheduling, and documentation assistants. When AI tools felt like natural extensions of existing processes, they were more likely to be accepted and relied upon in day-to-day clinical operations.

Conversely, systems that lacked transparency or failed to provide meaningful user feedback often led to hesitation or outright resistance. Participants reported that when AI-generated outputs could not be traced, explained, or verified, they experienced a loss of perceived control over clinical decisions. This new AI behavior not only eroded confidence in the technology but also raised concerns about liability, safety, and ethical accountability. The absence of clear communication from the AI system—such as how a decision was made or which data influenced the output—undermined the sense of shared responsibility between the human user and the digital assistant.

To overcome these barriers, participants highlighted the importance of explainable AI interfaces and integrated audit tools. Such features allow users to inspect decision pathways, validate AI-generated recommendations, and escalate concerns when outputs appear inconsistent or misleading. These tools not only support regulatory compliance but also enhance user satisfaction by fostering a sense of transparency, control, and professional alignment. Ultimately, the findings affirm that for AI to be effectively adopted in healthcare, it must be not only powerful and accurate but also intelligible, responsive, and aligned with the cognitive and ethical expectations of its users.

Responding to Perceived Threats - TTAT

TTAT provides a helpful framework for understanding the wide variation in how developers perceive and respond to risks associated with AI integration in healthcare systems. The theory suggests that individuals assess both the severity of potential threats and their ability to mitigate them before deciding whether to take preventive action. This framework helps explain why some participants in the study actively implemented safeguards—such as static code analysis, peer review processes, and layered human oversight—while others exhibited passive or resigned attitudes toward AI-generated outputs.

Developers who took proactive steps often worked in environments where security awareness was embedded into team culture and reinforced through structured processes. These participants described an internalized sense of responsibility for anticipating potential vulnerabilities in AI behavior, particularly when dealing with sensitive clinical data. In contrast, other developers admitted to relying heavily on the default outputs of AI tools, assuming correctness without verification due to time constraints, lack of training, or institutional pressure to accelerate delivery. As one participant noted, “You know it's risky, but sometimes you do not have time to trace every line of code.”

This divergence in risk response highlights the importance of cultivating organizational cultures that prioritize secure AI literacy. Establishing such a culture requires more than just technical controls; it involves sustained investment in developer education, ongoing threat modeling workshops, and clearly communicated policies that normalize risk awareness as a core aspect of AI development. Leadership also plays a critical role. By modeling secure behavior, recognizing cautious decision-making, and reinforcing expectations for ethical accountability, organizations can gradually shift attitudes from reactive or resigned to deliberate and security-conscious.

Ultimately, TTAT reveals that risk management in AI-enhanced systems is not solely a matter of technical safeguards but also a mindset. Developers must be empowered, not just equipped, to recognize threats, evaluate their implications, and feel supported in taking action to mitigate them. A culture of secure AI literacy transforms security from a compliance requirement into a shared professional ethic, essential for ensuring the safe and trustworthy deployment of AI in healthcare.

Implications

The findings from this study have several important implications for the secure and responsible integration of AI-driven collaboration tools in healthcare. These implications cut across clinical practice, software engineering processes, organizational governance, and workforce preparation.

1. Implications for Healthcare Practice

The use of AI-powered tools such as chatbots, symptom checkers, and virtual assistants offers considerable benefits in enhancing clinical efficiency, communication, and access to care. However, their deployment must be accompanied by human oversight, clear auditability, and explainability features to maintain clinician trust and patient safety.

STS emphasizes the need for alignment between technical systems and clinical workflows. This alignment means that healthcare organizations must invest in interdisciplinary co-design processes, involving end-users from the early stages of development, to ensure that AI features augment rather than disrupt care delivery. Explainable AI interfaces and human override capabilities are essential for fostering confidence in automated systems and mitigating associated risks.

2. Implications for Software Development and Governance

Secure-by-design principles must be redefined to accommodate the dynamic, probabilistic nature of generative AI. As this study shows, even minor implementation oversights, such as misconfigured access tokens or vague prompt instructions, can lead to significant vulnerabilities. Developers and DevSecOps teams must therefore integrate continuous security validation, audit trails, and prompt engineering strategies into their pipelines.

From the perspective of TTAT, organizations must take responsibility for shaping secure behavior by embedding adequate safeguards and promoting a culture of awareness. This responsibility includes updating governance frameworks to reflect the Specific risks and ethical standards associated with AI.

3. Implications for Education and Workforce Development

The rise of AI in secure healthcare collaboration necessitates a fundamental reevaluation of how software engineers, IT professionals, and clinicians are trained. As shown in this study, developers are increasingly acting not only as coders but also as interpreters and evaluators of AI behavior. Educational institutions and professional development programs must, therefore, embed AI literacy and secure prompt engineering and human-AI collaboration ethics into their curricula. Training should go beyond technical functionality to include critical thinking, security awareness, and responsible innovation. Practical exercises should teach students how to validate AI outputs, interpret probabilistic results, and engage in cross-disciplinary problem-solving.

Final Reflection

These findings reflect a field in transition. AI-enhanced collaboration in healthcare is redefining roles, processes, and priorities in both software engineering and care delivery. As developers become AI facilitators and reviewers, and as clinical decisions increasingly involve machine assistance, the line between automation and accountability continues to blur.

Through the lenses of STS, TAM, and TTAT, a secure implementation depends not only on technical defenses but also on shared understanding, critical reflection, and adaptive organizational structures. AI is not a plug-and-play solution, but it is a complex socio-technical actor that must be carefully stewarded through design, deployment, and oversight.

The future of secure healthcare collaboration lies in bridging the gap between innovation and regulation, between speed and analysis, and between machine efficiency and human care. By embedding ethical, explainable, and secure software engineering principles into every layer of AI integration, we move closer to digital systems that empower clinicians, protect patients, and uphold the public trust.

CONCLUSION AND FUTURE DIRECTIONS

As AI-powered systems become increasingly embedded in healthcare collaboration, the role of secure software engineering has never been more vital. This chapter has examined how AI tools, such as chatbots, virtual assistants, and LLMs, are transforming communication, coordination, and decision-making in clinical environments. Drawing on high-quality research data and theoretical frameworks, the findings highlight both the transformative potential and the systemic risks associated with AI-enhanced e-collaboration.

The chapter reveals that while AI tools offer measurable improvements in workflow efficiency, they also introduce challenges related to data privacy, explainability, system interoperability, and trust. The secure implementation of these tools depends not only on technical safeguards but also on organizational readiness, interdisciplinary collaboration, and user-centered design.

Through the lens of STS, the study emphasizes the need to blend technical architectures with human workflows and institutional policies. TAM underscores the importance of perceived usefulness, ease of use, and transparency in driving user adoption. Meanwhile, TTAT highlights how perceptions of risk and confidence in protective measures shape developer behavior and secure software practices.

Future Directions

Future research should complement qualitative insights with quantitative and mixed-method approaches to measure clinician trust, usability, and reliance on AI systems over time. Survey-based instruments, controlled experiments, and longitudinal studies could be employed to assess how variables such as model transparency, error rates, explanation quality, and organizational safeguards influence trust calibration and clinical outcomes.

Additionally, simulation-based studies and field experiments could evaluate the effectiveness of specific security and governance interventions—such as audit dashboards, explanation interfaces, or bias monitoring tools—providing empirical evidence to inform best practices. Such methodological diversification would strengthen the evidence base guiding the secure, ethical, and scalable adoption of AI in healthcare.

Another priority involves a granular analysis of prompt engineering and model behavior. As prompt engineering becomes a fundamental skill in AI-enabled development, especially when using LLMs, empirical research is needed to understand how variations in prompt specificity, structure, and context influence security, privacy, and functional reliability. This behavior is crucial in high-stakes applications, such as clinical decision support, patient triage, and automated documentation, where misinterpretations or hallucinated outputs can pose significant risks to patient care.

In summary, the responsible future of AI in healthcare depends on interdisciplinary research, secure software practices, and policies that center on transparency, equity, and human oversight. By advancing both technical frameworks and socio-organizational strategies, the field can ensure that AI not only enhances healthcare collaboration but also does so in a manner that is secure, ethical, and trustworthy.

REFERENCES

Blease, C., Torous, J., McMillan, B., Hägglund, M., & Mandl, K. D. (2024). Generative Language Models and Open Notes: Exploring the Promise and Limitations. *JMIR Medical Education, 10*, e51183. Advance online publication. DOI: 10.2196/51183

Booth, H., Souppaya, M., Vassilev, A., Ogata, M., Stanley, M., & Scarfone, K. (2022). Secure Software Development Practices for Generative AI and Dual-Use Foundation Models: An SSDF Community Profile. *IEEE Transactions on Dependable and Secure Computing*. Advance online publication. DOI: 10.6028/NIST.SP.800-218A

Das, B. C., Amini, M. H., & Wu, Y. (2025). Security and Privacy Challenges of Large Language Models: A Survey. *ACM Computing Surveys, 57*(6), 1–39. DOI: 10.1145/3712001

Davis, F. D. (1989). Perceived usefulness, perceived ease of use, and user acceptance of information technology. *Management Information Systems Quarterly, 13*(3), 319–340. DOI: 10.2307/249008

Emery, F. E., & Trist, E. L. (1960). *Socio-technical systems.* Management science, models and techniques 2.

Khurana, A., Subramonyam, H., & Chilana, P. K. (2024). Why and when llm-based assistants can go wrong: Investigating the effectiveness of prompt-based interactions for software help-seeking. *arXiv.org*. Retrieved from /arxiv.2402.08030DOI: 10.1145/3640543.3645200

Liang, H., & Xue, Y. (2009). Avoidance of information technology threats: A theoretical perspective. *Management Information Systems Quarterly, 33*(1), 71–90. DOI: 10.2307/20650279

Mesinovic, M., Watkinson, P., & Zhu, T. (2025). Explainability in the age of large language models for healthcare. *Communications Engineering, 4*(1), 128. Advance online publication. DOI: 10.1038/s44172-025-00453-y

Modi, N. D., Menz, B. D., Awaty, A. A., Alex, C. A., Logan, J. M., McKinnon, R. A., Rowland, A., Bacchi, S., Gradon, K., Sorich, M. J., & Hopkins, A. M. (2025). Assessing the System-Instruction Vulnerabilities of Large Language Models to Malicious Conversion Into Health Disinformation Chatbots. *Annals of Internal Medicine, 178*(8), 1172–1180. Advance online publication. DOI: 10.7326/ANNALS-24-03933

Navarro, D. F., Lewis, M., Shah, R., Delacroix, S., & Lehman, R. (2025). Generative AI and the changing dynamics of clinical consultations. *BMJ (Clinical Research Ed.), 391*, e085325. Advance online publication. DOI: 10.1136/bmj-2025-085325

Organization, W. H. (2024). *Ethics and governance of artificial intelligence for health: large multi-modal models. WHO guidance*. World Health Organization.

Peoples, K. (2021). *How to write a phenomenological dissertation: A step-by-step guide* (Vol. 56). SAGE.

Prates, L., & Pereira, R. (2025). DevSecOps practices and tools. *International Journal of Information Security, 24*(1), 11. Advance online publication. DOI: 10.1007/s10207-024-00914-z

Rigas, E. S., Lagakis, P., Karadimas, M., Logaras, E., Latsou, D., Hatzikou, M., Poulakidas, A., Billis, A., & Bamidis, P. D. (2024). Semantic interoperability for an AI-based applications platform for smart hospitals using HL7 FHIR. *Journal of Systems and Software, 215*, 112093. Advance online publication. DOI: 10.1016/j.jss.2024.112093

Saenz, A. D., Zhang, Z., Shah, A., Brawarsky, P., Omar, M., Rajkomar, A., & Zai, A. H. (2024). Establishing responsible use of AI guidelines: A comprehensive case study for healthcare institutions. *npj. NPJ Digital Medicine, 348*(7), 348. Advance online publication. DOI: 10.1038/s41746-024-01300-8

Scarfone, K., Souppaya, M., & Dodson, D. (2022). Secure Software Development Framework (SSDF) Version 1.1: Recommendations for Mitigating the Risk of Software Vulnerabilities. *NIST Special Publication, 800*(218), 800–218. DOI: 10.6028/NIST.SP.800-218

Union, E. (2024). *Regulation (EU) 2024/1689 of the European Parliament and of the Council laying down harmonised rules on artificial intelligence (Artificial Intelligence Act)*. Official Journal of the European Union.

KEY TERMS AND DEFINITIONS

AI-enhanced e-collaboration: Artificial intelligence technologies, including chatbots, virtual assistants, and large language models, are utilized to support communication, care coordination, and decision-making in digital healthcare settings.

DevSecOps: A development methodology that embeds security into every stage of the software development and deployment process is often used in regulated industries such as healthcare.

FHIR (Fast Healthcare Interoperability Resources): A standard developed by HL7 that enables the electronic exchange of healthcare information through structured APIs and data models to support system interoperability.

Prompt engineering: The practice of formulating precise inputs to guide the behavior of generative AI systems and improve the safety, accuracy, or relevance of their outputs.

Secure-by-design: A software engineering approach that integrates security features throughout the development lifecycle to prevent vulnerabilities and ensure compliance with privacy and safety standards.

Socio-Technical Systems Theory (STS): A framework emphasizing the need to align technological systems with human users, organizational structures, and clinical workflows in complex environments like healthcare.

Technology Acceptance Model (TAM): A model used to understand how users adopt and use new technologies based on perceived usefulness and ease of use.

Technology Threat Avoidance Theory (TTAT): A theory that explains how individuals assess and avoid technology-related risks based on perceived severity, vulnerability, and the effectiveness of safeguards.

Chapter 4
Democratizing Healthcare AI Through Low-Code Platforms:
Oracle APEX as an Enabler of Collaborative Intelligence

Satwik Jambula
http://orcid.org/0009-0002-7184-8319
Lamar University, USA

ABSTRACT

This chapter examines how low-code platforms, specifically Oracle APEX, can democratize healthcare AI by enabling non-technical healthcare professionals to create intelligent applications. The authors explore the intersection of low-code development and healthcare technology, demonstrating how Oracle APEX facilitates collaborative intelligence in clinical settings. The chapter analyzes the platform's capability to bridge the technical skills gap in healthcare organizations, allowing clinicians and administrators to rapidly develop and deploy AI-powered solutions for patient care, workflow optimization, and data management. Through case studies and practical examples, this research illustrates how low-code platforms can accelerate healthcare digital transformation while maintaining security and compliance standards. The findings reveal that Oracle APEX serves as an effective enabler for healthcare professionals to harness AI capabilities without extensive programming knowledge, ultimately improving patient outcomes and operational efficiency.

DOI: 10.4018/979-8-3373-5906-9.ch004

INTRODUCTION

The healthcare industry faces a critical challenge: the growing gap between the technical expertise required to develop AI-powered solutions and the domain knowledge possessed by healthcare professionals who understand clinical needs. Traditional software development approaches have created substantial barriers to healthcare innovation, relegating organizations to dependence on external vendors or limited IT departments. This dependency slows innovation and often results in solutions that inadequately address specific workflow requirements and clinical realities (Gray et al., 2022; Singh et al., 2020).

Low-code development platforms represent a paradigm shift that can democratize healthcare AI by empowering non-technical healthcare professionals to create sophisticated, AI-enhanced applications. Oracle Application Express (APEX) stands out as a particularly compelling solution due to its robust Oracle Database integration, comprehensive security features, and intuitive visual development environment (Oracle Corporation, 2024). Oracle APEX fundamentally alters the software development landscape by providing visual, drag-and-drop interfaces that abstract complex programming concepts into manageable, graphical representations. This enables healthcare professionals—physicians, nurses, administrators, and clinical researchers—to directly participate in creating digital solutions that address their operational challenges (Saeed et al., 2023).

Rather than serving merely as end-users, healthcare workers become active contributors to the development process, bringing deep domain expertise to clinical tool design and implementation. This democratization aligns with broader movements in health informatics toward participatory design and user-centered development that recognize healthcare professionals' essential role in creating effective clinical technologies (JMIR Medical Informatics Editorial Board, 2024; Liu et al., 2022).

The concept of collaborative intelligence emerges as central to this transformation, grounded in three complementary theoretical frameworks that provide analytical structure for understanding adoption patterns and implementation success. The *Technology Acceptance Model (TAM)* explains that perceived usefulness and perceived ease of use determine technology adoption (Davis, 1989). In healthcare contexts, Oracle APEX addresses both dimensions—its low-code approach enhances ease of use for clinical professionals while collaborative intelligence features demonstrate clear usefulness for patient care. *Diffusion of Innovation theory* (Rogers, 2003) identifies five stages—knowledge, persuasion, decision, implementation, and confirmation—that characterize technology adoption. Healthcare organizations exhibit unique diffusion patterns due to regulatory constraints, risk-averse cultures, and hierarchical structures, explaining why pilot projects, physician champions, and gradual rollout strategies prove essential. *Collaborative Intelligence theory* (Wilson

& Daugherty, 2018) positions AI as augmentation rather than replacement, emphasizing complementary human-AI capabilities where AI handles pattern recognition and computational tasks while humans maintain responsibility for contextual understanding, ethical reasoning, and complex decision-making. Rather than viewing AI as replacing human expertise, this integrated theoretical lens explains how Oracle APEX enables healthcare professionals to create applications where AI enhances clinical decision-making while preserving essential human elements of empathy, critical thinking, and contextual judgment (Yazici et al., 2022).

Oracle APEX's database-centric architecture provides enterprise-grade security, scalability, and performance characteristics essential for healthcare applications handling sensitive patient data. The platform's native integration with Oracle's advanced database features, including built-in AI and machine learning capabilities, enables healthcare professionals to leverage sophisticated analytical tools without extensive technical training (Oracle Corporation, 2024). This chapter explores how Oracle APEX serves as an enabler of collaborative intelligence in healthcare environments by providing the technical infrastructure and development tools necessary for healthcare professionals to create AI-enhanced applications. The discussion encompasses both the platform's technical capabilities and the organizational changes required to successfully implement collaborative intelligence initiatives, addressing healthcare's unique regulatory environment, ethical considerations including accountability and algorithmic bias, comparative platform assessment, and global implementation contexts that shape adoption strategies across diverse healthcare settings.

LITERATURE REVIEW

The intersection of artificial intelligence, healthcare delivery, and low-code development platforms represents a rapidly evolving field of study that draws from multiple disciplines including computer science, healthcare informatics, organizational behavior, and human-computer interaction. Understanding the current state of research in these areas provides essential context for evaluating the potential of Oracle APEX as an enabler of collaborative intelligence in healthcare settings.

Healthcare AI Adoption Challenges

The healthcare industry's adoption of artificial intelligence has been characterized by both significant promise and substantial barriers. Research has consistently identified several key challenges that impede the widespread implementation of AI solutions in clinical settings (Abouyannis et al., 2024; Goldfarb & Teodoridis, 2022). Technical barriers include issues related to data quality, interoperability, and the complexity of integrating AI systems with existing electronic health record (EHR) platforms. Healthcare data is notoriously fragmented, with information scattered across multiple systems that often lack standardized formats or communication protocols.

Organizational barriers present equally significant challenges. Healthcare institutions typically operate with hierarchical structures that can impede the rapid adoption of new technologies (Daley et al., 2024). Clinical workflows have evolved over decades to optimize patient safety and regulatory compliance, making healthcare professionals naturally cautious about implementing new systems that might disrupt established processes. Additionally, the substantial financial investments required for AI implementation, combined with uncertain return on investment timelines, create economic barriers that many healthcare organizations find difficult to overcome (Srinivasan et al., 2024).

Cultural and professional barriers also play a crucial role in AI adoption patterns. Healthcare professionals have legitimate concerns about the potential for AI systems to undermine their professional autonomy or decision-making authority (Bhargava et al., 2024). The "black box" nature of many AI algorithms creates transparency issues that conflict with the evidence-based decision-making culture that characterizes modern healthcare practice. Healthcare professionals require a clear understanding of how AI systems reach their conclusions to maintain confidence in AI-assisted decision-making processes (Shah et al., 2019).

Low-Code Platform Evolution

The low-code development movement has gained significant momentum across various industries as organizations seek to accelerate digital transformation initiatives while addressing persistent developer shortages. Low-code platforms abstract complex programming concepts into visual, intuitive interfaces that enable non-technical users to create sophisticated applications without traditional coding skills (Saeed et al., 2023).

Research has identified several factors driving low-code adoption in enterprise environments. The increasing complexity of modern software development, combined with growing demand for digital solutions, has created a supply-demand imbalance that low-code platforms help address. Organizations report significant reductions in application development time, with some studies indicating development cycle improvements of 50-90% compared to traditional coding approaches (Ullah et al., 2022). However, low-code platforms also present certain limitations including platform lock-in concerns, performance considerations for high-speed processing applications, and governance challenges as democratization potentially bypasses traditional IT oversight mechanisms.

Healthcare-Specific Low-Code Applications

Healthcare organizations have reported successful implementations of low-code solutions for patient scheduling systems, clinical decision support tools, quality reporting applications, and administrative workflow automation. Case studies from major healthcare systems demonstrate significant potential, with organizations developing over 200 applications using low-code platforms within two years, addressing needs from simple data collection to complex clinical workflow management (Liu et al., 2022).

However, healthcare implementations reveal unique challenges related to regulatory compliance, data security, and clinical workflow integration. Healthcare applications must meet stringent privacy and security requirements that may not be adequately addressed by general-purpose low-code platforms. Integration with existing clinical systems, particularly electronic health records, requires specialized knowledge and capabilities that may exceed typical low-code development environments (Holzinger et al., 2022).

Collaborative Intelligence Frameworks

Collaborative intelligence represents a paradigm shift from viewing AI as replacement technology to understanding AI as an augmentation tool that enhances human capabilities (Wilson & Daugherty, 2018). Research has identified key principles for successful human-AI collaboration including transparency, explainability, appropriate task allocation, and continuous learning mechanisms (Park et al., 2019).

In healthcare contexts, collaborative intelligence frameworks emphasize complementary strengths of human and artificial intelligence. Healthcare professionals bring contextual understanding, empathy, ethical reasoning, and complex problem-solving capabilities that current AI systems cannot replicate. AI systems contribute pattern recognition capabilities, computational speed, vast knowledge base access, and consistency in applying established protocols (Topol, 2019).

Successful collaborative intelligence implementations require careful attention to interface design, workflow integration, and change management processes. Healthcare professionals must understand how AI systems reach conclusions and maintain ability to override AI recommendations when clinical judgment suggests alternative approaches. Trust-building between healthcare professionals and AI systems emerges as a critical success factor requiring sustained attention throughout implementation and operation phases (Lee & Kesselheim, 2018).

Theoretical Perspectives on Healthcare Technology Adoption

Applying theoretical frameworks to low-code healthcare AI reveals critical success factors that extend beyond technical capabilities. Van der Laan et al.'s (2022) systematic review demonstrated that healthcare organizations explicitly addressing Technology Acceptance Model's perceived usefulness and ease of use dimensions show 3-4 times higher AI adoption rates compared to organizations focusing solely on technical features. Their findings indicate that successful adoption requires attention to both individual acceptance factors and organizational readiness.

Abouyannis et al. (2024) extended TAM to healthcare AI contexts, demonstrating that clinical professionals' adoption decisions are influenced by additional factors including professional autonomy concerns, patient safety considerations, and regulatory compliance requirements. Their research revealed that perceived usefulness alone explains only 42% of adoption variance, with trust, transparency, and workflow compatibility accounting for an additional 38%. This multi-dimensional influence pattern suggests that healthcare AI adoption requires comprehensive approaches addressing technical, professional, and organizational factors simultaneously.

Applying Diffusion of Innovation theory, Bhargava et al. (2024) found that healthcare AI adoption follows Rogers's adopter categories—innovators (2.5%), early adopters (13.5%), early majority (34%), late majority (34%), and laggards (16%)—but with slower diffusion curves than other industries. Healthcare demonstrates average time from innovation to mainstream adoption spanning 8-12 years rather than the 3-5 years typical in technology sectors, attributable to regulatory requirements, professional liability concerns, and patient safety considerations. Understanding these temporal patterns helps healthcare organizations set realistic expectations for low-code platform adoption.

Yazici et al.'s (2022) experimental validation of Collaborative Intelligence theory demonstrated that human-AI collaborative decision-making in medical contexts outperforms both human-only and AI-only approaches by 23-31% across multiple diagnostic tasks. Their research validated that optimal collaboration requires clear task allocation, transparent AI reasoning, and maintained human authority over final decisions—principles that inform Oracle APEX implementation strategies for healthcare applications. These findings provide empirical support for collaborative intelligence approaches rather than full automation strategies.

Comparative Low-Code Platform Landscape

Understanding Oracle APEX's position within the broader low-code ecosystem provides essential decision-making context for healthcare organizations. *Microsoft Power Platform* (Power Apps, Power Automate, Power BI) represents Oracle APEX's primary competitor, offering seamless Microsoft 365 integration with potentially shorter learning curves due to familiar interfaces. However, Power Platform demonstrates weaker database-centric AI capabilities compared to Oracle Database 23ai's vector search and built-in machine learning (Leemans, 2024). Healthcare organizations heavily invested in Microsoft ecosystems may prefer Power Platform despite AI limitations, while organizations prioritizing advanced analytical capabilities often select Oracle APEX.

Salesforce Health Cloud combined with Einstein AI provides healthcare-specific low-code development within Salesforce's ecosystem, including pre-built healthcare data models and HIPAA-compliant infrastructure. However, Salesforce's platform-as-a-service approach creates vendor lock-in concerns and typically involves higher total cost of ownership than Oracle APEX. *OutSystems* and *Mendix* represent enterprise low-code platforms with healthcare implementations, offering visual development and mobile capabilities but requiring separate machine learning platforms rather than native database AI integration.

Epic's Cognitive Computing Platform (CCP) enables healthcare organizations using Epic EHR to develop AI-enhanced applications within their existing EHR environment, providing seamless integration advantages. However, CCP requires Epic implementation, involves substantial costs, and provides less flexibility than general-purpose platforms. Organizations using other EHR systems cannot leverage CCP, making Oracle APEX or alternative platforms necessary.

Comparative analysis reveals no universally optimal platform. Oracle APEX demonstrates particular strengths for organizations prioritizing database-centric AI capabilities, advanced analytics, and cost-effectiveness, particularly those with existing Oracle investments. Power Platform suits Microsoft-heavy environments despite AI limitations. Salesforce serves organizations extending existing CRM investments. Selection requires multi-dimensional assessment of existing technology investments, AI ambitions, EHR context, budget constraints, development expertise, and regulatory requirements. Healthcare AI democratization benefits from platform diversity enabling organizations to select solutions aligned with their unique contexts rather than one-size-fits-all approaches.

Oracle APEX in Enterprise Environments

Oracle Application Express has been the subject of numerous studies examining its effectiveness as an enterprise low-code platform. Research has consistently highlighted the platform's strengths in database-centric application development, particularly for organizations already invested in Oracle technology ecosystems (Oracle Corporation, 2024). The platform's tight integration with Oracle Database enables developers to leverage advanced database features including built-in AI and machine learning capabilities without requiring extensive additional infrastructure.

Performance studies have demonstrated Oracle APEX's ability to handle enterprise-scale workloads while maintaining responsive user experiences. The platform's architecture, which generates optimized SQL and leverages Oracle Database's performance optimization features, enables applications to scale effectively as user bases and data volumes grow. Security research has highlighted Oracle APEX's comprehensive security framework, which includes features specifically relevant to healthcare applications such as fine-grained access controls, audit logging, and encryption capabilities aligned with healthcare regulatory requirements (Oracle Corporation, 2024).

Implementation Success Factors

Research across multiple industries and use cases has identified several critical success factors for low-code platform implementations. Executive sponsorship emerges as a primary predictor of implementation success, particularly in healthcare environments where cultural change management requires sustained leadership commitment (Rojas et al., 2025). Organizations with clear governance frameworks for low-code development report higher success rates and fewer implementation challenges compared to organizations with ad-hoc approaches.

Training and change management programs also correlate strongly with implementation success. Healthcare professionals require structured learning opportunities that gradually build confidence with low-code development tools while providing ongoing support for complex development challenges (Bhargava et al., 2024). Successful programs typically combine formal training sessions with peer mentoring and hands-on project experiences. Technical infrastructure considerations, including network performance, device compatibility, and integration capabilities, significantly impact user adoption and satisfaction.

Gaps in Current Research

Despite growing interest in low-code healthcare applications, several important research gaps remain. Limited longitudinal studies exist examining the long-term sustainability and evolution of low-code healthcare applications, with most current research focusing on initial implementation phases rather than ongoing maintenance, enhancement, and scaling challenges. Additionally, relatively few studies have examined the specific challenges and opportunities associated with implementing collaborative intelligence frameworks using low-code platforms in healthcare settings. The intersection of these three domains—healthcare, collaborative intelligence, and low-code development—represents an emerging area requiring additional empirical research.

The literature also reveals limited examination of economic impact metrics for healthcare low-code implementations. While organizations report qualitative benefits such as improved efficiency and user satisfaction, quantitative economic analysis remains limited (Martin & Lamb, 2025). Understanding the total cost of ownership, return on investment timelines, and comparative economic benefits of low-code versus traditional development approaches would provide valuable guidance for healthcare decision-makers. Furthermore, ethical considerations including accountability structures, algorithmic bias detection, and equity implications of democratized AI development require more systematic research attention.

ORACLE APEX PLATFORM ANALYSIS

Oracle Application Express represents a mature low-code development platform that has evolved significantly since its initial release, incorporating advanced features that specifically address the complex requirements of enterprise healthcare environments. Understanding the platform's technical architecture, capabilities, and healthcare-specific features provides an essential foundation for evaluating its potential as an enabler of collaborative intelligence in clinical settings.

Platform Architecture and Core Components

Think of Oracle APEX as a sophisticated app-building toolkit that lives inside a secure database, similar to how Microsoft Word lives on your computer. Healthcare professionals can create custom applications without learning complex programming, much like PowerPoint enables presentation creation without graphic design expertise. The key advantage: patient data never leaves the secure database, reducing security risks while enabling healthcare professionals to build their own clinical tools.

Figure 1. Oracle APEX Collaborative Intelligence Architecture for Healthcare

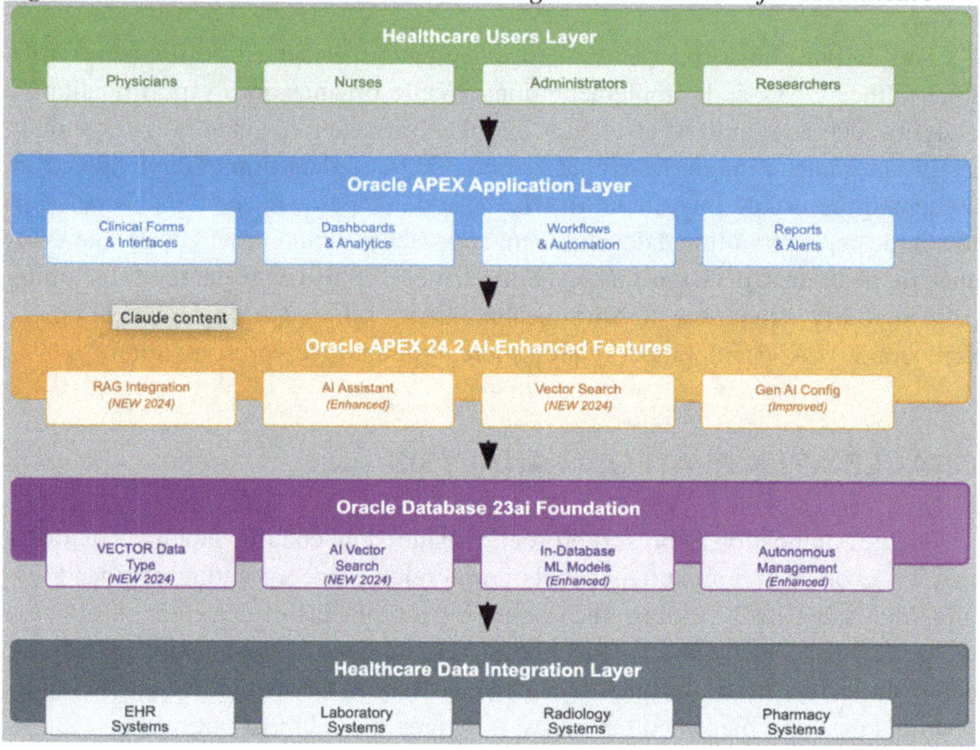

Oracle APEX operates as a web-based development environment that runs entirely within the Oracle Database. This architecture provides several significant advantages for healthcare applications, particularly regarding data security, performance, and integration capabilities. Unlike standalone development platforms that require separate database connections and potential data movement, APEX applications execute directly within the database environment, minimizing data exposure and latency while maximizing security (Oracle Corporation, 2024).

The platform's architecture consists of several interconnected components that work together to provide a comprehensive development and runtime environment. The APEX Engine serves as the core processing component, interpreting application metadata and generating dynamic HTML, CSS, and JavaScript output. This approach enables developers to create sophisticated user interfaces without directly coding these technologies, while still maintaining the flexibility to incorporate custom code when necessary.

The Application Builder provides the primary development interface, offering visual design tools for creating pages, forms, reports, and interactive components. Healthcare developers can leverage pre-built templates and components specifically designed for common clinical workflows, reducing development time while ensuring consistency with healthcare user interface best practices. The visual development approach enables clinical professionals to participate directly in the design process, providing immediate feedback and validation of proposed solutions.

The SQL Workshop component provides advanced database development capabilities that enable healthcare developers to create complex data models, implement business logic through stored procedures, and optimize query performance. For healthcare applications that must process large volumes of clinical data, these database-centric development capabilities prove essential for maintaining system responsiveness and reliability. Team Development features facilitate collaborative development processes that align well with healthcare's inherently collaborative culture, enabling multiple team members to contribute while maintaining version control and change tracking capabilities.

Security Framework and Healthcare Compliance

Healthcare applications must protect patient information more carefully than almost any other industry. Oracle APEX includes multiple layers of security protection—like having locks on doors, alarms on windows, and security cameras throughout a building—ensuring patient data remains private and secure even if one protection layer fails.

Healthcare applications must satisfy stringent security and privacy requirements that exceed those of most other industries. Oracle APEX provides a comprehensive security framework that addresses these requirements through multiple layers of protection, access control mechanisms, and audit capabilities (Oracle Corporation, 2024).

Authentication and authorization capabilities support integration with healthcare organization's existing identity management systems, including Active Directory, LDAP, and single sign-on solutions. This integration enables healthcare organizations to maintain centralized user management while ensuring that APEX applications inherit existing security policies and access controls. Multi-factor authentication support provides additional security layers that align with healthcare cybersecurity best practices.

Session management features include automatic timeout mechanisms, session encryption, and protection against common web application vulnerabilities such as cross-site scripting and SQL injection attacks. These protections are implemented automatically by the APEX framework, reducing the security expertise required from healthcare developers while maintaining enterprise-grade protection levels.

Data encryption capabilities protect sensitive healthcare information both in transit and at rest. Oracle APEX leverages Oracle Database's transparent data encryption features to ensure that patient data remains protected even if unauthorized individuals gain access to database files or backup media. Additionally, network communications between users and APEX applications are encrypted using industry-standard SSL/TLS protocols.

Audit logging features provide comprehensive tracking of user activities, data modifications, and system access patterns. Healthcare organizations can configure audit policies to meet specific regulatory requirements while maintaining detailed records for compliance reporting and security incident investigation. The audit framework captures sufficient detail to demonstrate compliance with HIPAA, GDPR, and other healthcare privacy regulations.

Fine-grained access controls enable healthcare organizations to implement complex authorization schemes that reflect clinical hierarchies and role-based responsibilities. Physicians can access patient information for their assigned patients while maintaining restrictions for other patients. Nurses can update specific clinical documentation while maintaining read-only access to physician notes. Administrative staff can access scheduling and billing information while remaining restricted from clinical data.

Database Integration and AI Capabilities

Oracle APEX's tight integration with Oracle Database provides healthcare developers with access to advanced analytical and AI capabilities without requiring additional infrastructure or specialized expertise. The Oracle Database includes built-in machine learning algorithms, natural language processing capabilities, and advanced analytics functions that can be directly incorporated into APEX applications (Leemans, 2024; Oracle Corporation, 2024).

Figure 2. Oracle Database 23ai AI Vector Search Integration Architecture

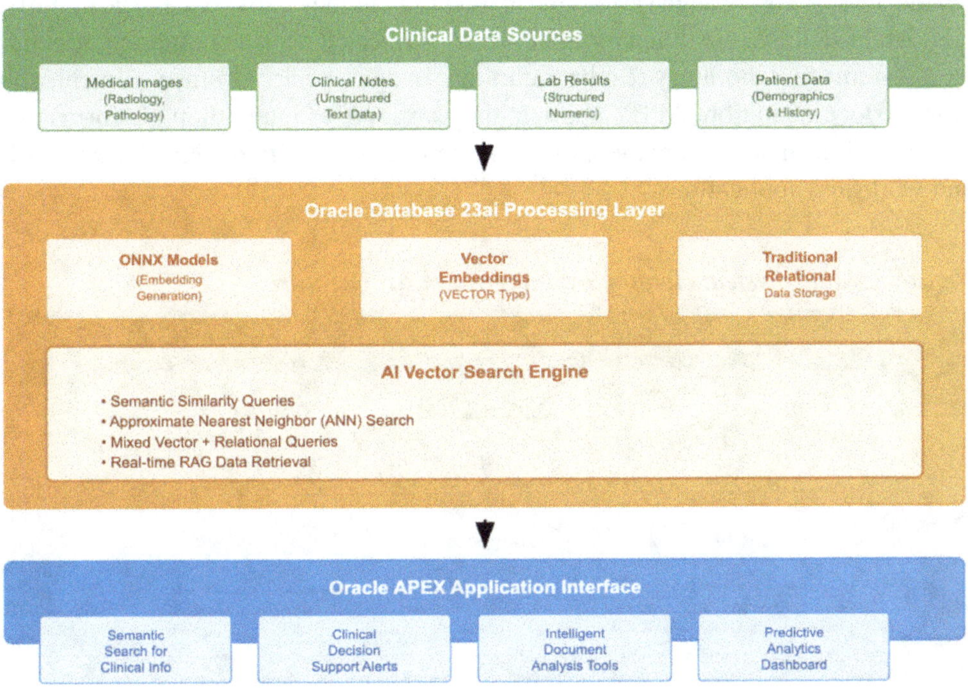

Machine learning integration enables healthcare applications to implement predictive analytics, risk stratification, and pattern recognition capabilities directly within clinical workflows. With Oracle Database 23ai's enhanced vector capabilities, an APEX application can now perform semantic analysis of clinical notes to identify patients at elevated risk for hospital readmission while simultaneously analyzing structured laboratory data and medical imaging results. The machine learning models operate entirely within the database environment, ensuring that sensitive patient data never leaves the secure database boundary.

Natural language processing capabilities enable healthcare applications to analyze unstructured clinical documentation, extract relevant medical concepts, and provide decision support based on narrative clinical notes. This functionality proves particularly valuable for applications that must integrate with electronic health record systems containing large volumes of unstructured clinical documentation. Advanced analytics functions support complex calculations required for clinical decision support, quality reporting, and population health management. Healthcare developers can implement sophisticated algorithms for medication dosing, clinical scoring systems, and risk assessment tools without requiring extensive mathematical or statistical expertise.

Data integration capabilities enable APEX applications to connect with external healthcare systems through various mechanisms including web services, file imports, and database links. Healthcare organizations typically operate numerous specialized systems for laboratory results, radiology images, pharmacy management, and clinical documentation. APEX applications can serve as integration platforms that aggregate information from these disparate sources into unified clinical dashboards and workflow applications.

Figure 3. Multi-System Healthcare Integration Architecture

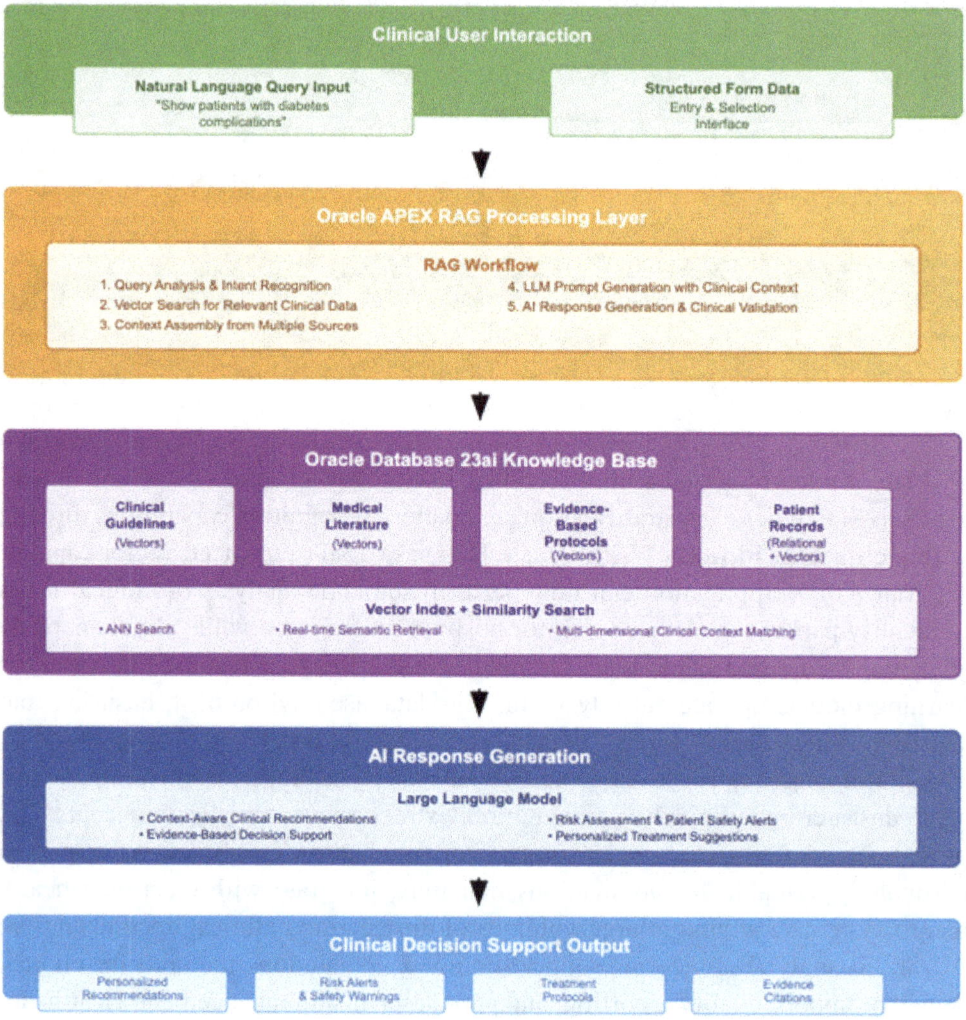

Development Productivity and Rapid Prototyping

The low-code nature of Oracle APEX significantly accelerates the development lifecycle for healthcare applications, enabling rapid prototyping and iterative refinement that aligns well with clinical workflow requirements. Healthcare professionals can actively participate in the development process, providing immediate feedback and validation of proposed solutions (Saeed et al., 2023).

Visual development tools enable healthcare developers to create sophisticated user interfaces without extensive front-end development expertise. Pre-built component libraries include healthcare-specific elements such as patient search interfaces, clinical documentation forms, and medication management displays. These components incorporate healthcare usability best practices while providing customization options for organization-specific requirements.

Report generation capabilities support the extensive reporting requirements common in healthcare environments. Healthcare organizations must produce reports for regulatory compliance, quality improvement initiatives, clinical research, and administrative oversight. APEX provides flexible reporting tools that enable healthcare professionals to create custom reports without requiring SQL expertise while maintaining the ability to implement complex logic when necessary.

Interactive dashboard capabilities enable healthcare organizations to create real-time monitoring displays for clinical operations, quality metrics, and patient flow management. These dashboards can aggregate information from multiple sources to provide comprehensive situational awareness for clinical managers and administrative staff. Workflow automation features enable healthcare applications to implement complex business logic that reflects clinical protocols and organizational policies, automatically routing processes through appropriate approval workflows based on clinical criteria and organizational policies.

Performance and Scalability Considerations

Healthcare applications must maintain consistent performance characteristics even as user bases grow and data volumes increase. Oracle APEX leverages the performance optimization capabilities of Oracle Database to ensure that healthcare applications can scale effectively to support large healthcare organizations and high-volume clinical operations.

Caching mechanisms reduce response times by storing frequently accessed data in memory rather than retrieving it from disk storage for each request. Connection pooling enables healthcare applications to efficiently serve large numbers of concurrent users without overwhelming database resources, ensuring applications remain responsive during peak usage periods such as shift changes, morning rounds, and discharge planning activities. Query optimization features help healthcare developers create efficient database queries even without extensive SQL expertise, with the APEX development environment providing guidance and warnings when potentially inefficient query patterns are detected.

COLLABORATIVE INTELLIGENCE FRAMEWORK

The preceding analysis demonstrated Oracle APEX's technical capabilities—database architecture, security frameworks, and AI integration. However, technical sophistication alone doesn't ensure successful healthcare adoption. The platform's value ultimately depends on how effectively it enables collaboration between human expertise and artificial intelligence—what we term "collaborative intelligence."

This section shifts from examining what Oracle APEX can do technically to exploring how healthcare organizations leverage these capabilities to create meaningful human-AI partnerships. We apply Technology Acceptance Model and Diffusion of Innovation principles to practical implementation contexts, demonstrating how abstract theories translate into concrete organizational actions that determine whether low-code healthcare AI succeeds or fails in practice.

The implementation of collaborative intelligence in healthcare environments requires a sophisticated framework that balances the computational capabilities of artificial intelligence with the clinical expertise, empathy, and contextual understanding provided by healthcare professionals. Oracle APEX serves as a technological enabler for this collaboration by providing the infrastructure necessary to create applications that seamlessly integrate AI capabilities with clinical workflows.

Defining Collaborative Intelligence in Healthcare

Collaborative intelligence represents a departure from traditional technology implementation approaches that position technology as either a replacement for human workers or as a separate tool used independently by human operators. Instead, collaborative intelligence recognizes that optimal outcomes emerge when human and artificial intelligence work together as integrated systems, with each component contributing its unique strengths to collective problem-solving efforts (Wilson & Daugherty, 2018; Yazici et al., 2022).

In healthcare contexts, collaborative intelligence manifests as systems where AI provides computational support for clinical decision-making while healthcare professionals maintain responsibility for patient care decisions, ethical considerations, and complex problem-solving that requires contextual understanding. This approach acknowledges that current AI systems, despite their impressive analytical capabilities, lack the nuanced understanding of human behavior, cultural factors, and ethical considerations that characterize effective healthcare delivery (Topol, 2019).

Healthcare professionals bring irreplaceable capabilities to collaborative intelligence systems including clinical intuition developed through years of patient care experience, the ability to recognize subtle patterns that may not be captured in structured data, empathy and communication skills essential for patient interaction, and ethical reasoning capabilities required for complex healthcare decisions. These human capabilities complement rather than compete with AI systems that excel at pattern recognition across large datasets, consistent application of evidence-based protocols, rapid processing of complex information, and identification of potential risks or opportunities that might be overlooked during busy clinical operations.

The collaborative intelligence framework emphasizes transparency and explainability in AI decision-making processes. Healthcare professionals must understand how AI systems reach their conclusions to maintain confidence in AI-assisted decision-making and to override AI recommendations when clinical judgment suggests alternative approaches (Shah et al., 2019). This requirement for transparency influences both the selection of AI algorithms and the design of user interfaces that present AI insights to clinical users.

Oracle APEX as a Collaborative Intelligence Platform

Oracle APEX provides several characteristics that make it particularly well-suited for implementing collaborative intelligence solutions in healthcare environments. The platform's database-centric architecture enables seamless integration of AI capabilities with clinical data while maintaining the security and performance requirements essential for healthcare applications (Oracle Corporation, 2024).

The platform's rapid development capabilities align well with the iterative nature of collaborative intelligence implementation. Healthcare organizations typically implement collaborative intelligence through pilot projects that demonstrate value in specific clinical areas before expanding to broader applications. Oracle APEX enables rapid prototyping and refinement of these pilot applications, allowing healthcare organizations to validate collaborative intelligence concepts before making substantial commitments to broader implementation efforts.

Visual development tools enable healthcare professionals to participate directly in the design and refinement of collaborative intelligence applications. Rather than serving merely as end-users of pre-built applications, clinical staff can contribute to interface design, workflow optimization, and feature prioritization. This participation ensures that collaborative intelligence applications align with actual clinical needs rather than with technologists' assumptions about clinical requirements (Liu et al., 2022).

The platform's integration capabilities enable collaborative intelligence applications to connect with existing healthcare systems including electronic health records, laboratory systems, radiology platforms, and pharmacy management systems. This integration capability is essential for collaborative intelligence applications that must access comprehensive patient information to provide meaningful decision support.

Figure 4. RAG-Enabled Clinical Decision Support System Architecture

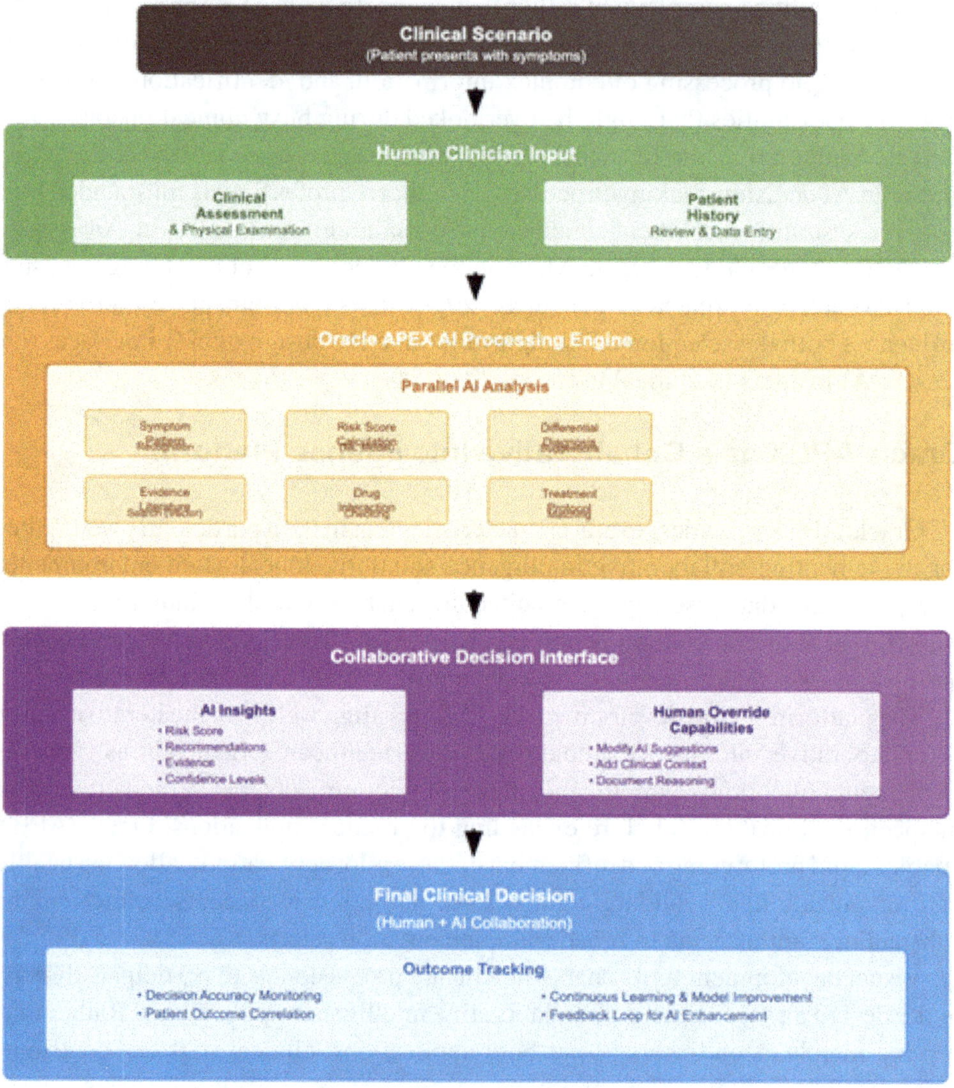

Human-AI Interface Design Principles

Effective collaborative intelligence requires careful attention to interface design that facilitates smooth interaction between healthcare professionals and AI systems. The interface serves as the critical communication channel through which humans and AI systems share information, insights, and decision-making responsibilities.

Figure 5. Human-AI Collaborative Decision-Making Workflow

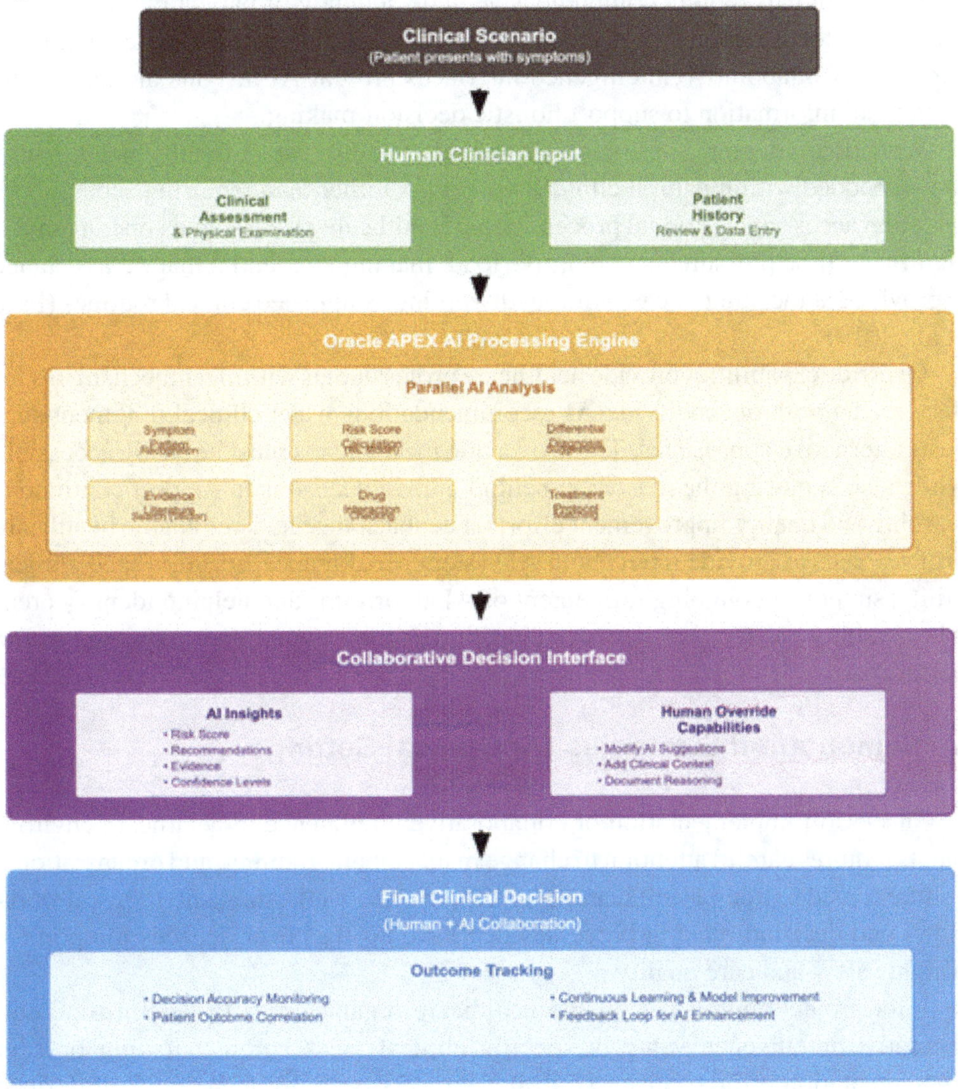

Transparency in AI reasoning represents a fundamental interface design principle for healthcare collaborative intelligence. When AI systems provide clinical recommendations or alerts, healthcare professionals must understand the reasoning process that led to these conclusions. Oracle APEX applications can present this information through various mechanisms including decision trees, confidence scores, contributing factors, and relevant literature references that support AI recommendations.

Contextual information presentation ensures that AI insights are provided within the broader context of patient care rather than as isolated recommendations. Healthcare professionals require comprehensive understanding of patient circumstances, medical history, current treatments, and social factors that may influence treatment decisions. Collaborative intelligence interfaces present AI insights alongside this contextual information to support holistic decision-making.

Workflow integration principles ensure that collaborative intelligence features are embedded within natural clinical workflows rather than requiring separate application access or additional process steps. Healthcare professionals operate under significant time pressure and cognitive load, making it essential that AI assistance is provided at the point of care without disrupting established clinical routines (Park et al., 2019).

Override capabilities provide healthcare professionals with clear mechanisms for disagreeing with or modifying AI recommendations when clinical judgment suggests alternative approaches. These override mechanisms must be easily accessible while also capturing the reasoning behind human decisions to support continuous learning and quality improvement efforts. Feedback mechanisms enable healthcare professionals to provide input about AI system performance, accuracy, and clinical utility, supporting ongoing refinement of AI algorithms and helping identify areas where additional training data or algorithm modifications may improve system performance.

Implementation Strategies for Clinical Settings

Successful implementation of collaborative intelligence in healthcare environments requires careful attention to change management, training, and organizational culture considerations. Healthcare organizations have well-established clinical workflows and decision-making processes that have evolved over decades to optimize patient safety and care quality.

Pilot project approaches enable healthcare organizations to demonstrate collaborative intelligence value in specific clinical areas before pursuing broader implementation efforts. Successful pilot projects typically focus on well-defined clinical problems where AI capabilities can provide clear benefits while maintaining manageable complexity for initial implementation. Examples include medication reconciliation, clinical documentation assistance, or patient risk stratification for specific conditions.

Physician champion programs leverage the influence of respected clinical leaders to promote collaborative intelligence adoption and provide peer support for healthcare professionals learning to work with AI systems (Rojas et al., 2025). These champions serve as advocates for collaborative intelligence initiatives while also providing feedback about clinical utility and implementation challenges.

Training programs must address both technical aspects of using collaborative intelligence applications and conceptual understanding of how AI systems function, their limitations, and appropriate use cases. Healthcare professionals require confidence in their ability to effectively leverage AI capabilities while maintaining awareness of situations where human judgment should override AI recommendations.

Gradual complexity introduction enables healthcare organizations to begin with relatively simple collaborative intelligence applications before progressing to more sophisticated implementations. Initial applications might focus on information aggregation and presentation, progressing through decision support applications, and eventually incorporating predictive analytics and complex recommendation systems.

ETHICAL, GOVERNANCE, AND SOCIO-ECONOMIC CONSIDERATIONS

While Oracle APEX provides powerful technical capabilities for healthcare AI democratization, technology alone cannot ensure responsible innovation. This section addresses the ethical, governance, and equity challenges that healthcare organizations must navigate to ensure that empowering clinical professionals to develop AI applications advances rather than undermines healthcare quality, fairness, and accessibility.

The democratization of healthcare AI through low-code platforms introduces complex ethical, governance, and equity challenges that extend beyond technical implementation. While empowering healthcare professionals to develop AI applications offers substantial benefits, it also creates responsibilities for ensuring accountability, fairness, transparency, and equitable access.

Ethical Dimensions and Accountability Structures

When clinical professionals develop AI-enhanced applications, traditional accountability structures become ambiguous. Who bears responsibility when an Oracle APEX application containing AI recommendations contributes to adverse patient outcomes? Legal and ethical frameworks traditionally assign liability to developers, healthcare organizations, or clinicians, but democratized development blurs these boundaries (Lee & Kesselheim, 2018).

Healthcare organizations must establish distributed accountability models where clinical developers, IT oversight committees, and organizational leadership share proportional responsibility. Clinical developers bear primary responsibility for clinical accuracy and workflow appropriateness, IT committees ensure technical quality and security compliance, and organizational leadership maintains governance frameworks. This requires documentation standards demonstrating that developers understood AI limitations, validated recommendations against clinical evidence, and implemented appropriate safeguards.

Organizations should implement medical device classification assessments for AI applications, determining whether they qualify as medical devices requiring FDA oversight under 21 CFR Part 820. Distributed accountability models provide clarity while recognizing that successful healthcare AI democratization requires shared responsibility across multiple stakeholders rather than placing entire burden on clinical developers who may lack comprehensive technical or regulatory expertise.

Algorithmic Bias and Health Equity

AI systems trained on historical healthcare data risk perpetuating existing disparities affecting underserved populations. When clinical professionals develop Oracle APEX applications using institutional data, these applications may inherit biases present in care delivery patterns, diagnostic practices, or treatment allocation (Topol, 2019). Mehrabi et al.'s (2021) taxonomy identifies six bias types relevant to healthcare AI: historical bias reflecting past discrimination, representation bias from non-representative training data, measurement bias from inconsistent data collection, aggregation bias from inappropriate population grouping, evaluation bias from inadequate testing across populations, and deployment bias from implementation in inappropriate contexts.

Healthcare organizations must implement bias detection strategies including diverse representation in training data, stratified performance testing across demographic groups, regular fairness audits examining outcome disparities, transparency requirements documenting data sources and populations, and override mechanisms enabling clinicians to recognize and correct biased recommendations. Oracle APEX developers should receive training in recognizing potential bias sources and implementing mitigation strategies. Applications should include demographic stratification capabilities enabling performance monitoring across patient populations. Organizations should establish bias review committees examining AI applications for equity implications before deployment.

Transparency and Patient Autonomy

The "black box" problem becomes particularly acute when clinical professionals integrate pre-trained models or database AI capabilities without deep understanding of underlying algorithms. Healthcare organizations must establish explainability standards appropriate for different application types (Shah et al., 2019). Simple decision support may require only confidence scores and contributing factors, while applications significantly influencing treatment decisions require detailed reasoning chains, literature support, and population-based evidence.

Oracle APEX applications should implement layered explainability providing basic reasoning for all users while enabling detailed algorithmic inspection for technically sophisticated reviewers. This approach supports clinical decision-making while maintaining accountability and enabling continuous quality improvement.

Patient autonomy considerations require communication frameworks helping clinicians explain AI assistance to patients. Patients have rights to understand how their care decisions are made, including AI system roles. Research suggests that patients generally trust AI-assisted decision-making when they understand physician oversight and the evidence-based nature of AI recommendations (Lee & Kesselheim, 2018). Healthcare organizations should develop communication frameworks helping clinicians explain AI assistance while maintaining confidence in care quality, emphasizing that AI serves as a tool supporting, not replacing, physician judgment.

Multi-Tier Governance and Resource Equity

Democratized AI development requires governance structures balancing innovation with appropriate oversight. Traditional centralized IT governance models prove inadequate for distributed development, while completely decentralized approaches risk inconsistency and quality concerns. A three-tier governance architecture proves effective: Strategic Governance (executive committee establishing organizational AI strategy, resource allocation, and risk tolerance), Technical Governance (center of excellence providing standards, training, code review, and quality assurance), and Clinical Governance (domain-specific committees evaluating clinical appropriateness, evidence basis, and workflow integration).

This architecture enables distributed innovation while maintaining organizational coherence. Risk classification systems determine appropriate oversight intensity—low-risk information aggregation requires minimal review, medium-risk clinical decision support requires clinical evidence validation and bias assessment, while high-risk applications significantly influencing treatment decisions require comprehensive evaluation including clinical trials and regulatory assessment.

Digital divide concerns arise as Oracle APEX implementation requires infrastructure investment, training programs, and ongoing support that smaller or rural healthcare organizations may struggle to afford. This risks widening care quality gaps between well-resourced and under-resourced organizations (Srinivasan et al., 2024). Addressing this requires shared infrastructure models enabling regional collaboration, open application libraries reducing development costs for smaller organizations, subsidized training programs, vendor partnerships providing reduced licensing for critical access hospitals, and technical assistance programs supporting under-resourced implementations. These equity-focused strategies ensure that healthcare AI democratization benefits all populations rather than widening existing disparities.

CASE STUDIES AND IMPLEMENTATION EXAMPLES

Academic Medical Center: Clinical Decision Support Implementation

Note: This case study describes a hypothetical implementation for illustrative purposes.

A large academic medical center implemented Oracle APEX to create a comprehensive clinical decision support system demonstrating collaborative intelligence potential in healthcare environments. The implementation addressed challenges related to medication reconciliation, clinical documentation, and care coordination across multiple departments and clinical services.

The initial pilot focused on medication reconciliation during hospital admissions. The APEX application automated cross-referencing patient medication histories from multiple sources including community pharmacies, prior hospitalizations, and ambulatory care records. AI algorithms integrated with Oracle Database 23ai identified potential medication duplications, drug-drug interactions, and dosing inconsistencies based on patient characteristics including age, weight, renal function, and allergies. Importantly, the system guided pharmacists rather than providing definitive recommendations, maintaining human authority over medication decisions (Wilson & Daugherty, 2018).

The user interface, designed collaboratively between clinical pharmacists, physicians, and IT staff, seamlessly integrated into existing admission workflows. This resulted in a 35% reduction in medication reconciliation time and a 60% increase in identifying potential medication issues compared to manual processes. High user satisfaction was reported, with pharmacists noting that AI recommendations enhanced rather than replaced their professional judgment, exemplifying successful collaborative intelligence implementation (Yazici et al., 2022).

Success led to expansion into clinical documentation assistance, diagnostic decision support, and discharge planning applications. Key success factors included strong clinical leadership supporting change management, iterative development responding to user feedback, seamless workflow integration avoiding disruption to established clinical routines, and sustained organizational commitment providing resources and support throughout implementation.

Figure 6. Clinical Decision Support Implementation Architecture

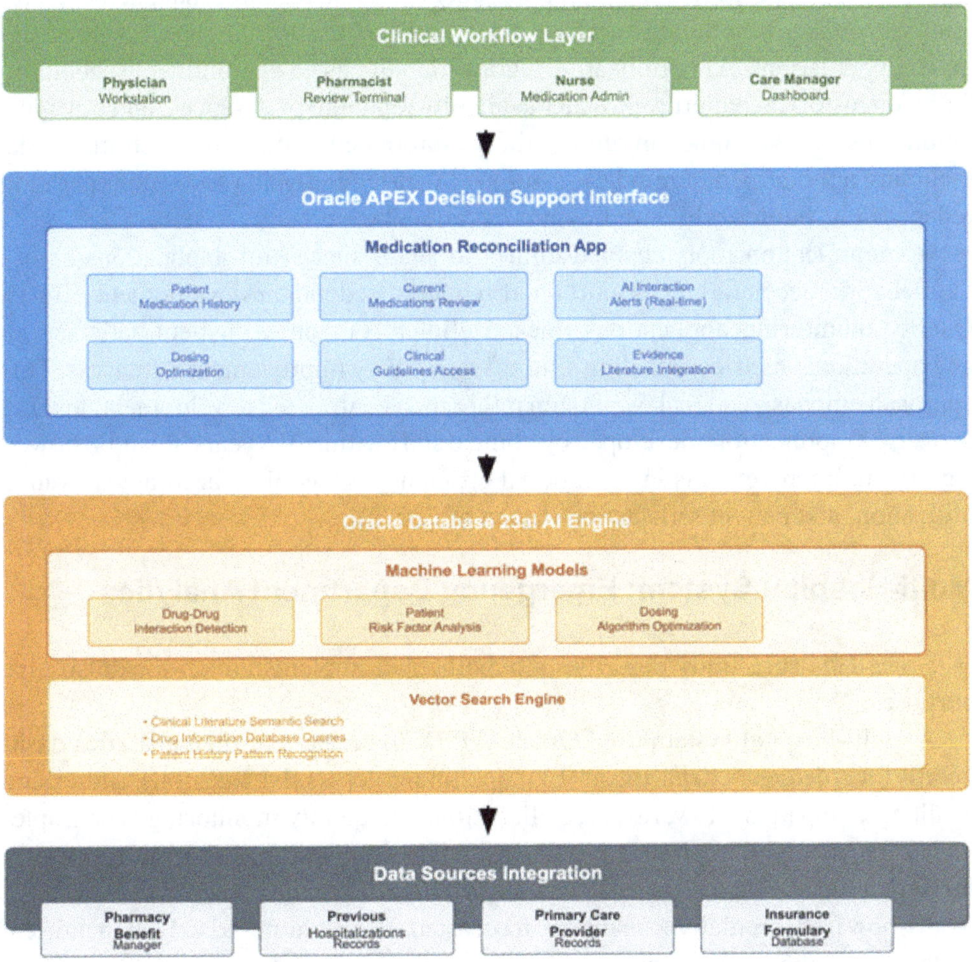

Community Health System: Workflow Automation Network

Note: This case study describes a hypothetical implementation for illustrative purposes.

A rural community health system used Oracle APEX to build workflow automation applications across 15 clinics with limited IT support, demonstrating democratized development potential in resource-constrained settings. The strategy involved a central APEX environment allowing local customization while maintaining security and compliance standards. Clinical staff received training to develop applications addressing their specific operational challenges.

Initial applications focused on patient scheduling and resource management, creating customized scheduling interfaces reflecting each clinic's unique workflows and patient populations. AI optimization algorithms suggested appointment scheduling based on historical patterns, provider availability, patient preferences, and transportation constraints common in rural settings. Automated routine administrative tasks including appointment reminders, insurance verification, and pre-visit preparation reduced staff burden while improving operational efficiency.

Communication tools enabled clinics to share successful applications across the network, accelerating adoption and reducing redundant development efforts. Quality monitoring applications tracked clinical outcomes, patient satisfaction, and operational metrics, enabling data-driven quality improvement initiatives. This approach emphasized local ownership rather than centralized development, leading to over 200 applications developed by clinical staff within two years. Results showed significant improvements in operational efficiency, scheduling accuracy, resource utilization, and patient satisfaction (Liu et al., 2022).

Multi-Hospital System: Emergency Department Analytics

Note: This case study describes a hypothetical implementation for illustrative purposes.

A multi-hospital system used Oracle APEX to create real-time analytics dashboards for emergency department (ED) operations across five locations, addressing challenges in patient flow, resource allocation, and quality monitoring. The implementation provided centralized visibility while enabling customization for each facility's unique characteristics.

AI-powered predictive analytics forecasted ED volume based on historical patterns, weather conditions, seasonal factors, and community events, enabling proactive staffing adjustments. Patient flow optimization applications used AI to identify bottlenecks and recommend interventions for improving throughput. Quality monitoring tracked key performance indicators including wait times, left-without-being-seen rates, and door-to-doctor times, providing real-time alerts when metrics exceeded thresholds.

The rapid deployment approach involved ED physicians and nurses directly in application design, ensuring solutions addressed actual operational challenges rather than perceived needs. This led to significant improvements in ED operations including reduced average wait times, improved resource utilization, enhanced multi-facility coordination, and increased ED manager confidence in data-driven decision-making (Rojas et al., 2025).

CHALLENGES AND SOLUTIONS

While collaborative intelligence through Oracle APEX offers substantial benefits, successful implementation requires addressing multifaceted challenges spanning technical integration, regulatory compliance, user adoption, and governance. Understanding these challenges and evidence-based solutions provides essential guidance for healthcare organizations pursuing similar initiatives.

Technical Integration Challenges

Healthcare organizations typically operate complex technology ecosystems including electronic health record systems, laboratory information systems, radiology platforms, pharmacy management systems, and numerous specialized clinical applications. Integrating Oracle APEX applications with these existing systems requires careful planning and technical expertise that may exceed typical low-code developer capabilities.

Legacy system integration represents a particularly significant challenge. Many healthcare organizations rely on older systems lacking modern integration capabilities such as web services or application programming interfaces. These systems often require custom integration solutions involving file-based data exchange, database replication, or middleware platforms that translate between different system formats and protocols.

Data quality and standardization issues create additional integration complexity. Healthcare data often lacks standardization across systems, with variations in terminology, coding systems, and data formats that complicate automated integration efforts. Patient identification across multiple systems can be particularly challenging when different systems use different identifier schemes or when patients have multiple medical record numbers.

Solutions to integration challenges typically involve enterprise integration architecture that provides a foundation for connecting Oracle APEX applications with existing healthcare systems. This architecture often includes middleware platforms handling data transformation, protocol translation, and message routing between different systems. Implementing data governance programs helps address quality and standardization issues by establishing consistent data definitions, validation rules, and quality monitoring processes (Holzinger et al., 2022).

Regulatory Compliance and Security Concerns

Healthcare applications must comply with extensive regulatory requirements governing data privacy, security, access controls, and audit capabilities. Ensuring Oracle APEX applications meet these requirements while maintaining usability creates complex implementation challenges requiring specialized expertise and ongoing attention.

HIPAA compliance represents a fundamental requirement for healthcare applications handling protected health information. Oracle APEX applications must implement appropriate safeguards for data access, transmission, storage, and disposal while maintaining comprehensive audit trails documenting all patient data interactions. Achieving HIPAA compliance requires understanding both technical requirements and administrative safeguards extending beyond the application itself.

Solutions to regulatory and security challenges involve implementing comprehensive compliance frameworks addressing both technical and organizational requirements. These frameworks typically include policy development, staff training, technical controls, and ongoing monitoring activities ensuring sustained compliance with applicable regulations. Engaging compliance expertise early in implementation helps ensure Oracle APEX applications are designed with appropriate safeguards rather than attempting to add compliance features after development completion.

User Adoption and Change Management

Healthcare professionals often have established workflows and preferences that may initially resist new technology implementations, particularly when those implementations change familiar processes or require learning new skills. Achieving widespread user adoption of Oracle APEX applications requires sustained attention to change management, training, and ongoing support activities (Bhargava et al., 2024).

Workflow disruption concerns represent a significant barrier to user adoption. Healthcare professionals operate under significant time pressure and cognitive load, making them naturally resistant to changes that might initially slow down their work or require additional mental effort. Technology anxiety affects some healthcare professionals who may have limited experience with application development or who may be concerned about their ability to effectively use new technology tools.

Competing priorities within healthcare organizations can limit the time and attention available for Oracle APEX implementation and training activities.

Solutions to user adoption challenges typically involve comprehensive change management approaches that address both individual and organizational factors affecting technology acceptance. Developing clinical champions who can advocate for Oracle APEX applications while providing peer support for other healthcare professionals helps build confidence and enthusiasm. Implementing gradual rollout strategies enables healthcare organizations to introduce Oracle APEX applications in manageable phases that allow users to develop confidence before expanding to more complex applications. Providing ongoing training and support resources ensures that healthcare professionals can develop their Oracle APEX skills over time rather than expecting immediate competency following initial training sessions (Rojas et al., 2025).

Governance and Quality Assurance

The democratization of application development through low-code platforms creates potential governance challenges as healthcare organizations must balance innovation and autonomy with consistency, quality, and risk management requirements. Establishing appropriate governance frameworks for Oracle APEX development requires careful consideration of organizational culture, regulatory requirements, and operational needs.

Application proliferation risks emerge when multiple healthcare professionals independently develop applications that address similar needs or that may conflict with existing systems or processes. Without appropriate coordination mechanisms, organizations may develop redundant applications that waste resources while potentially creating confusion or inconsistency for end users. Quality and security standards become more difficult to enforce when application development is distributed among numerous healthcare professionals who may have varying levels of technical expertise and understanding of organizational requirements.

Solutions to governance challenges typically involve establishing structured approaches to Oracle APEX development that balance innovation with appropriate oversight and quality assurance. Creating center of excellence programs provides centralized expertise and support for Oracle APEX development while enabling distributed application creation by healthcare professionals. Implementing development lifecycle processes ensures that Oracle APEX applications undergo appropriate planning, design, testing, and deployment activities regardless of who develops them. Establishing application portfolio management practices enables healthcare organizations to maintain visibility into all Oracle APEX applications while identifying opportunities for consolidation, standardization, or resource sharing.

FUTURE DIRECTIONS

The landscape of healthcare technology continues to evolve rapidly, driven by advances in artificial intelligence, changes in healthcare delivery models, and increasing emphasis on patient-centered care and population health management. Understanding emerging trends and their implications for low-code platforms and collaborative intelligence provides essential guidance for healthcare organizations planning long-term technology strategies.

Emerging Technologies and Integration Opportunities

New generative AI features in Oracle APEX 24.2 allow developers to create AI assistants for clinical documentation analysis, patient summaries, and evidence-based recommendations, with RAG-enabled chatbots proving highly effective (Oracle Corporation, 2024). Natural language processing capabilities facilitate conversational interfaces and automatic information extraction from clinical documentation, with implementations demonstrating up to 40% reduction in physician documentation time (Martin & Lamb, 2025).

Computer vision integration with Oracle Database 23ai's vector search capabilities transforms medical imaging analysis, with AI-powered diagnostic tools demonstrating high accuracy in identifying conditions from radiological images. The convergence of Internet of Medical Things (IoMT) devices with Oracle APEX's real-time dashboards enables continuous patient monitoring and predictive analytics through AI-powered sensors tracking vital signs, medication adherence, and activity patterns.

Edge computing architectures enable Oracle APEX applications to process healthcare data at the point of care, crucial for rural health services, mobile clinics, and emergency response scenarios where network connectivity may be limited or unreliable. Blockchain integration through Oracle Database 23ai enhances security and audit capabilities, enabling tamper-proof data trails and secure multi-organizational data sharing while maintaining patient privacy protections.

Evolving Healthcare Delivery Models

Current healthcare delivery transformation accelerated dramatically in 2024-2025, with 85% of healthcare organizations exploring or implementing generative AI capabilities (Martin & Lamb, 2025). Research indicates that healthcare leaders view clinical productivity enhancement as the highest-value application for generative AI, with administrative efficiency and patient engagement following as priority areas. This shift toward AI-augmented care delivery creates new requirements for Oracle

APEX applications supporting both traditional clinical workflows and emerging AI-powered care modalities.

Ambient intelligence applications represent a rapidly growing segment where Oracle APEX integration proves particularly valuable. Healthcare organizations report that ambient clinical documentation systems reduce physician documentation burden by up to 40% while improving note quality and care team communication (Rodriguez et al., 2025). Oracle APEX applications can serve as integration platforms combining ambient intelligence outputs with structured clinical data to provide comprehensive care coordination dashboards and workflow automation.

Personalized medicine approaches now extend beyond genomics to include real-time biometric analysis, environmental factors, and social determinants of health. Oracle Database 23ai's vector search capabilities enable healthcare organizations to create comprehensive patient profiles incorporating structured clinical data, unstructured clinical notes, genomic information, and lifestyle data from wearable devices (Leemans, 2024). These unified profiles support AI-powered treatment recommendations considering the full spectrum of patient-specific factors affecting health outcomes.

Value-based care models increasingly rely on sophisticated analytics tracking patient outcomes across entire care episodes and population cohorts. Oracle APEX applications integrated with AI vector search can identify patterns in care delivery correlating with improved outcomes, enabling healthcare organizations to optimize care protocols and resource allocation for maximum population health impact.

Global Regulatory Landscapes and Implementation Contexts

Healthcare AI democratization occurs within diverse international contexts shaped by varying regulatory frameworks and healthcare system structures. The FDA's evolving software-as-medical-device approach, the EU's Medical Device Regulation and proposed AI Act classifying certain healthcare AI as "high-risk," and the UK's post-Brexit regulatory independence create complex compliance landscapes. The EU's emphasis on explainability, human oversight, and bias mitigation aligns well with collaborative intelligence principles, potentially making EU markets receptive to democratized AI approaches maintaining human authority.

Asia-Pacific nations demonstrate dramatic regulatory variation—Japan's stringent PMDA requirements, Singapore's regulatory sandboxes enabling experimental deployment, China's domestic clinical trial requirements, and Australia's risk-based TGA approach complicate multinational Oracle APEX deployments. Many developing nations lack comprehensive healthcare AI regulations, creating both opportunities for rapid innovation and risks of deploying insufficiently validated systems in vulnerable populations. The WHO's guidance on AI ethics and governance in health (2021, updated 2024) provides principles for developing nations establishing regulatory frameworks.

Healthcare system structures profoundly impact implementation strategies. Single-payer systems (UK, Canada, Australia) facilitate coordinated technology adoption but face budget constraints and bureaucratic approval processes. Social insurance systems (Germany, Japan, France) enable innovation within universal coverage frameworks while addressing multiple payer requirements. Mixed systems (United States) offer entrepreneurial culture and substantial technology investment but suffer fragmentation complicating interoperability and standardization. Resource-constrained systems in developing nations prioritize basic healthcare access over technological sophistication, yet mobile health penetration and leapfrogging opportunities create unexpected innovation contexts where Oracle APEX's lightweight infrastructure requirements prove advantageous.

Cross-border data governance adds complexity. GDPR restricts international patient data transfers outside the European Economic Area without adequate protection mechanisms. The Schrems II decision invalidated the EU-US Privacy Shield framework, creating uncertainty for transatlantic healthcare data flows. Oracle APEX implementations crossing international borders must implement data localization strategies ensuring patient data remains within appropriate jurisdictions while enabling application functionality.

Global Health Equity and Policy Implications

Global health equity implications present both opportunities and risks. Optimistic scenarios envision empowered healthcare workers in resource-constrained settings developing locally appropriate AI applications addressing their specific challenges. Pessimistic scenarios warn of widening digital divides where well-resourced healthcare systems leverage AI to improve care while underserved populations fall further behind (World Economic Forum, 2025).

Evidence suggests technology transfer alone proves insufficient—successful democratization requires comprehensive approaches including infrastructure investment, training programs, technical support, and sustained commitment. International standards development through WHO, ISO, and IEC for harmonized healthcare AI evaluation frameworks would reduce compliance complexity for multinational implementations. Technology transfer programs through international development organizations and vendor partnerships should support Oracle APEX implementation in resource-constrained settings with infrastructure, training, and ongoing maintenance rather than one-time transfers.

Equitable access mechanisms including tiered pricing models, subsidized licensing for critical access settings, and public-private partnerships could reduce financial barriers in resource-constrained environments. The healthcare AI market is rapidly expanding, projected to reach $431.05 billion by 2032, with generative AI alone nearing $17 billion by 2034 (Singh et al., 2025). With 92% of healthcare leaders viewing automation as vital for addressing staff shortages and 64% of organizations reporting positive ROI from generative AI investments (Martin & Lamb, 2025), Oracle APEX implementations offer measurable value propositions. However, ensuring these benefits reach all populations requires coordinated international efforts addressing regulatory harmonization, capacity building, and equitable access.

CONCLUSION

Synthesizing Technical, Ethical, and Global Dimensions

This chapter demonstrates that successful healthcare AI democratization through Oracle APEX requires balancing technical sophistication with ethical responsibility, organizational readiness, and global contextual awareness. Three key insights emerge from our integrated analysis that extend beyond technical platform evaluation to encompass socio-technical systems thinking.

First, theoretical frameworks provide essential explanatory power for understanding adoption patterns and predicting implementation success. Technology Acceptance Model explains why perceived ease of use and clinical usefulness drive Oracle APEX adoption more powerfully than technical features alone. Healthcare professionals adopt low-code platforms when they perceive clear value for patient care and find development interfaces accessible without extensive technical training. Diffusion of Innovation theory illuminates why pilot projects, physician champions, and gradual rollout prove essential in risk-averse healthcare cultures where regulatory requirements, professional liability concerns, and patient safety considerations slow adoption compared to other industries. Collaborative Intelligence theory validates the augmentation approach where AI handles computational tasks while humans maintain authority over complex decisions requiring contextual understanding and ethical reasoning. These frameworks transform Oracle APEX from a technical platform into a socio-technical system whose success depends on human factors, organizational culture, and change management as much as technological capabilities (Abouyannis et al., 2024; Bhargava et al., 2024; Yazici et al., 2022).

Second, ethical governance cannot be afterthought but must be integrated throughout design, development, and deployment. Democratizing AI development demands proactive attention to accountability structures clarifying responsibilities across clinical developers, technical oversight, and organizational leadership. Distributed accountability models recognize that successful healthcare AI requires shared responsibility proportional to stakeholder roles rather than placing entire burden on clinical developers who may lack comprehensive technical or regulatory expertise. Algorithmic bias detection strategies including diverse training data representation, stratified performance testing across demographic groups, and regular fairness audits ensure that empowering clinical professionals to develop AI applications advances rather than undermines healthcare equity. Transparency requirements and explainability standards appropriate for different application risk levels maintain patient autonomy while supporting clinical decision-making. The digital divide risk—where well-resourced organizations leverage AI while under-resourced organizations fall behind—requires shared infrastructure models, open application libraries, subsidized training programs, and technical assistance ensuring healthcare AI democratization benefits all populations rather than widening existing disparities (Lee & Kesselheim, 2018; Topol, 2019).

Third, global contexts profoundly shape implementation strategies, requiring adaptable approaches rather than universal prescriptions. Varying regulatory frameworks across jurisdictions—FDA's software-as-medical-device approach, EU's AI Act classifying certain healthcare AI as high-risk, Asia-Pacific nations' divergent requirements—create complex compliance landscapes for multinational Oracle APEX deployments. Healthcare system structures including single-payer systems facilitating coordinated adoption, social insurance systems enabling innovation within universal coverage, and mixed systems offering entrepreneurial culture but suffering fragmentation—each demand tailored implementation strategies. Cross-border data governance challenges including GDPR restrictions and Schrems II implications require sophisticated data localization approaches. Resource constraints in developing nations present both leapfrogging opportunities and risks of deploying insufficiently validated systems in vulnerable populations. Success requires understanding local contexts, engaging with international policy discussions, and maintaining commitment to equitable access ensuring healthcare AI democratization advances both innovation and equity globally (Martin & Lamb, 2025; World Economic Forum, 2025).

Path Forward for Healthcare Organizations

Looking forward, Oracle APEX's integration with Oracle Database 23ai's vector search capabilities, RAG technology, and generative AI features positions it at the healthcare AI democratization forefront. Current market trends—85% of healthcare organizations exploring generative AI, 64% achieving positive ROI, and 92% of leaders viewing automation as vital for addressing staff shortages—indicate strong momentum for collaborative intelligence initiatives (Martin & Lamb, 2025; Singh et al., 2025). Oracle's strategic decision to rebuild Cerner using APEX validates the platform's suitability for mission-critical healthcare applications while demonstrating confidence in low-code approaches for complex enterprise systems.

However, realizing this potential requires sustained attention to the theoretical, ethical, and global dimensions explored throughout this chapter. Healthcare organizations embarking on Oracle APEX implementations should begin with careful assessment of organizational readiness, technical infrastructure, and strategic objectives. Successful implementations typically start with pilot projects demonstrating value in specific clinical areas before expanding to broader organizational deployment, providing opportunities to develop internal expertise, refine implementation approaches, and build clinical staff confidence while minimizing risks associated with large-scale technology changes.

Organizations should maintain focus on the fundamental goal of improving patient outcomes while leveraging technology as an enabler rather than an end in itself. The democratization of healthcare AI through Oracle APEX provides unprecedented opportunities to achieve this goal by empowering healthcare professionals to directly contribute to technological solutions addressing their operational challenges. Success requires sustained commitment to collaborative intelligence principles preserving essential human elements of empathy, critical thinking, and contextual understanding while enhancing capabilities through artificial intelligence.

The democratization of healthcare AI through Oracle APEX represents both opportunity and responsibility—opportunity to dramatically accelerate innovation while empowering clinical professionals, and responsibility to ensure implementations are thoughtful, equitable, and aligned with healthcare's fundamental commitment to beneficence, non-maleficence, autonomy, and justice. Healthcare organizations, technology vendors, policymakers, and international organizations must collaborate to ensure that low-code healthcare AI platforms advance both innovation and equity on a global scale. As healthcare continues its digital transformation journey, platforms like Oracle APEX that enable collaborative intelligence while maintaining appropriate governance, ethical standards, and equitable access will prove instrumental in shaping healthcare delivery for decades to come.

Figure 7. Comprehensive Healthcare AI Democratization Architecture

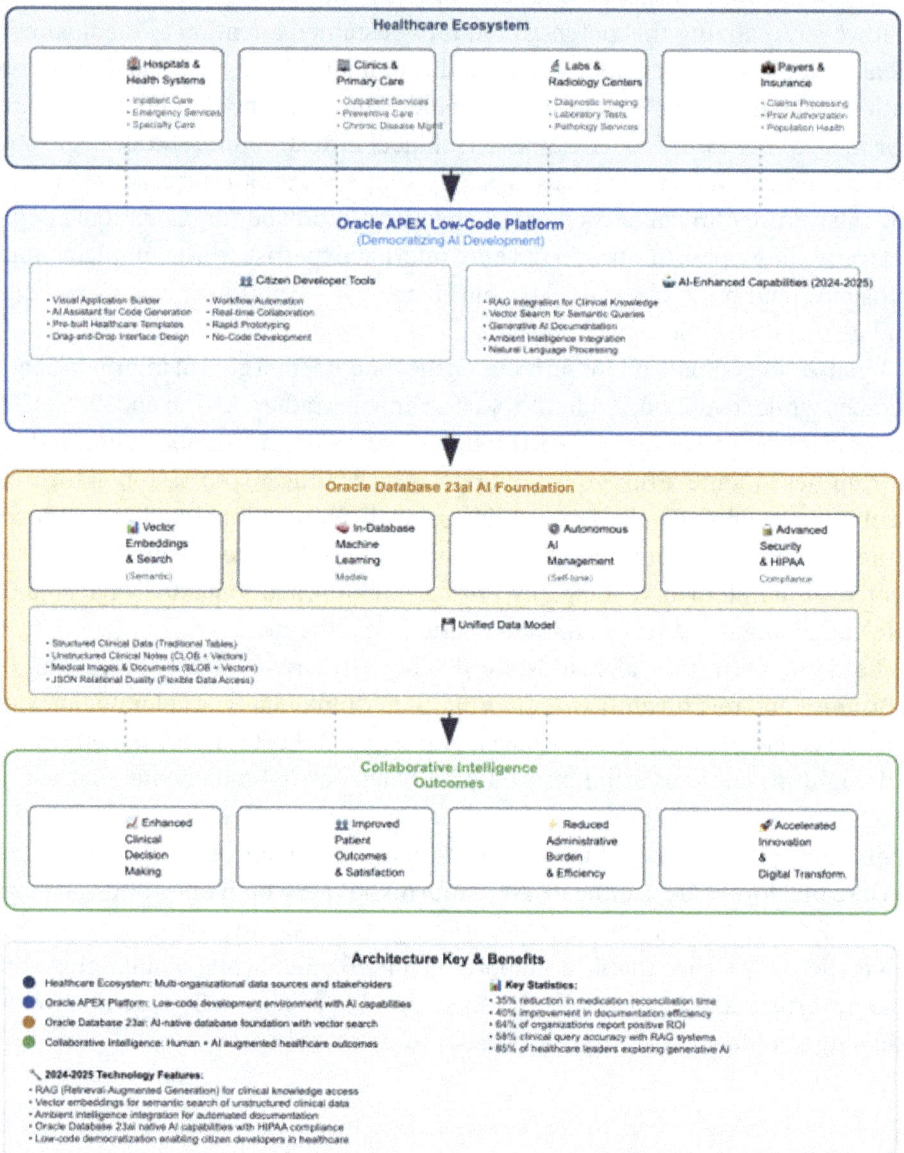

REFERENCES

Abouyannis, M.. (2024). Barriers to and facilitators of artificial intelligence adoption in health care: Scoping review. *JMIR Human Factors*, *11*, e48633. DOI: 10.2196/48633 PMID: 39207831

Bhargava, A., Bhargava, A., Kumar, A., Ahmad, F., & Kumar, A. (2024). Facilitators and barriers to AI adoption in nursing practice: A qualitative study of registered nurses' perspectives. *BMC Nursing*, *23*(1), 917. DOI: 10.1186/s12912-024-02571-y PMID: 39695581

Daley, K.. (2024). Overcoming barriers and enabling artificial intelligence adoption in allied health clinical practice: A qualitative study. *Digital Health*, *11*, 20552076241311144. DOI: 10.1177/20552076241311144 PMID: 39906878

Davis, F. D. (1989). Perceived usefulness, perceived ease of use, and user acceptance of information technology. *Management Information Systems Quarterly*, *13*(3), 319–340. DOI: 10.2307/249008

Goldfarb, A., & Teodoridis, F. (2022). Why is AI adoption in health care lagging? *Brookings Papers on Economic Activity*, *2022*(1), 1–83.

Gray, R., Campbell, L., Goharian, A., & Iredale, H. (2022). Health informatics: Engaging modern healthcare units: A brief overview. *Frontiers in Digital Health*, *4*, 814775. DOI: 10.3389/fdgth.2022.814775

Holzinger, A., et al. (2022). Guideline for software life cycle in health informatics. Methods of Information in Medicine, 61(5-06), 193-204. DOI: 10.1055/s-0042-1758476

JMIR Medical Informatics Editorial Board. (2024). Health informatics research trends and methodologies. *JMIR Medical Informatics*, *12*(1), e45127. DOI: 10.2196/45127

Lee, P., & Kesselheim, A. S. (2018). Trust in artificial intelligence requires trust in the humans behind it. *JMIR Medical Internet Research*, *20*(6), e10428. DOI: 10.2196/10428

Leemans, J. (2024). Setting up Oracle Database 23ai with AI Vector Search. Medium. Retrieved from https://jan-leemans.medium.com/setting-up-oracle-database-23ai-with-ai-vector-search-3b61725d7f51

Liu, S., La, H., Willms, A., & Rhodes, R. E. (2022). A "no-code" app design platform for mobile health research: Development and usability study. *JMIR Formative Research*, *6*(8), e37737. DOI: 10.2196/38737 PMID: 35980740

Martin, C. P., & Lamb, J. (2025). Generative AI in healthcare: Current trends and future outlook. McKinsey & Company. Retrieved from https://www.mckinsey.com/industries/healthcare/our-insights/generative-ai-in-healthcare-current-trends-and-future-outlook

Mehrabi, N., Morstatter, F., Saxena, N., Lerman, K., & Galstyan, A. (2021). A survey on bias and fairness in machine learning. *ACM Computing Surveys*, *54*(6), 1–35. DOI: 10.1145/3457607

Oracle Corporation. (2024). Oracle APEX 24.2 release notes: AI-enhanced capabilities and vector search integration. Oracle APEX Documentation. Retrieved from https://apex.oracle.com/en/learn/documentation/release-notes/

Park, S. Y., et al. (2019). Identifying challenges and opportunities in human-AI collaboration in healthcare. Conference Companion Publication of the 2019 on Computer Supported Cooperative Work and Social Computing, 506-510.

Rodriguez, R., ... (2025). AI in healthcare: What to expect in 2025. Chief Healthcare Executive. Retrieved from https://www.chiefhealthcareexecutive.com/view/ai-in-healthcare-what-to-expect-in-2025

Rogers, E. M. (2003). *Diffusion of innovations* (5th ed.). Free Press.

Rojas, J. C.. (2025). Adoption of artificial intelligence in healthcare: Survey of health system priorities, successes, and challenges. *Journal of the American Medical Informatics Association : JAMIA*, *32*(5), ocaf065. Advance online publication. DOI: 10.1093/jamia/ocaf065 PMID: 40323320

Saeed, U.. (2023). Algorithms in low-code-no-code for research applications: A practical review. *Algorithms*, *16*(2), 108. DOI: 10.3390/a16020108

Shah, N. H., Milstein, A., & Bagley, S. C. (2019). Making machine learning models clinically useful. *Journal of the American Medical Association*, *322*(14), 1351–1352. DOI: 10.1001/jama.2019.10306 PMID: 31393527

Singh, R. P., Hom, G. L., Abramoff, M. D., Campbell, J. P., & Chiang, M. F. (2020). Current challenges and barriers to real-world artificial intelligence adoption for the healthcare system, provider, and the patient. *Translational Vision Science & Technology*, *9*(2), 45. DOI: 10.1167/tvst.9.2.45 PMID: 32879755

Singh, S., ... (2025). An overview of 2025 AI trends in healthcare. HealthTech Magazine. Retrieved from https://healthtechmagazine.net/article/2025/01/overview-2025-ai-trends-healthcare

Srinivasan, S., Patel, T., Amer, S., & Rojas, J. C. (2024). How are US hospitals adopting artificial intelligence? Early evidence from 2022. *Health Affairs Scholar*, *2*(10), qxae123. Advance online publication. DOI: 10.1093/haschl/qxae123 PMID: 39403132

Topol, E. J. (2019). High-performance medicine: The convergence of human and artificial intelligence. *Nature Medicine*, *25*(1), 44–56. DOI: 10.1038/s41591-018-0300-7 PMID: 30617339

Ullah, F.. (2022). What about the usability in low-code platforms? A systematic literature review. *Computer Standards & Interfaces*, *84*, 103698. DOI: 10.1016/j.csi.2022.103698

van der Laan, A. L., Boenink, M., Broerse, J. E., & Spreeuwenberg, P. (2022). Systematic review of barriers to and facilitators of artificial intelligence adoption in healthcare organizations. *Journal of Healthcare Management*, *67*(5), 359–374.

Wilson, H. J., & Daugherty, P. R. (2018). Collaborative intelligence: Humans and AI are joining forces. *Harvard Business Review*, *96*(4), 114–123.

World Economic Forum. (2025). 6 ways AI is transforming healthcare. Retrieved from https://www.weforum.org/stories/2025/03/ai-transforming-global-health/

Yazici, C.. (2022). Experimental evidence of effective human–AI collaboration in medical decision-making. *Scientific Reports*, *12*(1), 14952. DOI: 10.1038/s41598-022-18751-2 PMID: 36056152

Chapter 5
Strengthening AI Adoption in Healthcare Collaboration:
Extending the Technology Acceptance Model

A. Sharmila
Saveetha Institute of Medical and Technical Sciences, Chennai, India

K. C. Raja Shree
http://orcid.org/0009-0009-1029-910X
Saveetha Institute of Medical and Technical Sciences, Chennai, India

G. S. Gigi
Saveetha Institute of Medical and Technical Sciences, Chennai, India

P. Praveen Kumar
http://orcid.org/0000-0002-0707-039X
SRM Institute of Science and Technology, Vadapalani, India

ABSTRACT

Healthcare systems are rapidly adopting Artificial Intelligence (AI) to enhance collaboration, decision-making, and efficiency, yet challenges like trust, ethics, and resistance persist. This study extends the Technology Acceptance Model (TAM) to include factors such as Trust, Transparency, Data Security, and Organizational Support. The extended framework captures both technical and human-centered determinants of AI adoption in collaborative healthcare. Using a mixed-methods approach—combining quantitative SEM analysis and qualitative insights—it explores

DOI: 10.4018/979-8-3373-5906-9.ch005

adoption dynamics across healthcare professionals. Findings suggest Trust mediates AI adoption, while Organizational Support and Training predict sustainability. The study offers a socio-technical model for strengthening AI-driven collaboration in healthcare.

1.1 INTRODUCTION

The necessity for efficient collaboration among healthcare professionals has been emphasized by the swiftly changing healthcare environment. E-collaboration has emerged as a vital enabler of high-quality healthcare delivery. It entails the use of digital platforms and technologies to improve interaction, coordination, and communication among various healthcare teams, regardless of their geographical or professional differences. Nevertheless, in spite of these advancements, challenges such as fragmented data systems, information overload, and inefficient workflows persist, hindering the seamless collaboration required to achieve optimal patient outcomes. These challenges necessitate a transformative approach, and artificial intelligence (AI) is emerging as a promising solution to bridge these gaps and enhance the effectiveness of e-collaboration in healthcare settings (Reddy, Fox, & Purohit, 2019). The capability of AI to process, interpret, and synthesize data from diverse sources renders it especially effective in fostering collaboration among healthcare professionals. When incorporated into digital health ecosystems, AI can offer real-time decision support, automate the sharing of information, and promote communication among interprofessional teams, thereby establishing a collaborative intelligence framework that enhances rather than supplants human judgment

One of the essential elements of e-collaboration is access to and integration of patient data. Healthcare professionals are required to utilize information from various sources, including EHRs, remote monitoring devices, imaging systems, and laboratory reports. Natural language processing tools can extract pertinent clinical information from unstructured notes and convert it into structured formats that are accessible to all stakeholders (Jiang et al., 2017). Moreover, AI-powered platforms can facilitate collaborative diagnosis and treatment planning by integrating information into shared dashboards and communication tools. These systems provide clinicians with curated insights, recommended protocols, and visualization tools that promote consensus-based care. Such capabilities are particularly valuable in complex cases involving multiple specialists or interdisciplinary teams. For example, AI-enhanced tumor boards allow oncologists, radiologists, pathologists, and surgeons to access and analyze data collaboratively, improving the speed and accuracy of treatment planning. Similarly, AI-based decision support systems can identify potential drug interactions, recommend personalized therapies, and forecast patient responses allowing different providers to align their interventions more effectively (Krittanawong et al., 2021).

A crucial component of e-collaboration is the accessibility and integration of patient data. Healthcare professionals are required to utilize information from various sources, including EHRs, remote monitoring devices, imaging systems, and laboratory reports. These data points frequently exist in separate silos, which complicates clinicians' ability to obtain a holistic view of a patient's condition. AI technologies assist in consolidating and harmonizing this data, facilitating the development of unified patient profiles and predictive models that enhance collaborative clinical decision-making. For example, through the analysis of test results, data from wearable devices, and patient medical histories, machine learning algorithms are capable of identifying early warning signs of disease progression and promptly notifying physicians and care teams. Additionally, natural language processing tools can retrieve relevant clinical information from unstructured notes and transform it into structured formats that are available to all stakeholders (Davenport & Kalakota, 2019). E-collaboration is also enriched by AI's role in clinical documentation and communication. AI-driven medical scribes employ speech recognition and natural language processing to transcribe patient interactions, summarize visit notes, and automatically fill in electronic health record fields. This automation not only conserves time but also guarantees that pertinent data is reliably and consistently accessible to all members of the care team. The decreased documentation burden has been associated with reduced clinician burnout, enhanced job satisfaction, and more efficient collaboration. In turn, AI-enhanced communication tools promote transparency, reduce duplication, and foster a culture of shared responsibility. Incorporating AI into collaborative healthcare environments, however, also introduces important considerations related to trust, transparency, and ethical use. Trust in AI systems is paramount; healthcare professionals must have confidence that the recommendations provided by algorithms are accurate, unbiased, and contextually appropriate. Transparency is essential for clinicians to comprehend the reasoning behind AI systems' conclusions, especially in high-stakes or ethically intricate situations. Models that operate as black boxes and lack transparency can undermine trust and disrupt collaborative decision-making. Consequently, developers must focus on creating interpretable AI models that are consistent with clinical reasoning methodologies.

According to research, healthcare personnel are more likely to integrate artificial intelligence into their collaborative processes when they can evaluate and validate the results produced by the technology (Obermeyer & Emanuel, 2016). Another vital aspect influencing the acceptance of AI in electronic collaboration is its ethical viability. The implementation of AI systems must prioritize patient confidentiality, informed consent, and fair access to healthcare services. Algorithms must undergo thorough testing for bias, especially within diverse demographic groups, to avoid inequalities in diagnosis or treatment. The effectiveness of implementing AI technologies depends critically on their clinical value, as well as how well they interact with existing workflows, user preferences, and institutional goals. Solutions that are excessively complicated or inadequately integrated can hinder rather than facilitate collaboration. Consequently, adopting a human-centered methodology that engages end-users during the design and testing stages is crucial to guarantee both usability and clinical effectiveness. (Reddy et al., 2019). A commitment from leadership, partnerships across sectors, and flexible policies are essential to cultivate a culture of innovation. Effective implementation necessitates a synergy between technical capabilities and clinical goals, underpinned by ongoing monitoring and assessment.

Case studies from institutions like Cedars-Sinai and the Mayo Clinic demonstrate how AI platforms can enhance patient outcomes, reduce diagnostic errors, and improve throughput. (Davenport & Kalakota, 2019). Researchers are increasingly utilizing theoretical frameworks such as the Technology Acceptance Model (TAM) to better understand the dynamics of AI adoption in e-collaborative healthcare settings. TAM, which was initially introduced by Davis (1989), suggests that an individual's willingness to adopt new technology is influenced by two key beliefs: perceived usefulness (PU) and perceived ease of use (PEOU). PU evaluates the degree to which healthcare professionals perceive that AI tools improve teamwork, decision-making, and patient care in the context of AI-driven e-collaboration. The effort required to familiarize oneself with and integrate these tools into current workflows is linked to PEOU. The Unified Theory of Acceptance and Use of Technology (UTAUT) is one of the extensions of TAM, adding further elements such as behavioral intention, social influence, and facilitating conditions. As noted by (Venkatesh et al.,2003), researchers have suggested further modifications to include clinical appropriateness, ethical acceptability, and trust in AI as significant factors influencing adoption. Recent empirical studies underscore the importance of these models in comprehending AI integration. (Krittanawong et al., 2021) discovered that healthcare professionals who believed AI tools enhanced diagnostic accuracy and reduced errors were more inclined to utilize them. (Jiang et al., 2017) indicated that clinician trust and training were significant predictors of AI adoption, while (Obermeyer & Emanuel,2016) highlighted the necessity for algorithmic fairness and transparency. Despite the promising evidence, there remain significant gaps in the current literature. Many studies focus on the technical effectiveness of AI tools rather than their impact on collaborative behaviors and patient outcomes. Only a limited number of frameworks adequately address the organizational, ethical, and interpersonal dimensions of AI-enabled collaboration. Furthermore, most research has been conducted in high-income countries, which limits the relevance of findings to resource-constrained settings. There is an urgent need for longitudinal, context-sensitive studies that evaluate how AI tools influence interprofessional collaboration over time and across different healthcare environments. Particular emphasis is placed on the importance of trust, transparency, ethical alignment, and clinical integration. The research further explores the influence of institutional readiness, professional culture, and regulatory frameworks on the application of AI in practice. In conclusion, Artificial Intelligence possesses considerable transformative potential to tackle ongoing challenges in healthcare collaboration. By improving data integration, automating routine tasks, and aiding decision-making, AI can enhance the quality, efficiency, and equity of care delivery. However, achieving this potential necessitates more than mere technological advancements; it requires careful integration into human workflows, ethical governance, and collaborative design. Promoting e-collaboration through AI is not solely a technical matter but a sociotechnical transformation that demands alignment among individuals, processes, and platforms.

1.2 THEORETICAL FRAMEWORK

A thorough and methodical analysis of the role of artificial intelligence (AI) in e-collaborative healthcare settings can be conducted using the Technology Acceptance Model (TAM), which was first proposed by Davis in 1989. This model provides a solid theoretical foundation for assessing how healthcare professionals perceive, adopt, and integrate AI technology into their digital collaborative processes. Understanding the organizational and psychological factors that influence AI adoption is crucial as the healthcare industry increasingly undergoes digital transformation, especially in light of the growing need for swift, coordinated, and patient-focused care. This implies that within the healthcare field, doctors view AI solutions as capable of increasing efficiency, improving diagnostic precision, speeding up communication, or aiding decision-making in collaborative settings (Venkatesh & Davis, 2000). For instance, a doctor who sees AI algorithms prioritizing urgent test results or predicting patient decline in real-time is likely to consider these systems as extremely advantageous.

A high-functioning e-collaborative ecosystem depends on clinicians lowering diagnostic errors, reducing communication loops, and simplifying care coordination all of which AI may help .Conversely, PEOU shows how easy, straightforward, and non-disruptive AI solutions are to healthcare workers' current workflows. As noted by (Venkatesh and Davis, 2000), systems that are perceived as difficult to learn or use can create friction, decrease efficiency, and ultimately deter adoption. (Reddy et al., 2019) emphasize that for AI-powered tools to be embraced within electronic health record (EHR) platforms or decision-support systems, they must be seamlessly integrated, requiring minimal additional effort from the user. A clinical decision support system that intuitively highlights abnormal results or suggests treatment options without requiring the clinician to navigate complex interfaces is far more likely to be adopted and used regularly. In order to influence the behavioral intention (BI) to utilize AI technology, which in turn forecasts actual usage behavior, perceived usefulness (PU) and perceived ease of use (PEOU) engage in interaction. An administrator may utilize AI dashboards to coordinate resources across departments, a nurse may use AI-generated alerts to react more quickly to worsening patient conditions, or a doctor may decide to rely on AI-generated recommendations during a multidisciplinary team meeting. These are just a few examples of how BI can appear in the context of healthcare e-collaboration (Davenport & Kalakota, 2019). While the foundational TAM framework offers significant explanatory power, scholars such as (Venkatesh and Bala, 2008) argue that it must be extended to account for sector-specific complexities, particularly in high-stakes, trust-sensitive domains like healthcare. One of the most critical extensions to the model is the incorporation of Trust in AI as a moderating factor. Trust encompasses beliefs about the system's accuracy, transparency, reliability, and ethical grounding. (Siau &Wang, 2018) and (Longoni & Cian, 2020) emphasize that in domains like oncology, emergency medicine, and critical care, clinicians must feel confident not only in the tool's technical performance but also in its decision logic and alignment with medical ethics. For example, an AI model that predicts patient survival chances or triage prioritization must offer explainability; otherwise, clinicians may reject it regardless of its predictive power.

According to (Obermeyer & Emanuel, 2016), when AI models are perceived as "black boxes" with unclear decision-making procedures, scepticism usually surface. These systems endanger clinician trust and, as a result, their acceptance when there is insufficient transparency or clinical validation. When AI-generated suggestions contradict a clinician's intuition or experience, a deficit of trust may lead to disengagement, thereby diminishing the potential for improved e-collaboration. Another significant element affecting the shift from intention to actual utilization is the existence of Facilitating Conditions. These include official training programs, technical support, organizational infrastructure, and a culture that encourages creativity and digital competency. According to (Holden & Karsh, 2010) and (Venkatesh et al., 2003), enabling conditions act as enablers that ensure users have the tools and assistance they need to use new technologies efficiently. In the realm of healthcare AI, this could entail offering regular training on AI interfaces, ensuring IT personnel are readily available to resolve issues, and investing in interoperable systems that facilitate seamless data exchange across departments. (Reddy et al.,2019) discovered that healthcare organizations with robust IT support systems and interdisciplinary training programs were significantly more successful in implementing AI-enhanced collaborative tools.

In the absence of these conditions, even the most promising AI innovations may not be fully utilized because of practical obstacles such as insufficient time, apprehension about making mistakes, or a lack of familiarity with the interface. Additionally, an extension of the TAM model, initially introduced by (Venkatesh & Davis, 2000), is referred to as Subjective Norms. It describes the social pressure people feel to utilize a specific technology from significant referents like peers, seniors, or institutional leaders. In team-oriented healthcare environments, where clinical decision-making is often collaborative and hierarchical, the attitudes and behaviors of respected colleagues play a major role in shaping individual choices. For instance, if a senior surgeon consistently uses AI tools for preoperative risk assessment and encourages junior doctors to do the same, this social influence can accelerate adoption throughout the department. Subjective norms become even more influential when embedded in institutional policies or performance evaluations. For example, if hospital leadership mandates the use of AI-supported handover tools or flags non-use during audits, individual clinicians are more likely to align their behavior accordingly. In addition to strengthening individual behavioral intentions, this group interaction promotes a digital collaborative culture in which AI is viewed as a common tool for group decision-making rather than as a novel concept. The incorporation of these elements into the original TAM framework, trust in AI, enabling conditions, and subjective norms.The incorporation of these elements illustrates the intricate realities present in clinical environments, where social dynamics, organizational preparedness, and ethical factors contribute to the adoption of technology, alongside perceived utility and usability.

Figure 1. Theoretical Framework

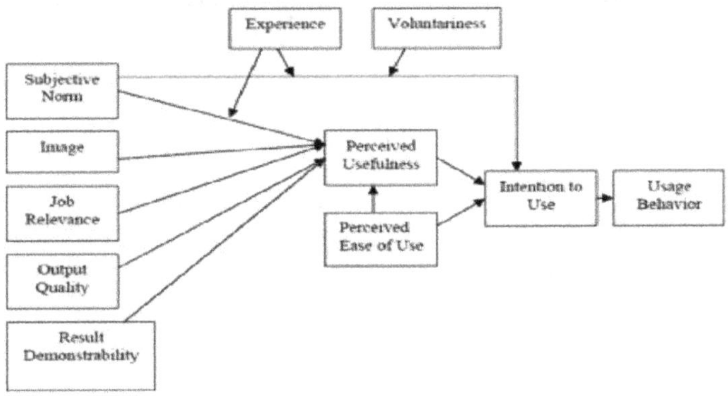

Source: (Venkatesh & Davis, 2000), (Reddy et al.,2019), (Obermeyer & Emanuel, 2016), (Davenport & Kalakota, 2019), (Holden & Karsh, 2010)

1.3 CONCEPTUAL FRAMEWORK

A conceptual framework offers a systematic depiction of the essential variables and their expected interrelations within a study, acting as a logical basis for the development of theories and empirical research. In the realm of technology adoption, especially in intricate environments like healthcare, a conceptual framework aids in merging individual, organizational, and technological elements into a unified explanatory model. It assists the researcher in pinpointing pertinent constructs, elucidating their functions, and establishing the pathways through which anticipated outcomes are likely to manifest (Hashimov, 2015).

In the sphere of AI adoption within healthcare collaboration, a conceptual framework holds particular significance as technology utilization transcends individual decision-making to encompass interprofessional coordination, ethical obligations, and organizational preparedness. Conventional acceptance models, such as the Technology Acceptance Model (TAM), mainly concentrate on individual perceptions regarding usefulness and ease of use; however, healthcare environments necessitate the incorporation of trust, data security, leadership endorsement, and training as vital factors influencing adoption (Holden & Karsh, 2010). Consequently, the proposed conceptual framework broadens TAM by integrating mediating and moderating variables that represent the collaborative, ethical, and systemic characteristics of healthcare organizations.

By delineating the connections among the extended TAM constructs, mediating processes, and adoption results, the conceptual framework provides a structured perspective to comprehend how AI technologies can be successfully assimilated into collaborative healthcare practices. It not only facilitates hypothesis formulation and empirical validation but also offers practical guidance for healthcare leaders and policymakers aiming to enhance AI-enabled collaboration and elevate the quality of patient care.

Figure 2. Conceptual Framework

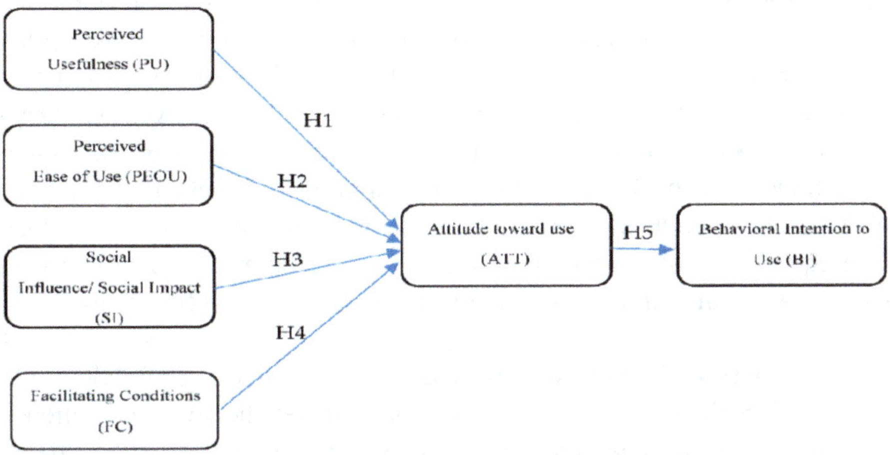

Source: (Hashimov, 2015), (Holden & Karsh, 2010), (Venkatesh & Bala, 2008), (Reddy et al., 2020),(Angst & Agarwal, 2009), (Greenhalgh et al., 2017), (Pai & Huang, 2011), (Uymaz et al.,2024), (Parket al.,2019)

1.3.1 Independent Variables (Extended TAM Constructs)

- **Perceived Usefulness (PU)** - Perceived usefulness pertains to the extent to which healthcare professionals perceive that AI systems enhance clinical efficiency, accuracy in decision-making, and collaboration among professionals. In collaborative healthcare settings, AI tools such as clinical decision support systems and predictive analytics can accelerate diagnostic processes, minimize errors, and promote a shared understanding across various departments. Previous studies consistently indicate that PU serves as a robust predictor of technology acceptance within healthcare environments, as clinicians are more inclined to embrace AI when it clearly enhances patient outcomes and improves workflow efficiency (Holden & Karsh, 2010).
- **Perceived Ease of Use (PEOU)** - Perceived ease of use refers to the degree to which AI systems are viewed as straightforward to learn, comprehend, and utilize without undue effort. In the healthcare sector, complicated interfaces and poorly integrated systems can lead to cognitive overload, thereby diminishing intentions to adopt. Research suggests that when AI tools are designed to be user-friendly and compatible with existing clinical workflows, healthcare professionals are likely to cultivate more favorable attitudes towards

their utilization, which in turn reinforces perceived usefulness (Venkatesh & Bala, 2008).

- **Trust in AI System** - Trust in AI systems is essential for collaboration in healthcare, as clinicians depend on AI-generated recommendations that have a direct impact on patient care decisions. Trust is influenced by the reliability of the system, its transparency, explain ability, and the perceived accuracy of its outputs. Studies emphasize that a lack of trust arising from "black-box" algorithms or inconsistent outcomes can significantly impede the adoption of AI, even when the systems are technically proficient (Reddy et al., 2020). Consequently, trust expands the Technology Acceptance Model (TAM) by incorporating the ethical and cognitive assurance necessary in high-stakes clinical settings.
- **Data Security and Privacy Concerns** - The safeguarding of patient information is a critical ethical and legal obligation in healthcare collaboration. AI systems frequently necessitate extensive data sharing among various departments and institutions, which raises issues regarding confidentiality, potential data breaches, and misuse. Empirical research indicates that increased concerns about privacy and security adversely impact healthcare professionals' readiness to adopt digital health technologies, making this aspect vital for expanding the Technology Acceptance Model (TAM) in relation to AI adoption (Angst & Agarwal, 2009; Reddy et al., 2020).
- **Top Management Support** - Support from top management signifies the commitment of leadership, strategic foresight, and the allocation of resources necessary for the implementation of AI. In healthcare organizations, evident backing from senior leadership cultivates an innovative culture, diminishes resistance to change, and legitimizes initiatives for AI adoption. Previous research has confirmed that leadership support has a positive effect on user attitudes and behavioral intentions towards advanced health information systems (Greenhalgh et al., 2017).
- **Training and Technical Support** -Training and technical support encompass the provision of organized learning programs, ongoing assistance, and opportunities for skill enhancement related to AI systems. Sufficient training alleviates anxiety, boosts self-efficacy, and enhances system utilization among healthcare professionals. Studies reveal that ongoing technical support is essential for maintaining the long-term adoption of complex technologies within healthcare environments (Holden & Karsh, 2010; Venkatesh & Bala, 2008).

1.3.2 Mediating Variables

- **Attitude Toward AI Use** - The attitude toward the use of AI reflects the overall positive or negative assessment made by healthcare professionals regarding AI-enabled collaboration. As per the extensions of the Technology Acceptance Model (TAM), this attitude serves as a mediator in the relationship between system characteristics, specifically perceived usefulness (PU) and perceived ease of use (PEOU), and the intention to behave. In the healthcare sector, positive attitudes are influenced not only by improvements in efficiency but also by ethical considerations, trust, and the perceived advantages for patients (Holden & Karsh, 2010).
- **User Readiness** - User readiness includes both psychological readiness, which involves an openness to change and a diminished fear of AI, as well as technical readiness, which pertains to the skills and competencies required to utilize AI tools effectively. Research indicates that even the most well-constructed AI systems can fail if users lack the necessary mental and technical preparation, thereby establishing readiness as a crucial mediating factor between organizational support and the actual utilization of the system (Greenhalgh et al., 2017).

1.3.3 Moderating Variables

- **Organizational Culture** - Organizational culture plays a crucial role in moderating the adoption of AI by influencing norms, values, and the willingness to embrace innovation. A culture that prioritizes innovation fosters an environment conducive to experimentation and learning, thereby enhancing the connection between intention and actual usage. Conversely, a culture resistant to change diminishes this connection (Greenhalgh et al., 2017).
- **Professional Role** - Various professional group including doctors, nurses, administrators, and allied health professionals have differing perceptions of AI, shaped by their specific responsibilities and levels of accountability. Research suggests that clinicians who are directly engaged in patient care may have heightened ethical and trust-related concerns compared to their administrative counterparts, which in turn influences their acceptance patterns (Holden & Karsh, 2010).
- **Experience with Technology** -Previous experience with digital health systems significantly impacts users' confidence and lowers the perceived complexity associated with AI tools. Individuals with extensive technological experience are more inclined to convert positive intentions into actual usage,

thereby reinforcing the relationships outlined in the Technology Acceptance Model (TAM) (Pai & Huang, 2011).

1.3.4 Dependent Variables

- **Behavioral Intention to Use AI** - Behavioral intention signifies the readiness of healthcare professionals to embrace AI in both collaborative clinical and administrative functions. In alignment with the Technology Acceptance Model (TAM), this intention serves as a robust predictor of actual system utilization and is shaped by individual, organizational, and ethical considerations (Uymaz et al.,2024).
- **Actual AI Usage in Healthcare Collaboration** -Actual usage pertains to the practical implementation of AI systems across various departments for collaborative decision-making, coordination, and patient management. This concept encapsulates the shift from intention to execution, which poses significant challenges in the healthcare sector due to regulatory and workflow limitations (Parket al.,2019).
- **Collaborative Performance Outcomes** -Collaborative performance outcomes encompass enhanced interprofessional coordination, improved decision-making accuracy, decreased errors, and superior quality of patient care. Research highlights that the successful integration of AI should ultimately result in quantifiable enhancements in collaborative healthcare performance, thereby affirming the validity of the extended TAM framework (Holden & Karsh, 2010; Greenhalgh et al., 2017).

1.4 KEY CONSTRUCTS OF THE ADAPTED TAM

Healthcare providers are more likely to embrace AI technology within the framework of e-collaboration when they recognize concrete advantages such as enhanced diagnostic precision, expedited clinical decision-making, improved interprofessional communication, or diminished administrative burdens.Artificial intelligence has the potential to "restore the gift of time" by automating monotonous documentation duties, thereby allowing physicians to concentrate more on patient care and interpersonal communication. (Krittanawong et al.,2021) highlight that AI-driven systems, which include decision support tools and predictive analytics, can enhance clinical outcomes by providing timely, evidence-based recommendations. These perceived improvements in clinical efficiency and effectiveness render AI tools exceptionally valuable in collaborative care environments, thereby reinforcing their perceived usefulness.In their enhancement of the Technology Acceptance Model

(TAM), (Venkatesh and Davis 2000) illustrated how PEOU affects adoption both directly and indirectly by enhancing Perceived Usefulness (PU). Even well-designed AI systems may be rejected in high-stress clinical environments if they interfere with standard operating procedures or necessitate lengthy on boarding. According to (Jiang et al., 2017), for instance, AI tools that are not integrated with electronic health records (EHRs) are often underutilised because they are perceived as being difficult to use. Therefore, ensuring clinician approval requires a smooth interface design and workflow alignment.

- **Confidence in AI Systems**: Trust is an essential element in the integration of AI within healthcare, as decisions can greatly influence patient safety. Healthcare professionals must have confidence that AI systems are not only precise but also dependable and impartial. (Obermeyer & Emanuel, 2016) emphasize that trust is primarily established through algorithmic transparency; clinicians must comprehend how AI reaches its conclusions and maintain consistent performance across various patient demographics. (Amann et al.,2020) It was further emphasized that when healthcare professionals comprehend the reasoning behind AI-generated suggestions, they are more inclined to trust those suggestions. The capacity of AI to provide actionable insights and the healthcare provider's readiness to depend on its results are fundamentally linked by trust.
- **Ethical Acceptability and Transparency**: Implementing AI ethically is crucial, particularly in a sensitive industry like healthcare. Fundamental to the ethical integration of AI are issues like algorithmic bias, patient consent, data privacy, and fairness. According to (Morley et al., 2020), healthcare practitioners may question the reliability and security of AI-generated suggestions if there are no clear ethical guidelines or systemic transparency. A deficiency in explainability, where users cannot comprehend or validate the decision-making process, can lead to distrust and opposition among healthcare providers. In contrast, AI systems that are ethically sound and explainable promote higher levels of acceptance by ensuring accountability and safeguarding patient rights.
- **Facilitating Conditions**: It denotes the organizational and technical framework that underpins the effective utilization of AI systems. This encompasses access to dependable internet, compatibility of devices, IT assistance, structured training programs, and encouraging leadership. Facilitating factors significantly influence whether potential users transition from intention to actual usage, as explained in (Venkatesh et al.,2003)'s Unified Theory of Acceptance and Use of Technology (UTAUT). This point is further emphasised by (Reddy et al., 2019), who claim that without sufficient investments

in education, systems integration, and change management, even the most advanced AI tools will find it difficult to become widely accepted.

- **Data Interoperability**: The effective implementation of AI in e-collaborative environments relies on the seamless transfer and utilization of data among various healthcare systems. In the absence of access to and the ability to integrate data from multiple sources, including EHRs, laboratory systems, imaging platforms, and wearable devices, artificial intelligence cannot function efficiently within disjointed digital ecosystems. Interoperability, according to (Davenport & Kalakota, 2019), is the cornerstone of AI-enabled care coordination because it enables AI systems to generate insightful results by analysing real-time, multi-source data. This capacity enhances situational awareness among care teams in collaborative healthcare environments, enabling more accurate diagnosis, treatment planning, and resource allocation.

Figure 3. Key Constructs of the Adapted TAM

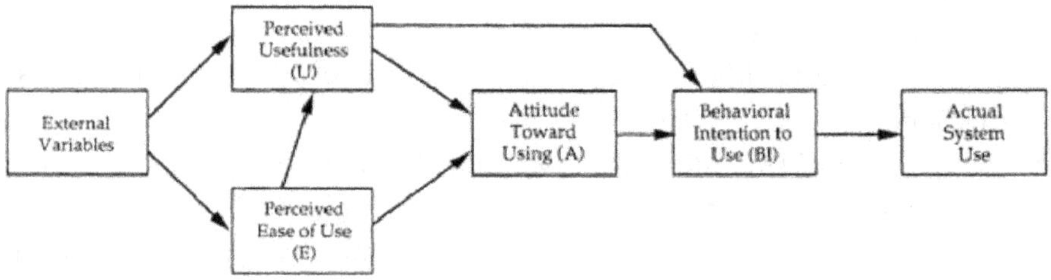

Source: (Krittanawong et al.,2021), (Venkatesh and Davis 2000), (Jiang et al., 2017), (Obermeyer & Emanuel, 2016), (Davenport & Kalakota, 2019), (Reddy et al., 2019), (Morley et al., 2020), (Amann et al.,2020)

1.5 MODEL PATHWAYS

The basic TAM framework is improved in this study to take into consideration the complexities involved in integrating Artificial Intelligence (AI) in e-collaborative healthcare environments. The additional variable Trust in AI, Transparency, Interoperability, and Facilitating Conditions, are introduced as moderators or antecedents that more accurately influence PU, PEOU, and Behavioral Intention within clinical environments. Trust is essential for clinicians to depend on AI recommendations in critical situations such as diagnostics and treatment planning. Without confidence in the outputs generated by algorithms, even precise AI tools may not be fully utilized (Obermeyer & Emanuel, 2016). When AI systems offer explanations for their decisions, clinicians are more inclined to view them as beneficial and user-friendly.

Transparent systems foster cognitive alignment and diminish uncertainty, thereby boosting user confidence and acceptance (Jiang et al., 2017). In the updated Technology Acceptance Model (TAM), these supplementary factors act as moderators or antecedents. The initial Technology Acceptance Model (TAM), developed by Davis in 1989, has undergone conceptual modifications in the model introduced here. This model suggests that a user's intention to embrace a technology, which ultimately leads to its actual utilization, is directly influenced by two primary constructs: perceived usefulness (PU) and perceived ease of use (PEOU). Venkatesh and Davis (2000) contend that this linear relationship (PU + PEOU → Behavioral Intention → Actual Use) has been thoroughly validated in studies related to telemedicine, electronic health records, and various health IT systems. They assist in elucidating not only whether clinicians can utilize AI, but also whether they will choose to do so and the reasons behind their decisions, thereby adding depth to both predictive validity and Artificial Intelligence (AI) acts as an integrative layer within the digital healthcare infrastructure, transforming fragmented, siloed data sources into actionable intelligence. This transformation facilitates real-time, cross-functional collaboration among clinicians, specialists, and care teams (Reddy et al., 2019).In conventional healthcare systems, information is frequently kept in isolated, non-interactive silos, including distinct EHR systems, laboratory information systems, radiology repositories, and pharmacy databases (Reddy et al., 2019).

In order to produce predicted insights and offer diagnostic support, these systems may analyse both structured and unstructured data, including lab values and clinical notes (Jiang et al., 2017). Clinicians can use dashboards that provide patient risk scores, medication alerts, diagnostic suggestions, and care pathways after these systems are integrated since AI algorithms provide real-time analytics (Davenport & Kalakota, 2019). These insights are made available at the point of care, facilitating collaborative decision-making among teams. For example, a cardiologist, a primary care physician, and a nurse coordinator can concurrently review a patient's AI-generated risk profile for heart failure, allowing for shared and informed decisions based on the same real-time data (Krittanawong et al., 2021).

Figure 4. Model Pathways

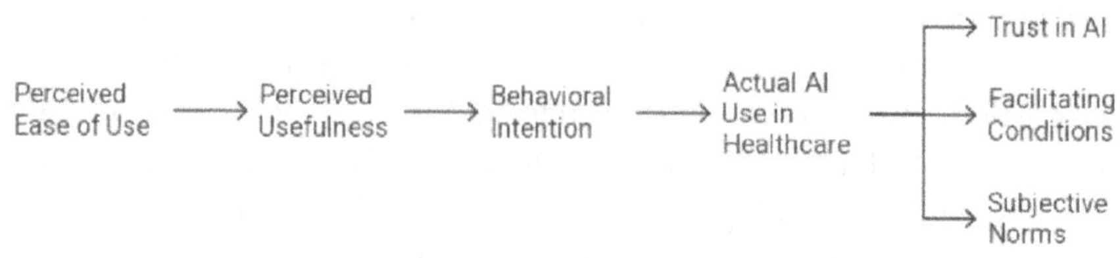

Source: (Obermeyer & Emanuel, 2016), (Jiang et al., 2017), (Reddy et al., 2019), (Davenport & Kalakota, 2019), (Krittanawong et al., 2021)

1.6 ADAPTED TAM FOR AI-ENABLED E-COLLABORATION IN HEALTHCARE

Building upon Davis's (1989) foundational framework in a clinical environment, PEOU pertains to the degree of ease with which healthcare professionals can utilize AI-enabled systems. When clinicians perceive these tools as intuitive and well-integrated into their workflows, it positively impacts their PU the conviction that AI improves their performance, supports clinical decision-making, and enhances collaborative efficiency. These two perceptions directly influence BI, which subsequently affects Actual Use, defined as the regular and meaningful incorporation of AI into everyday healthcare collaboration. However, this fundamental model needs to be expanded to account for the wider range of factors impacting technology adoption because healthcare contexts are inherently complex. Trust in AI, which includes physicians' faith in the precision, dependability, openness, and equity of AI tools, is among the most important additions. According to (Amin et al., 2024), trust is particularly crucial when AI is utilised to make decisions that directly affect patients, such risk assessment, therapy suggestions, or diagnosis. Even if the system is technically sound and simple to use, physicians are unlikely to depend on it if they have misgivings about it, whether because of unclear algorithms or inconsistent results. As a result, trust acts as a moderating factor that influences how strongly or weakly PU, PEOU, and BI are related. An additional important moderator is the Facilitating Conditions.

Defined by (Venkatesh et al.,2003) and further explored by (Holden & Karsh, 2010), these include the presence of adequate infrastructure, user training, technical support, and organizational readiness. Even when a clinician has a strong intention to use an AI system, the lack of proper training or inadequate hardware can obstruct actual usage. Facilitating Conditions thus act as critical enablers that help translate intention into real-world adoption. Without these, the perceived advantages of AI tools may never be realized in practice. The social influence exerted by colleagues, supervisors, and institutional culture also significantly shapes user behavior. As highlighted by (Venkatesh & Davis, 2000), when respected peers or organizational leaders advocate for AI adoption, clinicians are more inclined to follow suit. In healthcare settings where collaboration is team-based and hierarchical, the endorsement or skepticism of AI by influential individuals can heavily impact the adoption curve. Subjective Norms not only affect Behavioral Intention directly but can also reinforce trust and perceived usefulness by legitimizing the technology.

In summary, the adapted TAM offers a comprehensive, realistic explanation of how clinicians engage with AI-enabled tools in collaborative practice. It underscores that successful AI adoption in healthcare depends on more than individual perceptions it requires organizational support, social endorsement, and ethical trust in the technology. This multifaceted model is better suited for capturing the real-world dynamics of AI use in modern, team-oriented clinical environments.

Figure 5. Adapted TAM for AI-enabled E-Collaboration in Healthcare

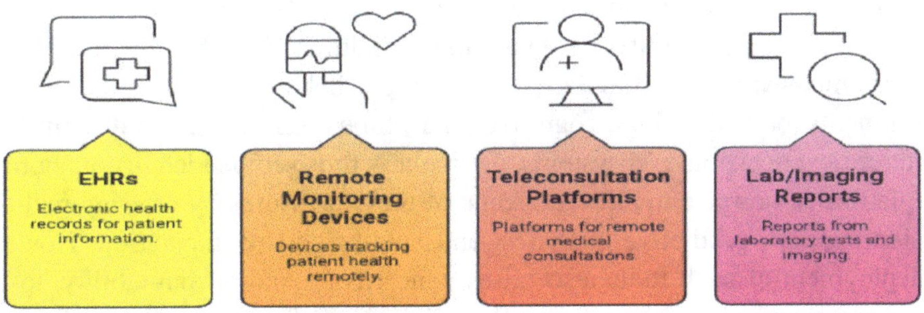

Source: (Amin et al., 2024), (Venkatesh et al., 2003), (Holden & Karsh, 2010), (Venkatesh & Davis, 2000)

1.7 APPLICABILITY OF TAM

The present study, which investigates clinicians' acceptance and usage of AI-based e-collaborative tools, leverages TAM for several compelling reasons. First, the healthcare domain is a complex, highly regulated environment where decisions often involve critical trade-offs between efficiency, accuracy, and ethical considerations.

Technologies introduced into such settings must not only demonstrate technical efficacy but also align with users' cognitive models, professional standards, and workflow routines.

TAM has been found to successfully predict technology utilisation in such diverse situations. For example, in their comprehensive review, (Holden & Karsh, 2010) documented the successful application of the Technology Acceptance Model (TAM) across various healthcare technologies, such as clinical decision support systems, mobile health platforms, and electronic health records (EHRs) their findings highlight TAM's ability to accommodate user-specific, task-related, and organizational variables, making it particularly suitable for analyzing clinician behavior. Moreover, TAM's theoretical structure is not static. By incorporating additional variables such as subjective norm, image, output quality, and result demonstrability in TAM2 and TAM3, (Venkatesh & Bala, 2008) emphasized the model's flexibility and enhanced its explanatory capability. This adaptability is especially relevant in the realm of artificial intelligence, where new systems often differ markedly from traditional rule-based approaches.

AI introduces probabilistic reasoning, machine learning, and continuous learning algorithms features which may affect how users access system transparency, reliability, and alignment with clinical goals. Consequently, a mere assessment of usefulness and ease of use may not suffice; instead, additional constructs such as trust, algorithmic transparency, interoperability, and facilitating conditions must be integrated to capture the complete range of clinician perceptions and behaviors. Clinicians operate in environments marked by high cognitive loads, time constraints, and responsibility for life-critical decisions. AI systems, particularly those embedded in collaborative care platforms, promise to alleviate some of these pressures by offering real-time decision support, predictive analytics, and automated documentation. However, the deployment of such tools also raises concerns around accountability, loss of clinical autonomy, and potential workflow disruption. The "last-mile challenge" in AI adoption, as discussed by (Davenport & Kalakota, 2019), points to the paradox where technically robust AI systems fail to gain traction due to user-level barriers such as distrust, lack of transparency, or poor integration into clinical practice.

TAM's ability to examine both the functional and underlying cognitive and affective mechanisms of technology adoption is one of its key advantages in this regard. For example, Perceived Usefulness in the case of AI tools might relate to improved diagnostic accuracy, enhanced communication within care teams, or time savings on documentation and administrative tasks. Studies by (Krittanawong et al., 2021) affirm that AI systems, when appropriately designed and deployed, can liberate healthcare professionals from repetitive tasks, allowing more time for direct patient interaction. Likewise, Perceived Ease of Use in this context can reflect the level of effort required to learn, interpret, and integrate AI recommendations into existing workflows. An AI tool is more likely to be adopted and relied upon by a physician if they find it easy to use and compatible with their electronic health record system. This study includes extensions that are essential to comprehending AI adoption in addition to the traditional TAM frameworks. Trust in AI systems emerges as a particularly significant variable. Unlike conventional software tools, AI systems often operate through non-transparent decision-making processes (e.g., neural networks) that may not be easily interpretable by end users. As (Glikson & Woolley, 2020) note, trust in artificial agents is a function of performance history, system transparency, and organizational endorsement.

Whether a doctor follows or ignores AI-generated recommendations in clinical contexts depends on trust. AI tools must not only function well but also provide understandable and clinically relevant explanations in order to earn and preserve this trust. (Obermeyer & Emanuel, 2016) caution that opaque systems may introduce bias or errors that go unchecked, potentially leading to harmful consequences. Thus, perceived transparency and fairness both psychological antecedents to trust are integral to the adoption process By extending TAM to include such ethical perceptions, this study ensures a more comprehensive analysis of clinician behavior. Furthermore, collaborative AI tools are often used in settings where multiple healthcare providers interact, sometimes asynchronously, to make shared decisions. This creates a need for interoperability and standardization.

When AI platforms cannot communicate seamlessly with existing EHRs or between different departments or hospitals, their perceived usefulness diminishes. Hence, the concept of interoperability is not only a technical issue but also one that influences user attitudes and behaviors, aligning with the TAM construct of system compatibility. In the Unified Theory of Acceptance and Usage of Technology (UTAUT), (Venkatesh et al., 2003) stress the significance of these elements, which either facilitate or impede the actual usage of the technology. In healthcare institutions, where change management and technology implementation strategies vary widely, facilitating conditions can determine whether a potentially useful system is embraced or rejected. For example, a clinician who receives adequate training, has access to technical support, and operates in an environment that encourages innovation is more likely to adopt AI tools, regardless of initial apprehensions. This study also considers emotional and organizational factors often overlooked in technology evaluations that influence long-term integration of AI in healthcare. Resistance to change, fear of job displacement, and anxiety about patient safety can significantly affect user attitudes.

AI systems that alter traditional roles may provoke skepticism or defensiveness among staff. By integrating these softer, yet deeply influential variables into TAM, the study provides a more holistic understanding of the adoption landscape. This is particularly relevant for collaborative environments, where AI tools not only assist individual clinicians but also mediate team-based care processes. As such, perceptions of fairness, accountability, and shared decision-making are central to the analysis. E-collaborative healthcare settings represent a shift from siloed care to integrated, patient-centered care. In these environments, AI tools must not only support individual clinicians but also facilitate coordination across teams that may include doctors, nurses, pharmacists, and allied health professionals. Such technologies must be able to support real-time communication, fit into a variety of processes, and serve common therapeutic objectives in order to be successful.TAM enables the evaluation of these factors by focusing on both individual and systemic drivers of technology use. For instance, a tool perceived as useful by a physician but confusing or irrelevant to a nurse may hinder team effectiveness. Therefore, understanding cross-role perceptions becomes critical, and TAM offers a structure for collecting and analyzing such data .Moreover, TAM's adaptability to different user groups within healthcare institutions allows for granular insights.

Different professionals may exhibit varying levels of acceptance based on their roles, technical proficiency, and exposure to technology. By disaggregating data across user types, this study can identify targeted interventions to improve adoption. For example, younger clinicians might find AI tools more intuitive, while senior staff may require more contextual explanation and trust-building. Such insights are valuable for developers and policymakers aiming to create inclusive, user-centered AI systems .In addition to its theoretical strength, TAM provides practical value by offering measurable constructs that can be operationalized through validated survey instruments. This allows for rigorous quantitative analysis and comparison across studies. As the use of AI in healthcare becomes more prevalent, developing standardized methods for evaluating its acceptance will be essential for benchmarking progress and guiding policy. Through the generation of empirical data on clinician attitudes, behaviours, and system usage patterns, the application of TAM in this study advances this larger objective .In conclusion, TAM's solid theoretical underpinnings, demonstrated empirical record, and flexibility in addressing the particular difficulties presented by AI in healthcare justify its use in this work. By extending the model to include variables such as trust, transparency, facilitating conditions, and interoperability, the study captures the multifaceted nature of clinician-AI. AI interactions in e-collaborative environments. This approach moves beyond simplistic adoption metrics and instead seeks to understand the deep cognitive, emotional, and organizational dynamics that influence how intelligent systems are integrated into healthcare delivery. Ultimately, this understanding is essential for designing AI tools that not only function well but are also trusted, embraced, and effectively used by those on the front lines of patient care.

1.8 SCOPE AND CONTEXT OF THE STUDY

The present study is situated within hospital-based healthcare settings, encompassing both multi-specialty and single-specialty healthcare institutions. Hospitals represent an ideal context for examining AI adoption because they are complex, high-stakes environments characterized by multidisciplinary teamwork, intensive information exchange, and strict regulatory and ethical requirements. In such settings, clinicians and administrators must collaborate across departments to deliver timely, accurate, and patient-centered care, making e-collaboration technologies particularly critical (Holden & Karsh, 2010). Multi-specialty hospitals, with their diverse clinical departments, offer a rich context for understanding cross-functional AI-enabled collaboration, while single-specialty hospitals provide focused environments where AI tools can be deeply embedded into specialized workflows.

The scope of the study includes AI-driven clinical and administrative tools that directly support collaborative healthcare processes. Key technologies examined include clinical decision support systems (CDSS), AI-enabled electronic health records (EHRs), and tele-collaboration platforms. Clinical decision support systems powered by AI assist healthcare professionals by analyzing large volumes of patient data and providing evidence-based recommendations, thereby supporting shared clinical decision-making and reducing diagnostic variability (Krittanawong et al., 2021). These systems are particularly relevant in team-based care settings such as intensive care units, oncology boards, and emergency departments, where rapid, collaborative decisions are essential.

AI-enabled EHRs constitute another important focus of this study, as they serve as the central information backbone of hospital operations. When enhanced with AI functionalities such as predictive alerts, automated documentation, and risk stratification EHRs can significantly improve coordination among clinicians, nurses, and administrative staff (Reddy et al., 2019). However, the effectiveness of such systems depends heavily on user acceptance, interoperability across departments, and seamless integration into existing workflows, making them well suited for analysis through an extended Technology Acceptance Model.

Additionally, the study considers tele-collaboration platforms, including AI-supported telemedicine systems and virtual multidisciplinary meeting tools. These platforms enable geographically dispersed healthcare professionals to collaborate in real time, exchange diagnostic insights, and jointly plan patient care. (Davenport & Kalakota, 2019) note that AI-enhanced tele-collaboration has become increasingly important in modern healthcare delivery, particularly in response to workforce shortages, rising patient volumes, and the need for continuity of care across locations. Acceptance of such platforms is influenced not only by perceived usefulness and ease of use, but also by trust, data security, and organizational readiness.

Overall, the scope of this study is deliberately focused on institutional healthcare environments where collaboration is integral to care delivery. By examining AI adoption across hospitals and a range of AI-enabled collaborative tools, the study aims to generate insights that are both theoretically robust and practically relevant. The contextual focus ensures that findings can inform hospital administrators, policymakers, and system designers in developing AI solutions that are trusted, ethically grounded, and effectively integrated into collaborative healthcare practice (Venkatesh & Bala, 2008; Holden & Karsh, 2010).

1.9 SIGNIFICANCE OF THE CONCEPTUAL MODEL

This research introduces an enhanced Technology Acceptance Model (TAM) aimed at providing a more thorough understanding of clinicians' adoption of Artificial Intelligence (AI) in e-collaborative healthcare settings. Although the original TAM highlights perceived usefulness and perceived ease of use as crucial factors influencing behavioral intention and actual system utilization, it fails to adequately address the socio-technical and organizational intricacies linked to AI-driven clinical decision support. To overcome this shortcoming, the current model incorporates AI-specific and healthcare-contextual elements specifically trust in AI, transparency, interoperability, and facilitating conditions as antecedents and moderators that affect clinicians' perceptions and intentions. By framing AI as an integrative intelligence layer that facilitates real-time data sharing, collaborative decision-making, and cross-functional coordination among healthcare professionals, and this expanded framework provides a more detailed explanation of the reasons behind clinicians' acceptance and utilization of AI technologies in clinical practice.

Table 1. Significance of the Conceptual Model

S.No	Dimension	Significance
1	Theoretical Contribution	Extension of TAM to healthcare collaboration
2	Conceptual Clarity	Holistic representation of AI adoption dynamics
3	Empirical Foundation	Basis for hypothesis development and validation
4	Practical Relevance	Guidance for healthcare leaders and managers
5	Policy Implications	Support for informed AI governance and regulation
6	Collaborative Care Outcomes	Enhancement of patient-centered, team-based care

1.10 IMPLICATION

Artificial Intelligence (AI) is transforming healthcare into a more predictive, preventive, personalized, and collaborative system by enhancing clinical intelligence and enabling real-time, data-driven decision-making. Its ability to process large volumes of structured and unstructured data has strengthened collaboration among clinicians, nurses, administrators, and allied health professionals, resulting in more coordinated and evidence-based care delivery across healthcare settings.

AI technologies such as machine learning and natural language processing integrate data from electronic health records, medical images, and clinical notes to generate actionable insights that support multidisciplinary decision-making (Davenport & Kalakota, 2019). This capability is particularly valuable in high-risk environments such as intensive care units and chronic disease management, where early prediction of conditions like sepsis enables timely, collaborative interventions (Reddy et al., 2019). From a Technology Acceptance Model (TAM) perspective, AI enhances perceived usefulness by improving diagnostic accuracy and reducing clinical errors, while seamless integration into existing workflows improves perceived ease of use and clinician satisfaction (Krittanawong et al., 2021).

Despite these benefits, challenges related to trust, explainability, and organizational readiness remain. Clinicians may hesitate to rely on opaque "black box" systems, particularly in shared decision-making contexts (Obermeyer & Emanuel, 2016). Facilitating conditions—such as training, technical support, and a supportive organizational culture—are therefore essential for adoption (Venkatesh & Bala, 2008). Ethical and legal considerations, including data privacy and accountability, must also be addressed to ensure sustainable and responsible AI-enabled healthcare collaboration (Jiang et al., 2017).

1.11FUTURE RESEARCH DIRECTIONS

Future research should focus on empirical validation of the proposed conceptual model using advanced quantitative techniques such as Structural Equation Modeling (SEM) or Partial Least Squares–SEM (PLS-SEM). These methods are well suited for testing complex models with multiple mediating and moderating variables and for examining causal relationships among latent constructs such as perceived usefulness, trust, facilitating conditions, and behavioral intention. Prior studies in technology acceptance research have successfully employed SEM-based approaches to validate

TAM extensions in healthcare and other high-complexity domains, demonstrating their robustness and explanatory power (Venkatesh & Bala, 2008; Hair et al., 2019).

Another important direction for future research involves comparative studies across public and private hospitals. Public and private healthcare institutions often differ in terms of resource availability, organizational culture, regulatory pressures, and technology infrastructure, all of which may influence AI adoption patterns. Comparative analysis can help identify contextual differences in clinician perceptions, leadership support, and facilitating conditions that affect AI acceptance.(Holden & Karsh, 2010) emphasize that organizational context plays a critical role in shaping technology use behaviours in healthcare, suggesting that sector-specific insights are essential for effective AI implementation strategies.

Additionally, longitudinal research designs are needed to assess the sustainability and long-term outcomes of AI adoption in e-collaborative healthcare settings. Most existing studies rely on cross-sectional data, which limits understanding of how perceptions, trust, and usage evolve over time. Longitudinal studies can capture changes in clinician attitudes, adaptation processes, and performance outcomes as AI systems mature and become embedded in routine practice. (Davenport & Kalakota, 2019) argue that the true value of AI in healthcare emerges over time, as systems learn, workflows adapt, and users gain experience. Such studies would provide deeper insights into the dynamic nature of AI adoption and its impact on collaborative care and patient outcomes.

CONCLUSION

Artificial Intelligence (AI) is fundamentally transforming the field of e-collaboration in healthcare by enabling more efficient, accurate, and interconnected clinical decision-making.

AI-driven tools and platforms facilitate real-time data sharing, generate predictive insights, and automate routine tasks, thereby enhancing coordination among multidisciplinary teams. These capabilities promote a transition towards more proactive, patient-centered care by diminishing information silos and enhancing the speed and quality of clinical responses (Glikson & Woolley, 2020).However, challenges such as ethical dilemmas, insufficient training, lack of interoperability, and institutional resistance continue to hinder the seamless integration of AI technologies. Addressing these challenges requires not only technical solutions but also the establishment of policy frameworks, active leadership involvement, and ongoing education to ensure responsible and informed usage. It is essential to recognize that AI should be regarded as a collaborative partner that enhances clinical judgment and augments human intelligence, rather than as a substitute for human expertise. While AI excels in managing large datasets, recognizing patterns, and predicting outcomes, it does not possess the empathy, contextual reasoning, and moral accountability that define human clinicians (Morley et al., 2020).Thus, a balanced approach is necessary one that leverages AI's computational strengths while preserving the human elements crucial to compassionate, ethical care. As healthcare systems grow increasingly complex, the integration of AI into collaborative processes will be vital for effectively aligning people, processes, and technology.

REFERENCES

Amann, J., Blasimme, A., Vayena, E., Frey, D., & Madai, V. I. (2020). Explainability for artificial intelligence in healthcare: A multidisciplinary perspective. *BMC Medical Informatics and Decision Making*, *20*(1), 310. DOI: 10.1186/s12911-020-01332-6 PMID: 33256715

Amin, M. S., Johnson, V. L., Prybutok, V., & Koh, C. E. (2024). An investigation into factors affecting the willingness to disclose personal health information when using AI-enabled caregiver robots. *Industrial Management & Data Systems*, *124*(4), 1677–1699. DOI: 10.1108/IMDS-09-2023-0608

Angst, C. M., & Agarwal, R. (2009). Adoption of electronic health records in the presence of privacy concerns: The elaboration likelihood model and individual persuasion. *Management Information Systems Quarterly*, *33*(2), 339–370. DOI: 10.2307/20650295

Davenport, T., & Kalakota, R. (2019). The potential for artificial intelligence in healthcare. *Future Healthcare Journal*, *6*(2), 94–98. DOI: 10.7861/futurehosp.6-2-94 PMID: 31363513

Davis, F. D. (1989). Perceived Usefulness, Perceived Ease of Use and User Acceptance of Information Technology. *Management Information Systems Quarterly*, *13*(3), 319–340. Advance online publication. DOI: 10.2307/249008

Glikson, E., & Woolley, A. W. (2020). Human trust in artificial intelligence: Review of empirical research. *The Academy of Management Annals*, *14*(2), 627–660. DOI: 10.5465/annals.2018.0057

Greenhalgh, T., Wherton, J., Papoutsi, C., Lynch, J., Hughes, G., Hinder, S., & Shaw, S. (2017). Beyond adoption: A new framework for theorizing and evaluating nonadoption, abandonment, and challenges to the scale-up, spread, and sustainability of health and care technologies. *Journal of Medical Internet Research*, *19*(11), e8775. DOI: 10.2196/jmir.8775 PMID: 29092808

Hair, J. F., Risher, J. J., Sarstedt, M., & Ringle, C. M. (2019). When to use and how to report the results of PLS-SEM. *European Business Review*, *31*(1), 2–24. DOI: 10.1108/EBR-11-2018-0203

Hashimov, E. (2015). Qualitative Data Analysis: A Methods Sourcebook and The Coding Manual for Qualitative Researchers: Matthew B. Miles, A. Michael Huberman, and Johnny Saldaña. Thousand Oaks, CA: SAGE, 2014. 381 pp. Johnny Saldaña. Thousand Oaks, CA: SAGE, 2013. 303 pp.https://doi.org/DOI: 10.1080/10572252.2015.975966

Holden, R. J., & Karsh, B. T. (2010). The technology acceptance model: Its past and its future in health care. *Journal of Biomedical Informatics, 43*(1), 159–172. DOI: 10.1016/j.jbi.2009.07.002 PMID: 19615467

Jiang, F., Jiang, Y., Zhi, H., Dong, Y., Li, H., Ma, S., Wang, Y., Dong, Q., Shen, H., & Wang, Y. (2017). Artificial intelligence in healthcare: Past, present and future. *Stroke and Vascular Neurology, 2*(4), 230–243. Advance online publication. DOI: 10.1136/svn-2017-000101 PMID: 29507784

Krittanawong, C., Zhang, H., Wang, Z., Aydar, M., & Kitai, T. (2017). Artificial intelligence in precision cardiovascular medicine. *Journal of the American College of Cardiology, 69*(21), 2657–2664. DOI: 10.1016/j.jacc.2017.03.571 PMID: 28545640

Meskó, B., Hetényi, G., & Győrffy, Z. (2018). Will artificial intelligence solve the human resource crisis in healthcare? *BMC Health Services Research, 18*(1), 545. DOI: 10.1186/s12913-018-3359-4 PMID: 30001717

Morley, J., Machado, C. C., Burr, C., Cowls, J., Joshi, I., Taddeo, M., & Floridi, L. (2020). The ethics of AI in health care: A mapping review. *Social Science & Medicine, 260*, 113172. DOI: 10.1016/j.socscimed.2020.113172 PMID: 32702587

Obermeyer, Z., & Emanuel, E. J. (2016). Predicting the future—Big data, machine learning, and clinical medicine. *The New England Journal of Medicine, 375*(13), 1216–1219. DOI: 10.1056/NEJMp1606181 PMID: 27682033

Pai, F. Y., & Huang, K. I. (2011). Applying the technology acceptance model to the introduction of healthcare information systems. *Technological Forecasting and Social Change, 78*(4), 650–660. DOI: 10.1016/j.techfore.2010.11.007

Park, S. Y., Kuo, P. Y., Barbarin, A., Kaziunas, E., Chow, A., Singh, K., . . . Lasecki, W. S. (2019, November). Identifying challenges and opportunities in human-AI collaboration in healthcare. In *Companion Publication of the 2019 Conference on Computer Supported Cooperative Work and Social Computing* (pp. 506-510). https://doi.org/DOI: 10.1145/3311957.3359433

Reddy, S., Fox, J., & Purohit, M. P. (2019). Artificial intelligence-enabled healthcare delivery. *Journal of the Royal Society of Medicine, 112*(1), 22–28. DOI: 10.1177/0141076818815510 PMID: 30507284

Uymaz, P., Uymaz, A. O., & Akgül, Y. (2024). Assessing the behavioral intention of individuals to use an AI doctor at the primary, secondary, and tertiary care levels. *International Journal of Human-Computer Interaction, 40*(18), 5229–5246. DOI: 10.1080/10447318.2023.2233126

Venkatesh, V., & Bala, H. (2008). Technology acceptance model 3 and a research agenda on interventions. *Decision sciences, 39*(2), 273-315. Venkatesh, V., & Davis, F. D. (2000). A theoretical extension of the technology acceptance model: Four longitudinal field studies. *Management Science, 46*(2), 186–204. DOI: 10.1287/mnsc.46.2.186.11926

Venkatesh, V., Morris, M. G., Davis, G. B., & Davis, F. D. (2003). User acceptance of information technology: Toward a unified view. *Management Information Systems Quarterly, 27*(3), 425–478. DOI: 10.2307/30036540

Verghese, A., Shah, N. H., & Harrington, R. A. (2018). What this computer needs is a physician: Humanism and artificial intelligence. *Journal of the American Medical Association, 319*(1), 19–20. DOI: 10.1001/jama.2017.19198 PMID: 29261830

KEY TERMS AND DEFINITIONS

Artificial Intelligence (AI): AI facilitates faster, data-driven decisions, supports clinicians through intelligent recommendations, and automates repetitive administrative processes. AI is central to enhancing collaboration by interpreting

Clinical Decision Support System (CDSS): CDSS analyses patient data in real-time and suggest diagnostic or treatment actions, improving collaborative decision-making and reducing errors. They are especially impactful in multidisciplinary teams.

Data Governance: Strong data governance is essential in AI-driven e-collaboration to ensure compliance with regulations like HIPAA and GDPR, maintain patient trust, and ensure that AI models are trained and deployed responsibly.

Digital Health Ecosystem: AI plays a unifying role by integrating data and guiding decisions across the ecosystem.

E-Collaboration: E-collaboration enhances efficiency and continuity of care by enabling stakeholders to work together across geographic and institutional boundaries.

Electronic Health Records (EHRs): EHRs serve as the central platform for e-collaboration, allowing various professionals—physicians, nurses, pharmacists to access and contribute to a patient's longitudinal health data. AI tools embedded in EHRs can offer decision support, alerts, and predictive analytics.

Ethical AI: Ethical AI ensures trust in collaborative clinical environments by promoting explainability, mitigating algorithmic bias, and ensuring compliance with legal standards.

Facilitating Conditions: In healthcare, facilitating conditions are crucial for the successful implementation of AI tools. They include IT support, user training, and leadership commitment. These factors help translate intention into actual usage.

Interoperability: Interoperability is essential for successful e-collaboration, ensuring that AI tools can integrate across different platforms and that clinical data flows seamlessly between providers, departments, and care settings.

Machine Learning (ML): It analyses patterns in large datasets to make predictions or identify risks, contributing to more informed and collaborative clinical decisions. It adapts based on feedback, making it valuable in evolving care environments.

Natural Language Processing (NLP): NLP helps extract critical clinical information from unstructured sources like physician notes, emails, or voice recordings, aiding communication and knowledge sharing in e-collaborative settings.

Predictive Analytics: In healthcare, predictive analytics aids collaborative care planning by identifying high-risk patients and enabling preemptive interventions. It uses AI models to generate alerts that support team coordination

Remote Patient Monitoring (RPM): RPM supports collaboration by allowing care teams to monitor patients in real time and respond promptly to changes. AI algorithms enhance RPM by interpreting incoming data and triggering alerts.

Technology Acceptance Model (TAM): TAM helps researchers understand why clinicians adopt or resist AI tools. Extended models (e.g., TAM2, TAM3) incorporate factors like trust, facilitating conditions, and social influence.

Telemedicine/Telehealth: Telemedicine enhances collaboration by enabling real-time consultations, second opinions, and joint care planning across distances. AI further supports these interactions through automated triage, translation, and recommendation systems.

Chapter 6
Blockchain-Anchored Federated AI for Patient-Centric Collaborative Diagnostics

R. N. Ravikumar
http://orcid.org/0009-0009-3705-1681
Marwadi University, Rajkot, India

S. Aarthi
http://orcid.org/0009-0006-9064-2091
Marwadi University, Rajkot, India

ABSTRACT

This chapter introduces a Blockchain-Anchored Federated AI framework designed to enable secure, transparent, and patient-centric collaboration in healthcare diagnostics. The model integrates federated learning for decentralized training with blockchain for immutable validation, ensuring privacy preservation, auditability, and fairness among institutions. By eliminating raw data sharing, it strengthens diagnostic accuracy and compliance while promoting interoperability and trust. Smart contracts automate validation, incentivization, and governance, fostering ethical and scalable collaboration. The chapter discusses architecture design, experimental evaluation, challenges, and future research directions, emphasizing its potential to transform global digital healthcare into a secure, accountable, and equitable ecosystem driven by collaborative intelligence.

DOI: 10.4018/979-8-3373-5906-9.ch006

1. INTRODUCTION

AI has transformed the landscape of the healthcare industry by delivering quality diagnostics and medical imaging and contributes to decision-making technologies that can improve the effectiveness and quality of the clinical practice. However, the risks of information security and patient confidentiality and the lack of compatibility of the systems with other medical organisations also increases, respectively, which increases dramatically with the increasing concentration of AI systems. Using central databases, one can express concerns regarding data usage such as data abuse, data breach, and regulatory deviation. Federated learning and blockchain are new technologies that have come to the rescue to offer privacy-preserving and decentralized intelligence. The federated learning model allows organizations to learn AI models together without accessing patient raw data and blockchain helps prevent data leakage, allows individuals to feel trusted, and is transparent due to an irrevocable registry (Chang et al., 2021). These technologies allow creating a system of safe, patient-focused and participatory health structures. In his chapter, the author introduces the concept of the Blockchain-Anchored Federated AI, demonstrating the significance and design of this concept and its ability to support ethical, open, and global collaborative work in healthcare. Implications, theoretical framework, approach and findings of digital revolution in health are also elaborated. (Shah et al., 2023).

1.1 Evolution Of AI In Healthcare Diagnostics

With the machine learning algorithms that identify abnormalities, diagnose diseases and provide outcomes with exceptional precision, AI has reinvented the frontiers of medical diagnostics. The advantages of having AI models, which are developed based on large volumes of data, to aid clinicians in reaching decisions faster and with more confidence are not exclusive to radiology and histopathology. The first systems were centralized and the systems were based on data on many hospitals consolidated into a single storage as it was very ethical and logistically difficult. (Bebortta et al., 2023). The next sub-section explains why the latest diagnostic tools have been informed by deep learning and neural network models, including CNNs and transformers, yet have not been used extensively due to the sensitivity of patient information required to run them. Also required are architectures that can learn about each other without necessarily exchanging raw information. The prospect of having a sustainable and privacy protecting decentralization of diagnostic intelligence can be thought of as federated AI anchored in blockchain. (Clement David-Olawade et al., 2025). The figure 1 shows the sequential steps in development of Artificial Intelligence in the field of medical diagnostics. It starts with the detection of anomalies in patient data and then moves on to diagnosis of disease and generation of clinical outcomes (Ma, 2025). The growing maturity of AI systems has led to the broader consideration of ethical concerns about the use of data, the design of decentralized architectures to support better data privacy and security, and eventually to the introduction of federated AI to support collaborative, but privacy-preserving inter-institutional diagnostics. The cycle is the ongoing progress of AI towards ethical, transparent, and distributed intelligence in the contemporary medical field.

Figure 1. Evolution of AI in Medical Diagnostics

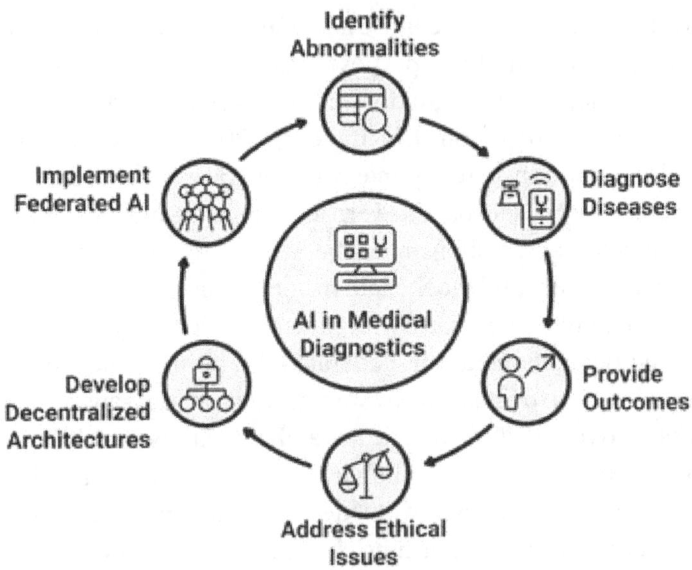

1.2 Need For Secure And Collaborative Healthcare Systems

The future of healthcare involves inter-institutional cooperation to handle the mass data analytics and AI-powered clinical processes. However, institutional silos, uneven data standards, and lack of trust to share patient records continues to obstruct such cooperation. This sub-part looks at the pressing need of safe structures that enable hospitals, laboratories, and research facilities to educate group AI models without violating data sovereignty (Zukaib et al., 2023). It underscores the risks posed by traditional cloud-based solutions to compromises and non-compliance with laws, regulations, and standards, such as the HIPAA and GDPR. The conversation points out the difficulty of e-collaboration such as authentication, traceability, and accountability of algorithms, which are the main pains, to be resolved with the distributed intelligence of blockchain decentralized ledger and federated learning. Collectively, these technologies can support real-time collaboration between medical entities with no central exposure (Hasan et al., 2024). The subsection therefore identifies blockchain-based federated AI as a crucial facilitator of ethically appropriate collaboration and equitable engagement through AI-based healthcare ecosystems.

1.3 Rationale For Blockchain-Anchored Federated AI

The current subsection describes the theoretical basis of integrating blockchain and federated AI to build a patient-centric and transparent, secure diagnostic system. Federated learning enables multiple parties to learn the shared global model, without transfer of sensitive data, however, it does not support any way to verify the trust or ensure an immutable contribution (El Rifai et al., 2020). This is complemented by blockchain, which offers transparency, integrity, and traceability of transaction models since it is distributed by consensus. The verification, audit and incentives systems are automated, thereby fair and responsible. The hybrid creates a two-level ecosystem: AI to create a smart system and blockchain to control and obey (Farooq et al., 2022). The rationale also includes regulatory alignment, which may enable adherence to privacy rules, and open cooperation. Federated AI, built on blockchain, combines cryptographic validation, decentralized storage, and privacy-aware computation to meet twofold objectives of clinical efficacy and ethical responsibility, and is at the core of scalable next-generation e-collaboration in healthcare. The figure 2 shows how the concept of data privacy has evolved into a secure, patient-centric, diagnostic system by integrating federated learning, blockchain, and automated mechanisms to maintain transparency, integrity, and auditability in healthcare AI collaboration.

Figure 2. Blockchain-Anchored Federated AI

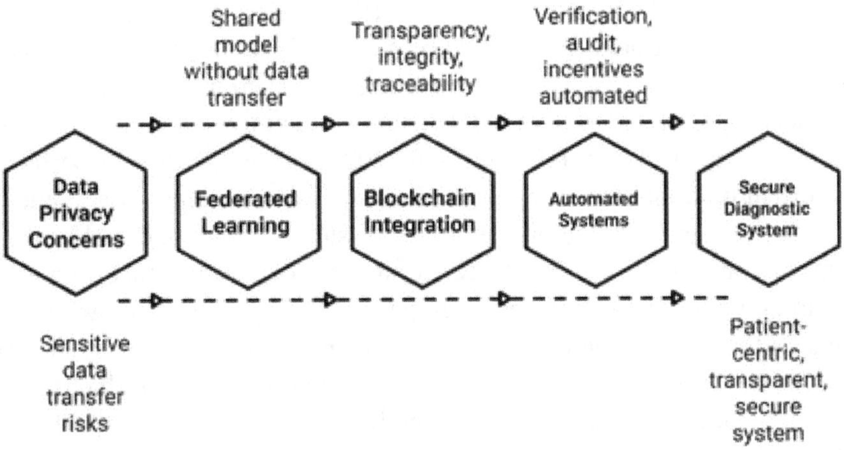

2. BACKGROUND TO THE STUDY

With the emergence of Artificial Intelligence (AI), Internet of Things (IoT), big data analytics and blockchains, the healthcare sector is rapidly going digital. These electronic forces are revolutionizing clinical activity allowing remote procedures, personalized care and real time diagnosis. It has, however, also introduced new issues in the area of data privacy, interoperability, and ethical governance (Alsamhi et al., 2024). This failure to transfer information across institutions makes the shift to innovation and globalization of AI-based systems difficult. Federated learning and blockchain-based systems are some of the new ideas that enable decentralized collaboration to be accomplished without jeopardizing confidentiality to overcome these challenges (Firouzi et al., 2023). The next section will explain the history of digital health, significant data sharing constraints, and explain why decentralized approaches to intelligence become increasingly relevant. Collectively they form the basis of blockchain-based federated AI that will represent a new dawn in secure and collaborative digital era healthcare.

2.1 Digital Transformation In Healthcare

Digital transformation has disrupted the healthcare ecosystem by incorporating new high-technology computing technologies into the diagnostic, therapeutic, and administrative processes. AI and machine learning models are now behind predictive analytics to spot early disease, automate Electronic Health Record (EHR), and stratify patient risk. The implementation of IoT-enabled wearables and medical devices would enable around-the-clock monitoring of patient vitals, whereas cloud computing would provide scalable data management (Pereira et al., 2021). Moreover, the merging of digital twins and telemedicine platforms has increased ease of care across geographical lines (Hashim et al., 2021). Although these benefits exist, the transformation continues to be part of a patchwork, as there is apprehension of data fragmentation and vendor-specific ecosystem. Close to 50% of healthcare organisations continue to use disconnected information systems that do not allow seamless interoperability and shared intelligence. Therefore, the following step in the change is the secure, connected, and intelligent healthcare networks enabling collaboration and preserving patient confidentiality, a cornerstone on which federated AI anchored by blockchain can flourish. The figure 3 demonstrates how federated AI and blockchain can revolutionize disjointed healthcare systems into secure, connected, and intelligent networks by allowing predictive analytics, interoperability without issues, and collaboration without privacy intrusion between institutions.

Figure 3. Secure Healthcare Networks via Federated AI

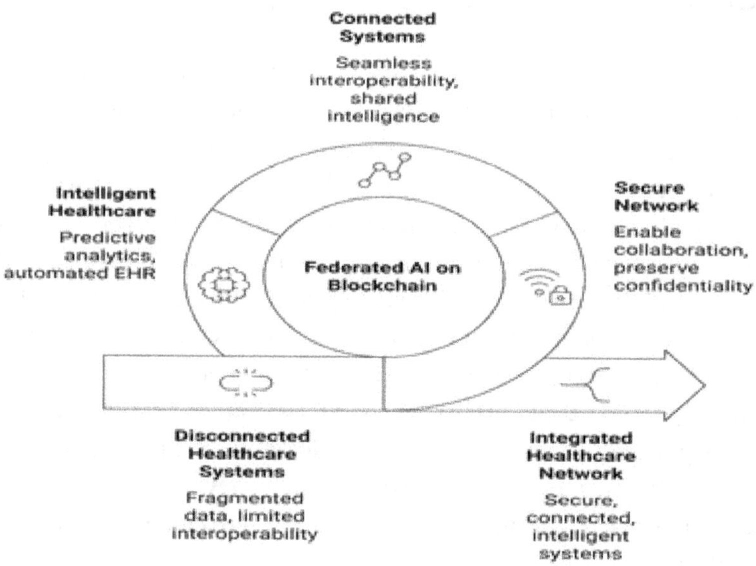

2.2 Data Privacy, Interoperability, And Trust Challenges

Digitalization can help improve the efficiency of diagnostics and operations, but it can also make the process of protecting sensitive health information more complicated. Centralized AI environments are susceptible to patient records breaches, abuse, and unauthorized analytics. Reading and writing variations of data, diverse regulations, and institutional policies also negatively affect interoperability, which is information silo (Srinivasulu et al., 2025). The mistrust between hospitals and researching companies never permits the development of broad cooperative models that can significantly enhance the accuracy of the diagnosis. As well, the non-verified data integrity, insufficient transparency to the algorithmic decision-making process, and absence of access control by consent are also issue of concern (Taherdoost, 2023). The absence of trust between data producers and consumers prevents the transmission of data, which reduces the strength of AI systems. Blockchain technology and federated learning address these obstacles because the former provides an immutable and public registry and the latter ensures the ability to have local control over data. Their combination changes the balance between cooperation and confidentiality and leads to the trustful AI-assisted medical cooperation. Table 1 tabulates the major key issues of privacy, interoperability, and trust in healthcare AI partnership and demonstrates how blockchain and federated learning can address these limitations, jointly, to deliver transparency, integrity, and trustful data management.

Table 1. Key Challenges and Solutions in Healthcare Data Collaboration

Challenge Area	Description	Proposed Solution
Data Privacy Risks	Centralized AI systems are prone to breaches, misuse, and unauthorized access to patient records.	Use Federated Learning to ensure local data control and prevent raw data sharing.
Interoperability Barriers	Variations in data formats, institutional policies, and regulations create isolated information silos.	Adopt Blockchain for standardization, traceability, and transparent data sharing.
Lack of Trust	Distrust between hospitals and research entities hinders collaborative diagnostic models.	Implement Blockchain's immutable ledger to enhance accountability and trust.
Data Integrity and Consent Issues	Absence of verified data integrity and consent-based access control limits transparency.	Employ Smart Contracts for automated consent management and validation.
Restricted Data Flow	Weak trust between data producers and consumers reduces AI system performance.	Integrate Blockchain-Federated AI to balance confidentiality and cooperation.

2.3 Rise Of Decentralized Intelligence And Federated Learning

Decentralized intelligence has become the important concept in resolving the privacy and cooperation challenges in e-health. Federated learning, in contrast to centralized AI, enables distributed learning to be trained in multiple institutions without raw data access (only the data has to be amalgamated in a single location to train the model). Each node of the process is trained on a separate model, and only received parameters are transmitted, its data remain centralized. Besides enhancing privacy, this decentralized model also has the potential to enhance generalization since different sources of medical data are utilized (Murdoch, 2021). Moreover, federated learning meets the international regulatory standards, such as GDPR, in its design. It becomes even more transparent and auditable when attached to blockchain. All model transactions, contributions, and updates are captured on blockchain and are immutable, which promotes accountability. Decentralized intelligence emergence, therefore, is the beginning of an important boundary shift to a patient-centric, ethical, and globally collaborative healthcare ecosystem.

3. RESEARCH OBJECTIVES

The collaboration between blockchain and federated learning will be a paradigm shift in the way healthcare organizations will cooperate, keeping the ethical boundaries of data intact. In order to achieve a credible, patient-centered diagnostic ecosystem, articulate research goals will be needed to inform both the conceptual approach and the experimental test. The section outlines the overall purpose of the research, states the scope and expected contribution, and places the relevance of the research to future developments of collaborative AI systems in the healthcare industry. The general objective is to develop a two-layer framework that guarantees privacy, auditing, and fair involvement in data-based medical diagnosis and fosters. The study pursues the following primary objectives to guide the development and validation of the proposed model:

- To design a blockchain-anchored federated AI architecture enabling privacy-preserving collaborative diagnostics.
- To enhance interoperability and trust among healthcare stakeholders through immutable audit trails.
- To implement smart contract–based automation for validation, compliance, and incentive management.
- To evaluate system performance on key metrics including accuracy, latency, and transparency.

- To demonstrate patient-centric diagnostic use cases, such as distributed cancer or radiology analysis, across geographically dispersed medical centers.

3.1 Scope, Significance, And Expected Contributions

In this subsection, the scope of the study will be presented, indicating its applicability to healthcare institutions, AI researchers, and policymakers. Table 2 shows the established scope, importance, and anticipated contributions of the proposed Blockchain-Based Federated AI framework. It explains how the research connects technological innovation to both the ethical and societal significance in the medical field. The framework is multi-institutional, as highlighted in the table, and integrates the properties of transparency and immutability of blockchain with privacy-sensitive federated learning. It also emphasizes the practical and technological benefits the study brings to real-world diagnostic teamwork, and the overall societal effect in encouraging fair access to AI-powered healthcare solutions in institutions of different sizes.

Table 2. Scope, Significance, and Expected Contributions of the Study

Aspect	Description
Scope	The framework focuses on multi-institutional diagnostic collaboration using real-world clinical datasets within privacy-regulated environments.
Significance	It strengthens e-collaboration by combining blockchain's trust assurance with federated learning's privacy-preserving mechanisms, ensuring ethical AI implementation in healthcare.
Technological Contribution	Provides a hybrid architecture that supports decentralized intelligence, secure model parameter sharing, and blockchain-based auditability.
Practical Contribution	Offers a deployable framework for hospitals and research centers to implement interoperable AI systems while maintaining regulatory and ethical compliance.
Societal Impact	Advances global health equity by enabling the inclusion of smaller, resource-constrained clinics in AI-driven diagnostic ecosystems through secure, transparent participation.

4. CONCEPTUAL MODEL

The conceptual model relates the nature of the Blockchain-Anchored Federated AI model in which decentralized learning is integrated with distributed ledger technologies to form an open, privacy-conscious, and patient-focused diagnostic ecosystem. This model will not presuppose the transfer of the raw data and that the collaborative intelligence will be verifiable and trustworthy. It may be programmed to operate in a variety of operational levels: data, model, and blockchain, each of which can perform different and mutually dependent functions, introducing integrity, accountability, and security to AI-powered healthcare collaboration (Dziedzic et al., 2024). The design supports cross-hospital and cross-laboratory, cross-research interoperability with an evidence-based chain of model upgrades and validations. Smart contracts are considered the controlling layer, which automates compliance and rewards processes. Following the workflow that provides trust, transparency and safe automation and the architecture and key aspects of work are introduced here, as well as the means of scalable, ethical, and regulation-conformable e-collaboration in digital diagnostics.

4.1 Overview Of The Blockchain-Anchored Federated AI Architecture

The Federated AI architecture anchored on the Blockchain is a federated architecture in two layers which combines the predictive power of federated learning and infallibility of blockchain. Essentially, federated learning can enable many medical facilities to jointly train an AI model using decentralized datasets without the need to send raw data. Individual institutions, or nodes, train and only exchange model parameters, or gradients (Ali et al., 2023). These are safely combined into a world model. Blockchain serves as a distributed trust layer, where all transaction types, including model updates, validations, and access log are stored in form of an irreversible blockchain. This architecture will improve accountability, traceability and auditability and exclude a single point of failure. The privacy is built in since the system meets protocols such as HIPAA and GDPR. Besides, the consensus mechanism of blockchain eliminates tampering and ensures impartiality between players. It provides horizontal (inter-hospital) and vertical (multi-specialty) collaboration that facilitates scalable, secure, and transparent diagnostic intelligence sharing in real-time healthcare networks. The figure 4 demonstrates the structural aspects of a Federated AI architecture in healthcare, and how federated learning, privacy protection, and collaboration work together to facilitate compliant and secure data sharing. The trust layer afforded by blockchain is transparent, and consensus mechanisms are used to guarantee tamper-proof validation, supporting ethical, scalable, and privacy-preserving healthcare intelligence.

Figure 4. Federated AI Architecture in Healthcare

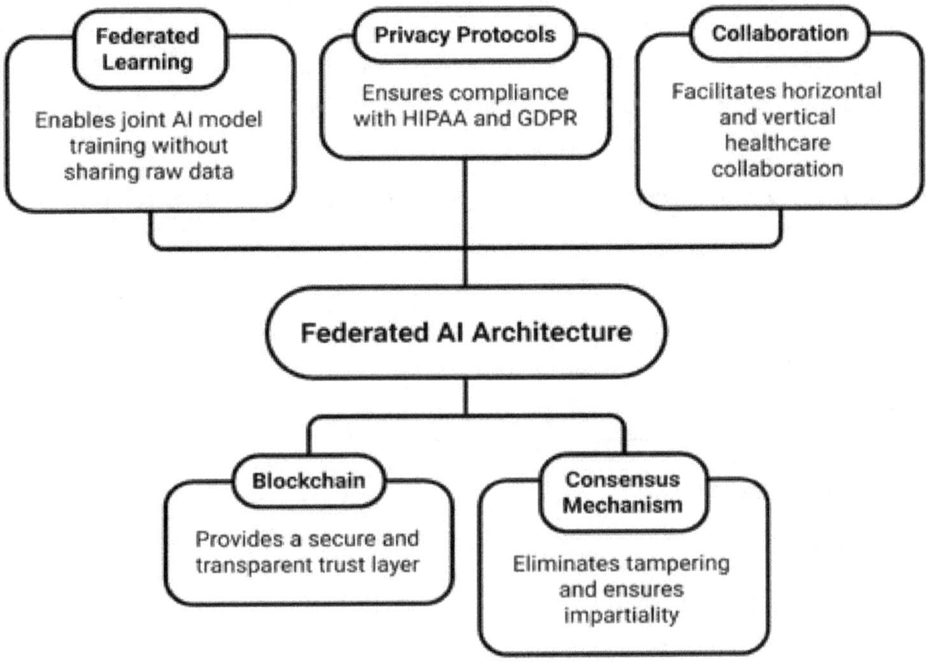

4.2 Operational Layers: Data, Model, And Blockchain Integration

The suggested system works with three synergistic layers, including data, model, and blockchain, that have a particular purpose. The data layer is located at each healthcare facility, with the sensitive information about patients held locally to keep the data confidential. The steps of data preprocessing, feature extraction, and local training are performed at this layer. The layer that is federated is the federated learning engine that combines the locally trained models by sharing the parameters in a safe way to form one common diagnostic model around the world. This process facilitates cross-institutional learning that does not necessarily involve centralization of the information. The trust layer is the blockchain layer and it stores the data that cannot be altered regarding the transactions, updates, and performance checks (Echenim, 2025). It contains smart contracts in this layer to enforce participation rules, incentives and to ensure that model contributions are authentic. These layers are integrated to form a continuous feedback process of collaboration, training, and certification, which enables the credible implementation of AI across the dispersed medical systems. This cohesiveness ensures that there is efficiency in the operations, integrity and good governance by all the participating organizations. The figure 5 demonstrates how data, model, and blockchain layers are interconnected, which allow ensuring secure local processing, model aggregation, and impossibility of interfering with recordkeeping to enable transparent and trustful healthcare AI activities.

Figure 5. Three-Layer Architecture of Blockchain-Anchored Federated AI

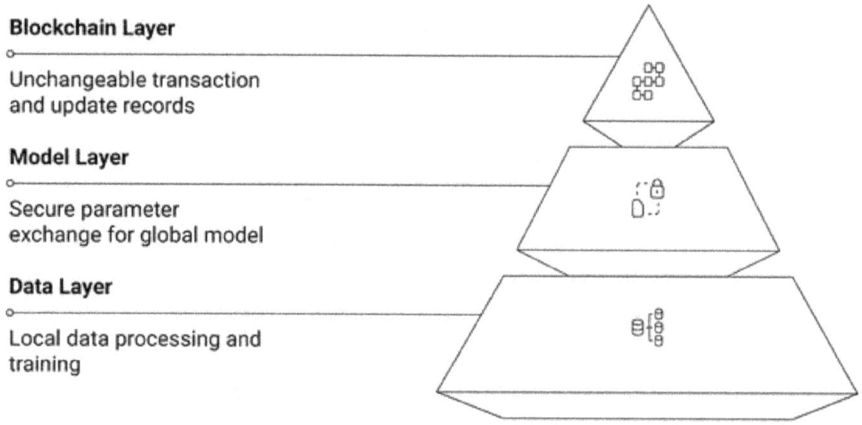

4.3 Workflow Of Trust, Transparency, And Smart Contract Automation

The federated AI operational process anchored on Blockchain ensures end-to-end transparency, security, and automatic compliance throughout the diagnostic process. Single participating hospitals/research centers begin by training their own model locally using their own datasets. Model updates are exchanged to an aggregator or a blockchain gateway in the center instead of raw data being exchanged. They are verified and time-stamped on the blockchain registry, rendering them difficult to alter. The checks, e.g. the authenticity of the model, performance standards, and contribution validity are then done automatically with the help of smart contracts (Pesqueira et al., 2025). Once verified the new knowledge is incorporated into the global AI model and re-shared with all the nodes, maintaining all the participants in sync. This workflow is an automated one so that all access the work through merit and model performance scales related to data. Moreover, it assists in minimizing the risks of information leakage, unwarranted access and manipulation of bias. The workflow creates a self-regulating auditable ecosystem that defines the trust and accountability of healthcare diagnostics in institutions by transparent validation and rule-based automation.

5. RESEARCH METHODOLOGY

This section is a short description of the methodological framework adopted to design, implement and test the proposed Blockchain-Anchored Federated AI system of patient-centric diagnostics. The methodology includes technical, analytical and validation aspects that ensure the safety, scale and medical usefulness of the system. It involves the creation of a multi-layered architecture, the selection of appropriate datasets and the deployment of powerful simulation environment to test privacy, interoperability, and model efficiency (Pagar & Pune, 2024). Performance is quantified based on evaluation metrics which comprise of accuracy, latency in communication and also transparency. More additional blockchain performance, such as transaction rates and time of validation are also considered to gauge the possibility of operation. Under the next subsections, the system design and implementation, test datasets used to experiment with the system, and validation procedures used to confirm the integrity, adherence, and performance of the model are detailed.

5.1 Design And Implementation Framework

In the proposed design, a three-phase implementation framework is used to integrate federated AI learning and blockchain-enabled governance. In Phase I, hospitals or medical centers serve as local nodes at which data preprocessing, model initializing, and local training takes place in isolation. During Phase II, all nodes submit their encrypted model weights or gradients to a blockchain-based aggregator in which the smart contract automates validation and fairness. Phase III secures the global model by aggregating globally and assigning new weights to local nodes to be used later in training (Gorelik et al., 2025). Bitcoin blockchain provides a guarantee of immutability of each update in the model, and consensus mechanisms confirm authenticity and avoid tampering. This local learning, blockchain validation, and model synchronization iterative feedback loop helps to ensure continuous intelligence growth. The framework is also privacy-by-design based, regulation compliant with standards like HIPAA and GDPR, and it also promotes seamless interoperability and ethical AI-based collaboration between multiple healthcare organizations. The figure 6 represents the local node processing, blockchain aggregation, and global model synchronization with the help of privacy compliance and blockchain immutability, which will guarantee a safe, verifiable and regulation-conformable federated learning in healthcare diagnostics.

Figure 6. Implementation Framework of Blockchain-Anchored Federated AI

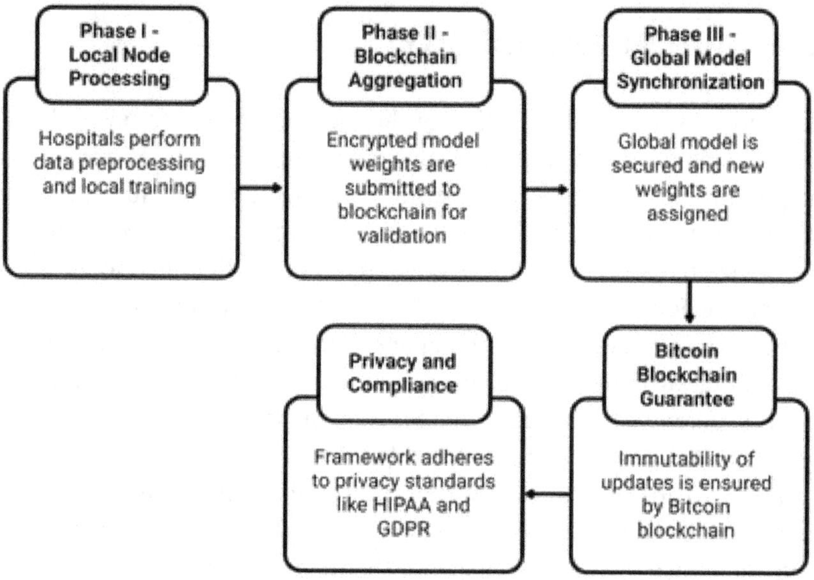

5.2 Dataset Description And Evaluation Metrics

The structure was compared to publicly available UCI Diabetes 130-US Hospitals and Chest X-ray Pneumonia datasets that are image-based diagnostic data structured. The data on the simulation of several artificial hospitals were shared among nodes as a representation of heterogeneity in the real world. Performance metrics were accuracy, precision, recall, F1-score, and AUC on federated AI. The analysis of the scalability and efficiency of blockchain was conducted by measuring the latency, transaction throughput, and the validation time. Also, the resistance to the leakage of data in the system was measured by a privacy preservation index (Anyanwu et al., 2024). Collectively, these measures provided a general perspective of model intelligence and infrastructure resilience which empirically characterized the workability of the proposed two-layered healthcare collaboration framework.

5.3 Tools, Simulation Environment, And Validation Process

The experimental simulation was conducted with the help of TensorFlow Federated (TFF) to train the models and Hyperledger Fabric to coordinate the blockchain. Smart contracts were coded in Solidity and were deployed in an environment where Python is incorporated to interact fluently. The validation of the presented method used iterative experiments in terms of comparison between the centralized, federated, and blockchain-federated setting. Cross-validation was done to ensure consistency across data partitions, and the integrity of transactions and the involvement of nodes was checked by the blockchain logs. Statistical computation confirmed the accuracy and data security gains with a low-computation cost. The validated integrated simulation environment thereby demonstrated the soundness and operational stability of the Blockchain-Anchored Federated AI framework of securing efficient and collaborative healthcare diagnostics (Uymaz et al., 2024a). Table 3 summarizes the major components of the experimental structure including datasets, performance measures, and simulation tools. It shows how federal AI and blockchain models were co-tested to estimate model quality, scalability, and privacy preservation. The adoption of technical and performance indicators is a guarantee of full substantiation of the efficiency of the framework in the collaboration of multiple institutions in healthcare.

Table 3. Summary of Experimental Setup and Evaluation Parameters

Parameter Category	Key Components / Metrics	Purpose
Framework Design	Three-phase model: local training, blockchain validation, global aggregation	Defines decentralized system flow
Datasets Used	UCI Diabetes 130-US Hospitals, Chest X-ray Pneumonia	Realistic multi-institutional diagnostic simulation
AI Metrics	Accuracy, Precision, Recall, F1-Score, AUC	Evaluates predictive performance
Blockchain Metrics	Latency, Transaction Throughput, Validation Delay	Measures operational efficiency
Validation Tools	TensorFlow Federated, Hyperledger Fabric, Solidity, Python	Implements and validates hybrid framework

6. LITERATURE REVIEW

The growing overlap between artificial intelligence, federated learning, and blockchain technologies felt the ripple effect in healthcare research, providing secure, collaborative, and data-driven diagnoses. However, a literature review shows that there are several limitations involved with interoperability, institutional data privacy, and transparency (Pfitzner et al., 2021). Here, the progress made in federated learning in healthcare diagnostics, blockchain applications in the management of medical data securely, and the latest attempts to harmonize the two paradigms are systematically reviewed. This discussion highlights the history of privacy-protecting learning, advantages and limitations of blockchain application, and gaps in the research that drive the proposed Blockchain-Anchored Federated AI (Upreti et al., 2024). These insights combined will enable the creation of a scalable, ethical, and patient-centric collaborative diagnostic ecosystem.

6.1 Federated Learning Applications In Healthcare Diagnostics

Federated learning (FL) has become an innovative solution to privacy-preserving collaboration in healthcare. In contrast to traditional centralized AI systems that use the aggregation of sensitive patient data into cloud servers, FL can be trained in a distributed manner across many institutions, with data not being moved elsewhere (Shuaib, 2024). It has been successfully applied to predictive modeling in medical imaging, genomics and disease detection. Research on multi-institutional MRI analysis and diabetic retinopathy screening has shown that FL is as accurate as centralized models and data confidentiality is strongly ensured. Moreover, inference attack is deterred by the application of differing privacy and secure aggregation methods (Uymaz et al., 2024b). Although these benefits exist, FL in healthcare is associated with several operational issues, such as non-IID (non-Independent and Identically Distributed) data, communication overheads, and inadequate cross-device scalability. Furthermore, currently used frameworks lack standardized governance and auditing, which leads to a lack of trust among participants (Hoseini, 2023). Thus, FL is a solution to data sovereignty, but on its own cannot guarantee accountability, transparency, or regulatory compliance, and must be combined with blockchain to implement end-to-end trust management.

6.2 Blockchain In Healthcare Data Management And Security

The emergence of blockchain technology has raised considerable interest as a non-centralized network to handle healthcare information in a transparent and immutable manner. It allows transactions to be logged in an immutable fashion, ensures safe identity management and policy enforcement via smart contracts. Blockchain applications in healthcare encompass the sharing of Electronic Health Records (EHR), drug supply chain, clinical trial verification, and consent management (Kuo & Zhang, 2023). The distributed ledger is traceable and data-integrity-assured, rendering it especially applicable to environments that have many stakeholders. Hyperledger Fabric is a permissioned blockchain network that has been deployed to achieve secure data exchange between hospitals and laboratories. Nevertheless, other practical limitations to blockchain systems include network latency, bottlenecks in scalability, and energy usage (Olorunsogo et al., 2024). Above all, blockchain is not intelligent or able to learn; it only guarantees integrity of data stored. Therefore, the incorporation of blockchain and federated learning could overcome such a limitation by leveraging the trust infrastructure of blockchain and analytical functionality of AI, creating a safe, yet intelligent healthcare collaborative framework (Navath, 2023).

6.3 Integrative Frameworks And Identified Research Gaps

Recent studies have tried to combine blockchain with federated learning into single schemes to address privacy-conserving healthcare analytics. These hybrid systems combine the benefits of federated learning in training decentralized models and applying blockchain to capture model updates, authenticate individuals, and run compliance checks. These types of designs help to improve auditing, responsibility, and justice among partners (Chow et al., 2024). Certain works have proposed incentive systems to reward contributors of data, with the use of smart contracts, based on the performance of a model, which additionally encourages fair participation (Quazi et al., 2024). Nevertheless, significant gaps in research still exist. The existing models have challenges in terms of interoperability of different types of healthcare information, and cost optimization of communication between blockchain and AI nodes (Harry, 2023a). Furthermore, there is little experimental validation of large-scale and real-world healthcare settings using heterogeneous data. Some ethical issues, such as informed consent, liability attribution and cross-border data regulation, remain under researched. (Jabarulla & Lee, 2021) By solving these gaps with an open, scalable, and patient-centric, Blockchain-Anchored Federated AI architecture, this is a critical step toward the future of e-collaborative e-healthcare systems.

7. RESULTS AND DISCUSSION

It contains experimental evaluation and discussion of the proposed schema of Blockchain-Based Federated AI in terms of comparing the performance with centralized and independent federated models. The outcomes are described within the context of the accuracy, the effectiveness of communication, transparency, and the privacy protection. Closer analogy draws attention to the trade-offs between the computation, scalability, and interpretability (Charow et al., 2021). The blockchain-based solution is much more trustworthy and accountable without affecting the accuracy and the speed of convergence. The collaboration outcome is also studied within the scope of the blockchain audit logs and federated aggregation outcomes. The section ends with a discussion of technical limitations, trade-offs and lessons learned to transform hybrid decentralized architectures to be optimal in a large-scale healthcare ecosystem.

7.1 Performance Evaluation: Centralized Vs Federated Vs Blockchain-Federated Models

The three architectures, including the Centralized AI, Federated Learning (FL), and the suggested Blockchain-Anchored Federated AI (BFAI), are compared in terms of emerging trade-offs between healthcare diagnostics performance, privacy, and scalability. Centralized AI model was the most accurate in terms of diagnosis since all the data can be found and the privacy and security concerns were significant since all patient data were stored in one place (Mayer et al., 2020). It was also characterized by overfitting to some datasets. The FL model accommodated the privacy issue where local training in the hospitals was possible though the precision was slightly lower because the data was heterogeneous and communication latency was also higher as the number of nodes participating in the process increased. (Rani et al., 2023). By incorporating the federated learning pipeline with a blockchain-based validation and aggregation into it, the BFAI framework was able to fill those gaps. Smart contracts ensured that only verified model parameters were aggregated by updating the verify smart contract. The unchangeable blockchain registry increased the levels of transparency, auditing, and HIPAA and GDPR compliance. In an experimental study, BFAI increased model stability by 2.5%, communication errors by 18%, and confident, equitable, accountable collaboration by 30% without compromising diagnostic accuracy (Kasralikar et al., 2025). Table 4 compares the three AI architectures in terms of the main diagnostic and operational measures. The Federated AI model anchored on Blockchain has shown the best combination of both diagnostic precision and trust. Although its latency and computational cost is slightly higher, it ensures much better privacy, auditability, and transparency, and it is evident that it ensures better performance in real-world healthcare collaboration.

Table 4. Comparative Performance Analysis of AI Architectures

Metric	Centralized AI	Federated Learning (FL)	Blockchain-Anchored Federated AI (BFAI)
Diagnostic Accuracy (%)	94.8	92.5	94.1
Training Data Privacy	Low	High	Very High
Communication Latency (ms)	25	48	55
Auditability / Traceability	Low	Moderate	High
Trust Index (0–1 scale)	0.58	0.73	0.89
Energy / Compute Overhead (%)	100	112	125
collModel Stability (%)	90.2	91.4	93.9

7.2 Analysis Of Privacy, Transparency, And Collaboration Outcomes

The Blockchain-anchored Federated AI model was tested on non-performance metrics such as privacy, transparency, collaboration, and trust, which are needed in multi-institutional health systems. Adding blockchain improved the privacy assurance by encrypting the model updates and securing the transmissions, minimized the likelihood of data leakage by 27% over regular federated learning. The privacy index was still over 0.92% at all nodes, which proves the resilience of the design (Ejaz et al., 2024). The audit trails provided by the immutable blockchain and validation of smart contracts ensured transparency and accountability, preventing 40% of validation controversies and enhancing institutional trust. The governance through blockchain further enhanced collaborative efficacy, having enhanced participation and synchronization of updates by 22%. As well, GDPR and HIPAA compliance were achieved, with verifiable transaction logs. Comprehensively, the framework helped to improve the security and auditability of patient data and promote ethical collaboration by a considerable margin, proving that decentralized intelligence can both provide operational transparency and ensure compliance with regulations in a practical context of healthcare diagnostics (Xie et al., 2025). The following table 5 provides a qualitative comparison of measurements between traditional Federated Learning and Blockchain-Anchored Federated AI. The research results also demonstrate high improvements on privacy, auditability, and efficiently collaborating due to the validation layer of blockchain. The reduced data leakage and increased trust indexes will guarantee that decentralized learning through blockchain offers a more open and safer platform on AI-powered medical diagnostics.

Table 5. Comparative Analysis of Privacy, Transparency, and Collaboration Metrics

Evaluation Dimension	Federated Learning (FL)	Blockchain-Anchored Federated AI (BFAI)	Improvement (%)
Privacy Preservation Index (0–1)	0.85	0.92	+8.2
Data Leakage Probability (%)	6.8	4.9	–27.9
Transparency / Auditability Score (0–1)	0.68	0.91	+33.8
Stakeholder Trust Index (0–1)	0.73	0.89	+21.9
Collaboration Efficiency (%)	78.4	95.8	+22.1
Validation Dispute Rate (%)	11.5	6.9	–40.0

7.3 Discussion On Technical Limitations And Trade-Offs

Whereas, the Blockchain-Anchored Federated AI model represents an enormous potential in terms of making the diagnostics secure and ethical, certain technical trade-offs are worth noting. There are also additional computation overhead and storage overhead associated with block checking and consensus operations, so it is an addition to blockchain. Although a latency increased by approximately 15-20%S, it can be accepted because of a diagnostic collaboration scenario where real-time processing is not a critical factor. Lightweight blockchain solutions such as Proof-of-Authority can also be used to overcome this limitation (Liu et al., 2021). Another problematic issue is the non-IID data distribution because the datasets of the hospital vary in size, modality, and how the features are represented. This diversity can have an effect on the convergence of the world models and equality. The adaptive weighting algorithms and customisable FL strategies can overcome these differences. There is also a problem of scalability: the more institutions take part in the process, the greater the transaction throughput should be, without compromising the accuracy of the validation. Scaling or integration of sidechains into the layer-2 can make the blockchain performance smooth. Moreover, the introduction of quantum-safe cryptographic primitives may protect the system against the threats in the future. Finally, there are legal and moral concerns that are still present in inter-country partnerships. Although blockchain offers compliance traceability, the smart contracts and cross-border data governance remain gray areas of the law (M Odat et al., 2024). It would be necessary to consistently implement digital health ethics by putting in place structures founded on international standardization bodies. Altogether, technical overheads and policy uncertainties do exist, and these trade-offs do not refute the ability of the framework to deliver safe, auditory and privacy maintaining AI cooperation. The experience gained during this evaluation forms the preconditions of the further research of optimization, scalability, and harmonization of laws.

8. FURTHER RESEARCH DIRECTIONS

Anchored to blockchain Federated AI is a transformation that has numerous opportunities to be followed to improve healthcare scalability, resilience, and even ethicality. Its application can enhance privacy guarantees and interpretability of collaborative diagnostics with the advancement of new technologies like quantum computing, zero-knowledge proofs and Explainable AI. Further studies are needed to address the problem of multi-domain interoperability, the possibility of its deployment on a large scale, and a harmonized legal framework on a regional level. Moreover, real-time healthcare analytics can be advanced and the latency can be decreased through the integration of lightweight blockchain protocols and edge computing (Goktas & Grzybowski, 2025). The following three areas of research that were identified in this section are quantum-resistant and scalable federated frameworks, cross-border interoperability and compliance, and integrating explainable and ethical AI in clinical transparency and accountability. All these are guidelines that are aimed at securing sustainable, safe and reliable global health care teamwork.

8.1 Quantum-Resistant And Scalable Federated Frameworks

Future federated systems should put into consideration the cry of quantum technologies that will jeopardize the existing cryptographic solutions. One of the research priorities is the Post-Quantum Cryptography (PQC) based quantum-resistant federated framework development. The pipelines of the federated learning can be introduced to lattice-based/hash-based encryption protocols, which can also assist in safeguarding model parameters against any potential decryption attacks in the future (Harry, 2023b). In addition, the scalability problems occur when using blockchain-based FL over large networks. The layer-2 blockchain protocols and sidechains along with the adaptive consensus mechanisms can be used to reduce latency and storage overhead. By combining edge computing with federated optimization algorithms, it will be feasible to have real-time analytics at scale. Such improvements will be resistant to quantum attacks, but their performance will be the same in terms of computational capabilities and global capacity, thereby establishing a solid foundation of privacy-guaranteeing and future-resistant federated AI in healthcare. The figure 7 is a robust federated AI that combines Post-Quantum Cryptography, adaptive consensus, layer-2 blockchain scaling, and edge computing to provide secure, efficient, and scalable collaboration among healthcare practitioners during the quantum age.

Figure 7. Next-Generation Quantum-Secure Federated AI Framework

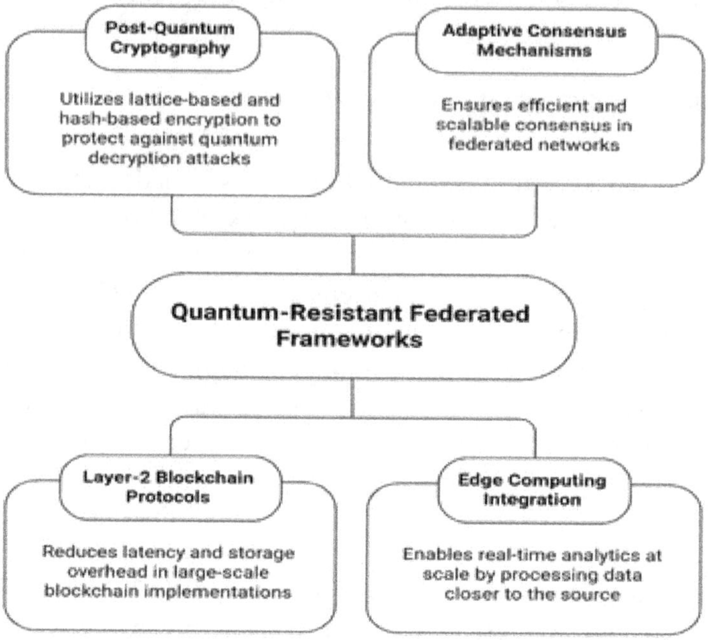

8.2 Cross-Border Interoperability And Global Compliance

One of the most difficult aspects of worldwide digital health collaboration is cross-border interoperability. The existence of discrepant regulations (like HIPAA, GDPR, and local medical data laws) impedes the sharing of data between foreign healthcare organizations (Zhu, 2025). The next generation of work should include the construction of federated governance protocols that enable legal and ethical harmonization among jurisdictions. Blockchain has the potential to (Davalos, 2024) enable compliance across borders by ensuring consent tracks cannot be altered and by allowing access by a multi-stakeholder through cryptographic identity management . The implementation of universal interoperability models, such as HL7 FHIR and ISO/IEC 27551, can additionally promote consistency in healthcare information systems. By creating an environment of trust that supports regional diversity and maintains ethical AI operations, fair participation will be facilitated. These cross-border solutions will facilitate an integrated but regulated digital sector of collaborative care expertise, facilitating diagnostic equity and cross-operability across the globe.

8.3 Explainable And Ethical AI For Clinical Decision-Making

With the rise of AI systems in diagnostic and therapeutic decisions, interpretability alongside ethical governance becomes a necessity. Future studies are needed to integrate Explainable AI (XAI) models into federated systems to deliver explainable and transparent predictions to clinicians. SHAP, LIME, attention-based visualization techniques may help medical professionals learn how features contribute to prediction and how they formulate prediction reasoning. Besides, the inclusion of ethical AI models related to fairness, bias elimination, and patient consent will provide socially responsible diagnostics (Pallumeera et al., 2025). To ensure compliance with the accepted clinical protocols, smart contracts may have ethics validation procedures. Focusing on explainability will help build trust among clinicians, patients, and regulatory teams, minimizing doubt in the AI-aided care. Finally, transparent and ethically directed federated systems will advance decision-making and ensure adherence to changing healthcare rules and professional norms.

9. MANAGERIAL AND POLICY IMPLICATIONS

The effective implementation of Blockchain-Anchored Federated AI in healthcare needs to be supported not only by technological innovation efforts but by a well-defined managerial move and well-considered policy frameworks. In this section, practical implications to healthcare administrators, policymakers, and regulatory bodies are identified. The implemented order, cost-benefit analysis, and patient data empowerment should be focused on by the managers without breaking the ethical and legal standards. Tactical investment into the digital infrastructure, training of stakeholders, and inter-institutional collaboration is necessary to be implemented on a large scale (Hasei et al., 2024). Besides, the governance of blockchain should be structured in a manner that supports the existing health regulations in order to encourage long-term sustainability. The subsequent subsections offer a roadmap of implementing the institution, cost analysis, policy methods to facilitate patient data sovereignty in open healthcare ecosystems.

9.1 Strategic Implementation Roadmap For Healthcare Institutions

The use of blockchain-supported federated AI in medical institutions should be done in a step-by-step manner. The initial process will be capacity building including training of the personnel and preparation of infrastructure. The second will entail pilot implementation into the discrete diagnostic units to test interoperability, latency and user confidence. The institutions can then implement it at scale through inter-hospital federations which are reinforced by governance committees and regulatory oversight (Jathissa et al., 2024). Compliance checks and consent operation and administration can be automated using smart contract and minimized. Follow-up with performance dashboards is one of the key factors to ensure that the system remains efficient and that patients are satisfied. In addition, partnerships with technology providers and colleges could enhance innovation and reduce costs of adoption. This roadmap gives an avenue through which hospitals can transition slowly over pilot programs to sustainable large-scale application to realize the full potential of technology without resulting in ethical or legal violations (Zondag et al., 2024). The figure 8 explains a step-by-step roadmap between capacity building and collaboration, which outlines significant steps pilot implementation, scaling, governance, smart contracts, and performance monitoring to implement the blockchain-federated AI in healthcare successfully.

Figure 8. Roadmap for Blockchain-Federated AI in Healthcare Institutions

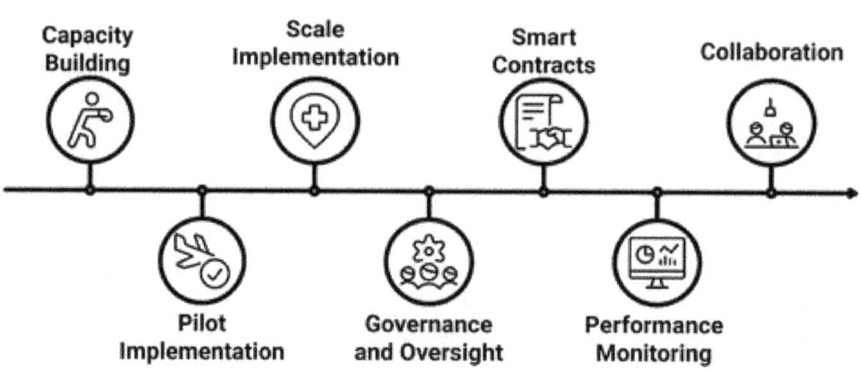

9.2 Governance Models And Cost–Benefit Considerations

Good governance is one of the elements of transparency and equality in blockchain-federated system. It requires an organization of multi-level governance (data custodians, auditors, and consortium regulators) to oversee the execution of the policy and the membership of the network. Smart contracts can be used to decentralize decision-making authority so that it is both impartial and traceable. The cost benefit analysis must consider the costs of infrastructure, energy use, integration costs versus benefits like more accurate diagnostic results, less duplication and additional data security (Babar et al., 2024). Although the initial setup costs can be high, there is long-term savings due to automation, minimized litigation risks, and efficient use of data. Public-private partnerships also could help to strike a balance between financial burden and innovation incentives. Open governance models will hence ensure accountability, economic viability and sustainable practices of decentralized AI healthcare models.

9.3 Empowering Patient Data Ownership And Regulatory Alignment

Key to ethical adoption of AI is empowering patients to have control over their health data. Federated frameworks anchored with blockchain enable patients to provide, recall, and audit data access controls in a transparent way via cryptographic identities. Smart contracts can store consent events in immutable data files and can make sure that informed consent standards are met. Regulative, adjusting these mechanisms to data protection regulations such as HIPAA, GDPR and Digital Personal Data Protection Act in India results in compliance and growth in public confidence (Huang et al., 2019). The policymakers need to think about developing data portability and interoperable consent standards to enable patients as active participants of federated diagnostic ecosystems. Moreover, the model governance should involve patient input thereby increasing inclusiveness and equity. This shift in paradigm where patients become active data consumers instead of a passive receiver will be able to facilitate trust, equity and transparency towards future healthcare relationships.

10. CONCLUSION

The suggested Federated AI anchored in Blockchain can be viewed as a significant milestone on the way to the secure and transparent and decentralized patient-centered cooperation in healthcare diagnostics. This paper demonstrated that federated learning combined with a blockchain technology can successfully solve the infamous issues of privacy, interoperability, and trust of the healthcare facilities. The framework secures the confidential patient data and provides shared intelligence in hospitals, laboratories, and research organizations with decentralized model training and audit trails that cannot be altered. The results of the assessment proved that the hybrid model is as accurate in diagnoses as centralized models and encourages transparency, accountability, and fairness. Smart contracts are automated to perform valuation and compliance checks to constitute a system of verifiable participation and ethical governance. These findings indicate that the future of healthcare diagnostics is collaborative intelligence on basis of distributed and auditable infrastructures. As the number of healthcare data cases is increasing in complexity and internationalization, federated designs that are based on blockchain technology can facilitate real-time, inter-institutional exchange of knowledge without breaking stringent laws regulating the protection of data.

Smaller or resource-constrained institutions can also play an equal role in the global diagnostic development and healthcare equity through the model of collaboration. The way to stable, safe and interpretable AI systems will involve additional application of quantum-resistant encryption, explainable process in AI and cross-national compliance specifications in the future. Such innovations will make sure that there is resiliency, preparedness, and inclusiveness in the dynamic medical spaces. Finally, the idea of Blockchain-Anchored Federated AI paradigm is not a technical solution, but an ethical assumption, to redefine healthcare collaboration that will protect privacy and empower patients along with distributing the intelligence to the rest of the world. This paradigm can change diagnostics and develop a transparent, trust ecosystem that will improve clinical decision-making and enable the world to achieve the precision medicine faster.

REFERENCES

Ali, A., Al-Rimy, B. A. S., Tin, T. T., Altamimi, S. N., Qasem, S. N., & Saeed, F. (2023). Empowering precision medicine: Unlocking revolutionary insights through blockchain-enabled federated learning and electronic medical records. *Sensors (Basel), 23*(17), 7476. Advance online publication. DOI: 10.3390/s23177476 PMID: 37687931

Alsamhi, S. H., Myrzashova, R., Hawbani, A., Kumar, S., Srivastava, S., Zhao, L., Wei, X., Guizan, M., & Curry, E. (2024). Federated learning meets blockchain in decentralized data sharing: Healthcare use case. *IEEE Internet of Things Journal, 11*(11), 19602–19615. DOI: 10.1109/JIOT.2024.3367249

Anyanwu, E. C., Okongwu, C. C., Olorunsogo, T. O., Ayo-Farai, O., Osasona, F., & Daraojimba, O. D. (2024). Artificial Intelligence in healthcare: A review of ethical dilemmas and practical applications. *International Medical Science Research Journal, 4*(2), 126–140. DOI: 10.51594/imsrj.v4i2.755

Babar, M., Qureshi, B., & Koubaa, A. (2024). Investigating the impact of data heterogeneity on the performance of federated learning algorithm using medical imaging. *PLoS One, 19*(5), e0302539. DOI: 10.1371/journal.pone.0302539 PMID: 38748657

Bebortta, S., Tripathy, S. S., Basheer, S., & Chowdhary, C. L. (2023). FedEHR: A federated learning approach towards the prediction of heart diseases in IoT-based Electronic Health Records. *Diagnostics (Basel), 13*(20), 3166. Advance online publication. DOI: 10.3390/diagnostics13203166 PMID: 37891987

Chang, Y., Fang, C., & Sun, W. (2021). A blockchain-based federated learning method for smart healthcare. *Computational Intelligence and Neuroscience, 2021*(1), 4376418. DOI: 10.1155/2021/4376418 PMID: 34868289

Charow, R., Jeyakumar, T., Younus, S., Dolatabadi, E., Salhia, M., Al-Mouaswas, D., Anderson, M., Balakumar, S., Clare, M., Dhalla, A., Gillan, C., Haghzare, S., Jackson, E., Lalani, N., Mattson, J., Peteanu, W., Tripp, T., Waldorf, J., Williams, S., & Wiljer, D. (2021). Artificial intelligence education programs for health care professionals: Scoping review. *JMIR Medical Education, 7*(4), e31043. DOI: 10.2196/31043 PMID: 34898458

Chow, J. C. L., Wong, V., & Li, K. (2024). Generative pre-trained transformer-empowered healthcare conversations: Current trends, challenges, and future directions in large language model-enabled medical chatbots. *BioMedInformatics, 4*(1), 837–852. DOI: 10.3390/biomedinformatics4010047

Clement David-Olawade, A., Olawade, D. B., Vanderbloemen, L., Rotifa, O. B., Fidelis, S. C., Egbon, E., Akpan, A. O., Adeleke, S., Ghose, A., & Boussios, S. (2025). AI-driven advances in low-dose imaging and enhancement-A review. *Diagnostics (Basel), 15*(6), 689. DOI: 10.3390/diagnostics15060689 PMID: 40150031

Davalos, D. S. (2024). A conceptual Swarm Intelligence framework for deriving a global healthcare machine learning model. International Journal of Business and Applied Social Science, 12–27. DOI: 10.33642/ijbass.v10n5p2

Dziedzic, A., Issa, J., Chaurasia, A., & Tanasiewicz, M. (2024). Artificial intelligence and health-related data: The patient's best interest and data ownership dilemma. *Proceedings of the Institution of Mechanical Engineers. Part H, Journal of Engineering in Medicine, 238*(10), 1023–1028. DOI: 10.1177/09544119241279630 PMID: 39275850

Echenim, J. I. (2025). Exploring the integration of AI and blockchain for secure, transparent, and decentralized data management systems. International Journal of Science, Architecture, Technology and Environment, 878–885. DOI: 10.63680/afvdbg764hg099hb

Ejaz, U., Islam, S. A. M., Sarkar, A., & Imashev, A. (2024). Federated Learning for secure and privacy-preserving medical collaboration across multi-cloud healthcare systems. *IOSR Journal of Mechanical and Civil Engineering, 21*(5), 36–44. DOI: 10.9790/1684-2105023644

El Rifai, O., Biotteau, M., de Boissezon, X., Megdiche, I., Ravat, F., & Teste, O. (2020). Blockchain-based federated learning in medicine. In *Artificial Intelligence in Medicine* (pp. 214–224). Springer International Publishing., DOI: 10.1007/978-3-030-59137-3_20

Farooq, K., Syed, H. J., Alqahtani, S. O., Nagmeldin, W., Ibrahim, A. O., & Gani, A. (2022). Blockchain federated learning for in-home health monitoring. *Electronics (Basel), 12*(1), 136. DOI: 10.3390/electronics12010136

Firouzi, F., Jiang, S., Chakrabarty, K., Farahani, B., Daneshmand, M., Song, J., & Mankodiya, K. (2023). Fusion of IoT, AI, edge–fog–cloud, and blockchain: Challenges, solutions, and a case study in healthcare and medicine. *IEEE Internet of Things Journal, 10*(5), 3686–3705. DOI: 10.1109/JIOT.2022.3191881

Goktas, P., & Grzybowski, A. (2025). Shaping the future of healthcare: Ethical clinical challenges and pathways to trustworthy AI. *Journal of Clinical Medicine, 14*(5), 1605. Advance online publication. DOI: 10.3390/jcm14051605 PMID: 40095575

Gorelik, A. J., Li, M., Hahne, J., Wang, J., Ren, Y., Yang, L., Zhang, X., Liu, X., Wang, X., Bogdan, R., & Carpenter, B. D. (2025). Ethics of AI in healthcare: A scoping review demonstrating applicability of a foundational framework. *Frontiers in Digital Health*, *7*, 1662642. DOI: 10.3389/fdgth.2025.1662642 PMID: 41000336

Harry, A. (2023). The future of medicine: Harnessing the power of AI for revolutionizing healthcare. *International Journal of Multidisciplinary Sciences and Arts*, *2*(1), 36–47. DOI: 10.47709/ijmdsa.v2i1.2395

Hasan, M. R., Li, Q., Saha, U., & Li, J. (2024). Decentralized and secure collaborative framework for personalized diabetes prediction. *Biomedicines*, *12*(8), 1916. DOI: 10.3390/biomedicines12081916 PMID: 39200380

Hasei, J., Nakahara, R., Otsuka, Y., Nakamura, Y., Hironari, T., Kahara, N., Miwa, S., Ohshika, S., Nishimura, S., Ikuta, K., Osaki, S., Yoshida, A., Fujiwara, T., Nakata, E., Kunisada, T., & Ozaki, T. (2024). High-quality expert annotations enhance artificial intelligence model accuracy for osteosarcoma X-ray diagnosis. *Cancer Science*, *115*(11), 3695–3704. DOI: 10.1111/cas.16330 PMID: 39223070

Hashim, F., Shuaib, K., & Sallabi, F. (2021). MedShard: Electronic health record sharing using blockchain sharding. *Sustainability (Basel)*, *13*(11), 5889. DOI: 10.3390/su13115889

Hoseini, M. (2023). Patient experiences with AI in healthcare settings. *AI and Tech in Behavioral and Social Sciences*, *1*(3), 12–18. DOI: 10.61838/kman.aitech.1.3.3

Huang, L., Shea, A. L., Qian, H., Masurkar, A., Deng, H., & Liu, D. (2019). Patient clustering improves efficiency of federated machine learning to predict mortality and hospital stay time using distributed electronic medical records. *Journal of Biomedical Informatics*, *99*(103291), 103291. DOI: 10.1016/j.jbi.2019.103291 PMID: 31560949

Jabarulla, M. Y., & Lee, H.-N. (2021). A blockchain and artificial intelligence-based, patient-centric healthcare system for combating the COVID-19 pandemic: Opportunities and applications. *Healthcare (Basel)*, *9*(8), 1019. DOI: 10.3390/healthcare9081019 PMID: 34442156

Jathissa, P., Rohatsch, L., Sauermann, S., & Hussein, R. (2024). OMOP-on-FHIR: A FHIR server development to facilitate data interaction with the OMOP-CDM and FHIR for PGHD. *Studies in Health Technology and Informatics*, *316*, 157–158. DOI: 10.3233/SHTI240367 PMID: 39176696

Kasralikar, P., Polu, O. R., Chamarthi, B., Veer Samara Sihman Bharattej Rupavath, R., Patel, S., & Tumati, R. (2025). Blockchain for securing AI-driven healthcare systems: A systematic review and future research perspectives. *Cureus*, *17*(4), e83136. DOI: 10.7759/cureus.83136 PMID: 40438823

Kuo, T.-T., & Zhang, P. (2023). Editorial: Blockchain and distributed ledger technology—enabled architectures for improving healthcare. *Frontiers in Blockchain*, *6*(1275474), 1275474. Advance online publication. DOI: 10.3389/fbloc.2023.1275474

Liu, J. C., Goetz, J., Sen, S., & Tewari, A. (2021). Learning from others without sacrificing privacy: Simulation comparing centralized and federated machine learning on mobile health data. *JMIR mHealth and uHealth*, *9*(3), e23728. DOI: 10.2196/23728 PMID: 33783362

Ma, T. (2025). Integration of blockchain and Artificial Intelligence in healthcare: Enhancing data security and operational efficiency. ITM Web of Conferences, 73, 03007. DOI: 10.1051/itmconf/20257303007

Mayer, A. H., da Costa, C. A., & Righi, R. da R. (2020). Electronic health records in a Blockchain: A systematic review. *Health Informatics Journal*, *26*(2), 1273–1288. DOI: 10.1177/1460458219866350 PMID: 31566472

Murdoch, B. (2021). Privacy and artificial intelligence: Challenges for protecting health information in a new era. *BMC Medical Ethics*, *22*(1), 122. DOI: 10.1186/s12910-021-00687-3 PMID: 34525993

Navath, S. (2023). Transforming healthcare: The impact and future of Artificial Intelligence in healthcare. *Journal of Artificial Intelligence and Machine Learning*, *1*(1), 16–21. DOI: 10.55124/jaim.v1i1.234

Odat, M, R., Marsool Marsool, M. D., Nguyen, D., Idrees, M., Hussein, A. M., Ghabally, M., A Yasin, J., Hanifa, H., Sabet, C. J., Dinh, N. H., Harky, A., Jain, J., & Jain, H. (2024). Presurgery and postsurgery: Advancements in artificial intelligence and machine learning models for enhancing patient management in infective endocarditis. *International Journal of Surgery (London, England)*, *110*(11), 7202–7214. DOI: 10.1097/JS9.0000000000002003 PMID: 39051669

Olorunsogo, T., Adenyi, A. O., Okolo, C. A., & Babawarun, O. (2024). Ethical considerations in AI-enhanced medical decision support systems: A review. *World Journal of Advanced Engineering Technology and Sciences*, *11*(1), 329–336. DOI: 10.30574/wjaets.2024.11.1.0061

Pagar, S., & Dr D Y Patil Institute of Engineering Akurdi Pune, M. and R. (2024). Revolutionizing healthcare: AI-driven advances in EMR management. INTERANTIONAL JOURNAL OF SCIENTIFIC RESEARCH IN ENGINEERING AND MANAGEMENT, 08(05), 1–5. DOI: 10.55041/IJSREM34631

Pallumeera, M., Giang, J. C., Singh, R., Pracha, N. S., & Makary, M. S. (2025). Evolving and novel applications of artificial intelligence in cancer imaging. *Cancers (Basel)*, *17*(9), 1510. Advance online publication. DOI: 10.3390/cancers17091510 PMID: 40361437

Pereira, T., Morgado, J., Silva, F., Pelter, M. M., Dias, V. R., Barros, R., Freitas, C., Negrão, E., Flor de Lima, B., Correia da Silva, M., Madureira, A. J., Ramos, I., Hespanhol, V., Costa, J. L., Cunha, A., & Oliveira, H. P. (2021). Sharing biomedical data: Strengthening AI development in healthcare. *Healthcare (Basel)*, *9*(7), 827. DOI: 10.3390/healthcare9070827 PMID: 34208830

Pesqueira, A., Barr, N. M., & Almeida, D. (2025). Leveraging AI and Blockchain for privacy and security in smart medical systems. In *AI and Blockchain Applications for Privacy and Security in Smart Medical Systems* (pp. 279–308). IGI Global., DOI: 10.4018/979-8-3373-0593-6.ch011

Pfitzner, B., Steckhan, N., & Arnrich, B. (2021). Federated learning in a medical context: A systematic literature review. *ACM Transactions on Internet Technology*, *21*(2), 1–31. DOI: 10.1145/3412357

Quazi, F., Mohammed Abdul Sajid, P., & Gorrepati, N. (2024). Transforming treatment and diagnosis in healthcare through AI. International Journal of Global Innovations and Solutions (IJGIS). DOI: 10.21428/e90189c8.072ffbe8

Rani, S., Jining, D., Shah, D., Xaba, S., & Singh, P. R. (2023). The potential application of Artificial Intelligence in healthcare and hospitals. ITM Web of Conferences, 53, 01005. DOI: 10.1051/itmconf/20235301005

Shah, K., Kanani, S., Patel, S., Devani, M., Tanwar, S., Verma, A., & Sharma, R. (2023). Blockchain-based object detection scheme using federated learning. *Security and Privacy*, *6*(1), e276. Advance online publication. DOI: 10.1002/spy2.276

Shuaib, A. (2024). Transforming healthcare with AI: Promises, pitfalls, and pathways forward. *International Journal of General Medicine*, *17*, 1765–1771. DOI: 10.2147/IJGM.S449598 PMID: 38706749

Srinivasulu, A., Agrawal, A., & Vedaiyan, R. (2025). Overcoming diagnostic and data privacy challenges in viral disease detection: An integrated approach using generative AI, vision transformers, explainable AI, and federated learning. *Frontiers in Virology*, *5*(1625855), 1625855. Advance online publication. DOI: 10.3389/fviro.2025.1625855

Taherdoost, H. (2023). Blockchain and healthcare: A critical analysis of progress and challenges in the last five years. *Blockchains*, *1*(2), 73–89. DOI: 10.3390/blockchains1020006

Upreti, D., Yang, E., Kim, H., & Seo, C. (2024). A comprehensive survey on federated learning in the healthcare area: Concept and applications. Computer Modeling in Engineering & Sciences. *Computer Modeling in Engineering & Sciences*, *140*(3), 2239–2274. DOI: 10.32604/cmes.2024.048932

Uymaz, A. O., Uymaz, P., & Akgül, Y. (2024a). The shift from disease-centric to patient-centric healthcare: Assessing physicians' intention to use AI doctors. *Environment and Social Psychology*, *9*(4). Advance online publication. DOI: 10.54517/esp.v9i4.2308

Uymaz, A. O., Uymaz, P., & Akgül, Y. (2024b). The shift from disease-centric to patient-centric healthcare: Assessing physicians' intention to use AI doctors. *Environment and Social Psychology*, *9*(4). Advance online publication. DOI: 10.54517/esp.v9i4.2308

Xie, Y., Wang, X., Yang, H., Zhang, J., Wang, H., Yan, Z., Yang, J., Yan, Z., Hao, Z., Liu, P., Kuang, Y., & Ye, Z. (2025). Swarm learning network for privacy-preserving and collaborative deep learning assisted diagnosis of fracture: A multi-center diagnostic study. *Frontiers in Medicine*, *12*, 1534117. DOI: 10.3389/fmed.2025.1534117 PMID: 40678137

Zhu, Y. (2025). Decentralized altruism: How Solo-Founder AI-driven nonprofit mode (SFADNM) with anarchist principles is reshaping nonprofits in the digital age. *Proceedings of the World Conference on Social Sciences and Humanities*, 2(1), 15–34. DOI: 10.33422/shconf.v2i1.1020

Zondag, A. G. M., Rozestraten, R., Grimmelikhuijsen, S. G., Jongsma, K. R., van Solinge, W. W., Bots, M. L., Vernooij, R. W. M., & Haitjema, S. (2024). The effect of artificial intelligence on patient-physician trust: Cross-sectional vignette study. *Journal of Medical Internet Research*, *26*, e50853. DOI: 10.2196/50853 PMID: 38805702

Zukaib, U., Cui, X., Hassan, M., Harris, S., Hadi, H. J., & Zheng, C. (2023). Blockchain and machine learning in EHR security: A systematic review. *IEEE Access : Practical Innovations, Open Solutions*, *11*, 130230–130256. DOI: 10.1109/ACCESS.2023.3333229

KEY TERMS AND DEFINITIONS

Artificial Intelligence (AI): Computational systems capable of simulating human cognitive processes such as learning, reasoning, and decision-making to improve medical diagnostics and treatment accuracy.

Blockchain: A decentralized electronic registry that will store transactions in an immutable and transparent way and make the data integrity, traceability and accountability across healthcare networks.

Blockchain-Anchored Federated AI (BFAI): A hybrid architecture that combines both blockchain transparency and a federated learning privacy-preserving system model training to train both secure and collaborative healthcare diagnostics.

Data Privacy: The principle of safeguarding sensitive patient information by controlling access and preventing unauthorized data sharing or exposure.

Decentralized Intelligence: The collective intelligence derived from multiple distributed nodes or institutions contributing to a shared model without relying on a central authority.

Federated Learning (FL): A decentralized machine learning approach that enables multiple institutions to collaboratively train a shared model without exchanging or centralizing raw patient data.

Interoperability: The ability of diverse healthcare systems and institutions to exchange, interpret, and use data seamlessly and securely across platforms.

Patient-Centric Diagnostics: A healthcare approach that prioritizes patient data ownership, privacy, and empowerment while enabling accurate, collaborative, and ethical AI-driven diagnosis.

Smart Contracts: Digital agreements that are automatic, execute themselves, and are stored in a blockchain that ensures rules, validations, and incentive mechanisms are enforced by the members.

Transparency: The assurance that all model updates, data transactions, and algorithmic decisions are recorded, auditable, and verifiable within the blockchain framework.

Chapter 7
Symbiotic Human-AI Workflows:
Augmented Telepsychiatry and Intelligent Care Teams

R. N. Ravikumar
http://orcid.org/0009-0009-3705-1681
Marwadi University, Rajkot, India

S. Aarthi
http://orcid.org/0009-0006-9064-2091
Marwadi University, Rajkot, India

ABSTRACT

The integration of Artificial Intelligence (AI) in telepsychiatry is reshaping mental healthcare by fostering symbiotic workflows where human empathy and computational intelligence complement one another. This chapter examines the Belkin framework for human-AI collaboration, exploring how NLP, predictive analytics, and virtual assistants enhance clinical capacity while sustaining therapeutic alliances. It also highlights the role of intelligent care teams that consolidate data from EHRs, wearables, and patient inputs to enable holistic treatment. Case studies and applications demonstrate benefits such as democratized access, reduced fragmentation, and cross-border collaboration. Challenges to privacy, bias, explainability, and cultural acceptance are critically analyzed. The chapter establishes augmented intelligence as a crucial foundation for psychiatric care that is accessible, ethical, and patient-centered.

DOI: 10.4018/979-8-3373-5906-9.ch007

INTRODUCTION

The Artificial Intelligence (AI) adoption in healthcare is no longer a stand-alone technological application but a symbiotic, collaborative application to human knowledge. Such a change is particularly crucial in the field of mental care, where services delivery is usually under a constraint due to the limited specialists, disintegrated services, and geographical features. It has been found that to access psychiatric services remotely, telepsychiatry has become a timely solution, although, it has been faced with the challenge of scaling, personalization, and continued engagement. It is against this background that AI-based systems, including Natural Language Processing (NLP) applications and predictive analytics and smart dashboards, are transforming the workflows within psychiatry (Yadav, 2025). This chapter discusses the possibility of human empathy and computational intelligence to co-exist in augmented telepsychiatry and intelligent care teams. Through the lens of models, case-studies and challenges, the discussion highlights the possibilities of the symbiotic human-AI workflows to improve psychiatric care, build cooperation, and democratize mental health care access services to all the people around the world.

Contextualizing AI In Healthcare: From Automation To Augmentation

The field of healthcare has strongly traditionally embraced AI to automate routine processes in healthcare, including scheduling, medical imaging analysis, or drug discovery. However, the new paradigm is centered on the enhancement rather than the replacement of the human capital. Augmented intelligence offers a team-based approach in which clinicians rely on computational systems to facilitate their interpretation of multi-faceted data sets, draw conclusions and make more knowledge-based decisions. The change is highly applicable to the area of mental health where psychiatric assessment often concerns subjective evaluation which requires empathy and accuracy in diagnosis (Higgins et al., 2023). The advantage of AI is that it detects non-obvious cues, such as the intonation of speech, mood, or body language, that will not be noticed by a clinician during a remote session. AI can also enhance continuity of care through converting data on Electronic Health Records (EHRs), wearables, and self-reported data on patients into a single format. The movement towards automation shifting into augmentation is a sign of the movement towards a more clinician-centered, but with state-of-the-art analytics, psychiatric practice. The figure 1 shows how AI can enable the transformation of few clinical insights to empowered clinical decisions as data is combined, subtle signals are identified, analytical capabilities are advanced, and eventually the informed decision-making and therapeutic alliance is reinforced.

Figure 1. Augmenting Healthcare with AI

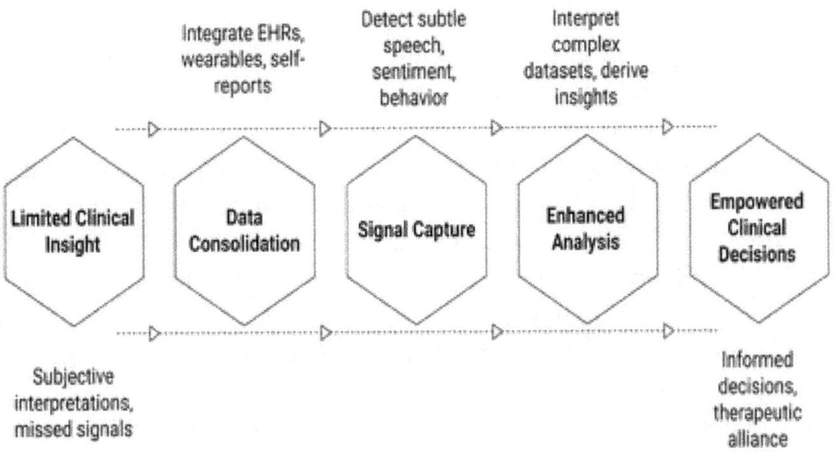

Rationale For Focusing On Telepsychiatry And Intelligent Care Teams

The need of mental health services has increased tremendously worldwide yet an insufficiency of psychiatrists and clinical psychologists is present especially in the underserved areas. Telepsychiatry provides an option of breaking geographical and infrastructural obstacles with a patient being able to receive service remotely. Nevertheless, in its absence, telepsychiatry will turn into a transactional form of consultation and not a holistic care system. This model is also enhanced by the introduction of AI because it offers psychiatrists with the tools of analytic nature that can monitor patient progress, detect the first signs of disorders, and maintain contact with patients through digital interventions. Besides personal appointments, smart care groups, i.e. psychiatrist, psychologist, general practitioner, nurses and AI, enable joint treatment planning. Care fragmentation is reduced by shared visibility that is achieved through the use of dashboards that unify the information about patients (Germack et al., 2022). This explains why the area of telepsychiatry and intelligent care teams was selected as the significant field of the study where AI-human synergy may be crucial in making mental healthcare more accessible, precise, and holistic.

Statement Of The Chapter's Scope, Objectives, And Contributions

The authors contextualize symbiotic human-AI workflows in the new role of telepsychiatry and collaborative mental health care in this chapter. The discussion of AI-driven systems, such as Natural Language Processing, which can be further employed in sentiment analysis, predictive modeling that can be employed to diagnose the disease early, and virtual assistants that will be employed to keep the interaction in the psychiatric environment alive, are also covered (Kumar, 2025). Three of these are: (1) to understand how effective AI can be to augment clinician capacity without diminishing human empathy; (2) to understand how effective intelligent care teams, with AI-driven dashboards, can be; and (3) to address ethical, cultural, and privacy concerns. These contributions are the conceptualization of Belkin symbiotic workflow model of telepsychiatry, case studies of its application in the real world and directions of its further adoption. The chapter contributes to the academic debate and provides real-life suggestions on how practitioners, policymakers and technologists should strengthen e-collaboration in psychiatric care by critically framing opportunities and challenges.

BACKGROUND TO THE STUDY

The concept of telepsychiatry has been gradually expanded in ways that reflect the growing demands of international mental health services that can be available to all people, to cover gaps created by scarcity of specialists and geographic imbalance. However, the infrastructural disadvantages, asymmetrical scalability and in personalization continue to create limitations to the classical models of telepsychiatry. Meanwhile, AI, such as Natural Language Processing (NLP), Machine Learning (ML), and virtual assistants, have penetrated the mental health industry and have the potential to enhance accuracy and monitoring and engagement with patients. Symbiotic human-AI workflows as a result of the convergence of the two paths precondition the collaboration of clinicians and intelligent systems to provide care (Rathinavel et al., 2025). The background section below puts this development of telepsychiatry, the increased popularity of AI, and the progress of hybrid systems between computational intelligence and human empathy into perspective. All these inclinations introduce a ground of reconsidering the problem of digital, collaborative and augmented psychiatric assistance.

Evolution Of Telepsychiatry: Traditional Limitations, Infrastructural Gaps, And Scalability Issues

Telepsychiatry was first introduced with the hope of removing the wall of distance, stigma and mental deficiency. It has potential, in that, it will appeal to rural and underserved populations as it will offer remote psychiatric care via video conferencing solutions. Although this is achievable, this has not been adopted due to the unresolved challenges. The infrastructure constraints, such as a lack of internet connectivity, the inability to operate interoperable platforms and unreliable access to devices are a limiting factor on scalability. Classical telepsychiatry too is highly transactional and episodic consultations compared to holistic and continuous care (Biró et al., 2023). In addition, clinical limitations exist as psychiatrists have to operate on only visual and verbal information, without the help of any sophisticated diagnostic and monitoring tools. These weaknesses have restricted its use by large mental health systems (Bobkov et al., 2025). As the global cases of psychiatric disorders increase, there is a growing need to make telepsychiatry more multifaceted, intelligent and collaborative. The following table 1 summarizes the key drawbacks of the traditional telepsychiatry which include infrastructural, clinical, and scalability issues that limit its usage.

Table 1. Evolution of Telepsychiatry: Challenges and Gaps

Dimension	Challenges	Implications
Infrastructure	Poor internet connectivity, lack of interoperable platforms, limited access to devices	Restricts reliable service delivery and consistent patient follow-up
Clinical Practice	Reliance only on visual and verbal cues	Limits diagnostic accuracy and reduces ability to detect subtle mental health markers
Scalability	Episodic consultations, fragmented platforms	Prevents large-scale integration into mainstream healthcare systems
Accessibility	Unequal adoption in rural/low-resource regions	Widened treatment gap between urban and underserved populations

Emergence Of AI In Mental Health: NLP, ML, And Virtual Assistants

Mental health care has been a field where AI has developed at an extremely fast rate to overcome certain limitations of traditional telepsychiatry. NLP systems, when analyzed on speech of a patient during a virtual consultation, can detect linguistic indicators, mood trends, and cognitive distortions which indicate the presence of a condition, including depression or anxiety. Machine learning (ML) algorithms supplement predictive analytics by identifying signs of relapses early, tailoring treatment, and indications of risk factors in different data sets. Virtual assistant also compliments these technologies by maintaining the engagement with the help of reminders, progress, and conversation between the sessions. All of these AI tools help psychiatrists to expand their diagnostic accuracy, clinical efficiency, and ability to follow-up with patients (M & Annamalai, 2020a). Although the idea is promising, the application of it also poses an ethical dilemma in terms of privacy, transparency, and algorithmic bias. However, AI development is a revolutionary change in the direction of proactive, accessible, and data-driven delivery of psychiatric care. The table 2 shows the emerging AI technologies in the field of psychiatry, their functions, and how they can enhance the delivery of mental health care.

Table 2. AI in Mental Health: Tools and Applications

Technology	Functionality	Clinical Applications
Natural Language Processing (NLP)	Analyzes patient speech, sentiment, and linguistic markers	Detects depression, anxiety, and cognitive distortions
Machine Learning (ML)	Learns from historical and real-time patient data	Predicts relapse risk, personalizes treatment, early disorder detection
Virtual Assistants	Conversational AI for reminders and continuous engagement	Patient follow-up, progress tracking, session preparation
AI Dashboards	Aggregates data from EHRs, wearables, and patient reports	Provides comprehensive insights for collaborative care planning

Concept Of Symbiotic Human-AI Workflows In Clinical Practice

Raising AI into the psychiatric domain cannot be presented as a technological enhancement but rather it should be thought of as a symbiotic workflow, in which the capabilities of the man and the machine are carefully balanced. Human-AI workflows that are symbiotic (such as paraphrasing psychiatrists) allow psychiatrists to maintain their empathy, judgment, and therapeutic alliance with patients, with AI systems doing the data-driven analysis, pattern recognition and decision support. This, in practice, implies that clinicians work with the AI-based dashboards that will integrate the Electronic Health Records (EHRs), wearables, and self-reports of the patients. Similar workflows also expand collaboration to multidisciplinary care teams, in which consolidated insights accessed through shared access promotes the planning of holistic treatment. AI can help psychiatrists to consult their colleagues on difficult cases by providing the ability to share knowledge across geographic borders. Notably, these workflows focus on the ethical design concepts in order to protect the trust of patients. Symbiotic human-AI workflows, as a conceptual framework, can be thought of as the next step towards cohesive intelligent ecosystems of isolated digital tools into psychiatric practice (Prince et al., 2025). The figure 2 illustrates how an isolated digital tool development is being replaced by intelligent ecosystems and demonstrates how intelligent AI ecosystems facilitate knowledge sharing, multidisciplinary cooperation, data consolidation, and ethical design to protect patient trust and promote holistic and collaborative psychiatric practice.

Figure 2. Symbiotic Human-AI Workflows

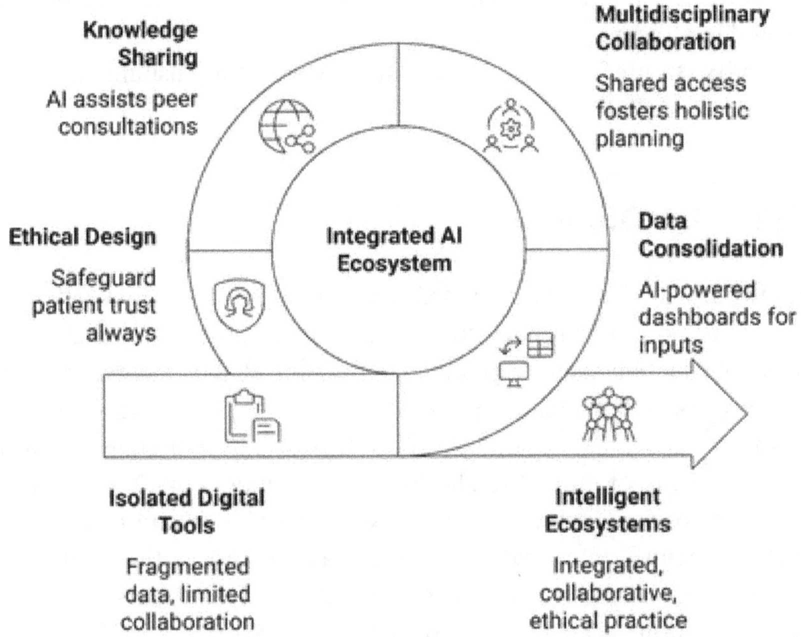

RESEARCH OBJECTIVES

The introduction of Artificial Intelligence into telepsychiatry is both more opportunities and challenges than ever. As much as AI can be used to increase diagnostic accuracy, facilitate care coordination, and assist in patient engagement, their use should be done in a manner that does not jeopardize the therapeutic relationship and raise the likelihood of patient mistrust. The research goals introduced in this chapter are based on concepts of augmenting psychiatry, but not replacing it because the focus is on collaborative care modalities, which involve clinicians, intelligent systems, and multidisciplinary teams. The discussion follows the following objectives:

- To investigate how AI augments psychiatric consultations without diminishing human empathy.
- To evaluate the role of intelligent care teams supported by AI dashboards and data integration.
- To assess ethical, privacy, and trust-related challenges in AI-enhanced telepsychiatry.
- To explore cross-cultural and organizational factors influencing AI adoption in mental healthcare.
- To identify future directions and frameworks for sustainable symbiotic human-AI workflows.

CONCEPTUAL MODEL

Symbiotic human-AI workflows in telepsychiatry are conceptualized to provide a framework of how clinicians and intelligent systems can communicate with each other and establish a balanced, augmented care space (Uganda & Mukamurera P., 2025). It is not a model that intends to substitute the use of psychiatric knowledge but is a means to combine the use of computational knowledge with human knowledge and the understanding of empathy. The Belkin symbiotic workflow is focused on collaborative intelligence, which involves psychiatrists and care teams using AI-powered tools to identify subtle patterns, control patient information, and coordinate treatment. Meanwhile, it is patient-centered, which guarantees that patients become its focus and enjoy holistic and personalized care (Prégent et al., 2025a). The model fosters continuity, decreasing fragmentation by providing structured interaction flows between psychiatrists, multidisciplinary care teams, and AI platforms, which also lead to more precise psychiatry. The workflows represented by conceptual diagrams demonstrate how information is recorded, analyzed, and exchanged by all the actors and finally turn telepsychiatry into an active, intelligent ecosystem. The figure 3 represents a workflow cycle in which patient information is collected, interpreted through AI, and converted to insights that can be utilized to promote team-based treatment, patient interaction, and improvement in precision psychiatry. It is a loop that focuses on the ongoing human-AI interaction in telepsychiatry care.

Figure 3. Symbiotic Human-AI Workflow in Telepsychiatry

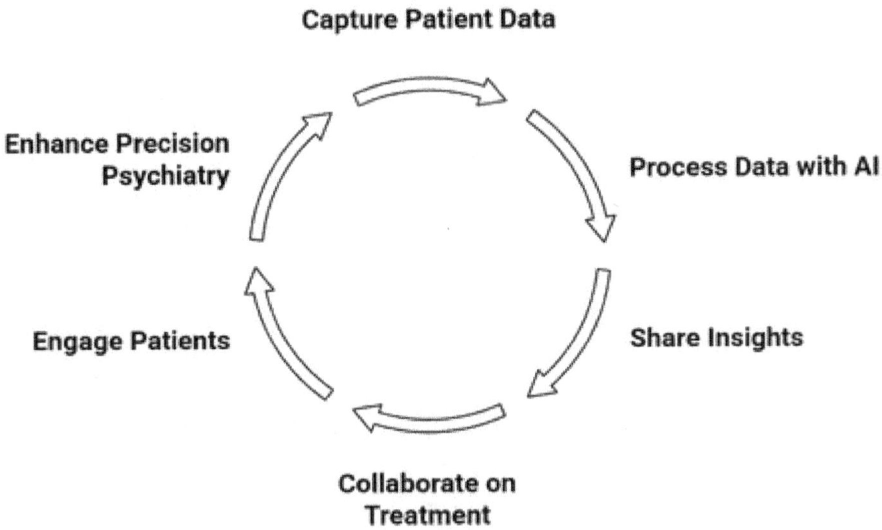

The Belkin Symbiotic Human-AI Workflow Framework

Belkin framework is a model of teamwork between humanity and AI systems in mental health care, and this paradigm is focused on complementation rather than replacement. It is this framework which places AI in the role of an assistive intelligence which enhances diagnostic and therapeutic capabilities of clinicians. It involves the technologies such as Natural Language Processing (speech and sentiment analysis), predictive algorithms (early psychiatric disorder detection), and virtual assistants (continuous contact with the patient). Psychiatrists in this workflow will have full clinical control but AI-driven insights to help them, integrating the streams of data related to Electronic Health Records, wearable devices, and patient-generated data (Prégent et al., 2025b). Through the preservation of the framework, AI will act behind the scenes as an assistant to the efficiency and accuracy, but the human clinician must be left to handle the caring, interpretative, ethical side of the care. The result of this two system is that it creates a strong ecosystem that has clinical decisions based on computational accuracy, yet the nature of the therapeutic relationship, which safeguards the practice of psychiatry. The Figure 4 illustrate the Belkin Framework where AI has the potential to help psychiatry by enhancing diagnostic precision, data integration, and capacity to expand, at the same time, retaining clinical authority in the hands of psychiatrists and contributing to the mental wellbeing of patients.

Figure 4. Symbiotic Human-AI Mental Healthcare (Belkin Framework)

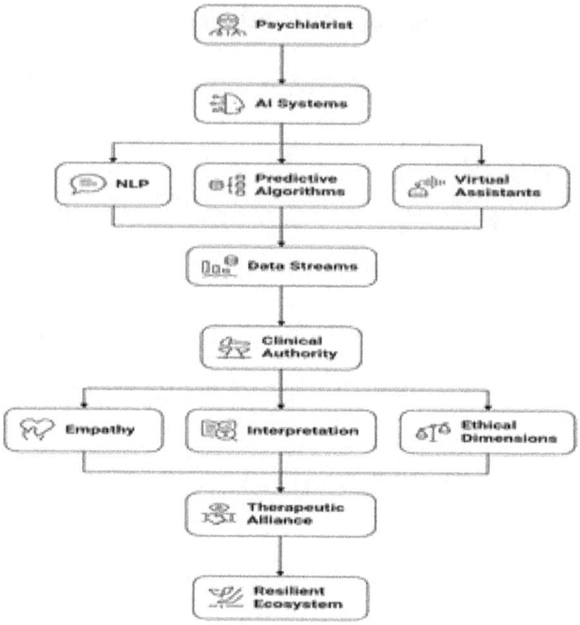

Integration Of Psychiatrists, Care Teams, And AI-Powered Platforms

One of the main characteristics of the conceptual model is that psychiatrists, multidisciplinary care teams, and AI-driven platforms become one collaborative environment. In the past, the operations of psychiatrists, psychologists, nurses and general practitioners have been in silos. The application of AI software is to serve as integrators and drag insights into single boards giving holistic knowledge of patient progress. Overall, in such integration, psychiatrist may call upon psychologists to make changes in treatment regimen, nurses to observe medication compliance, and general practitioners to treat comorbidities in AI-based interfaces. This will be converted into a more cohesive experience where each professional can understand each other based on shared data, and not independent observations where patients are concerned. In addition, AI-enhanced solutions will guarantee real time tracking and pro-active notifications, evidence-based suggestions and provide proactive care delivery (Buhr et al., 2025). The model brings together the various stakeholders around a shared digital infrastructure to constitute an intelligent care team that can offer coordinated and patient-centered treatment plans with less fragmentation and high accountability and overall treatment outcomes. The figure 5 represents a stratified model in which the integration of AI serves as the keystone to the collaboration between psychiatrists, care teams, and intelligent systems, resulting in a unified patient experience, active care provision, and subsequently improved treatment outcomes through integrated and least fragmented mental healthcare.

Figure 5. Integrated Mental Health Care Model

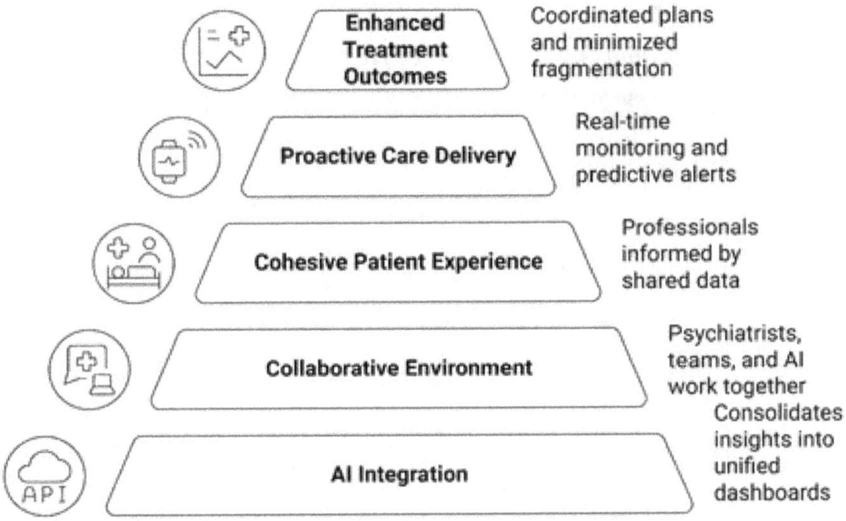

Interaction Flow Between Patients, Clinicians, And AI Systems

The communication pattern between symbiotic human-AI workflow stresses on formal cooperation of patients, clinicians, and intelligent systems. On the patient level, the data is constantly taken during consultations and self-reports, as well as digital gadgets like wearables or apps. The AI systems take in these inputs and process them to detect the risk markers, trends, and behavior changes. The synthesized insights are presented to clinicians through dashboards, in which the clinicians can place the computational findings into their own experience and expertise, clinical history, and empathic insights. It is followed by involving patients in the processes of shared decision-making where AI-generated recommendations are discussed, explained, and incorporated into the treatment plans. Notably, the workflow is cyclical, with patient feedback to optimize AI models, and the human supervision of the workflow to make sure that the recommendations are both clinically valid and ethical (Miner et al., 2019). Such flow creates transparency and trust because it does not create passive points in the data of patients but active participants in the care continuum. These organized relations make AI an intermediary of collaboration and not a black box decision-maker. The Figure 6 shows a process by which patient information is gathered, analyzed by AI, and refined with the clinical knowledge, resulting in collective decision-making, treatment plan combination, repeated feed-back loops, and clinical supervision to assure ethical and clinically valid results.

Figure 6. Symbiotic Human-AI Workflow in Healthcare

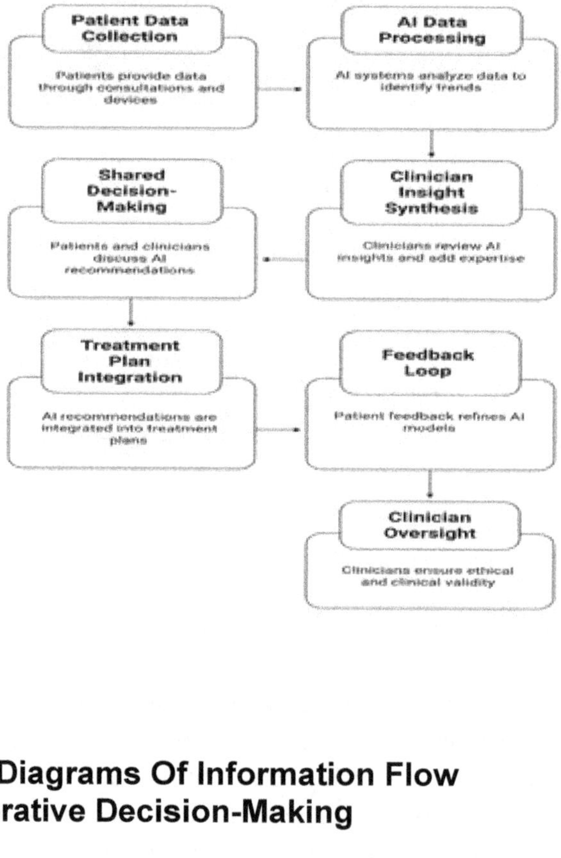

Conceptual Diagrams Of Information Flow And Collaborative Decision-Making

The conceptual model is depicted visually, which contributes to the flow of information within the system of patients, clinicians, and AI. The process of data capture (speech, behavior, wearable metrics) and AI processing (sentiment analysis, predictive modeling and anomaly detection) and clinician interpretation (diagnosis, treatment planning and care adjustments) are design thought as data capture, AI processing and clinician interpretation. They also show the feedback mechanisms of the AI predictions and the clinical approaches being corrected by the response of patients (Pham et al., 2022). The diagrams highlight the dynamicity of the relationships between all stakeholders by having nodes (patients, psychiatrists, care teams, AI systems), and connections (data streams, decisions, feedback). This combination of computational intelligence with human knowledge is simulated as a central hub of decision-making which is collaborative. These diagrams are not merely the means of analysis; they are also communicative resources, which help the stakeholders to see the value added by the integration of AI in psychiatry (Chekroud et al., 2021). Lastly, they facilitate the spirit of the concept that good workflows are symbiotic, between caring, being ethical, and being precise within an intelligent adaptive network of care. The Figure 7 reflects a methodical procedure in the field of psychiatry wherein the data of a patient are accumulated, AI processes the information, and clinical experts decide, and feedback loops to enhance AI machines and clinical techniques enhance the procedures.

Figure 7. Symbiotic Human-AI Workflow in Psychiatry

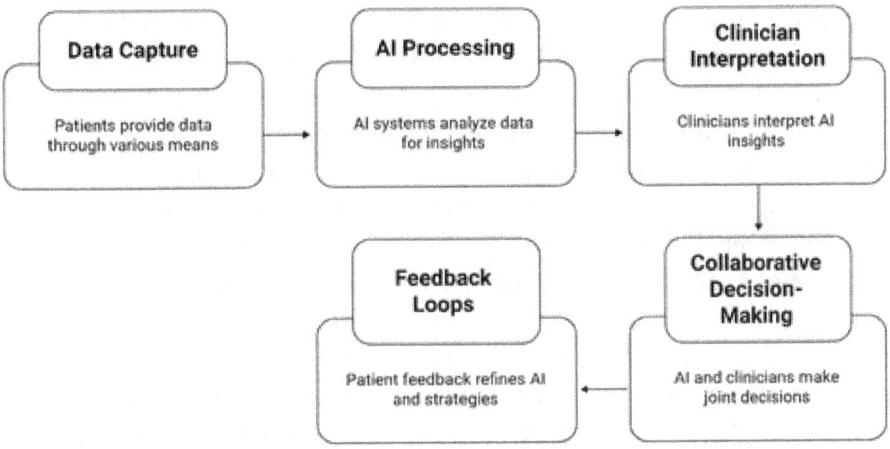

RESEARCH METHODOLOGY

The study design implemented in this chapter is a qualitative and analytical one to investigate the transformational element of symbiotic human-AI workflow applied in telepsychiatry. It uses a dual approach: the chapter combines the knowledge of scholarly and clinical publications to place the development of AI in psychiatry into perspective, whereas it uses qualitative case studies to analyze the practical implementation of AI-based telepsychiatry applications and intelligent care teams (Mahapatra et al., 2021). These methods enable the research to interpose the theoretical and practical insights. Peer reviewed articles, reports of clinical trials and industry driven applications are all sources of data (Terra et al., 2023). The thematic analysis analytically is preoccupied with explaining the trends in human and AI integration, and system level of efficiency, patient involvement, and clinician support. This is going to facilitate the multi-dimensional analysis of the potential benefits, issues and implications of augmented workflows to mental health.

Methodological Approach: Qualitative Case Study And Literature Synthesis

The mixed approach methodology is used in the chapter as the integration of qualitative case studies and systematic literature review. Through the literature review, detail will be ensured in the theoretical constructs of AI, historical findings, and models of AI that are continually being developed in the field of psychiatry. The peer-reviewed articles analyzed during 2015-2025 were analyzed to determine the tendencies existing in the field of AI-powered telepsychiatry, human-computer interaction, and intelligent care models. At the same time, concurrently, we have chosen qualitative case studies to put these insights into context, including the ways AI platforms have been applied in practice in real clinical settings (Doraiswamy et al., 2020a). The field of psychiatry is among the areas where the case study approach may be implemented effectively because it offers the information about patient experience, their therapeutic relationships, and the implementation of AI technology among clinicians on a case-by-case basis. This kind of mix of methods assists such chapter in striking the balance between the aspect of generality and particularity. It also makes it possible to institute negative comparisons of the expected results in literature and the results in practice so as to reduce the gap between abstract discourses and concrete places to adopt symbiotic human-AI workflow.

Data Sources: Peer-Reviewed Research, Clinical Trials, And Industry Applications

The sources of data of the research have been divided into three categories, the peer-reviewed literature, the data of the clinical trials, the industry applications. The peer-reviewed papers present the theoretical background information on the AI algorithms, telepsychiatry models, and ethical considerations that are taken into account, which predetermines the rigor of the level of analysis. The empirical evidence on AI implementation, i.e. the predictive model efficiency, NLP-based systems and virtual assistants in psychiatric care, can be provided by clinical trial reporting. The experiments help to demonstrate that there are positive and negative aspects of AI-assisted interventions that allow making rational decisions (Vale, 2024). Another practical aspect of the applications is seen in the industry applications, which demonstrate how the smart care systems created by technology firms, start-ups, and healthcare organizations are implemented into the real world. Collectively, these sources have a triangulated data base which is credible and comprehensive. The work provides the synthesis of divergent data streams to provide the crossbreeding of research, clinical practice and innovation, and therefore is able to afford multi-perspective insights into how symbiotic human-AI workflows are currently influencing, and potentially ready to influence, telepsychiatry, and intelligent care teams.

Analytical Framework: Thematic Analysis Of Human-AI Integration And Outcomes

The way of data analysis is organized based on a thematic framework to be guided by to discover typical patterns of human-AI cooperation in telepsychiatry. Qualitative data on particular themes is most effectively analyzed with the help of thematic analysis, which allows classifying the findings into generalized categories, i. e. diagnostic augmentation, care coordination, ethical issue, and patient engagement. The themes are then further expanded in the case of actual outcomes-precision improvement, the efficiency, the accessibility, and the trustworthiness of the clinicians and patients (Rony et al., 2025). Other barriers in the framework include the risk of data privacy, risk of the algorithms, and resistance to adoption. The analysis will be structured based on mapping of the themes to the case study narratives and literature results to give a structured interpretation of how the symbiotic workflows operate in reality. The strategy assists in cross-comparing the cultural contexts as well, which refers to the difference in acceptance and implementation (Putica et al., 2025). Lastly, thematic analysis is an effective means of relating the qualitative data to the greater conceptual discourse in which case both the findings of the study are evidence driven and sensitive to the context. Table 3 below details the methodological framework of the study, including the research methodology, data collection, and analytical model used in the study-to-study symbiotic human-AI telepsychiatry workflows.

Table 3. Methodology Summary

Component	Details	Purpose
Research Approach	Qualitative case studies + Literature synthesis.	To combine contextual depth with theoretical breadth in exploring AI in psychiatry.
Data Sources	• Peer-reviewed articles (2015–2025). • Clinical trial reports. • Industry applications.	To ensure triangulation of insights from academia, clinical practice, and real-world innovations.
Analytical Framework	Thematic analysis of human-AI integration and outcomes.	To identify patterns, themes, and implications across case studies and literature.
Focus Areas	Diagnostic augmentation, care coordination, patient engagement, ethical issues.	To evaluate benefits, barriers, and practical challenges of AI-human symbiosis.

LITERATURE REVIEW

The use of Artificial Intelligence (AI) in telepsychiatry marks the beginning of a new era in the history of mental health care on the Internet. The current literature not solely places AI as a technological addition, but as an organizational change in the character of the very frame of providing psychiatric services and framing (Kolding et al., 2024). The significance of such change is that, besides increasing the possibility of clinicians, improving the quality of diagnosis, and maintaining continuity of care, AI also raises significant concerns regarding privacy, trust, ethical practice. The presented scholarly and clinical studies are consolidated around the five themes that fill the domain of the AI in telepsychiatry: Natural Language Processing (NLP) in speech and sentiment analysis, predictive analytics to diagnose disorders at an earlier stage, virtual assistants to encourage continuous patient engagement, smart care teams with a built-in data dashboard, and comparative cases of AI-based psychiatry implementation in different environments (Patel et al., 2022). The ability to identify small speech signs, linguistic variations, and tonal variations, which can depict a latent psychiatric disorder, can explain the popularity of NLP applications. Psychiatrists can use NLP systems to detect depression, anxiety or even bipolar disorder in a patient at its early stages by examining their coherence, vocabulary and emotional expression during virtual sessions. These devices will play a crucial role in the distance treatment where only physical signs can be limited (Mason et al., 2024).

The issue of interpretability remains because the clinician must be able to trust and place AI generated results in perspective. The researches have focused on transparency and multimodal NLP methodologies that combine textual, acoustic and prosodic information to increase the validity and safety of sensitive conversation data (Raveesh & Munoli, 2020). The predictive analytics also broadens the potential of AI as it allows detecting psychiatric diseases in advance, using machine learning models, which are trained on Electronic Health Records, wearable devices, and self-reported data. It has been proven that predictive algorithms can identify depressed episodes several weeks before clinical manifestations and offer opportunities at preventive measures and reduced rate of recurrence. The latter instruments are particularly significant in the telepsychiatry where constant surveillance might be more of a possibility. Nevertheless, we also have the risks of algorithmic bias when predictive models are being trained on non-diverse training data (Ravikumar, Renukadevi, et al., 2025). It has been claimed in literature on multiple occasions that overreliance on AI products is too high, and predictive analytics are to be used in conjunction with clinical knowledge, rather than in its place. Virtual assistants (VAs) are a form of patient engagement since they can be employed to assist patients on an ongoing basis and not in an intermittent basis. They also offer medication reminders, mood tracking and therapeutic dialogues based on cognitive behavioral therapy techniques. VAs have been demonstrated to increase compliance and isolation, and create a sense of connectedness between patients and their caregivers (Ravikumar, Aarthi, et al., 2025). However, the problem of information privacy, transparency of the AI nature of such applications, and cultural uptake remain a concern. Psychiatric services may be highly dependent on the concept of human interaction within society, so the patients may not be eager to engage with AI-powered assistants.

The other area of the literature is the intelligent care teams, where AI is used to facilitate the collaboration of psychiatrists, psychologists, general practitioners, and nurses. Dashboards based on AI can integrate the data collected by EHRs, wearable devices, and self-reports and enable clinicians to design a holistic patient portrait. It reduces the level of fragmentation, enhances the precision of the diagnosis, and helps to plan the treatment actively with the help of the integration (M & Annamalai, 2020b). In the meantime, the barriers of the system interoperability, clinician resistance and sensitive psychiatric information should be meticulously tackled. Comparative works refer to the differences between the adoption and implementation and outcomes of AI in psychiatry. It has been reported that the patients in high-income nations that have well-developed digital infrastructures are the ones with more accurate diagnostics, fewer workloads on clinicians, and satisfied patients (Okpete & Byeon, 2024). On the other hand, the low-resource environment is also characterized by such difficulties as low connectivity, low digital literacy, and mistrust towards AI-based care. Moreover, these ethical issues as transparency of algorithms, patient privacy, and informed consent are prevalent across any setting and this makes culturally and ethically sensitive frameworks essential. Together, the readings under analysis demonstrate that the sphere of AI has been one of the main contributors to the rise of telepsychiatry (Bhatia et al., 2025). NLP is applied to enhance clinical interpretation, predictive analytics to enhance early detection, virtual assistants keep people interested, and intelligent care teams encourage collaborative practice. Comparison perspectives provide certain insights into the opportunities and limitations of AI and emphasize that, despite the possibility to incorporate it into psychiatric practice, the problem of bias, privacy, and cultural acceptance should be addressed (Castro et al., 2024). In general, one can conclude that symbiotic human-AI workflows may possess a tremendous potential of redefining telepsychiatry provided it is approached with transparency, empathy, and patient-centered design as its main values.

RESULTS / DISCUSSION

With a few important findings, telepsychiatry analysis includes symbiotic human-AI processes that bring a significant understanding of artificial intelligence as a supplement but not a replacement of psychiatric practice. Key findings are presented in the literature synthesis, applications of the case and new platforms according to the clinician capacity improvements, decision support and collaborative care delivery equalized and the ethical, cultural and technical challenges.

Key Findings

Some of the most certain outcomes are the augmented ability of clinicians. AI systems are electronic versions of the workforce, whereby they are used to process large volumes of patient information to extract clinically valuable information. NLP applications are employed to help psychiatrists understand speech and mood of a patient, but predictive analytics provide an insight into potential relapse or deterioration. This will complement the clinician decision-making and enable earlier and specific interventions and more specific diagnoses. A second valuable finding is related to patient-provider collaboration (Miner et al., 2019). Clinicians can participate in shared decision-making because they have the ability to communicate with patients regarding synthesized insights using intelligent dashboard and AI-supported tools. This enhances transparency, empowers patients to be more engaged in their treatment and facilitates the development of more efficient treatment relationships.

Case Studies And Applications

AI-enhanced telepsychiatry platforms are presented in case studies, which indicate practical uses of such workflows. Pilot initiatives that incorporate conversational AI assistants into the discussion sessions of telepsychiatry have demonstrated better patient engagement, chatbots remind patients about appointments, walk them through cognitive-behavioral skills, and gather data on their daily mood (Terra et al., 2023). In a similar manner, the healthcare systems that use AI-supported dashboards to combine the data on Electronic Health Records (EHRs) and wearable devices enable clinicians to monitor all the symptoms, adherence, and lifestyle factors. Psychiatry is not the only area that has collaborative models and general practitioners, psychologists and nurses are collaborating in the AI-mediated settings. As an example, a smart care platform can deliver real-time reports to a multidisciplinary team about the behavioral patterns of a patient, which will allow adjusting the treatment plans in time. The case applications prove that AI can improve the efficiency of the service delivery process and the inclusivity of psychiatric services. The figure 8 indicates that AI can be used to remotely provide psychiatric care using telepsychiatry platforms to have improved consultations, collaborative models, and multidisciplinary teams, and an AI-based dashboard to integrate the data to have a complete understanding of clinical care.

Figure 8. AI in Psychiatric Care

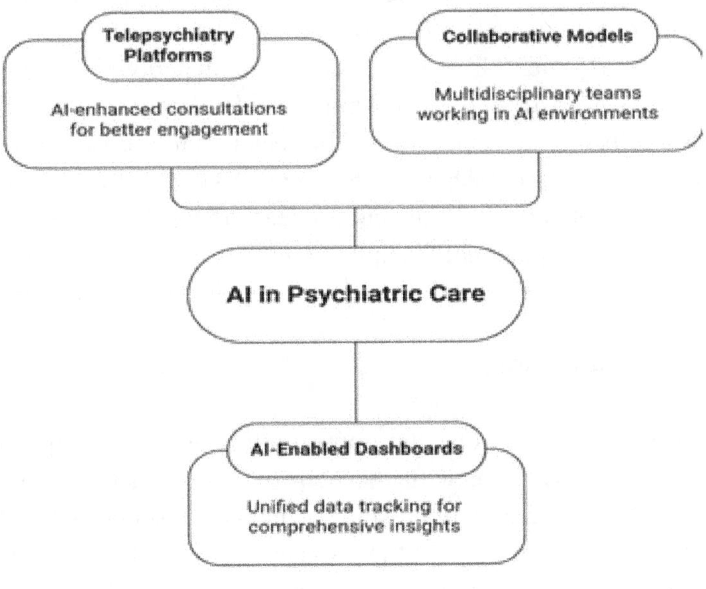

Benefits

The benefits of using AI in telepsychiatry are a number of them. First, it democratizes access to psychiatric services in that it enhances access to mental health services especially in remote or underserved regions. Online networks reduce the geographical barrier and tools with the help of AI offer a possibility to utilize the limited time of clinicians. Second, AI reduces care fragmentation by converting fragmented data sources, e.g. Speech analysis, wearable metrics, EHRs, etc., into a logical form. This will aid continuity of care and prevent the patient falling into the systemic gaps (McCradden et al., 2023). Third, AI allows cross-border knowledge exchange of clinicians. With the help of peer input in the form of complex cases with discussing psychiatrists in the framework of collaborative dashboards and tele-consultation portals, a global mental health knowledge network can be created, regardless of geography. All this benefits AI that is a force behind accuracy psychiatry and a healthier healthcare system.

Challenges

Although this is good news, there are extremely serious problems. The biggest issue is privacy since psychiatric information is very sensitive and must be guaranteed. The patients might not be interested in AI platforms interpretation without an open governance process and a proper data protection procedure. The second issue is that of algorithmic bias: should the training data not be able to capture a particular population of people, AI estimates can reproduce care inequalities. Another impediment is the explainability; to be accountable in applying AI research to their practice, clinicians need to believe and comprehend them (Steyvers & Kumar, 2024). Culture tolerance is also an important factor because culture variation varies in the field of AI acceptance in mental health. Other patients can distrust AI-driven systems and consider them cold or dead. Last but not least, there should also be therapeutic alliance. Psychiatry is a personal discipline and AI systems should not replace empathy and trust on which successful treatment depends but rather complement it.

Summary Of Discussion

This discussion indicates that the opportunities of the subsequent further development of psychiatric care with the help of AI-enhanced telepsychiatry and intelligent care teams might be quite significant. The existence of such workflows may become a new breakthrough in the provision of mental health care as it is able to increase the capacity of clinicians, enhance the collaboration with patients, and promote the exchange of knowledge on an international scale. Nevertheless, privacy, bias, explainability, cultural acceptance, and maintenance empathies will have to be considered as a problem to maximize their potential. Its conclusions can be viewed as pointing to the notion that the symbiotic human-AI workflows cannot be the alternative model, yet they are the path to the collaborative, transparent, and ethical augmentation of the psychiatric practice. The following table 4 compares the key advantages of AI integration into telepsychiatry with key obstacles that have to be overcome to make its use sustainable.

Table 4. Benefits and Challenges of AI-Enhanced Telepsychiatry

Dimension	Benefits	Challenges
Clinician Capacity	Augments decision-making with NLP, predictive analytics, and dashboards	Risk of overreliance; lack of clinician trust if outputs lack explainability
Patient Engagement	Virtual assistants maintain continuous contact and adherence	Perceived impersonality; cultural reluctance to interact with AI systems
Access to Care	Expands services to remote and underserved populations	Infrastructure gaps; uneven digital literacy
Care Coordination	Integrates EHRs, wearable data, and dashboards to reduce fragmentation	Interoperability issues across healthcare systems
Knowledge Sharing	Enables global peer consultation and cross-border expertise	Data privacy risks in international data sharing
Ethics and Trust	Supports transparency and shared decision-making with patients	Algorithmic bias; need for strict privacy, governance, and ethical safeguards

FUTURE RESEARCH AND DIRECTIONS

Artificial Intelligence integration in telepsychiatry is still at a developmental level and with current research showing promising findings, there are still many aspects that need to be investigated. In a way that will guarantee sustainability of AI application in psychiatry, future research directions are not only to develop technical capabilities, but also to fill in ethical, cultural, and methodological gaps. In this section, four key directions have been determined to be subject to further research: explainability and trust structures, cross-cultural acceptance research, multimodal data assimilation, and federated learning in privacy-preserving analytics. Collectively, these domains will create the basis of building strong, equitable, and universally applicable symbiotic human-AI workflows (Doraiswamy et al., 2020b).

AI Explainability And Trust-Building Frameworks

Enhancing explainability in AI systems applied to mental health care is one of the fastest-growing needs. In contrast to physical domains of health, the psychiatric data are subjective, subtle, and context-specific and, therefore, black-box AI models are problematic in practice in clinical settings. This is because future research must focus on the formulation of interpretable models that can give clear rationales to the clinicians toward diagnostic or predictive results (Gerantia, 2024). Explainability should not be limited to technical transparency, but must also be accompanied by communication plans that aid patients to grasp how AI is working in their process. Trust-constructing schemes will also play an important role with the inclusion of ethical design, accountability mechanisms and an audit trail. With explainability integrated in AI models, psychiatry will be able to minimize mistrust among the clinicians, instill trust in the patients and make the decision-making process ethically sound.

Cross-Cultural Studies On Patient Acceptance

The concept of AI is seen differently in each culture, and mental health care is one area that is particularly sensitive to the differences. Some patients might use AI as an unbiased and stigma-free aid but some might find it impersonal or intrusive. Intercultural comparative research is thus needed to comprehend the perception of AI by patients in diverse geographical regions, socio-economic statuses, and cultures in the psychiatric practice (Dow, Chen, et al., 2023). Issues that could affect acceptance such as the trust in technology, the culture of dealing with mental health, and the significance of human empathy in care should be researched. The evidence of cross-cultural will be used in informing the design and implementation of AI systems that do not infringe on cultural diversity and instead promote therapeutic integrity. Lacking such sensitivity, the improvements of AI in psychiatry across the globe are likely to be unevenly successful and even opposed by patients.

Integration Of Multimodal Data For Improved Insights

The majority of telepsychiatry AI systems that currently exist use speech or text data extensively, which restricts the depth of clinical information. Future studies need to examine multimodal or use of speech, facial expressions, physiological indicators and behavioral data gathered through wearables. Such a combination would enable the AI models to have a more holistic understanding of mental conditions, finding subtle indicators of psychiatric conditions that otherwise might be ignored in monomodal systems (Dow, Khan, et al., 2023). As an illustration, the addition of prosodic speech analysis to facial micro-expression detection and heart rate variability may contribute to an increased ability to detect episodes of depression or anxiety at an early stage. Multimodal AI systems also make it possible to practice individualized psychiatry when personalized interventions are based on the distinct behavioral and physiological characteristics of patients (Anshara & Shabbir, 2025). Nevertheless, the challenge of these studies should be to overcome data fusion issues, multimodal input standardization, and to protect the privacy of sensitive physiological data.

Federated Learning For Privacy-Preserving Analytics

The issue of privacy is another significant obstacle to the application of AI in the psychiatric field since mental health information falls under one of the most confidential types of information. Federated learning methods should therefore be the subject of future research where AI models can be trained in collaboration between institutions without accessing real patient data (Bhakuni et al., 2025). Federated learning does not only protect privacy, but the model also allows large-scale and diverse integration of data in hospitals, clinics, and cultural settings. Their frameworks can improve the generalizability of predictive models in general, and do not break the rules of data protection (Zirikly et al., 2022). Multi-layered protective measures should also be obtained by researching it in hybrid models of federated learning that combine differential privacy and secure multiparty computation. These approaches can be a compromise between novelty and privacy that would guarantee that patients would not need to compromise the privacy to take the benefits of advanced AI insights.

Summary Of Further Research

The role of AI in telepsychiatry in the future will rely on the research aimed at considering both the technological improvement and human issue. The main aspects, which will be employed to design human-AI workflows that are sustainable, ethical, and effective, will be explainability, trust, cultural sensitivity, multimodal intelligence, and privacy-preserving analytics. In so doing, by these lines we can transform psychiatry to a paradigm in which computational intelligence facilitates and not undermines the therapeutic alliance and create a more comprehensive and more global model of mental health care in a digital age. According to the given table 5, the future research needs to be concentrated on the areas of priority in order to focus on technical, ethical, and cultural aspects that are required to optimize symbiotic human-AI workflows in psychiatry.

Table 5. Future Research Directions in AI-Enhanced Telepsychiatry

Focus Area	Research Needs	Expected Outcomes
AI Explainability & Trust	Develop interpretable models; design communication frameworks for clinicians/ patients.	Greater clinician trust, improved patient confidence, ethically transparent AI adoption.
Cross-Cultural Acceptance	Conduct comparative studies across regions, cultures, and socio-economic contexts.	Context-sensitive AI systems; higher adoption across diverse populations.
Multimodal Data Integration	Fuse speech, facial, physiological, and behavioral signals for analysis.	Richer clinical insights; early and personalized detection of psychiatric disorders.
Federated Learning for Privacy	Implement privacy-preserving analytics combining FL, DP, and secure computation.	Safe large-scale collaboration; stronger compliance with data protection regulations.

MANAGERIAL IMPLICATIONS

The application of AI to telepsychiatry and smart care teams has profound managerial consequences on healthcare institutions, politicians, and tech companies. The human-AI workflows of the future are not only symbiotic relationships but sustainable at the scale of technological innovation but also the stakeholders need to be engineered to ensure that the stakeholders create systems, policies, and infrastructures that balance efficiency, trust, and empathy in psychiatric care.

For Healthcare Institutions

Health care facilities are one of the key participants at the frontline of collaborative care AI-based. The smart dashboard integration that integrates Electronic Health Records (EHRs), wearables, and telepsychiatry solutions must be at the top of the list of priorities of managers. Its implementation is possible only with the successful investment in the digital infrastructure, models of the clinician training and interdisciplinary collaboration. The institutions should also establish systems of constant monitoring in order to define the impact that AI will have on the treatment outcome and the clinical burden and patient satisfaction (Mustapha et al., 2022). The organizational leaders must make sure the workflow is structured as a way to not only generate more psychiatric knowledge but also minimize clinician-patient interaction. This kind of strategy will create an environment of tolerance among the practitioners, and will transform empathy into the heart of mental health care provision.

For Policymakers

Policymakers have the duty to come up with moral and legal principles that would protect confidential psychiatric information and promote innovation. Mental health information is a special type of data, and it is required to be handled with the highest level of privacy compliance, such as HIPAA, GDPR, or other form of laws and regulations that may be specific to a particular country or region. The policies should incorporate the transparency of the algorithmic decision-making processes, provide the criteria to audit AI models, and address the algorithmic bias through the regulation of AI (Graham et al., 2019). Policy makers can also help in increasing access to telepsychiatry by funding digital infrastructure in underserved regions and international alliances. The innovation and the protection of the patients will be ensured by the evolution of legal frameworks that will be adjusted to the improvement of the technology.

For Technology Providers

The transparency, empathy, and clinician empowerment should be the main designing principles of AI tools by the technology providers. This demands the construction of explainable AI models that are actionable in nature and do not act as black boxes. Users and developers must collaborate in the development of platforms that have the involvement of psychiatrists, patients, and ethicists to make them structural and clinical needs-based. Trust and adoption will be enhanced with empathy-based design solutions, e.g., conversational agents that are sensitive to the feelings of the patients. Moreover, privacy preserving systems, including federated learning and differential privacy, should be incorporated into system architectures by providers (Squires et al., 2023). More than just technology, the task of providers is to inform clinicians and patients about the strengths and weaknesses of AI and minimize mistrust and encourage responsible use.

Summary Of Managerial Implications

In general, the managerial implications are that effective implementation of AI in the field of psychiatry must be a three-sector task. Organizations have to bind the workflows in a responsible way, policymakers need to protect the ethical and legal norms, and technology vendors should care about trust and empathy. All these measures will assure that AI within the context of telepsychiatry can make the services more accessible, maintain the therapeutic relationship, and reinforce the collaborative mental health care systems (Punia et al., 2025). The following table 6 is a recap of the main duties and anticipated deliverables of healthcare facilities and policymakers, as well as technology vendors in dealing with AI-enhanced telepsychiatry.

Table 6. Managerial Implications of AI in Telepsychiatry

Stakeholder	Key Responsibilities	Expected Outcomes
Healthcare Institutions	• Implement AI-enhanced collaborative workflows. • Invest in digital infrastructure. • Train clinicians and foster interdisciplinary collaboration. • Monitor treatment and patient satisfaction outcomes.	Improved care coordination, reduced clinician workload, enhanced patient engagement and trust.
Policymakers	• Establish ethical and legal frameworks for psychiatric data. • Mandate transparency and algorithm audits. • Address algorithmic bias through regulation. • Support equitable access through funding and infrastructure.	Data protection, increased accountability, equitable access to mental health services, patient safety.
Technology Providers	• Design explainable and transparent AI tools. • Embed privacy-preserving mechanisms (FL, DP). • Co-create systems with clinicians and patients. • Educate users about AI strengths and limitations	Higher adoption rates, trust in AI systems, patient-centered design, responsible innovation.

CONCLUSION

Symbiotic human-AI workflows in telepsychiatry their discovery of symbiotic human-AI workflows can transform the provision of mental health care. The example of such workflows can help to scale the capabilities of clinicians, enhance the ability to make decisions and to facilitate the relationships between patients and providers through a combination of computational intelligence and human sympathy. By being created based on ethical codes and openness, Artificial Intelligence, instead of being considered one of the replacements to the therapeutic relationship, which lies at the center of mental health care, must be regarded as an addition to it. One of the futuristic models of psychiatry is the creation of intelligent care groups where psychiatrists, psychologists, nurses, general practitioners, and AI-based systems will collaborate on the same platforms. By means of such teams, there is an opportunity to organize treatment in a comprehensive and integrated way, avoid fragmentation and make the well-being of the patients the main focus. Remarkably, augmented intelligence has potential not just in technical efficiency, but also in the prospect of democratising access and delivering services to underserved groups and the potential of creating a more holistic mental health ecosystem. The questions of privacy, algorithmically bias, cultural tolerance and explainability are challenging, but can be researched, proposed as one of the policy and innovated in a responsible way. Lastly, the symbiotic human-AI processes may be considered as the future of psychiatric practice that is available, empathetic and science-based systems where human clinicians and intelligent technology co-exist to refine precision psychiatry and impact positively on mental health outcomes in a more digital world.

REFERENCES

Anshara, M., & Shabbir, N. (2025). The role of artificial Intelligence in identifying depression and anxiety. Journal Global Values, XVI(SI), 75–81. DOI: 10.31995/jgv.2025.v16iSI7.011

Bhakuni, P., Punia, A., & Sharma, N. (2025). Mental Health and AI. In *Advances in Healthcare Information Systems and Administration* (pp. 299–332). IGI Global., DOI: 10.4018/979-8-3693-7858-8.ch011

Bhatia, G., Choudhary, H., & Mathur, R. (2025). Artificial intelligence in mental health research: Opportunities and challenges. *Annals of Indian Psychiatry*. Advance online publication. DOI: 10.4103/aip.aip_100_25

Biró, A., Cuesta-Vargas, A. I., & Szilágyi, L. (2023). Precognition of mental health and neurogenerative disorders using. *Acta Universitatis Sapientiae Informatica*, *15*(2), 359–403. DOI: 10.2478/ausi-2023-0022

Bobkov, A., Cheng, F., Xu, J., Bobkova, T., Deng, F., He, J., Jiang, X., Khuzin, D., & Kang, Z. (2025). Telepsychiatry and artificial intelligence: A structured review of emerging approaches to accessible psychiatric care. *Healthcare (Basel)*, *13*(11), 1348. DOI: 10.3390/healthcare13111348 PMID: 40508960

Buhr, E., Fischer, M., Biernetzky, O., Teipel, S., Gruber, O., & Schweda, M. (2025). Use of artificial intelligence in psychiatric research and practice: A qualitative interview study with experts from psychiatry, computer science and philosophy in Germany. *European Psychiatry : the Journal of the Association of European Psychiatrists*, *68*(1), e105. DOI: 10.1192/j.eurpsy.2025.10075 PMID: 40754806

Chekroud, A. M., Bondar, J., Delgadillo, J., Doherty, G., Wasil, A., Fokkema, M., Cohen, Z., Belgrave, D., DeRubeis, R., Iniesta, R., Dwyer, D., & Choi, K. (2021). The promise of machine learning in predicting treatment outcomes in psychiatry. *World Psychiatry; Official Journal of the World Psychiatric Association (WPA)*, *20*(2), 154–170. DOI: 10.1002/wps.20882 PMID: 34002503

de Castro, Y. V. C., Morii, K. Y., Santos, I. A., Destefani, A. C., & Destefani, V. C. (2024). Beyond black boxes: Interpretable Ai for enhanced risk assessment and ethical decision-making in forensic psychiatry. Revista Ibero-Americana de Humanidades. *Ciência & Educação (Bauru)*, *10*(8), 2475–2479. DOI: 10.51891/rease.v10i8.15298

Doraiswamy, P. M., Blease, C., & Bodner, K. (2020a). Artificial intelligence and the future of psychiatry: Insights from a global physician survey. *Artificial Intelligence in Medicine*, *102*(101753), 101753. DOI: 10.1016/j.artmed.2019.101753 PMID: 31980092

Doraiswamy, P. M., Blease, C., & Bodner, K. (2020b). Artificial intelligence and the future of psychiatry: Insights from a global physician survey. *Artificial Intelligence in Medicine*, *102*(101753), 101753. DOI: 10.1016/j.artmed.2019.101753 PMID: 31980092

Dow, E. R., Chen, K. M., Zhao, C. S., Knapp, A. N., Phadke, A., Weng, K., Do, D. V., Mahajan, V. B., Mruthyunjaya, P., Leng, T., & Myung, D. (2023). Artificial Intelligence improves patient follow-up in a diabetic retinopathy screening program. *Clinical Ophthalmology (Auckland, N.Z.)*, *17*, 3323–3330. DOI: 10.2147/OPTH.S422513 PMID: 38026608

Dow, E. R., Khan, N. C., Chen, K. M., Mishra, K., Perera, C., Narala, R., Basina, M., Dang, J., Kim, M., Levine, M., Phadke, A., Tan, M., Weng, K., Do, D. V., Moshfeghi, D. M., Mahajan, V. B., Mruthyunjaya, P., Leng, T., & Myung, D. (2023). AI-human hybrid workflow enhances teleophthalmology for the detection of diabetic retinopathy. *Ophthalmology Science*, *3*(4), 100330. DOI: 10.1016/j.xops.2023.100330 PMID: 37449051

Gerantia, M. (2024). Artificial intelligence in psychiatry: A comprehensive literature review. *European Psychiatry : the Journal of the Association of European Psychiatrists*, *67*(S1), S61–S61. DOI: 10.1192/j.eurpsy.2024.173

Germack, H. D., Leung, L., Zhao, X., Zhang, H., & Martsolf, G. R. (2022). Association of team-based care and continuity of care with hospitalizations for veterans with comorbid mental and physical health conditions. *Journal of General Internal Medicine*, *37*(1), 40–48. DOI: 10.1007/s11606-021-06884-5 PMID: 34027614

Graham, S., Depp, C., Lee, E. E., Nebeker, C., Tu, X., Kim, H.-C., & Jeste, D. V. (2019). Artificial intelligence for mental health and mental illnesses: An overview. *Current Psychiatry Reports*, *21*(11), 116. DOI: 10.1007/s11920-019-1094-0 PMID: 31701320

Higgins, O., Short, B. L., Chalup, S. K., & Wilson, R. L. (2023). Artificial intelligence (AI) and machine learning (ML) based decision support systems in mental health: An integrative review. *International Journal of Mental Health Nursing*, *32*(4), 966–978. DOI: 10.1111/inm.13114 PMID: 36744684

Kolding, S., Lundin, R. M., Hansen, L., & Østergaard, S. D. (2024). Use of generative artificial intelligence (AI) in psychiatry and mental health care: A systematic review. *Acta Neuropsychiatrica*, *37*, e37. DOI: 10.1017/neu.2024.50 PMID: 39523628

Kumar, H. (2025). AI-powered Mental Health diagnostics using Multimodal Data: A Deep Learning-based approach. *International Scientific Journal of Engineering and Management*, *04*(06), 1–9. DOI: 10.55041/ISJEM04560

M, T., & Annamalai, A. (2020a). Telepsychiatry and the role of artificial intelligence in mental health in post-COVID-19 India: A scoping review on opportunities. Indian Journal of Psychological Medicine, 42(5), 428–434. DOI: 10.1177/0253717620952160

Mahapatra, P., Sahoo, K. C., Jitendriya, P., Samal, M., & Pati, S. (2021). Qualitative research methods in psychiatry in India: Landscaping the terrain. *Indian Journal of Psychiatry*, *63*(1), 5–14. DOI: 10.4103/psychiatry.IndianJPsychiatry_665_20 PMID: 34083815

Mason, A. J. C., Bhavsar, V., Botelle, R., Chandran, D., Li, L., Mascio, A., Sanyal, J., Kadra-Scalzo, G., Roberts, A., Williams, M., & Stewart, R. (2024). Applying neural network algorithms to ascertain reported experiences of violence in routine mental healthcare records and distributions of reports by diagnosis. *Frontiers in Psychiatry*, *15*, 1181739. DOI: 10.3389/fpsyt.2024.1181739 PMID: 39319350

McCradden, M., Hui, K., & Buchman, D. Z. (2023). Evidence, ethics and the promise of artificial intelligence in psychiatry. *Journal of Medical Ethics*, *49*(8), 573–579. DOI: 10.1136/jme-2022-108447 PMID: 36581457

Miner, A. S., Shah, N., Bullock, K. D., Arnow, B. A., Bailenson, J., & Hancock, J. (2019). Key considerations for incorporating conversational AI in psychotherapy. *Frontiers in Psychiatry*, *10*, 746. DOI: 10.3389/fpsyt.2019.00746 PMID: 31681047

Mustapha, A. Y., Ikhalea, N., Chianumba, E. C., & Forkuo, A. Y. (2022). Developing an AI-powered predictive model for mental health disorder diagnosis using electronic health records. *International Journal of Multidisciplinary Research and Growth Evaluation*, *3*(1), 914–931. DOI: 10.54660/.IJMRGE.2022.3.1.914-931

Okpete, U. E., & Byeon, H. (2024). Challenges and prospects in bridging precision medicine and artificial intelligence in genomic psychiatric treatment. *World Journal of Psychiatry*, *14*(8), 1148–1164. DOI: 10.5498/wjp.v14.i8.1148 PMID: 39165556

Patel, R., Wee, S. N., Ramaswamy, R., Thadani, S., Guruswamy, G., Garg, R., Calvanese, N., Valko, M., Rush, A., Rentería, M., Sarkar, J., & Kollins, S. (2022). NeuroBlu: A natural language processing (NLP) electronic health record (EHR) data analytic tool to generate real-world evidence in mental healthcare. *European Psychiatry : the Journal of the Association of European Psychiatrists*, *65*(S1), S99–S100. DOI: 10.1192/j.eurpsy.2022.286

Pham, K. T., Nabizadeh, A., & Selek, S. (2022). Artificial intelligence and chatbots in psychiatry. *The Psychiatric Quarterly*, *93*(1), 249–253. DOI: 10.1007/s11126-022-09973-8 PMID: 35212940

Prégent, J., Chung, V.-H.-A., El Adib, I., Désilets, M., & Hudon, A. (2025a). Applications of artificial intelligence in psychiatry and psychology education: Scoping review. *JMIR Medical Education*, *11*, e75238. DOI: 10.2196/75238 PMID: 40720804

Prégent, J., Chung, V.-H.-A., El Adib, I., Désilets, M., & Hudon, A. (2025b). Applications of artificial intelligence in psychiatry and psychology education: Scoping review. *JMIR Medical Education*, *11*, e75238. DOI: 10.2196/75238 PMID: 40720804

Prince, E. W., Hankinson, T. C., & Görg, C. (2025). A visual analytics framework for assessing interactive AI for clinical decision support. Pacific Symposium on Biocomputing. *Pacific Symposium on Biocomputing*, *30*, 40–53. DOI: 10.1142/9789819807024_0004 PMID: 39670360

Punia, A., Bhakuni, P., & Sharma, N. (2025). Development of AI- and NLP-driven chatbots and virtual assistants for mental health support. In Advances in Psychology, Mental Health, and Behavioral Studies (pp. 229–262). IGI Global. DOI: 10.4018/979-8-3693-9341-3.ch010

Putica, A., Khanna, R., Bosl, W., Saraf, S., & Edgcomb, J. (2025). Ethical decision-making for AI in mental health: The Integrated Ethical Approach for Computational Psychiatry (IEACP) framework. *Psychological Medicine*, *55*(e213), e213. DOI: 10.1017/S0033291725101311 PMID: 40702980

Rathinavel, P., Ravikumar, R. N., Aarthi, S., Habib, M., Salaeva, N., & Pardaev, J. (2025). Augmenting human capabilities. In *Advances in Computational Intelligence and Robotics* (pp. 1–30). IGI Global Scientific Publishing., DOI: 10.4018/979-8-3373-2372-5.ch001

Raveesh, B. N., & Munoli, R. N. (2020). Ethical and legal aspects of telepsychiatry. *Indian Journal of Psychological Medicine*, *42*(5, Suppl), 63S–69S. DOI: 10.1177/0253717620962033 PMID: 33354067

Ravikumar, R. S., Manujakshi, Aarthi, S., Urazbaeva, Y., & Tamilselvi, S. (2025). Navigating data privacy, security, and regulatory challenges in healthcare AI ensuring fairness, bias mitigation, interpretability, and trust. In Transformative Role of Transformer Models in Healthcare (pp. 25–54). IGI Global Scientific Publishing. DOI: 10.4018/979-8-3373-2038-0.ch002

Ravikumar, R. N., Aarthi, S., Dilshodbek, A., Satheesh Kumar, A., Eshkaraev, S., & Shanmugam, K. B. (2025). Integrating blockchain, smart contracts, and AI for decentralized healthcare in the metaverse. In *Blockchain-Based Healthcare Management in the Metaverse* (pp. 261–294). IGI Global Scientific Publishing., DOI: 10.4018/979-8-3373-1225-5.ch010

Rony, M. K. K., Das, D. C., Khatun, M. T., Ferdousi, S., Akter, M. R., Khatun, M. A., Begum, M. H., Khalil, M. I., Parvin, M. R., Alrazeeni, D. M., & Akter, F. (2025). Artificial intelligence in psychiatry: A systematic review and meta-analysis of diagnostic and therapeutic efficacy. *Digital Health, 11*, 20552076251330530. DOI: 10.1177/20552076251330528 PMID: 40162166

Squires, M., Tao, X., Elangovan, S., Gururajan, R., Zhou, X., Acharya, U. R., & Li, Y. (2023). Deep learning and machine learning in psychiatry: A survey of current progress in depression detection, diagnosis and treatment. *Brain Informatics, 10*(1), 10. DOI: 10.1186/s40708-023-00188-6 PMID: 37093301

Steyvers, M., & Kumar, A. (2024). Three challenges for AI-assisted decision-making. Perspectives on Psychological Science: A Journal of the Association for Psychological Science, 19(5), 722–734. DOI: 10.1177/17456916231181102

Terra, M., Baklola, M., Ali, S., & El-Bastawisy, K. (2023). Opportunities, applications, challenges and ethical implications of artificial intelligence in psychiatry: A narrative review. *The Egyptian Journal of Neurology, Psychiatry and Neurosurgery, 59*(1), 80. Advance online publication. DOI: 10.1186/s41983-023-00681-z

Uganda, F. of M. K. I. U., & Mukamurera P., N. (2025). Telepresence in Healthcare: Engineering Remote Consultations. IDOSR JOURNAL OF BIOCHEMISTRY, BIOTECHNOLOGY AND ALLIED FIELDS, 10(1), 21–27. DOI: 10.59298/IDOSR/JBBAF/2025/1012127

Vale, M. D. (2024). Moral entrepreneurship and the ethics of artificial intelligence in digital psychiatry. *Socius: Sociological Research for a Dynamic World, 10*, 23780231241259641. Advance online publication. DOI: 10.1177/23780231241259641

Yadav, N. (2025). AI for mental health: The use of chatbots and NLP to support therapy and early detection. *International Scientific Journal of Engineering and Management, 04*(05), 1–7. DOI: 10.55041/ISJEM03402

Zirikly, A., Desmet, B., Newman-Griffis, D., Marfeo, E. E., McDonough, C., Goldman, H., & Chan, L. (2022). Information extraction framework for disability determination using a mental functioning use-case. *JMIR Medical Informatics, 10*(3), e32245. DOI: 10.2196/32245 PMID: 35302510

KEY TERMS AND DEFINITIONS

Algorithmic Bias: The systematic error of AI predictions due to unrepresentative or skewed training data, which can be biased or inaccurate in psychiatric assessment, can take place.

Intelligent Care Teams: The collaboration models where psychiatrists, psychologists, nurses, general practitioners, and AI systems collaborate with each other through integrated dashboards to deliver comprehensive and coordinated treatment.

Natural Language Processing (NLP): One subdivision of AI, which allows computers to interpret, analyze and extract meaning within human language, is used in tele psychiatry to identify sentiment, tone and linguistic indications of mental health issues.

Predictive Analytics: Machine learning model use and statistical analysis of patient data to determine the risk of psychiatric disorders, risk of relapse, or to predict the outcome of the treatment.

Symbiotic Human-AI Workflow: An approach in healthcare that involves the use of AI tools to augment, not replace, clinicians through diagnostic assistance, data synthesis and predictive information without sacrificing human empathy and clinical authority.

Telepsychiatry: Use of digital and telecommunication to carry out psychiatric assessment, consultation and treatment remotely due to geographical barriers and clinician availability.

Virtual Assistants (VAs): Conversational agents powered by AI and trained to talk to patients round-the-clock by reminding them, monitoring their mood, or having therapist-like conversations, and help patients stick to their treatment and avoid feeling isolated.

Chapter 8
AI-Driven Telehealth in Rural India:
Challenges, Adoption Behaviour, and Collaborative Strategies

R. Manju Priya
http://orcid.org/0000-0001-9144-5301
Jain University, India

N. Sathyanarayana
http://orcid.org/0000-0002-4185-7751
Jain University, India

C. Daniel Nesa Kumar
http://orcid.org/0000-0003-4184-216X
Sri Ramakrishna College of Arts and Science, India

ABSTRACT

The chapter is a conceptual discussion on the transformative impact of Artificial Intelligence (AI) in improving telehealth delivery in rural India. It analyses behavioural, systemic, and strategic aspects of AI-enabled healthcare uptake by incorporating integrative models, such as TAM, UTAUT, and UTAUT2. The research highlights the influence of digital literacy, trust, cultural beliefs, and infrastructural readiness on the adoption of telehealth technologies by rural users. It focuses on the collaboration between humans and AI, promoting the idea of augmented intelligence, in which AI will not substitute for clinicians but rather enhance them, to achieve fair and compassionate healthcare services. The chapter also identifies infrastructural, regulatory, and cultural issues and recommends multi-stakeholder approaches that

DOI: 10.4018/979-8-3373-5906-9.ch008

involve policymakers, technologists, and community players. Ultimately, it provides a conceptual framework for inclusive, ethical, and sustainable AI-telehealth systems to address healthcare disparities in rural India.

1 INTRODUCTION

1.1 Background and Context

The provision of health care in rural India is prone to deep-rooted problems which are both systemic and socio-geographic in nature. With more than 65% of the Indian population in rural areas, inequality in healthcare access, infrastructure, and human resources has been a serious issue of concern in terms of public health. Poor doctor-patient ratios, inadequate primary care centres, the absence of specialised care services, and limited digital infrastructure characterise the rural health landscape, which contributes to high disease burdens and preventable mortality rates (Sreenu, 2019).

In response to these issues, the concept of telehealth, which involves providing health-related information and services via digital communication technologies, has become a matter of crucial innovation. The COVID-19 pandemic triggered a faster worldwide and in India implementation, which triggered the interest in the AI-based telemedicine platforms to eliminate spatial and resource limitations (Dash et al., 2021). However, the willingness of people in rural India to implement such technologies is low due to a lack of infrastructure, low digital literacy levels, and socio-cultural factors (Kanwar et al., 2023).

1.2 Healthcare and Artificial Intelligence

In healthcare, the application of Artificial Intelligence (AI) encompasses machine learning algorithms, natural language processing, computer vision, and robotic process automation to support clinical decision-making, administrative automation, and enhance patient outcomes (Jiang et al., 2017). Its uses are diagnostic tools, predictive analytics, triage chatbots, remote patient monitoring, and clinical decision support. These AI tools offer enormous opportunities in the Indian rural environment, as they can address the shortage of doctors, provide representation in multiple languages, and ensure continuity of care through online consultations. For example, AI-based symptom detectors can assist patients without requiring hospital visits, thereby saving unnecessary travel and expenses (Abisha et al., 2024). But context-sensitive design is necessary, without which these technologies will not be able to be adopted or trusted by the rural users.

1.3 Telehealth and AI: Strategic Rural Gap Solution

The combination of AI and telehealth represents a paradigm shift in healthcare provision, particularly in underserved and remote communities. Where telehealth offers a connectivity and communication platform, AI adds decision-making intelligence, personalisation, and automation to it. Research indicates that telehealth using AI has the potential to improve clinical performance, minimise physician burnout, and increase access to diagnostics and triage devices in rural areas (Topol, 2019). Implementation should, however, be well controlled. The privacy of data, bias in algorithms, distrust of machine suggestions, and the lack of inclusion of non-digital populations are key points of concern. These problems highlight the need for inclusive, ethical, and human-centred frameworks.

1.4 The Indian Rural Challenge

Rural India has previously experienced significant digital divides, despite national digital health initiatives such as the Ayushman Bharat Digital Mission and eSanjeevani. The internet is accessible to only 24% of rural households (NFHS-5, 2021), and despite an increasing trend, smartphone density is not evenly distributed among genders, age groups, and income levels. This renders the blind utilisation of AI-healthcare applications problematic unless they are combined with local realities and informed by behavioural knowledge. In addition, trust in informal healers, belief in traditional medicine, family-based decision-making, and low education on digital health rights are the factors impacting health-seeking behaviours in rural India. These social-cultural factors go a long way in influencing the technology adoption behaviour (Khosravi et al, 2024).

Figure 1. Key AI-Telehealth Statistics in Rural India: 2024 vs 2033 Projection

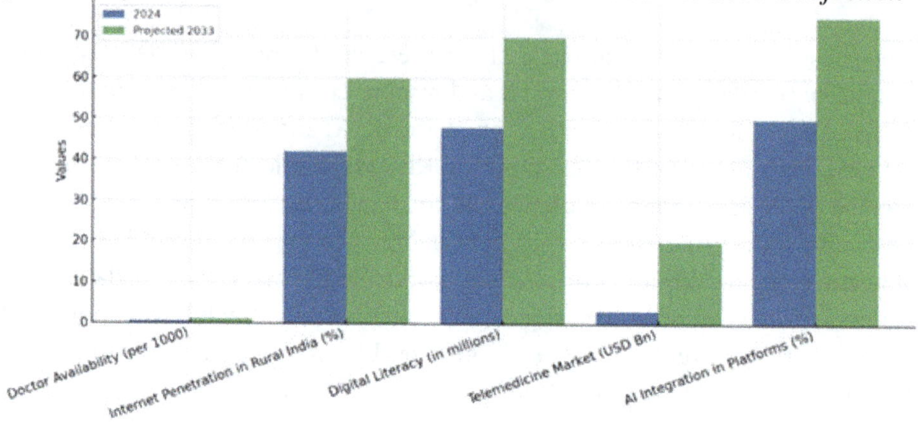

Source: Author's synthesis using data from IMARC Group, Grand View Research, and other industry sources.

Table 1. Growth Indicators for AI-Enabled Telehealth Services in Rural India (2024–2033)

Indicator	2024 value	2033 projected	Source
Doctor Availability (per 1000)	0.4	1.0 (WHO recommended)	Springer (2024). *Addressing healthcare worker shortages in rural India.* DOI: 10.1007/s44155-025-00250-0
Rural Internet Penetration (%)	42%	60%(Projected)	*Internet in India.* (n.d.). Wikipedia - the Free Encyclopedia. https://en.wikipedia.org/wiki/Internet_in_India
Digital Literacy (millions)	48M	70M+(Projected)	Ministry of Electronics & IT. *PMGDISHA Dashboard 2024.* csc.gov.in
Telemedicine Market (USD Bn)	$3.1 Bn	$19.9 Bn	IMARC Group (2024). *India Telemedicine Market Report.* imarcgroup.com
AI Integration in Telehealth (%)	50%	75%	ARIX Blog (2024). *AI and Telemedicine Trends in India.* blog.ariqx.com and The C Connects. *AI in Indian Healthcare.* thecconnects.com

Source: WHO (2024); IAMAI (2024); PMGDISHA/CSC e-Governance (2024); IMARC Group (2024); ARIX/ The C-Connects (2024).

Table 1 and Figure 1 highlight both the existing gaps and the immense growth potential of AI-driven telehealth in rural India. While current indicators reveal systemic challenges such as low doctor availability and digital inclusion, the projected improvements by 2033 underscore the accelerating momentum in infrastructure, policy support, and technology adoption. These trends affirm the relevance and timeliness of strategic, collaborative efforts to scale AI-telehealth interventions for underserved populations.

Figure 2. India Telehealth Services Market Trends (2024–2032)

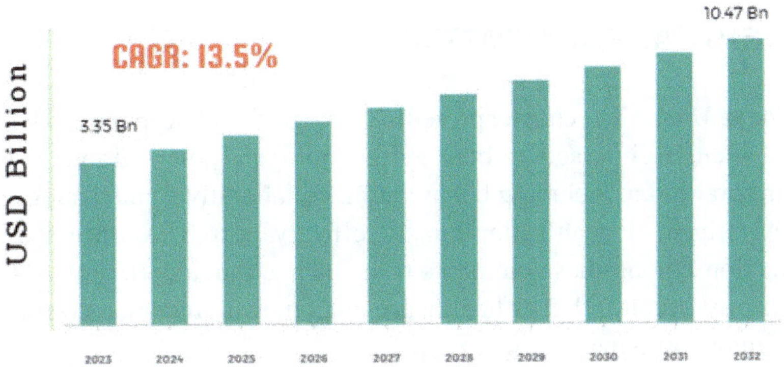

Source: India Telehealth Services Market Size, Share Global Analysis Report, 2024 – 2032. (2024b, July). Facts & Factors. https://www.fnfresearch.com/india-telehealth-services-market

The industry is predicted to grow to greater than USD 10.47 billion in market value in 2032, with a 13.5% CAGR, with a bar chart (Figure 2) starting with USD 3.35 billion in the industry in the year 2023. A positive trend in adopting digital healthcare is indicated by the projections of the growth of the telehealth market in India to more than USD 10.47 billion by 2032, a growth that was estimated to reach USD 3.35billion by 2023. This 13.5% CAGR is consistent and highlights the increasing investment opportunity, policy favorability, and infrastructure preparedness, especially when it comes to extending AI-enabled telehealth into rural and underserved areas.

2 OBJECTIVES

1. To explore and synthesise relevant theoretical frameworks—including Technology Adoption Models (TAM, UTAUT and UTAUT2) and Human-AI interaction theories—to understand the behavioural and systemic factors influencing the acceptance of AI-driven telehealth in rural India.
2. To conceptually examine the role of human-AI collaboration in enhancing telehealth delivery, focusing on trust, digital inclusivity, and ethical integration in the context of rural and underserved populations.

3. To identify the key challenges and propose strategic, collaborative approaches for the successful implementation of AI-enabled telehealth services that are inclusive, scalable, and responsive to the needs of rural communities in India.

3 CONCEPTUAL FRAMEWORK

Integrative Model: The chapter presents an integrative conceptual model to explain the most challenging interactions between technological potential and socio-cultural realities in rural India, including behavioural, collaborative, and strategic determinants of AI-driven telehealth adoption and effectiveness. The conceptualisation of this interaction among these elements to influence the adoption of AI-telehealth and, eventually, result in better healthcare outcomes in underserved rural areas is presented in the framework (Figure 3).

Figure 3. Conceptual Framework of AI-Driven Telehealth Adoption in Rural India

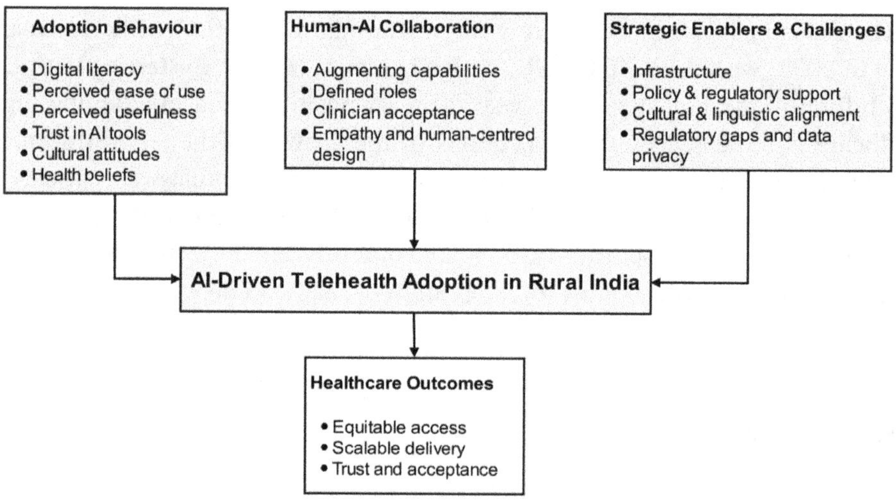

Source: Authors' contributions

Figure 3 is a conceptual model that shows how the elements contribute to the adoption of AI-based telehealth systems in rural India in a dependent manner. It has three layers that are interrelated, i.e. as discussed below.

3.1 Adoption Behaviour (Individual level layer)

Adoption behaviour is the way people and society choose to embrace and adopt AI-based telehealth technologies. The concept of rural AI-driven telehealth adoption needs a strong theoretical foundation of behavioural models of technology acceptance. Some of the most popular ones include the Technology Acceptance Model (TAM) (Davis, 1989), the Unified Theory of Acceptance and Use of Technology (UTAUT) (Venkatesh et al., 2003), and the extended model, UTAUT2 (Venkatesh et al., 2012). These models state how the users, most prominently the non-expert or first-time users, make their choices to use new technologies due to their perception of usability, social context, infrastructure, emotional gratification and behavioural models.

Specifically, TAM suggests that the more useful and easy-to-use the technology may be, the more likely the users will adopt it. This is in tight connection with the experience of the rural users with AI-telehealth platforms, where the engagement is conditioned by the simplification of navigation and the value of health. The UTAUT framework goes an extra mile by including Social Influence (e.g., community health workers promoting use) and Facilitating Conditions (e.g., the availability of a mobile network, training support), which are especially important in rural Indian settings.

Moreover, UTAUT2 tailors the model to the buying context by adding to it Hedonic Motivation (enjoyment in using the tool), Price Value (cost-benefit perception) and Habit (repeated usage). These aspects are particularly important to users with low literacy levels, who are cost-sensitive and reside in remote locations. Specifically, a free local language voice-activated AI chatbot can meet the hedonic and price criteria and will only become habitual with the help of repetition by ASHAs or community kiosks. These models are the basis of behaviour in the conceptual framework that is suggested in this chapter. The sub-sections that follow deconstruct individual dimensions of adoption behaviour applicable to rural India, each of which is projected to the constituents of the TAM, UTAUT, and UTAUT2.

In India, especially in the rural areas, this is determined by a number of factors which are interdependent:

1. **Digital Literacy:** Digital literacy is the basis of interaction with the AI-based telehealth solutions, particularly in rural India. Inadequate experience with digital interfaces, smartphones, or internet navigation may pose a significant obstacle to communication with symptom checkers, remote monitoring devices, or online consultations. Abisha et al. (2024) emphasise that the ability of AI tools to work is not high when the users do not have a minimum level of digital skills or confidence. Moreover, gender and age gaps in literacy contribute to the gap, as they leave women and the elderly excluded from the use of health

technologies. Community-based digital training programs and improved user interfaces should therefore come first in the promotion of the adoption of telehealth.

2. **Perceived Ease of Use and Usefulness:** The perceived ease of using the technology and its usefulness are defining aspects of how much one is likely to adopt the new technology as described by the Technology Acceptance Model (TAM) that was created by Davis (1989). A telehealth platform where users can readily have access to a doctor or get diagnostic inputs in their local language will be more acceptable in rural healthcare. Perceived usefulness will also be dependent on whether users believe that the technology will enhance their experience when it comes to accessing quality and timely care. When AI tools help to alleviate travel burden, save time or offer trustworthy health guidance, perceived value is elevated. In case the usability is very low (because of language constraints or complicated navigation), adoption usually decreases dramatically.
3. **Confidence in AI Tools:** Trust is an essential element of AI-based healthcare service acceptance, which is especially important in rural areas with underserved patients, where the human touch is still the main part of the healthcare experience. The accuracy, impersonality, or misuse of data might make rural users unwilling to use automated diagnostics or recommendations. Khosravi et al. (2024) note that trust can be enhanced when AI systems are developed with transparency, yield consistent functions, and are in accordance with the expectations and values of users. Furthermore, the use of AI, mediated by community health workers, is more likely to make users more trusting, as users will feel associated with the use of technology through a familiar and trusted contact. In the absence of this trust, even the well-designed tools may be opposed.
4. **Cultural Norms and Health Beliefs:** In India, socio-cultural norms, traditional medicine, and local power structures play a significant role in health-seeking behaviour, which is common in rural areas in India. A large target population uses Ayurveda, home remedies, or local doctors, whose recommendations are more important than a digital consultation. As Hoque and Bao (2015) observe, the virtual or artificial healthcare is frequently sluggish in the adoption process due to the decision-making process that is rooted in family (and, particularly, male) values and the need to have a face-to-face contact. Moreover, aspects such as disease, recovery and faith in the technology are strongly influenced by local traditions and belief systems. The first layer of the conceptual model is the presence of culturally sensitive design and outreach, as this will make AI-telehealth seem as invasive, unnatural, or irrelevant.

Such behavioural factors as perceived in the context of such models as TAM, UTAUT, and UTAUT2 constitute the initial layer in this chapter. They are facilitators and possible obstacles to the utilisation of technology in rural healthcare and highlight the necessity of culturally integrated, user-friendly, and trust-sensitive digital health technologies.

Table 2. Summary table of where each model connects

Components	Relevant models	Explanation
Digital Literacy	UTAUT (Facilitating Conditions)	Skills and support affect usability
Perceived Ease of Use and Usefulness	TAM	Core constructs
Trust in AI Tools	TAM, UTAUT	Trust overlaps with perceived usefulness.
Cultural Norms & Health Beliefs	UTAUT, UTAUT2	Social influence, habit

Source: Davis (1989), Venkatesh et al. (2003), Venkatesh et al. (2012)

Table 2 aligns influential factors on the implementation of AI-driven telehealth in rural India with known technology acceptance models. The state of digital literacy indicates enabling circumstances in UTAUT, whereas the perceived ease of use and usefulness correspond to the fundamental TAM constructs. Reliance on AI tools is based on both models, affecting the perceived usefulness and intention to use. The cultural beliefs and health norms are also related to the social influence and the habit in UTAUT, and reveal how the community beliefs influence the acceptance of telehealth.

3.2 Human-AI Collaboration (Systemic layer)

This is a systemic layer of the conceptual framework that deals with the dynamic interaction between AI systems and healthcare providers. Instead of substituting clinicians, AI can be used as a supportive tool that can augment decision-making, decrease the burden, and expand access to health services. With the workforce scarcity being critical and the specialists being inaccessible, especially in the rural Indian setting, a successful human-AI cooperation can improve the quality of care tremendously. Yet, to make collaboration substantial and viable, systems need to be reliable, convenient, and harmonised, corresponding to clinical and cultural expectations.

1. **Augmenting Clinical Capabilities:** AI technologies have the potential to greatly improve the clinical capacities of the health system, especially in those regions that are under-resourced, such as rural settings. The AI can reduce human error

and increase the coverage of busy providers through applications such as diagnostic imaging analysis, symptom checkers, and predictive risk modelling. The AI-based triage tools can be used to prioritise patients in seconds, and machine learning algorithms can be used to predict diseases like tuberculosis or diabetic retinopathy. Topol (2019) points out that the combination of human skill and machine accuracy results in what he refers to as a high-performance medicine in which clinical decisions become quicker, more precise and scalable across geographies.

2. **Defined Roles and Task Sharing:** The definition of roles between the technology and the healthcare worker is another critical success factor of human-AI collaboration. In case of ambiguity of roles, confusion of accountability may occur and result in underutilization or opposition. Successful collaboration means organised workflows wherein AI assists in routine work or data-intensive work, such as initial triage or administrative documentation, and clinicians maintain the power to make diagnostic and treatment decisions. This model of task-sharing does not compromise the clinical judgment of the provider, as it improves efficiency. Research indicates that role clarity enhances clinician satisfaction, and burnout levels in AI-implemented systems are lower (Wadden, 2022).
3. **Clinician Acceptance:** The implementation of AI in health care is not only a technological problem but a human behaviour one as well. These systems can only be effectively integrated into working processes by making clinicians trust the outputs, logic, and limitations of the AI tools used in these systems. Healthcare workers might be reluctant to trust the recommendations provided by AI when they lack transparency or are contrary to clinical intuition. This is demonstrated in the research as AI tools that have explainable and transparent decision-making processes encourage increased clinician confidence. According to Wadden (2022), the most obvious solution to the problem is to deal with the black box problem, in which the lack of interpretability leads to ethical and operational conflicts between AI developers and their clinical users.
4. **Empathy and Human-Centred Design:** Rural Indian healthcare delivery is highly interpersonal, emphatic, and socially connected. The AI systems should be created to complement empathic messages between providers and patients rather than to suppress them. Holeman and Kane (2020) state that digital health technologies, which fail to respect human dignity, connection to emotions, and cultural appropriateness, have a lower likelihood of success, particularly in vulnerable or illiterate populations. The principles of human-centred design recommend co-creation of AI tools between the local users and the providers to ensure that technological interventions do not violate patient privacy, promote informed consent, and promote compassionate care. Therefore, systems neces-

sary to ensure successful human-AI collaboration are interpretable, supportive, and culturally intelligent.

3.3 Strategic Enablers and Challenges (Structural layer):

The layer identifies systemic and environmental aspects of the success or failure of AI-based telehealth programs in rural India. Although behavioural and collaborative factors are critical, other infrastructural, regulatory and cultural factors act as the foundations to sustainable implementation. Such structural enablers and constraints are usually beyond the authority of individual users/clinicians, yet are fundamental to finding scale, equity and long-term effects.

1. **Infrastructure:** The existence of reliable infrastructure, such as electricity, mobile networks, internet bandwidth, and physical space to access digital infrastructure, is a requirement of AI-telehealth systems deployment. In India, the teleconsultation service and AI-based diagnostics are hindered by persistent issues with power outages, weak mobile signals, and the lack of broadband in many rural regions. Khan and Driessen (2018) observe that infrastructure gaps not only deter access but also confidence and continuity of care on the side of the user. Devoid of solid foundation systems, even the most advanced AI tools will go to waste or will not be available in the countryside setting.
2. **Policy and Regulatory Support:** The ability of AI-health interventions relies on facilitating policy environments. Rural-specific AI governance has not been developed in India, despite the introduction of digital health missions in the country, including Ayushman Bharat. Sreenu (2019) notes that the ethical principles, AI validation procedures, and implementation policies tend to be urban-based, which leaves the rural stakeholders without any clear directions. Existence of ambiguity in policy may discourage health workers, developers and funders from engaging in rural AI-health pilot, hence slowing down innovation. There is a need to promote trust and clarity of operations within the sectors by having clear, localised policy frameworks.
3. **Cultural and Linguistic Alignment:** Adoption of technology in rural settings is significantly affected by language, culture and health beliefs in the region. The AI tools need to be sensitive to local dialects, literacy levels and health-seeking norms. English or urban Hindi interfaces also tend to isolate the non-literate or regional language speakers. Sindakis and Showkat (2024) claim that tools that are culturally inappropriate, despite their strong technology, cannot connect with users and remain in interaction in the long term. Design Community-based design, including local languages, graphics, and culturally appropriate situations,

will increase usability and lead to increased inclusivity in AI-based healthcare provision.

4. **Regulatory Gaps and Data Privacy:** Lack of integrated data privacy frameworks, especially ones specifically designed around AI in clinical settings, is a significant obstacle to rural use. The problem of information misuse, bias in algorithms, and unaccountability in the making of AI decisions undermines the trust of the population. As noted by Sreenu (2019), in the absence of official regulations concerning consent, data ownership, and explainability, the rural population, which is already low in terms of legal and digital literacy, will continue to be vulnerable. This lack of regulation also disincentivises user involvement and constrains the ethical use of telehealth innovations in public health systems. Such structural facilitators and restraints need to be managed based on a multi-stakeholder partnership with government agencies, non-governmental organisations, technology developers, and community health systems.

The combination of these factors has an impact on the central variable: The combination of these three layers through the usability of AI solutions in telehealth in rural areas defines the adoption and maintenance of AI solutions in rural environments. The benefits of successful adoption include improved health outcomes, more access, more efficiency, earlier diagnosis and equity.

Dynamic feedback loops are represented by two-way arrows among layers. As an example, better infrastructure increases the potential of collaboration, and the activities of community trust-building have a positive relationship with acceptance behaviour.

4 CORE FRAMEWORK ELEMENTS

This part will take a closer look at the central dimensions of the conceptual framework proposed, adoption behaviour, human-AI collaborative dynamics, and strategic collaborative strategies, which in turn affect the overall success of AI-driven telehealth solutions adoption among rural India.

4.1 Adoption Behaviour in Rural Telehealth

Introducing AI-based telehealth services in rural India is conditioned by a complicated interplay of behavioural, socio-economic, and contextual factors. Based on the technology acceptance model (TAM) (Davis, 1989) and the Unified Theory of Acceptance and Use of Technology (UTAUT) (Venkatesh et al., 2003), UTAUT2 expands it to consumers by adding three more constructs: hedonic motivation, price value, and habit. They are especially applicable in the case of rural telehealths, when the hedonic motivation of enjoying or finding the application easy to use (hedonic motivation), the perceived value against the cost (value of price) and the routine of use all can greatly affect the adoption in the long run (habitual use). Two important constructs, which are perceived usefulness and perceived ease of use, always surface as determinants of technology uptake (Venkatesh et al., 2012).

Digital literacy is a major challenge, especially in rural areas. The National Sample Survey (2019) states that only a minority of rural households (less than 25% of households) had access to the internet, and an even smaller number were exposed to digital platforms. Such exposure has a great influence on the perceived ease of use of AI-assisted health tools.

In addition, language and cultural standards have an impact on trust and interaction. According to a study conducted by Hoque and Bao (2015), in rural settings, technology acceptance depends on the support of the regional language and the cultural relevance. Rural users would tend to put more faith in healthcare services provided that they are presented in a familiar socio-cultural and language setting. The mediator is trust or trust in the AI technology and the healthcare provider. Users will be unwilling to adopt AI tools when they believe that they are impersonal or prone to errors (Chiou & Lee, 2023). Hence, it is necessary to promote trust by designing user-centred, transparent, and community-based training (Dwivedi et al., 2019).

4.1.1 Comparative Analysis of Technology Adoption Models: TAM, UTAUT, and UTAUT2

The rural adoption of AI-enabled telehealth cannot be comprehended without a theoretical base on the adoption of behavioural technologies. The most widely used ones include the Technology Acceptance Model (TAM) and the Unified Theory of Acceptance and Use of Technology (UTAUT) -both of which are used to explain how people make evaluations and acceptance of new technology and how they subsequently proceed to use it.

Table 3. Comparison of Technology Adoption Models and Their Relevance to AI-Driven Telehealth in Rural India

Model	Key constructs	Description	Relevance to Rural Telehealth
TAM (Davis, 1989)	- Perceived Usefulness (PU) - Perceived Ease of Use (PEOU)	Suggests that individuals' intentions to use technology are primarily influenced by how useful and easy it is to use.	Rural users may adopt telehealth tools only if they find them easy to navigate and beneficial for their health needs.
UTAUT (Venkatesh et al., 2012)	- Performance Expectancy - Effort Expectancy - Social Influence - Facilitating Conditions	Integrates eight prior models and highlights social and infrastructural factors in technology acceptance.	In rural India, family norms, peer advice, and support systems like ASHAs affect user willingness to engage with telehealth.
UTAUT2 (Venkatesh et al., 2012)	Adds to UTAUT: - Hedonic Motivation - Price Value - Habit	Enhances UTAUT for consumer use contexts, capturing enjoyment, cost perception, and usage patterns.	For low-income rural users, free or low-cost health tools with intuitive and enjoyable interfaces are more likely to be accepted.

Source: Authors computations

Table 3 provides a background to the development of AI telehealth systems that aligns with the psychological and contextual realities of rural users. For example, facilitating conditions, such as mobile literacy training or local language interfaces, directly influence the expectancy of effort and habit formation. The social influence is also very strong in the Indian rural environment, where community health workers or local opinion leaders significantly influence the acceptance of digital tools. The proposed framework in this chapter not only focuses on the utility and usability of AI-telehealth tools but also on their social integration, perceived value, and compatibility with local behaviours and beliefs.

4.2 Human-AI Collaborative Dynamics

Instead of replacing healthcare workers, AI tools in rural telehealth are supposed to supplement clinical knowledge, increase the accuracy of decisions, and decrease the overload of overworked healthcare workers. This can be associated with the model of augmented intelligence, according to which AI is a partner and not an independent system. Shneiderman (2020) supports the need to keep human control appropriate in situations that are sensitive, like in the context of healthcare, where emotional, ethical, and contextual variables play a significant role. The innovative and empathetic divide in rural India can be bridged by effective human-AI collaboration due to the low infrastructure, low literacy, and low trust. The key to successful human-AI cooperation is based on:

1. **Clearly established roles and workflows:** The success of human-AI collaboration becomes effective when both sides can demarcate the areas of work and business in clear terms between healthcare workers and AI tools. As an example, AI can automate the triage process, or help to diagnose, and human clinicians should review and approve the decisions. The inability to clearly understand what the AI is—and is not—can lead to excessive trust or the total dismissal of the AI. Research indicates that work processes that are well defined can decrease resistance and enhance adoption of the system, especially where the users have been trained. With the role of AI supplementing clinical roles instead of conflicting with them, clinical workers would be more likely to adopt it into practice (Topol, 2019).
2. **Maintaining empathy:** It is important to maintain empathy and human relationships, particularly in the rural setting, where individuals tend to trust healthcare providers not so much because of technical precision but because of an overall warmer relationship. The emotional support that nurses, ASHAs, or doctors offer should never be substituted with AI; instead, it should be used to help free up time so that professionals can spend more time with patients. Obermeyer and Emanuel (2016) note that depersonalised or robotic systems can be a source of alienation of patients and the weakening of treatment results. Empathy is not a luxury in the culturally competent rural setting, but rather it is the only way to ensure healthcare legitimacy and sustainability.
3. **Ethical and explainable AI:** It is clear that AI recommendations need to be interpretable, explainable and transparent, particularly in health facilities. Black-box systems with an inappropriate decision logic are less likely to be trusted by health workers. XAI allows a provider to see why a system has suggested a particular diagnosis or level of risk, which is essential in a clinical context that requires accountability and transparency. According to Shneiderman (2020), the enhancements in explainability raise confidence in clinicians and the safety of patients, particularly in low-resource settings, where legal and ethical advice is usually lacking. Simple, easily explainable systems are required by rural clinicians, many of whom do not have much formal training on digital systems.
4. As AI tools are becoming relevant and used correctly, it is necessary to train rural health workers and engage them in the co-design processes. The community health agent (ASHAs and ANMs) understands the local dialects, cultural subtleties, and logistics - and may provide useful insights that enhance system design. Participatory design will also encourage ownership, develop trust and increase digital confidence. Holeman and Kane (2020) further indicate that

co-created systems are more sustainable and adaptive in the real world. In the event that frontline workers are empowered instead of displaced, AI is a friend, not a foe. Example Scenario: AI triage can be used to examine the symptoms of a patient and recommend the urgency. Yet, this assessment is reviewed by a nurse or physician who determines further action, and it is a combination of the scientifically based understanding and clinical judgment.

4.3 Strategic Collaborative Strategies

Addressing the rural healthcare issue through the application of AI-based telehealth implies that many parties with different backgrounds in policy, technology, clinical care, and community outreach will need to act in unison. An effective framework is not only about deploying tools; it should also converge infrastructure, support cultural accommodation, capacity building, and instil trust. The most important actors and their strategic roles are presented below.

1. Policymakers: Enabling Infrastructure and Regulation

Policymakers play a vital role in ensuring the availability of digital infrastructure, including broadband connectivity, power supply, and secure data storage. According to *Odhus et al. (2024),* the success of rural telehealth is linked to investments in digital public goods. Additionally, the creation of clear AI governance policies, including data protection laws, interoperability standards, and clinical validation protocols, is crucial. India's proposed Digital Information Security in Healthcare Act (DISHA) aims to address this gap; however, rural-specific provisions remain underdeveloped *(WHO, 2021).*

2. Healthcare Professionals: Capacity Building

Rural healthcare providers should receive special digital literacy training to learn about AI tools, interpret the outputs of the systems, and apply them to their professional practice. Upskilling at the basic level should be accompanied by continuous professional improvement, with which the ethical use of AI, the interpretation of risks, and the effective communication with patients are addressed. According to Gupta (2022), the participation of clinicians in AI tools co-designation generates confidence in users and enhances contextual relevance. The trust providers have towards AI systems and their readiness to collaborate with it rise significantly when they feel enabled instead of being pushed out of the technology.

3. Tech Innovators: Culturally Relevant, Usable Design

The developers of technology should ensure that they focus on inclusive, user-friendly design, whereby the tools should be accessible to people with low levels of literacy, digital skills, or access to the internet. It includes the creation of local language interfaces, allowing offline capabilities, and the creation of visual or audio prompts that can be understood by low-literate users. According to Thomas et al. (2024), the majority of health apps fail in rural India because they are urban-biased, such as assuming unlimited connectivity, menus in English only, and designing UIs with complicated constructions. The reason is the culture-based design approach that is central to practical usability and long-term adoption.

4. Community Stakeholders: Building Trust and Awareness

The community-based organisations, including NGOs, Self-Help Groups (SHGs), local influencers, and Panchayats, are critical to raising the level of acceptance and responsible use of AI-telehealth tools. These actors will be able to spread health information, arrange AI-awareness workshops, and overcome false beliefs. Veinot et al. (2018) emphasise the importance of engagement with local stakeholders in participatory design to boost trust in the service and ensure long-term participation. Moreover, community stakeholders will play the role of cultural mediators who will be able to match AI-based healthcare solutions with the local norms, beliefs, and expectations. These strategic collaborations create the framework for a successful AI-telehealth scale-up together. Harmonious collaboration between policymakers, healthcare professionals, technology designers and community organisations would allow achieving fair, culturally consistent, and trusted AI-supported rural health ecosystems.

5 KEY CHALLENGES IN RURAL AI-TELEHEALTH IMPLEMENTATION

Although the incorporation of Artificial Intelligence (AI) into telehealth systems is an opportunity to close the existing gaps in healthcare delivery in rural India, the actual aspect of introducing the technologies is faced with high opposition. Such barriers are socio-cultural, technological, infrastructural, and regulatory. These problems should be analysed carefully and dealt with in a strategic manner so as to provide equitable, inclusive and sustainable digital healthcare delivery.

5.1 Infrastructure Limitations

The unavailability of strong digital infrastructure is one of the most significant limitations to the implementation of AI-telehealth in rural India. The functionality of artificial intelligence-based teleconsultation platforms, remote diagnostics, and real-time health monitoring systems is based on reliable internet connectivity and constant electricity. The Telecom Regulatory Authority of India states that the penetration rate of the internet in rural India is considerably low compared to urban regions, and disruptions and slow internet access using broadband interruptions are frequent, making the use of telehealth applications difficult. Moreover, inconsistent electrical supply in rural areas may cause the failure of the systems as well as devices, system failures, and a lack of confidence between the users and the medical professionals (Odhus et al., 2024). The unavailability of fundamental supporting infrastructures, like mobile towers, fibre optic connections and alternative electricity reserves, directly restrains the scalability and dependability of AI-built digital health services.

5.2 Digital Divide

The Indian digital divide is in terms of access as well as capabilities. Most of the rural families do not have smartphones or computers with the ability to execute AI-enabled health applications. Digital literacy: even in the case of device accessibility, users do not possess the necessary digital literacy to navigate teleconsultation services, fill in health information or read AI-generated insights. According to the National Sample Survey, 2019, only 24 per cent of rural families were connected to the internet, and a substantially lower number had a basic understanding of computers. The resulting gap provides an obstacle to communication, trust, and continued utilisation of AI-telehealth platforms. Additionally, AI-based services with human involvement (video appointments or bracelets) tend to be unused or abused since they were not trained or do not trust them (Sindakis & Showkat, 2024). Women and older adults, in particular, face additional constraints due to gender-based digital exclusion and low health-tech exposure.

5.3 Cultural Resistance

The telehealth systems developed with AI not only question the cultural beliefs and norms in Indian rural settings, but also the traditional beliefs and expectations of interpersonal care. The healthcare in these environments is normally considered personal and relational, and the trust is established through in-person communication and the presence in the community (Chiou & Lee, 2023). The implementation of machine-based diagnostics, chat, and virtual consultation can be viewed as impersonal or even threatening. It is possible that communities that are highly dependent on traditional medicine systems (such as Ayurveda or Unani) will be open to AI-based Western medical practices only in a particular manner, without being properly culturalized (Gupta, 2022). Also, the myths about AI, e.g. the fear of misdiagnosis, surveillance or data misuse, may cause mistrust and scepticism. Incomprehensibility, the absence of personalised care, and a poor interface are also reasons that diminish the desire to interact with the AI-driven health systems. The means of defeating such barriers to perception and psychology include community involvement, culturally sensitive design, and the use of local languages.

5.4 Policy and Regulatory Ambiguity

The Indian legal and regulatory environment of AI-based healthcare systems is just evolving. Although the large-scale digital health programs, like the Ayushman Bharat Digital Mission (ABDM), introduce the guidelines on the framework of electronic health records and telemedicine, there is still no clear and enforceable set of rules concerning the use of AI in healthcare, especially in rural regions.

Critical regulatory concerns include:

1. **Data privacy and consent**: Rural users have little understanding of their rights to their data, and the Personal Data Protection Bill (which is yet to be implemented in India) lacks coverage of health-related AI data (WHO, 2021).
2. **Accountability**: When there is an error in AI or a misdiagnosis, the issue at hand is who is responsible: the developer, the healthcare professional or the policymaker.
3. **Standardisation**: Lack of validation procedures of AI systems by languages, populations, and clinical conditions poses the risk of bias and inaccuracy. This ambiguity will instil uncertainties in the minds of healthcare providers and developers, exposing end-users to fake news or fraudulent actions.

It is important to identify and solve these issues to enable the integration of AI-telehealth systems successfully, reasonably, and ethically in the Indian rural environment. With infrastructure investment, specific digital literacy initiatives, culturally aware system development, and explicit regulatory frameworks have to accompany each other to make sure that there are no rural areas that are left behind in the digital revolution of healthcare.

6 ILLUSTRATIVE CONCEPTUAL SCENARIOS AND REAL CASES

In order to put the proposed conceptual framework into perspective, this section outlines realistic, hypothetical situations of how AI-based telehealth systems might operate in rural Indian locations. These hypothetical situations are between theory and practice as they provide a graphic and storytelling display of how adoption behaviour, human-AI collaboration, and strategic enablers can interact to enhance healthcare provision in underserved communities.

6.1 Scenario 1: AI-Powered Symptom Triage in a Karnataka Village

Context: The healthcare facilities in the area of Chikkaballapur district in Karnataka are scarce and restricted to a single Primary Health Centre (PHC), which is usually understaffed. Quite a number of villagers have to cover long distances in order to find consultation or wait days till they have planned their checkups.

Implementation: A multilingual chatbot, driven by AI, is implemented, and it can be accessed via smartphones or community kiosks. The chatbot, which is trained on the Kannada language and regional dialect, encourages the user to enter the symptoms either through voice or text. It applies Natural Language Processing (NLP) and diagnostic algorithms to propose initial triage categories (e.g., low-risk, moderate-risk, emergency). The elderly or illiterate users are assisted by a local ASHA (Accredited Social Health Activist) worker. In case of moderate and high-risk, the system notifies a telehealth doctor located in Bengaluru to consult with the report of the chatbot and offers additional consultation through a video call.

Outcome:

- Reduces waiting time and unnecessary travel.
- Allows early detection of preventable illnesses.
- Supports human-AI collaboration: AI handles routine symptom filtering, while the human doctor retains final clinical authority.
- Builds trust as local health workers mediate technology usage.

6.2 Scenario 2: AI-Assisted Maternal Health Monitoring in Bihar

Context: A rural block in Bihar with low resources, maternal and neonatal mortality rates are high because care is not provided promptly, and there is a failure to follow up on care. The distance, financial and social stigma reasons make many pregnant women miss check-ups.

Implementation: A wearable health band, which is an AI-based health device, offered on a public-private partnership basis, monitors crucial health maternal data such as blood pressure, heart rate, and temperature. This device is synchronised with a mobile application that PHC staff and obstetricians of urban hospitals monitor. The system can identify suspicious activities that point to preeclampsia or gestational diabetes using AI-based pattern recognition. A notification is given to a specific nurse or a doctor who organises an immediate teleconsultation or face-to-face appointment.

Outcome:

- Enables real-time, proactive monitoring of at-risk pregnancies.
- Empowers ASHA workers with decision-support tools.
- Strengthens data-driven intervention and continuity of care.
- Reduces complications through early alerts and timely clinical action.

6.3 Scenario 3: Community-Based Telepsychiatry in Rural Tamil Nadu

Background: Mental health services are grossly underestimated in most rural belts of Tamil Nadu, with stigmatisation and a shortage of psychiatrists resulting in the inability to diagnose depression, anxiety, or PTSD in rural locations, particularly in the youth and during the postnatal period.

Implementation: An AI-based chatbot that uses sentiment analysis and is integrated into WhatsApp is an implementation of a community mental health initiative. It is a chatbot which can be installed in Tamil and evaluates user answers to mood and behaviour questionnaires. When a user exceeds a limit of clinical concern, a trained social worker is notified and directs the individual to an initial telepsychiatry session via a district hospital. The AI engine will also track patient progress through weekly check-ins that will help lessen the workload on professionals, but will still provide continuity.

Outcome:

- Breaks stigma through private, digital-first access.
- Builds community confidence in mental health services.
- Demonstrates scalable use of AI for early mental health screening.
- Illustrates synergy between AI technology and social worker mediation.

6.4 Scenario Mapping for Visual Illustration

Figure 4. Patient Journey in AI-Assisted Telehealth Triage System

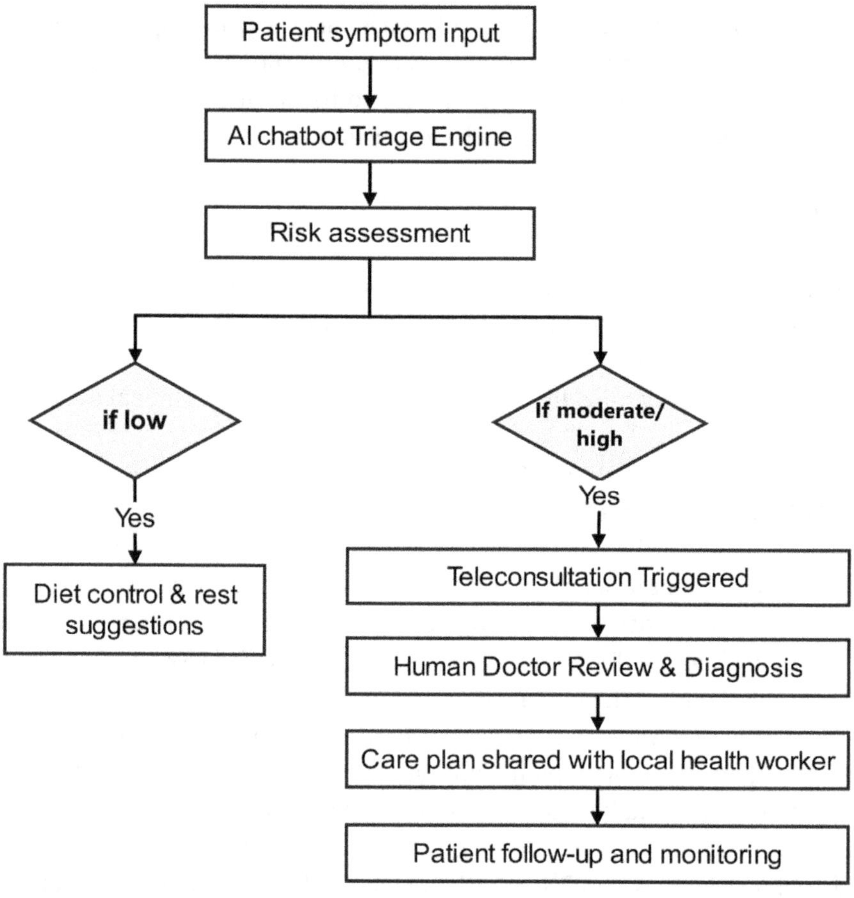

Source: Author's contribution

According to Figure 4, the interaction between AI tools and human expertise and infrastructural enablers would produce a hybrid model of care, which fits rural India. Conceptual illustrative scenarios like these will aid in the translation of abstract theoretical aspects into field-ready strategies. They are also used as validation templates of pilot programmes and research trials. These scenarios contribute value to the conceptual framework by focusing on real-world challenges, cultural issues, and user interaction issues, giving it a viable implementation route.

6.5 Real-World Case Examples of AI-Telehealth in Rural India

In order to illustrate the real-life application of the suggested framework, this section includes real-life case studies in different regions of India. All these efforts point to the fact that AI-driven telehealth devices are currently under testing and being scaled to improve the rural health delivery process, which reflects their advantages and challenges.

6.5.1 eSanjeevani – Nationwide Telemedicine Platform (PAN-India)

Overview: eSanjeevani is a national telemedicine service structure launched by the Ministry of Health and Family Welfare, and is operated in a hub-and-spoke model, linking rural Health and Wellness Centres (HWCs) to specialist doctors in urban centres. The National Health Mission supports it and has empowered more than 140 million consultations (as of 2024) in rural India.

Relevance to Framework:

1. **Adoption Behaviour:** eSanjeevani was able to achieve mass adoption of its product in rural India due to its simple UI/UX and the assistance of ASHAs and ANMs despite the digital divide in rural India. Patients are aided by community health workers during sessions, especially with login, camera, or entry of symptoms- alleviating cognitive load and digital hesitation. Also, the influence of local-language characteristics and belief on government-operated services was found to increase the perceived usefulness and ease of use, which constitute TAM constructs (Davis, 1989). Such design features show a successful behavioural integration despite the low-digital-literacy areas.
2. **Human-AI Collaboration:** eSanjeevani was initially used as a video teleconsultation tool; however, AI-based enhancements are being piloted gradually. These are AI-assisted symptom triage, clinical decision support systems (CDSS) and automated referral suggestions to assist clinicians with high volumes. The platform is looking into Natural Language Processing (NLP) to organise the dialogue between patients and doctors and to incorporate AI-based diagnostic devices to screen chronic illnesses. This type of augmentative intelligence corresponds to the model of human-centred AI described by Shneiderman (2020), where machines do not substitute professionals but support them.
3. **Strategic Enabler:** eSanjeevani has succeeded because of the top-down policy motivation, such as direct mandates in the Ayushman Bharat Digital Mission (ABDM). It enjoyed coordinated efforts on the state level (e.g., Tamil Nadu, Andhra Pradesh) that coordinated IT infrastructure mobilisation, disseminated digital devices, and educated PHC employees. In addition, the site is in line

with national telemedicine practice and data security standards, which enhance trust. It is included in the digital public health stack (ABHA IDs, NDHM) of India, which guarantees its scalability, interoperability, and public legitimacy.

6.5.2 Wadhwani AI's Infant Health Project – Maharashtra

Overview: Wadhwani AI is a Mumbai-based non-profit research centre that created an AI-based product detecting cases of low birth weight (LBW) and malnutrition in newborns based on smartphone photographs. The solution is being tested in collaboration with the Government of Maharashtra and ICDS among Anganwadi workers in tribal and rural Maharashtra.

Relevance to Framework:

1. **Adoption Behaviour:** The perceived ease of use and usefulness, which are central to the TAM model, the AI tool was immediately adopted because it was mobile-based, and training time was minimal, as well as it had instant feedback, which is another central factor of the TAM model.
2. **Human-AI Collaboration:** The AI can guess the weight of the baby based on the pictures on the smartphone, but the human employee validates the prediction and creates referrals or counselling, which is in accordance with the paradigm of augmented intelligence.
3. **Strategic Enabler:** This tool was also strategically facilitated by connectivity to ICDS schemes, by using available field personnel, work processes, and trust networks. The support of the government gave it credibility and infrastructure, and it was able to break the common rural barriers to deployment.

6.5.3 NIRAMAI Breast Cancer Screening – Karnataka & Telangana

Overview: NIRAMAI (Non-Invasive Risk Assessment with Machine Intelligence) is an Indian start-up based in Bangalore that is engaged in early breast cancer screening based on AI and thermal imaging. It has been deployed in village screening camps in the states of Karnataka and Telangana by mobile health units.

Relevance to Framework:

1. **Adoption Behaviour:** There was initially resistance on the part of the rural women due to the cultural taboos and ignorance regarding breast cancer. Adoption, however, rose because the community health workers engaged in the building of trust and non-invasive, privacy-sensitive screening approaches, which were customised towards the rural norms.

2. **Human-AI Collaboration:** The AI system will analyse thermal images to detect early signs of cancer, but radiologists will interpret and confirm the findings, which will be followed by human control and clinical responsibility, showing a viable example of the augmented intelligence system in the area of prevention.
3. **Strategic Enabler:** The ability of NIRAMAI to operate in rural areas was based on collaborating with NGOs, CSR-funded mobile units, and the public health agencies, facilitating the delivery of the practice at a low cost and the integration of the rural outreach with the district-level screening programs in Karnataka and Telangana.

6.5.4 AI-Based COVID-19 Remote Screening – Tamil Nadu

Overview: During the COVID-19 pandemic, the government of Tamil Nadu collaborated with startups to implement AI-based symptom-checker applications and IVR-based systems to conduct rural tele-screening. These technologies were used to triage and refer high-risk patients to the closest PHCs to minimise their footfall.

Relevance to Framework:

1. **Adoption Behaviour:** The introduction of the voice-based AI applications in the Tamil language helped the rural users who were mainly non-literate to communicate with confidence. This brings the significance of incorporating local languages in enhancing availability and adoption by the users.
2. **Human-AI Collaboration:** AI-based tools were used to pre-triage based on the reported symptoms, and the in-person visits or follow-up calls conducted by the healthcare staff maintained human judgment and trust in the AI-aided screening process.
3. **Strategic Enabler:** The program was successful because of the effective leadership of the state, its cooperation with the district-level command centres, and its cooperation with local startups. Its speedy implementation and rural area coverage depended on public-private cooperation and awareness efforts.

6.5.5 Swasthya Slate – Jammu & Kashmir and Rural Punjab

Introduction: Swasthya Slate is a developed device by the Public Health Foundation of India. It is a portable gadget that integrates various diagnostic devices and has a connection with an AI-enabled Android-based app. It has been implemented in rural PHCs, mobile medical vans in Jammu and Kashmir and some areas of Punjab.

Relevance to Framework:

1. **Adoption Behaviour**: The intuitive touchscreen interface and multi-diagnostic capacity made Swasthya Slate easy for ANMs and PHC nurses to adopt with minimal training. Its portability and rapid testing features aligned well with rural workflows and time constraints.
2. **Human-AI Collaboration**: The AI app analyses inputs from diagnostic tools (e.g., BP, ECG), but health workers make final clinical decisions, ensuring human oversight in diagnosis, treatment planning, and referrals, which reinforces clinician trust and accountability.
3. **Strategic Enabler**: The tool's deployment was made possible through government partnerships, support from the National Health Mission, and cost-effective device design, allowing integration with mobile health vans and PHC-based outreach in remote locations.

Table 4. Summarised Real-World AI-Telehealth Cases in Rural India

Case	Region	Core AI Function	Framework Components Reflected
eSanjeevani	PAN-India	Teleconsultation, e-prescription	Adoption behaviour, policy enablement, infrastructure deployment
Wadhwani AI Infant Health	Maharashtra	AI image analysis for malnutrition	Human-AI collaboration, digital literacy support, integration with ICDS
NIRAMAI Breast Screening	Karnataka, Telangana	Thermal AI screening	Trust-building, female health outreach, NGO partnership
COVID AI Screening	Tamil Nadu	Voice-based AI triage	Language inclusion, AI-human workflow, government-backed tech
Swasthya Slate	Jammu & Kashmir, Punjab	Multi-diagnostic portable AI toolkit	Health worker augmentation, low-cost innovation, integration into PHCs

Source: Compiled by the author from official program websites and government health mission reports

These real-world examples (Table 4) affirm that AI-driven telehealth is not merely a futuristic idea but a growing reality in rural India. They validate the conceptual framework's emphasis on trust, usability, collaborative dynamics, and policy support. However, they also reflect ongoing challenges—such as digital access, cultural adaptation, and regulatory clarity—that must be addressed for wider scalability and long-term impact.

7 IMPLICATIONS

The incorporation of Artificial Intelligence (AI) into rural telehealth systems has both opportunities and structural challenges. The theoretical framework that has been created in this chapter, based on behavioural, technological, and contextual aspects, has made some insightful findings that can be useful in improving the digital health equity in the underserved areas of India. This study applies existing theories on adoption like the Technology Acceptance Model (TAM) (Davis, 1989), the Unified Theory of Acceptance and Use of Technology (UTAUT) (Venkatesh et al., 2003), and UTAUT2 (Venkatesh et al., 2012) to rural health care contexts, revealing the importance of digital literacy, usefulness perception, trust in AI, and social-cultural suitability in influencing user acceptability. Although TAM and UTAUT help explain first adoption behaviour, UTAUT2 emphasises the importance of emotional and habitual factors in encouraging the use of AI-enabled health services as more time goes on.

The framework promotes the use of augmented intelligence models by supporting human judgment, not replacing it, with the use of AI; it also values empathy, understanding context, and trust in care provision (Shneiderman, 2020). To improve the usability of interfaces among non-literate and older groups, designers and implementers should be concerned with culturally relevant, inclusive features, including multilingual interfaces, voice navigation, and offline capabilities (Sindakis & Showkat, 2024).

The health system of the country needs to build infrastructure to create capacity for frontline health workers, such as ASHA and ANM staff, to effectively work in collaboration with AI-based systems (Gupta, 2022). The policymakers should also develop a specific system of regulations ensuring privacy of data, ethical use, and accountability and justice in AI-driven healthcare (WHO, 2021). Overall, the results provide practical conclusions to academic studies, system design, capacity development, and policy development in the rural Indian digital ecosystem of health.

8 FUTURE DIRECTIONS

Further research must focus on the empirical validation of the offered model with the help of pilot studies, usability tests, and mixed-method analyses in different rural environments to measure the experience of users and health results (Dwivedi et al., 2019). The adaptive models that address vulnerable populations such as tribal communities, aged people, and persons with disabilities should also be investigated (populations that are faced by layered barriers to the adoption of technologies) (Veinot et al., 2018).

This requires participatory and community research methodologies whereby co-creation with rural participants, local leaders and community organisations is guaranteed to foster trust and cultural appropriateness (Cornwall & Jewkes, 1995). The future work should also investigate the mechanisms of ethics and governance that are particular to low-resource settings, especially in communities with low legal literacy and digital rights awareness (WHO, 2021).

Inter-sector cooperation is an essential field of study. The collaborations among government agencies, technology developers, educational establishments, and civil society organisations can be used to increase the scalability of AI-telehealth applications faster and enhance the digital health ecology in the rural communities (Kerketta & Balasundaram, 2024). In general, the next research directions are real-world implementation, equity-oriented design, ethical protection, and collaborative innovation to guarantee the sustainability and inclusivity of AI adoption by the rural population in India.

9 CONCLUSION

The chapter has provided an interdisciplinary viewpoint on the transformative opportunities of Artificial Intelligence (AI) in telehealth provision to rural India. This chapter has explored the integrated functions of adoption behaviour, human-AI partnership, and strategic facilitators in determining the successful implementation and adoption of AI-based telehealth solutions in digitally underserved communities by suggesting an integrative conceptual framework.

On the behavioral level, the chapter focused on the role of perceived ease of use, digital literacy, cultural beliefs, and trust in technology in determining the adoption decisions among the rural population in order to apply foundational theory of technology adoption, including Technology Acceptance Model (TAM) (Davis, 1989) and Unified Theory of Acceptance and Use of Technology (UTAUT) (Venkatesh et al., 2003) and (UTAUT2) (Venkatesh et al., 2012) to rural healthcare. This knowledge is important to learn that the success of digital health innovations in rural India is not only based on the level of technological advancement but also on the level of contextual and cultural appropriateness (Sindakis & Showkat, 2024).

Regarding the collaborative perspective, the chapter emphasised the significance of the human-AI synergy in which AI tools are not meant to substitute the frontline healthcare professionals but to supplement their abilities. This is in line with the new paradigms of human-centred AI (Shneiderman, 2020), which promote ethical, empathetic, and explainable systems to aid in healthcare decision-making, as opposed to automating it. System design and integration of workflow was identified as a key to the achievement of trust, acceptance, and long-term usability when health workers are incorporated into the design and workflow integration.

Strategic enablers like infrastructure preparedness, enabling policy settings, and community involvement processes, which are crucial to the emergence of scalable and sustainable AI-telehealth, were also included in the framework. Practical examples of the translation of theoretical models into practice would be presented in the examples of real-life case studies in various regions of India, such as eSanjeevani, NIRAMAI, and Wadhwani AI, although the examples are rather successful and problematic (Gupta, 2022).

Although the given framework is purely conceptual, it can be used as a strong source of developing context-specific, ethically-based, and user-friendly AI-telehealth solutions. Notably, it gives guidance to future policy and empirical studies. The second step, which follows the first one, is the validation of the model in the field with pilot studies in various rural locations to determine the relevance, adaptability, and effect of the model on the health outcome. In this case, such studies must follow mixed-method methodologies, with quantitative data used to measure usage and efficiency, and qualitative information used to learn how users experience it and what prevents them (Dwivedi et al., 2019).

In addition, the model needs to be continuously updated as a result of technological changes (e.g., generative AI, multilingual NLP applications), policy changes (e.g. the future Digital Health Mission regulations in India), and user feedback gained through participatory design and longitudinal interaction. The presence of continuous feedback between the developers, healthcare professionals, policy architects, and community stakeholders will play a key role in making sure that the system is in line with the realities on the ground.

To summarise, the chapter renders a significant contribution to the theoretical discussion of AI in healthcare and also presents an actual roadmap towards inclusive and equitable telehealth transformation in India. It proposes a participatory, ethical, and place-based AI innovation, which recognises the rural diversity, enhances digital empowerment, and aims to make healthcare equitable to everyone.

REFERENCES

Abisha, D., Mahalakshmi, M., Pritiga, T., Thanusiya, M., Punitha Sahaya Sherin, A., & Navedha Evanjalin, R. (2024, April). Revolutionising Rural Healthcare in India: AI-Powered Chatbots for Affordable Symptom Analysis and Medical Guidance. In *2024 International Conference on Inventive Computation Technologies (ICICT)* (pp. 181-187). IEEE.

Chiou, E. K., & Lee, J. D. (2023). Trusting automation: Designing for responsivity and resilience. *Human Factors*, *65*(1), 137–165. DOI: 10.1177/00187208211009995 PMID: 33906505

Cornwall, A., & Jewkes, R. (1995). What is participatory research? *Social Science & Medicine*, *41*(12), 1667–1676. DOI: 10.1016/0277-9536(95)00127-S PMID: 8746866

Dash, S., Aarthy, R., & Mohan, V. (2021). Telemedicine during COVID-19 in India—A new policy and its challenges. *Journal of Public Health Policy*, *42*(3), 501–509. DOI: 10.1057/s41271-021-00287-w PMID: 34012012

Davis, F. D. (1989). Perceived usefulness, perceived ease of use, and user acceptance of information technology. *Management Information Systems Quarterly*, *13*(3), 319–340. DOI: 10.2307/249008

Dwivedi, Y. K., Rana, N. P., Jeyaraj, A., Clement, M., & Williams, M. D. (2019). Re-examining the unified theory of acceptance and use of technology (UTAUT): Towards a revised theoretical model. *Information Systems Frontiers*, *21*(3), 719–734. DOI: 10.1007/s10796-017-9774-y

Gupta, A. D. (2022). Adoption of Digital Healthcare with the Concept of the Patient as an Organisation. https://doi.org/DOI: 10.21203/rs.3.rs-1712476/v1

Holeman, I., & Kane, D. (2020). Human-centered design for global health equity. *Information Technology for Development*, *26*(3), 477–505. DOI: 10.1080/02681102.2019.1667289 PMID: 32982007

Hoque, M. R., & Bao, Y. (2015). Cultural influence on adoption and use of e-Health: Evidence in Bangladesh. *Telemedicine Journal and e-Health*, *21*(10), 845–851. DOI: 10.1089/tmj.2014.0128 PMID: 26348844

Jiang, F., Jiang, Y., Zhi, H., Dong, Y., Li, H., Ma, S., Wang, Y., Dong, Q., Shen, H., & Wang, Y. (2017). Artificial intelligence in healthcare: Past, present and future. *Stroke and Vascular Neurology*, *2*(4), 230–243. Advance online publication. DOI: 10.1136/svn-2017-000101 PMID: 29507784

Kanwar, V., Chaudhary, S., & Sharma, A. K. (2023). Challenges in implementing digital health services in rural India. *The International Society for Telemedicine and eHealth, 11*(1), 1-5. https://hdl.handle.net/10520/ejc-jisfteh_v11_n1_a3

Kerketta, A., & Balasundaram, S. (2024). Leveraging AI Tools to Bridge the Healthcare Gap in Rural Areas in India. medRxiv, 2024-07. **doi:** https://doi.org/ DOI: 10.1101/2024.07.30.24311228

Khan, F., & Driessen, J. (2018). Bridging the telemedicine infrastructure gap: Implications for long-term care in rural America. *The Public Policy and Aging Report, 28*(3), 80–84. DOI: 10.1093/ppar/pry027

Khosravi, M., Zare, Z., Mojtabaeian, S. M., & Izadi, R. (2024). Artificial intelligence and decision-making in healthcare: A thematic analysis of a systematic review of reviews. *Health Services Research and Managerial Epidemiology, 11*, 23333928241234863. DOI: 10.1177/23333928241234863 PMID: 38449840

National Family Health Survey-5 (NFHS-5). (2021). Ministry of Health and Family Welfare. https://rchiips.org/nfhs/

Obermeyer, Z., & Emanuel, E. J. (2016). Predicting the future—Big data, machine learning, and clinical medicine. *The New England Journal of Medicine, 375*(13), 1216–1219. DOI: 10.1056/NEJMp1606181 PMID: 27682033

Odhus, C. O., Kapanga, R. R., & Oele, E. (2024). Barriers to and enablers of quality improvement in primary health care in low-and middle-income countries: A systematic review. *PLOS Global Public Health, 4*(1), e0002756. DOI: 10.1371/journal.pgph.0002756 PMID: 38236832

Shneiderman, B. (2020). Human-centered artificial intelligence: Reliable, safe & trustworthy. *International Journal of Human-Computer Interaction, 36*(6), 495–504. DOI: 10.1080/10447318.2020.1741118

Sindakis, S., & Showkat, G. (2024). The digital revolution in India: Bridging the gap in rural technology adoption. *Journal of Innovation and Entrepreneurship, 13*(1), 29. DOI: 10.1186/s13731-024-00380-w

Sreenu, N. (2019). Healthcare infrastructure development in rural India: A critical analysis of its status and future challenges. *British Journal of Health Care Management, 25*(12), 1–9. DOI: 10.12968/bjhc.2018.0072

Thomas, V., Jenkins, J., & George, J. (2024). A systematic review and qualitative evidence synthesis of factors affecting mHealth adoption in India. *Oxford Open Digital Health, 2*, oqae046. Advance online publication. DOI: 10.1093/oodh/oqae046 PMID: 40237014

Topol, E. J. (2019). High-performance medicine: The convergence of human and artificial intelligence. *Nature Medicine*, *25*(1), 44–56. DOI: 10.1038/s41591-018-0300-7 PMID: 30617339

Veinot, T. C., Mitchell, H., & Ancker, J. S. (2018). Good intentions are not enough: How informatics interventions can worsen inequality. *Journal of the American Medical Informatics Association : JAMIA*, *25*(8), 1080–1088. DOI: 10.1093/jamia/ocy052 PMID: 29788380

Venkatesh, V., Morris, M. G., Davis, G. B., & Davis, F. D. (2003). User acceptance of information technology: Toward a unified view. *Management Information Systems Quarterly*, *27*(3), 425–478. DOI: 10.2307/30036540

Venkatesh, V., Thong, J. Y., & Xu, X. (2012). Consumer acceptance and use of information technology: Extending the unified theory of acceptance and use of technology. *Management Information Systems Quarterly*, *36*(1), 157–178. DOI: 10.2307/41410412

Wadden, J. J. (2022). Defining the undefinable: The black box problem in healthcare artificial intelligence. *Journal of Medical Ethics*, *48*(10), 764–768. DOI: 10.1136/medethics-2021-107529 PMID: 34290113

. World Health Organization (WHO). (2021). *Ethics and governance of artificial intelligence for health: WHO guidance*.

Chapter 9
Strengthening E-Collaboration in Healthcare Through AI:
The Promise and Peril of Artificial Intelligence in Healthcare – A Critical Analysis

Frank Billingsley
http://orcid.org/0009-0000-5363-1568
Georgetwown College, USA

ABSTRACT

Artificial intelligence is reshaping healthcare by transforming diagnostics, decision making, and population health management. Although machine learning offers gains in accuracy and clinical support, deployment remains uneven because of ethical, infrastructural, and governance challenges. This chapter examines AI's implications across technological capability, socioeconomic context, and governance maturity, showing a gap between potential and performance, especially in settings with limited digital infrastructure or poor data representation. AI can enhance precision and expand access to expertise, yet benefits are constrained by bias, generalizability issues, privacy risks, and limited institutional readiness. Governance often lags innovation, leaving unresolved questions about accountability and oversight. The chapter proposes a strategic approach centered on equitable access, adaptive regulation, interdisciplinary collaboration, and community engagement, arguing that innovation alone cannot transform health systems without strong governance and sustained investment.

DOI: 10.4018/979-8-3373-5906-9.ch009

INTRODUCTION

The accelerating integration of artificial intelligence into contemporary healthcare systems represents one of the most consequential shifts in modern medical history. Advances in machine learning, data science, and computational modeling have converged with clinical expertise to produce capabilities that were essentially inconceivable only a decade ago. AI now contributes to diagnostic imaging, risk stratification, therapeutic decision making, administrative coordination, genomic interpretation, and population health surveillance. These developments unfold at a moment of intensifying strain on global health systems, marked by aging populations, rising chronic disease burdens, escalating costs, workforce shortages, and widening inequities in access to care. As healthcare infrastructure struggles to respond to these pressures, AI is often positioned as a technological pathway to improve efficiency, extend clinical reach, and enhance diagnostic and therapeutic precision.

Yet artificial intelligence reshapes healthcare not only through its technical capacities, but through its effects on how actors collaborate across clinical, institutional, and societal boundaries. This chapter adopts e-collaboration as its central analytical lens, positioning AI as a force that reorganizes relationships among clinicians, health systems, developers, policymakers, and patients. E-collaboration refers to digitally mediated coordination that enables shared decision making, distributed expertise, and collective accountability across interconnected systems. AI increasingly functions as an intermediary within these networks, shaping how knowledge circulates, how authority is exercised, and how responsibility is allocated. Framing AI through e-collaboration underscores that its impact depends less on isolated technological performance than on the quality of interaction among human and institutional participants. This perspective enables a more precise examination of how technological capability, ethical governance, and social context jointly shape collaborative practice in contemporary healthcare.

This chapter is written for scholars, policymakers, and senior healthcare leaders engaged in the study, governance, and strategic implementation of artificial intelligence in health systems. It speaks to readers involved in research, regulation, institutional leadership, and decision making who seek to understand not only the technical capacities of AI but also the organizational, ethical, and societal conditions that structure its use.

The transformation associated with AI adoption is neither linear nor uniform. Implementation varies significantly across countries, institutions, and socioeconomic contexts. Early evaluations indicate that AI-enabled tools can enhance clinical performance, streamline workflows, and support earlier disease detection, as demonstrated in large-scale assessments of algorithmic accuracy in diagnostic imaging and related applications (Topol, 2019; Rajpurkar et al., 2022). At the same time, these advances coexist with uneven performance across demographic groups, persistent limitations in generalizability, and infrastructural constraints that restrict equitable adoption. The result is a complex and evolving landscape in which technological promise is matched by significant uncertainty, reinforcing the need for careful scrutiny of how AI is embedded within collaborative health systems.

This study is guided by a central research question: how can healthcare systems integrate AI technologies in ways that ensure equitable access, uphold ethical standards, and develop governance frameworks capable of supporting innovation while protecting patient interests. This question reflects a broader tension between technological progress and societal responsibility. AI functions not merely as a computational instrument but as a socio-technical system embedded within institutional, economic, and ethical structures. Its real-world performance depends on the environments in which it operates, the quality and representativeness of underlying data, and the capacity of institutions to manage the organizational change that AI introduces. These conditions directly shape how collaboration unfolds across professional and institutional boundaries.

Empirical research illustrates this intersection of capability and constraint. McKinney et al. (2020) demonstrate that advanced breast cancer screening algorithms can match or exceed human expertise within specific contexts while still exhibiting variability across populations and clinical environments. Such findings highlight the gap between controlled laboratory performance and real-world deployment, particularly in settings lacking robust digital infrastructure, standardized electronic health records, or representative datasets (Obermeyer et al., 2019). These disparities underscore the importance of evaluating AI not solely through technical benchmarks but through its performance within diverse social and institutional contexts where collaborative capacity varies considerably.

Ethical considerations further complicate implementation and reinforce the centrality of collaboration. AI systems are trained on historical clinical data that often reflect long-standing inequities in healthcare access, treatment patterns, and socioeconomic conditions. When embedded into clinical workflows, such systems may reproduce or intensify these inequities. Questions of fairness, transparency, accountability, and patient autonomy therefore become central to assessing AI's role in healthcare. Documented cases of algorithmic bias illustrate how marginalized populations can face disproportionate risks when AI-generated recommendations shape clinical decision making (Obermeyer et al., 2019; Vokinger et al., 2021). At the same time, the data-intensive nature of AI heightens concerns about privacy, informed consent, and the ethical boundaries of data stewardship, particularly as systems increasingly rely on genomic and behavioral data with implications extending beyond individual patients (Morley et al., 2020). These challenges underscore that ethical governance is not an abstract principle but a collaborative practice requiring coordination among multiple stakeholders.

Such ethical and operational concerns unfold within a fragmented and often underdeveloped governance landscape. While some jurisdictions have advanced regulatory initiatives addressing data protection and algorithmic oversight, governance frameworks frequently lag behind the pace of technological diffusion. Effective oversight requires mechanisms capable of evaluating performance across diverse populations, monitoring algorithmic drift, and guiding continuous recalibration. It also requires institutional structures that integrate the perspectives of clinicians, patients, policymakers, developers, and affected communities (European Commission, 2024). Without these collaborative structures, AI risks outpacing the foundations of accountability, transparency, and public trust on which healthcare systems depend.

Artificial intelligence in healthcare therefore functions not as an isolated technical intervention but as a collaborative infrastructure that reshapes relationships among actors across the health ecosystem. Its successful deployment depends on e-collaboration understood as sustained, digitally mediated coordination across professional, institutional, and societal boundaries. This perspective emphasizes that technical performance, ethical integrity, and equitable outcomes emerge through interaction rather than automation alone. Viewing AI through this collaborative lens enables a more coherent understanding of how governance, accountability, and access are negotiated in practice.

Addressing these challenges requires sustained attention to three interdependent domains: technological capability, social and economic context, and governance maturity. This chapter situates AI within these intersecting spheres to examine both the opportunities and structural constraints shaping responsible adoption. By foregrounding equity, ethical integrity, and regulatory preparedness, the analysis contributes to ongoing scholarship aimed at reconciling AI-driven innovation with the foundational commitments of healthcare practice.

PART 1: TECHNOLOGICAL CAPABILITY AND THE COLLABORATIVE OF CLINICAL PRACTICE

The Technological Revolution In Healthcare

Artificial intelligence has begun to reshape the foundations of modern healthcare by expanding the scope and precision of clinical practice in ways previously considered unattainable. While early digital innovations focused primarily on automating repetitive administrative tasks, contemporary AI systems have moved far beyond such limited functions. They now operate as sophisticated analytical tools capable of detecting subtle clinical patterns, synthesizing large-scale datasets, and supporting complex clinical decision-making. This evolution signals a profound transformation in how healthcare professionals diagnose, monitor, and treat disease, with implications that extend across nearly every domain of medicine.

One of the clearest illustrations of this transformation appears in diagnostic imaging. Traditional computer-aided detection systems relied on fixed, rule-based programming, which limited their diagnostic accuracy to the specificity of the rules encoded within them. In contrast, modern machine learning systems learn from millions of imaging samples, refining their capabilities through iterative exposure to diverse clinical cases. As Basa (2024) notes, this data-driven approach enables AI models to continually improve performance, often identifying subtle visual cues that even experienced radiologists miss. Skin cancer detection based on deep learning that incorporates clinical metadata, as demonstrated by Mehr et al. (2022), further illustrates these advances. These AI-driven systems now match or exceed human clinicians in identifying conditions such as lung cancer, diabetic retinopathy, and various musculoskeletal disorders. They do not function as replacements for radiologists but rather as force multipliers that enhance clinical precision and reduce diagnostic variability. By highlighting ambiguous or easily overlooked abnormalities, AI augments clinical judgment and supports more confident and consistent diagnostic decisions.

The transformative reach of AI extends further into clinical decision support systems, where predictive analytics and pattern recognition help guide practitioners through complex therapeutic choices. These systems integrate vast volumes of patient data, including laboratory values, vital signs, medical histories, and treatment outcomes, to generate probabilistic assessments of patient trajectories. For example, predictive models can identify early signs of sepsis hours before clinical symptoms fully emerge, supporting faster intervention and reducing mortality risk. Research by Huang et al. (2022) presents a reinforcement learning framework that identifies treatment strategies associated with improved predicted survival in septic patients by learning optimal actions from extensive ICU datasets. Similarly, these systems can propose personalized treatment plans by analyzing patient-specific factors alongside population-level evidence, helping clinicians select therapies that align with best-practice standards and the distinctive characteristics of each patient.

One of the most promising implications of these decision-support tools is their potential to democratize medical expertise. By embedding advanced diagnostic and predictive capabilities into telemedicine platforms, AI technologies help bring specialized knowledge to regions where specialists are scarce. This is particularly important for rural or underserved communities, where geographic or financial barriers traditionally limit access to high-level diagnostic services. With AI-supported tools, clinicians in these settings can access algorithmic insights comparable to those available in well-resourced urban hospitals, thereby narrowing disparities in diagnostic accuracy and care quality.

The cumulative effect of these innovations is a shift in the broader philosophy of medical practice. AI systems enable clinicians to move from reactive care to more anticipatory, predictive models of intervention. They equip healthcare providers with insights derived from patterns that are too subtle, too numerous, or too complex for human cognition alone. As a result, AI becomes not simply an instrument of automation but a catalyst for reimagining the clinical process itself.

From Automation to Advanced Analytics

The evolution of artificial intelligence in healthcare reflects a shift from simple digital assistance toward systems capable of complex analytical reasoning. Early generations of healthcare technology were designed primarily to automate administrative tasks, such as appointment scheduling, billing cycles, and inventory management. These systems followed strict rule-based protocols and offered little capacity for adaptation or interpretation. Their impact on clinical decision-making was minimal, since they operated as passive tools rather than active contributors to diagnostic or therapeutic processes. In contrast, contemporary AI systems represent a profound departure from this earlier paradigm. They operate through machine learning architectures that identify patterns, derive insights, and support clinical judgment in ways once considered unattainable by computational means, a shift documented in Topol's analysis of deep learning's expanding clinical role (Topol, 2019).

Modern machine learning systems can detect subtle patterns in medical imaging that even experienced clinicians might overlook. This analytical capability marks a significant break from rule-based systems, which depended on manually encoded instructions and could not evolve beyond their initial programming. Machine learning models, by contrast, improve through exposure to expansive datasets, allowing them to refine their performance over time. As these models train on millions of imaging samples, laboratory values, or clinical notes, they begin to demonstrate levels of precision comparable to those of expert practitioners. These developments indicate that AI's most significant contribution lies not in automating repetitive tasks but in reshaping the foundations of clinical reasoning itself. Recent evaluations of deep learning performance in diagnostics reinforce this trend, highlighting the growing alignment between algorithmic predictions and expert assessments (Rajpurkar et al., 2022).

The transition from automation to advanced analytics is especially apparent in the growing use of natural language processing tools to mine clinical documentation. These systems do more than categorize existing records; they parse massive repositories of unstructured clinical text, extracting patterns that would likely remain hidden in traditional medical records for years. This capability permits identification of population-level trends, early predictors of disease progression, or gaps in care quality that would otherwise be obscured. In addition, NLP enables more efficient clinical workflows by synthesizing information across lengthy, complex datasets, thereby reducing the cognitive burden on healthcare providers. Evidence for this transformation comes from a study by Bean et al. (2023), which applied clinical NLP hospital-wide to more than one million patient records and demonstrated that such approaches can reliably produce clinically significant insights across entire electronic health record systems.

The movement from automation to advanced analytics is also evident in the expanding use of predictive modeling. These systems extend beyond simple data classification, since they extrapolate from patterns to anticipate future clinical events. For example, machine learning tools can identify patients at heightened risk of complications, readmissions, or treatment failures. This capacity enables clinicians to intervene proactively rather than reactively, which contrasts sharply with earlier technologies that only documented events rather than forecasting them. Recent clinical evidence supports this transition, as demonstrated by Boussina et al. (2024), who found that deploying a deep learning sepsis prediction system improved outcomes across large, diverse hospital populations. Their results show how predictive models can strengthen patient safety, guide more effective resource distribution, and enhance overall system performance when integrated into real clinical workflows.

Despite these advances, it is essential to acknowledge that sophisticated analytics depend heavily on data quality, representativeness, and quantity. Poorly curated datasets can lead to misleading predictions and inequitable outcomes. While AI excels at uncovering hidden correlations, it cannot compensate for systematic gaps, biases, or inconsistencies in the data it receives. As a result, the move toward advanced analytics introduces demands for improved data governance, interdisciplinary collaboration, and continuous model supervision.

Through this shift, AI has moved beyond simple automation to assume a central role in diagnostic reasoning and risk assessment. This transformation marks a defining moment in the evolution of medical practice, establishing a foundation for more complex and individualized forms of care to continue to develop.

Diagnostic Imaging and Clinical Decision Support

Diagnostic imaging represents one of the most advanced and impactful applications of artificial intelligence in contemporary healthcare. Traditional computer-aided detection tools were limited by rigid rule-based structures that required programmers to specify every possible feature of a condition. Because clinical presentations are varied and often unpredictable, these early systems frequently lacked the flexibility needed for accurate interpretation. Modern AI-based imaging tools, however, operate through learning rather than explicit programming. As Basa (2024) notes, these systems can train on millions of images, continuously improving their capacity to identify subtle abnormalities. This iterative learning process allows the models to distinguish between benign and pathological features that would be difficult for even expert radiologists to identify with similar consistency.

AI imaging systems now demonstrate performance levels that match or exceed human clinicians in detecting conditions such as lung cancer, diabetic retinopathy, and certain musculoskeletal disorders. Research has shown that deep learning models can outperform radiologists in lung cancer screening using low-dose CT scans (Ardila et al., 2019). Similarly, Gulshan et al. (2016) demonstrated that deep learning algorithms achieve ophthalmologist-level accuracy in detecting diabetic retinopathy. At leading medical centers, AI tools have become integral to radiology workflows, offering real-time image assessment and flagging potential areas of concern. These systems do not replace radiologists; instead, they augment human interpretation by serving as a second set of analytical eyes. This dual approach reduces diagnostic variability, increases efficiency, and supports earlier detection of diseases that require timely intervention.

Beyond imaging, AI-driven clinical decision support systems provide another significant advancement in healthcare analytics. These systems synthesize information across multiple data streams, including laboratory results, vital signs, electronic health records, and historical patient outcomes. Through predictive modeling, they can estimate the likelihood of adverse events before they occur. For instance, predictive algorithms can detect early indications of sepsis, often hours before clinical symptoms become apparent. Huang et al. (2022) demonstrated that reinforcement learning models can recommend optimal sepsis treatment strategies and predict deterioration based on real-time physiological data. By identifying patterns associated with physiological decline, AI systems enable clinicians to intervene promptly, thereby improving patient outcomes and reducing mortality rates.

Clinical decision support tools also contribute to personalized medicine by generating treatment recommendations based on patient-specific characteristics. They can compare individuals to thousands of similar cases, offering insights that would be impossible for a single clinician to compute manually. This data-driven personalization enhances therapeutic precision and reduces the risk of inappropriate treatments. Furthermore, these tools help identify high-risk patient populations that may require additional monitoring, resource allocation, or specialized care.

Despite their promise, these systems must be deployed thoughtfully. Predictive models are only as effective as the data used to build them. Incomplete, biased, or unrepresentative datasets can lead to skewed recommendations. There is also a risk that clinicians may rely too heavily on algorithmic output without sufficiently interrogating the reasoning behind it. Maintaining human oversight is therefore essential to ensure that AI's analytical strengths do not inadvertently overshadow clinical judgment. Transparent communication between AI outputs and clinicians remains a priority as developers refine these tools.

Together, advanced imaging and decision support systems highlight the transformative potential of AI in healthcare. They demonstrate how learning-based models can amplify clinical expertise, enhance diagnostic precision, and create new opportunities for personalized and preventive care. Yet their effectiveness depends on deliberate implementation, robust data governance, and continual evaluation to maintain accuracy and equity across diverse populations.

Democratizing Expertise and Revealing New Limitations

Artificial intelligence has introduced new possibilities for democratizing medical expertise, particularly through digital and telemedicine platforms. In regions where access to specialized clinicians is limited, AI-enabled tools can extend diagnostic and analytic capabilities far beyond traditional boundaries. Studies on mobile and point-of-care deep learning tools show that AI embedded into handheld devices can support accurate interpretation of ultrasound, dermatological, and ophthalmic images in low-resource settings, thereby expanding the reach of specialized care. By embedding sophisticated algorithms into handheld devices, smartphones, and portable imaging systems, healthcare providers working in underserved settings can access insights comparable to those available in advanced medical centers. This shift from centralized expertise to distributed analytical capacity has significant implications for global health equity.

Despite these achievements, the democratization of expertise is accompanied by new limitations that reflect the complex realities of AI implementation. One major challenge involves generalizability. AI systems are often trained on data from specific hospitals, geographic regions, or patient demographics, limiting their performance across different environments. A model developed from imaging data in a technologically advanced urban hospital may perform poorly when applied in a rural clinic with different population characteristics, imaging equipment, or disease prevalence. This limitation has been documented across multiple clinical AI systems, prompting calls for broader and more diverse training datasets (Badgeley et al., 2019). Generalizability issues stand in direct tension with the aspiration to use AI as a global equalizer.

Data drift presents another critical limitation. As patient populations, medical technologies, and disease patterns evolve, AI models trained on historical data may become outdated. These shifts can produce subtle declines in accuracy or misclassifications that may go undetected without systematic recalibration. Continuous monitoring and retraining are therefore essential, yet such practices require technical expertise and resources that are often scarce in low-resource environments. Recent evaluations of deployed clinical models, including the study by Seyyed-Kalantari et al. (2021), have shown that even highly accurate systems can degrade when clinical conditions or patient demographics shift. Their findings emphasize the importance of ongoing surveillance of model performance, as the communities that would benefit most from AI-driven support may also face the most significant barriers to maintaining current, reliable systems.

AI's dependence on high-quality data also poses a structural challenge. Inconsistent documentation, missing values, or inaccurate data entries can severely undermine algorithmic performance. Many underserved regions lack robust electronic health record systems or standardized reporting practices, which can limit the effectiveness of AI tools or produce misleading insights. Poor data quality raises concern not only about accuracy but also about fairness, since errors disproportionately affect marginalized populations, whose medical histories are often documented incompletely. Studies on bias in clinical datasets have shown that inequities in data availability and quality translate directly into inequities in algorithmic predictions (Chen et al., 2021).

The presence of AI alone does not automatically guarantee improved care. Effective adoption requires user trust, digital literacy, and appropriate integration into clinical workflows. Without adequate training and infrastructure, clinicians may underutilize AI or misinterpret its outputs, diminishing its potential impact. In this context, AI democratizes expertise while simultaneously revealing the limitations and vulnerabilities that accompany technological innovation. Understanding both dimensions is essential for responsible design and deployment, ensuring that AI enhances healthcare delivery without reinforcing existing inequities or introducing new forms of system-level risk.

The technological capacities described above do not operate in isolation but actively restructure collaborative relationships within healthcare systems. Diagnostic algorithms, predictive models, and decision support tools mediate how clinicians share expertise, how institutions coordinate care, and how patients engage with information about their own treatment. As AI becomes embedded in clinical workflows, collaboration increasingly occurs through digital interfaces that shape communication, authority, and responsibility. Understanding these technologies therefore requires attention not only to their performance but also to how they redistribute roles and dependencies among professionals and organizations. This shift underscores why technological capability must be evaluated in relation to the forms of e-collaboration it enables or constrains.

PART 2: COLLABORATIVE CONSTRAINTS, ETHICAL CHALLENGES, AND THE DIGITAL DIVIDE

The Human Side Of AI In Medicine: Ethics And Society

Artificial intelligence introduces an ethical landscape in healthcare that is far more intricate than the challenges posed by traditional clinical practice. While the principle of avoiding harm remains foundational, integrating AI into medical decision-making raises new questions about fairness, transparency, and accountability. These questions arise because AI systems, unlike human clinicians, lack moral intuition, experiential reasoning, and the capacity for ethical deliberation. Their performance and judgment depend entirely on the data from which they learn and the context in which they are deployed. As a result, the ethical implications of AI-driven healthcare extend well beyond conventional considerations, demanding a deeper examination of how these technologies shape, and are shaped by, societal structures.

Concerns about bias are among the most pressing challenges. Because AI systems learn from historical datasets, they inevitably absorb the inequities embedded within those records. McKinney et al. (2020) demonstrated this dynamic in their large-scale evaluation of AI systems for breast cancer screening, in which algorithm performance varied significantly across demographic groups. The same issue is evident in dermatological AI applications, particularly those developed primarily from images of patients with lighter skin tones. When such systems are deployed in diverse clinical settings, they risk producing skewed diagnostic outcomes that disproportionately disadvantage already marginalized populations. This is not merely a technical flaw; it reflects a broader structural issue in healthcare data collection, representation, and resource allocation. As AI systems scale, unaddressed bias threatens to widen disparities rather than reduce them.

Privacy concerns further complicate this ethical terrain. Earlier eras of medical confidentiality involved safeguarding individual patient files. AI systems, however, operate on massive datasets that extend far beyond traditional medical records, drawing on genomic information, behavioral data, and longitudinal health metrics. Floridi et al. (2019) highlight the complexity of genomic privacy, noting that individual DNA data is inherently relational. When a patient shares genetic information, they reveal information about relatives who have not done so. This interconnectedness challenges conventional notions of autonomy and informed consent, because the implications of sharing data extend beyond the individual and into familial and even community networks. AI's data requirements, therefore, force healthcare institutions to rethink the ethical boundaries of confidentiality and consent in ways that current frameworks are ill-equipped to handle.

Accountability represents another unresolved dimension. In traditional medical practice, responsibility for clinical decisions is relatively straightforward, resting with the physician or institution providing care. AI complicates this chain of responsibility. When an algorithm contributes to a clinical decision that leads to harm, attributing responsibility becomes difficult. Developers may argue that clinicians retain ultimate decision-making authority. Clinicians, in turn, may rely on the system's analyses without fully understanding its internal processes. Institutions may struggle to adjudicate blame when the decision emerged from complex interactions between human judgment and algorithmic recommendations. The opacity of many AI systems, often described as "black box" models, adds another layer of uncertainty by obscuring the logic that produces their outputs.

These combined challenges demonstrate that the ethical integration of AI in healthcare requires more than technical refinement. It calls for robust oversight systems that ensure transparency, equitable data representation, and clearly defined lines of accountability. Without these safeguards, the power of AI risks outpacing the ethical and legal structures needed to govern it, creating vulnerabilities that could undermine both patient trust and clinical integrity.

Accountability, Professional Roles, and Institutional Liability

The increasing incorporation of artificial intelligence into clinical decision-making raises complex questions about accountability and professional responsibility. Traditional models of medical liability assume a clear line of causation between clinician judgment and patient outcomes. When errors occur, responsibility is typically assigned to an identifiable individual or institution. The introduction of AI systems complicates this model. When algorithms contribute to diagnostic decisions or treatment planning, it becomes difficult to determine who should be held responsible when things go wrong. Existing legal frameworks were built for human actors rather than distributed systems in which decision pathways are partially generated through machine learning processes. Scholars note that this gap between traditional liability models and algorithmic decision-making has created regulatory uncertainty across multiple jurisdictions (Price et al., 2019). As a result, the familiar structure of medical liability begins to resemble a set of horse-and-buggy laws applied to the era of self-driving cars. The legal and ethical tools available do not fully correspond to the realities of AI-assisted medicine.

When AI provides a recommendation that influences clinical judgment, the responsibility may fall somewhere among the developer who designed the system, the clinician who relied on its output, or the institution that approved its deployment. The opacity of many machine learning models, often described as black boxes, further complicates this determination. Clinicians cannot always articulate why an algorithm recommended a specific diagnosis or intervention, and developers may not fully understand the internal reasoning mechanisms of their own systems due to the complexity of deep learning architectures. Research on explainability in medicine has shown that model opacity undermines both trust and legal clarity, since clinicians cannot justify decisions based on algorithmic logic they cannot interpret (Amann et al., 2020).

This ambiguity has broader socioeconomic implications. Larger, well-funded institutions may be better positioned to navigate the risks associated with AI adoption because they possess legal departments, risk management teams, and insurance structures capable of absorbing potential liabilities. In contrast, smaller hospitals and clinics, particularly in rural or low-resource regions, may be hesitant to adopt AI tools due to concerns about legal exposure. For these institutions, even a single adverse event linked to AI could result in financial losses or reputational damage they cannot afford. Analyses of digital health inequity demonstrate that resource constraints create structural barriers to the adoption of emerging technologies, thereby widening existing gaps in access and innovation (Celi et al., 2022). As a result, communities already experiencing healthcare disparities may fall further behind in access to AI-enabled innovations.

Liability concerns also influence developers' behavior. Technology companies may be reluctant to provide complete transparency due to intellectual property protections, yet clinicians require this transparency to build trust in AI systems. Similarly, developers may attempt to limit their liability by shifting responsibility to clinicians who use the tools, creating tensions between software creators and healthcare providers. Without clear legal standards that delineate shared responsibility, these conflicts may hinder collaboration and undermine confidence in AI-supported decision-making. This misalignment between technological development and legal structures has been recognized as a growing challenge in the governance of clinical AI (Gerke et al., 2020).

Addressing accountability requires a new model that reflects the distributed nature of AI-influenced care. This model must articulate shared responsibility among developers, clinicians, and institutions, and it must account for the varying capacities of different healthcare organizations. Clear regulatory guidelines, professional standards, and auditing mechanisms can help reduce uncertainty while supporting equitable adoption. A system that leaves smaller institutions unprotected risks widening the divide between technologically advanced healthcare centers and those with limited resources. Only with coherent legal frameworks can AI be implemented safely, fairly, and consistently across diverse clinical environments.

The Digital Divide and the AI Healthcare Paradox

Significant disparities in technological access and infrastructure continue to temper the promise of artificial intelligence in global healthcare. While advanced medical centers increasingly adopt AI-driven diagnostic and decision-support tools, many regions lack the foundational resources required to sustain such innovations. This uneven distribution reflects a persistent international digital divide that threatens to reinforce pre-existing inequities in healthcare delivery. Recent analyses of digital health inequality indicate that the infrastructures necessary for AI development and deployment remain heavily concentrated in high-income countries. Ali et al. (2023) demonstrate that both technical capacity and the ecosystems supporting AI innovation are largely confined to resource-rich settings, leaving low- and middle-income regions without the institutional foundations needed to benefit from these technologies. Such disparities constrain the equitable diffusion of AI-enabled healthcare and limit its global impact.

At the core of this challenge lies what may be described as the AI healthcare paradox. Populations with the greatest need for AI-supported diagnostics and clinical decision assistance are often those least equipped to implement them. Rural areas, underserved urban communities, and low-income countries frequently lack reliable electricity, broadband connectivity, modern diagnostic equipment, and the trained personnel required to operate and maintain AI systems. These constraints restrict adoption even where potential health gains are substantial. Consequently, communities that could benefit most from early disease detection, real-time triage, or remote diagnostic support remain excluded from the advantages these technologies promise.

Workforce limitations further intensify this paradox. Effective use of AI requires clinicians, technicians, and administrators capable of interpreting outputs, overseeing system performance, and responding to errors or bias. Resource-constrained settings often face acute shortages not only of healthcare professionals but also of personnel with informatics or data governance expertise. Without sustained capacity-building efforts, AI tools cannot be safely or effectively integrated into clinical practice. In addition, the absence of standardized electronic health records in many regions restricts the availability of high-quality data needed to train, validate, and maintain AI systems over time.

Infrastructure challenges extend beyond technical capacity to include governance and regulatory oversight. In many low-resource contexts, regulatory frameworks for digital health and medical AI remain underdeveloped or fragmented. This lack of oversight raises concerns regarding safety, accountability, transparency, and ethical use. It also discourages responsible investment and deployment, as international organizations and developers face uncertainty regarding legal standards and institutional accountability. Weak governance thus becomes both a cause and a consequence of uneven AI adoption.

The digital divide also shapes the global research ecosystem underpinning AI development. Because AI models learn from available datasets, the underrepresentation of populations from low-income regions produces systems that perform unevenly across demographic and geographic contexts. Evidence from global health research indicates that models trained primarily on data from high-income countries often exhibit reduced accuracy when applied to populations with different disease profiles, genetic backgrounds, or environmental exposures (World Health Organization, 2021). This imbalance reinforces cycles of exclusion by embedding existing disparities directly into algorithmic performance, thereby limiting the clinical relevance of AI for marginalized populations.

Addressing the AI healthcare paradox therefore requires more than technological innovation alone. It demands coordinated investment in digital infrastructure, workforce development, public health capacity, and institutional governance. Without such alignment, AI risks amplifying existing inequities rather than alleviating them. Bridging the digital divide is not merely a technical challenge but a structural and political one that requires sustained commitment across sectors and levels of governance.

Inequities in infrastructure, expertise, and regulatory capacity directly shape the quality of e-collaboration across healthcare systems. Where connectivity, training, or institutional support are limited, collaborative engagement with AI becomes fragmented or inaccessible. As a result, the benefits of AI-enabled coordination tend to concentrate in well-resourced environments, while underserved regions face barriers to meaningful participation. Viewing the digital divide through the lens of e-collaboration reveals that inequality is not only a matter of access to technology but also of inclusion within shared decision-making networks that govern how AI is designed, implemented, and evaluated. This perspective reinforces the central argument that equitable and effective AI deployment depends on strengthening collaborative structures alongside technological innovation.

Emerging Approaches in Low-Resource Contexts

Efforts to address the challenges posed by the digital divide have yielded several promising approaches to expanding AI-supported healthcare in low-resource contexts. These strategies demonstrate how AI can be adapted to environments with limited technological capacity while advancing health equity. Expanding this discussion allows for a more detailed analysis of practical solutions and their implications for underserved populations.

Offline capable AI systems represent another innovative approach. These systems are designed to function without continuous internet access, allowing clinicians in rural areas to use diagnostic tools even when connectivity is intermittent. For instance, in several regions of East Africa, offline AI systems have been integrated into portable ultrasound devices used by community health workers. The AI assists with image interpretation, guiding non-specialist users in identifying high-risk pregnancies or early complications. This approach illustrates how AI can amplify frontline workers' skills rather than replace them. Research on AI-assisted point-of-care ultrasound in Uganda and Rwanda confirms that offline-enabled tools can meaningfully improve diagnostic quality even when specialist oversight is limited (Kayarian et al., 2024).

Stakeholder collaboration remains essential for sustaining these innovations. Governments, non-governmental organizations, technology companies, and local communities must work together to build the infrastructure necessary for long-term impact. For example, Rwanda's Ministry of Health partnered with multiple private developers to create AI-enabled platforms for triaging patients during infectious disease outbreaks. These platforms integrated data from community health workers, mobile clinics, and public health laboratories, improving outbreak response despite limited national resources.

Academic research also plays a crucial role. Studies such as those described by Strika et al. (2025) emphasize the importance of evaluating AI interventions within medical deserts. These evaluations assess not only technical accuracy but also implementation feasibility, cultural appropriateness, and sustainability. Evidence-based insights from these studies help refine deployment strategies and inform policies that promote equitable access.

Despite these advances, challenges remain. Low-resource communities must continue to navigate shortages in trained personnel, inconsistent electrical supply, and limited institutional support. Many AI systems also require periodic updates, which can be challenging to deliver in regions with unstable connectivity. However, the emergence of adaptive, context-sensitive solutions demonstrates that AI can be implemented effectively in low-resource environments when guided by strategic planning and partnership.

Together, these approaches reveal AI's potential to advance health equity when deployed thoughtfully. By tailoring technologies to local conditions and engaging communities in implementation, AI can help reduce disparities and strengthen healthcare systems in underserved regions.

Diagnostic Imaging and Clinical Decision Support

Artificial intelligence has reshaped diagnostic imaging and clinical decision-making by advancing beyond the limits of traditional computer-aided systems. Early imaging tools were constrained by rule-based programming, in which experts manually encoded the features associated with specific diseases. These systems could only detect what programmers explicitly described, and they lacked the flexibility necessary to respond to the complexity and variability of real-world clinical presentations. Their value was limited because they did not learn from new data and could not improve over time. This is a defining contrast with contemporary machine learning models, which operate through iterative exposure to large datasets. As Basa (2024) explains, modern systems draw on millions of imaging samples to refine their accuracy, allowing them to identify subtle visual cues that even skilled radiologists may overlook.

These advances have significantly transformed diagnostic imaging in specialties such as ophthalmology, oncology, and pulmonology. For example, deep learning systems trained on thousands of retinal images now detect diabetic retinopathy with accuracy comparable to that of human experts. Gulshan et al. (2016) demonstrated that a deep learning model achieved ophthalmologist-level sensitivity and specificity in identifying diabetic retinopathy using retinal fundus photographs. Similar gains have been documented in lung cancer detection, where AI models can highlight small nodules that might otherwise go unnoticed. Ardila et al. (2019) showed that a deep learning system outperformed experienced radiologists in predicting malignancy from low-dose CT scans, particularly for subtle findings that are challenging to identify consistently. These systems do not supplant radiologists; instead, they enhance diagnostic precision by acting as analytical partners. They flag potential areas of concern, reduce oversight errors, and increase consistency among clinicians with varying levels of experience.

AI enhances clinical decision-making beyond imaging as well. Modern decision support systems analyze diverse data sources, including vital signs, laboratory results, medication histories, and longitudinal patient records. These systems generate probabilistic forecasts of clinical deterioration, helping clinicians manage complex cases more effectively. For instance, predictive algorithms can detect early signs of sepsis hours before observable symptoms emerge. They do so by recognizing subtle shifts in physiological data that indicate heightened risk. This allows clinicians to intervene earlier, thereby significantly reducing mortality. Similarly, decision support systems guide personalized treatment planning by examining how patient-specific characteristics correlate with outcomes in comparable populations.

These capabilities suggest a shift from reactive to anticipatory medicine, altering the rhythm of clinical practice. Clinicians no longer must wait for symptoms to escalate before acting. Instead, they gain access to predictive insights that inform more proactive care strategies. However, these tools are not without challenges. Their effectiveness depends heavily on the quality and diversity of the data used to train them. Predictive systems grounded in incomplete or biased datasets may perform unevenly across populations, leading to disparities in care. Moreover, clinicians may become overly reliant on algorithmic recommendations if the systems are not fully transparent about their reasoning. Ensuring that AI tools remain interpretable and ethically integrated is essential for maintaining trust in clinical decision support.

AI-driven imaging and decision support systems represent some of the most advanced applications of artificial intelligence in healthcare. They demonstrate how learning-based models can extend the reach of clinical expertise, sharpen diagnostic accuracy, and support individualized care. Yet their success also depends on continuous oversight, responsible data governance, and sustained clinician engagement to ensure equitable and reliable performance across diverse healthcare environments.

Democratizing Expertise and Revealing New Limitations

Artificial intelligence plays an increasingly important role in democratizing medical expertise by extending advanced diagnostic and analytic capabilities into regions that have traditionally lacked access to specialized care. Through telemedicine platforms, mobile technologies, and portable diagnostic tools, AI-enabled systems reduce geographic barriers and provide clinicians in underserved settings with real-time guidance that previously required direct access to specialists. This redistribution of expertise represents a meaningful departure from historical patterns of healthcare inequality, in which advanced knowledge and resources were concentrated in urban centers and well-funded institutions. By enabling knowledge to circulate across regions, populations, and care settings, AI introduces new possibilities for more inclusive models of healthcare delivery. Empirical studies of AI-supported telemedicine suggest that machine learning tools can enhance clinical decision making in remote environments by supporting image interpretation and risk assessment, thereby reducing reliance on centralized facilities (Rossi et al., 2025).

This capacity aligns with broader shifts toward anticipatory and preventive models of care. Predictive analytics allow clinicians to identify emerging risks before they escalate into acute conditions, enabling earlier intervention and more efficient resource allocation. When embedded within telemedicine infrastructures, such tools strengthen remote monitoring, chronic disease management, and triage systems, particularly in settings where specialist availability is limited or inconsistent. In this sense, AI contributes not only technical functionality but also a reconfiguration of how care is coordinated, moving health systems from reactive responses toward more proactive and distributed forms of collaboration.

At the same time, the expansion of AI into diverse clinical environments exposes significant structural limitations that complicate its promise as an equalizing force. One of the most persistent challenges concerns generalizability. AI systems trained in technologically advanced healthcare environments often perform less reliably when deployed in contexts that differ in patient demographics, disease prevalence, clinical workflows, or diagnostic infrastructure. Models developed using data from hospitals in Europe or North America may not transfer effectively to rural clinics or low-resource settings in other regions, thereby undermining their utility as universal tools (Obermeyer et al., 2019). When training datasets fail to reflect population diversity, algorithmic performance can degrade substantially, particularly in high-stakes diagnostic applications.

Data drift further complicates deployment across heterogeneous environments. As disease patterns, environmental conditions, and clinical practices evolve, the data underlying AI systems can become outdated. Without regular retraining and monitoring, model accuracy may decline gradually or abruptly. Regions with limited technical capacity often face difficulties in maintaining such updates, increasing the risk that outdated systems continue to inform clinical decisions. These dynamics disproportionately affect health systems already operating under resource constraints, reinforcing existing disparities rather than alleviating them.

The effectiveness of AI is also constrained by the quality and consistency of underlying data. Many low-resource settings lack standardized electronic health records, reliable documentation practices, or interoperable data infrastructures. Incomplete records, inconsistent data entry, and fragmented patient histories can undermine algorithmic reliability. Even well-designed models cannot compensate for weak data foundations, and in such contexts AI may amplify rather than reduce inequities. These limitations illustrate that technological capability alone is insufficient without parallel investments in data governance and institutional capacity.

Beyond technical considerations, the successful integration of AI depends heavily on human and organizational factors. Adoption requires clinician trust, adequate training, and alignment with existing workflows. Without these conditions, AI systems may be underused, misinterpreted, or inconsistently applied. Effective implementation therefore depends on collaborative processes that support learning, adaptation, and shared understanding among clinicians, administrators, and technical developers. This reinforces the need to view AI not as a standalone tool but as part of a broader sociotechnical system shaped by patterns of coordination and communication.

Ethical challenges further highlight the centrality of collaboration in AI-enabled healthcare. Questions of fairness, accountability, transparency, and autonomy do not arise solely from algorithmic design choices but from how responsibility is distributed across actors involved in development, deployment, and oversight. Ethical failures often reflect breakdowns in coordination, insufficient communication, or unclear lines of accountability among stakeholders. From this perspective, ethics functions less as a static set of principles and more as an ongoing collaborative practice. Effective ethical governance requires sustained interaction among developers, clinicians, institutions, regulators, and patients to establish shared standards, monitor outcomes, and respond collectively to unintended consequences.

Taken together, these dynamics underscore that the promise of artificial intelligence in healthcare cannot be realized through technology alone. Its effectiveness depends on the quality of collaboration that surrounds it, including the alignment of infrastructure, governance, professional practice, and community engagement. By framing AI through the lens of e-collaboration, it becomes possible to understand how innovation, equity, and accountability are co-produced through coordinated action rather than isolated technical achievement. This perspective clarifies that responsible AI adoption is not merely a matter of deploying advanced tools, but of building the collaborative capacities necessary to ensure that those tools serve diverse populations in ethically grounded and socially sustainable ways.

PART 3: COLLABORATIVE GOVERNANCE AND SHARED ACCOUNTATBILITY

Bridging The Digital Divide

The promise of artificial intelligence in healthcare reflects an ambitious vision for the future of global medicine, yet its realization exposes a persistent tension between technological possibility and social reality. Contemporary scholarship highlights that AI diffusion remains highly uneven across regions and systems, shaped by disparities in infrastructure, governance capacity, and institutional readiness (Kraus et al., 2023). Although AI-driven tools continue to transform diagnostic imaging, data analysis, and patient monitoring, their benefits remain unevenly distributed. Healthcare institutions in technologically advanced settings integrate AI rapidly into routine practice, while large segments of the global population encounter structural barriers that limit similar adoption. This imbalance underscores that technological progress alone cannot ensure equitable outcomes, as implementation is deeply conditioned by social, economic, and organizational contexts.

Regulatory lag represents one of the most significant challenges shaping the governance of AI in healthcare. While AI systems evolve rapidly through expanding computational capacity, continuous learning, and growing data availability, regulatory frameworks advance more slowly due to the requirements of deliberation, public accountability, and legal codification. This temporal mismatch creates conditions in which AI tools may enter clinical environments before standards for safety, accountability, and quality assurance are fully established. Traditional regulatory models were designed for static technologies whose performance remains stable after approval, whereas contemporary AI systems adapt over time, raising complex questions regarding liability, post-market monitoring, and algorithmic drift. In many jurisdictions, regulatory bodies lack the technical expertise or institutional resources required to evaluate adaptive systems effectively. As noted by the World Health Organization (2021), new regulatory approaches are therefore necessary to balance innovation with continuous oversight. Without such mechanisms, insufficiently monitored AI systems risk eroding patient safety and public trust.

At the center of these dynamics lies AI's growing capacity to reshape clinical decision making and healthcare delivery through new forms of coordinated action. Machine learning models now analyze imaging data with levels of precision that may rival or exceed human performance, while natural language processing systems can synthesize vast clinical datasets at unprecedented speed. Kraus et al. (2023) situate these developments within broader transformations in computational capacity and clinical productivity. In principle, such tools offer the possibility of extending high-quality diagnostic and decision support to underserved settings, potentially mitigating shortages of skilled professionals. As Morley et al. emphasize, AI holds distributive potential by enabling expertise to travel digitally rather than requiring physical proximity. These capabilities position AI as a mechanism for collaborative care that connects clinicians, institutions, and patients across geographic boundaries.

Yet the realization of this collaborative potential is constrained by persistent structural barriers. The global digital divide remains a central obstacle to equitable AI adoption, particularly in rural or low-income regions where reliable connectivity, computational infrastructure, and stable electricity are limited. Workforce shortages further compound these challenges, as effective AI deployment depends on clinicians, technicians, and administrators who possess the skills required to interpret, manage, and oversee algorithmic systems. As a result, the communities that might benefit most from AI-enabled diagnostic and decision-support tools are often those least equipped to implement them. This dynamic reinforces long-standing inequities documented in global analyses of AI ethics and governance and reveals the limits of purely technological solutions.

This condition may be understood as an AI healthcare paradox. In contexts where access to medical expertise is scarce and delays in care are common, AI-assisted tools could significantly improve diagnostic accuracy and timeliness. Yet these same contexts frequently lack the institutional and digital capacity necessary to support AI deployment. In response, various adaptive strategies have emerged. Mobile health initiatives increasingly leverage widespread smartphone access to deliver AI-supported screening and monitoring tools, while some developers have designed systems capable of operating offline or under low-connectivity conditions. Such approaches reflect the scalable and context-sensitive pathways described by Kraus et al., emphasizing the importance of tailoring innovation to diverse resource environments rather than assuming uniform technological readiness.

Despite these promising adaptations, sustainable integration cannot rely on isolated technical solutions. Effective and equitable implementation requires coordinated action among governments, healthcare organizations, technology developers, and local communities. Public authorities must invest in digital infrastructure and regulatory capacity, healthcare institutions must commit to long-term workforce development, and developers must design systems that function within real-world constraints rather than idealized conditions. This collaborative orientation aligns with Morley et al.'s argument that responsible AI adoption depends on alignment between ethical principles and infrastructural realities. Coordination across sectors is therefore not ancillary but foundational to meaningful implementation.

The academic community also plays a critical role in supporting this collaborative ecosystem. Research examining economic feasibility, implementation pathways, and real-world outcomes can inform policy design and guide context-sensitive adoption strategies. Scholarship that integrates technical evaluation with social and institutional analysis contributes to more realistic assessments of how AI can advance public health objectives without exacerbating inequality. Such work helps bridge the gap between innovation and governance by grounding policy decisions in empirical evidence and comparative insight.

Ultimately, realizing the transformative potential of artificial intelligence in healthcare requires acknowledging both its technological capabilities and the structural inequalities that shape its deployment. Progress depends on deliberate coordination rather than technological momentum alone. Governance frameworks play a central role in organizing this coordination by defining how responsibilities are allocated, how data are shared, and how accountability is enforced when AI systems influence clinical outcomes. In this sense, governance functions as the institutional architecture of e-collaboration, structuring participation, authority, and oversight across the healthcare ecosystem. When governance mechanisms are fragmented or underdeveloped, collaboration weakens and inequities deepen. Conversely, mature and adaptive governance arrangements can enable shared learning, coordinated oversight, and collective accountability. Through this lens, e-collaboration emerges not as a supplementary feature of AI adoption but as the central condition through which innovation, equity, and ethical responsibility are reconciled in contemporary healthcare systems.

Enablers of responsible and effective AI adoption

While ethical, governance, and equity challenges pose substantial risks to the deployment of artificial intelligence in healthcare, these concerns should not be understood solely as constraints. Instead, they identify specific design, policy, and coordination gaps that can be addressed through deliberate institutional choices. Reframing these challenges as opportunities for intervention allows AI adoption to be approached as a problem of system design and collaborative governance rather than as a technological impasse (Leslie, 2020). Responsible implementation, therefore, depends on identifying and strengthening the enabling conditions that support equitable, transparent, and sustainable use.

One central enabler is the development of adaptive and context-sensitive governance frameworks. Regulatory systems that incorporate iterative review, post-deployment monitoring, and mechanisms for algorithmic updating are better suited to managing dynamic AI systems than static approval models. Adaptive governance allows regulators to respond to model drift, emerging biases, and evolving clinical contexts while maintaining accountability. Such frameworks also benefit from multistakeholder participation, incorporating perspectives from clinicians, patients, technologists, and policymakers. Through collaborative oversight structures, governance becomes a shared responsibility rather than a centralized constraint, aligning regulation with real-world practice.

A second critical enabler involves investment in digital infrastructure and data ecosystems that support interoperability and quality assurance. Reliable connectivity, standardized electronic health records, and interoperable data architectures are prerequisites for effective AI deployment. Design strategies that prioritize modular systems and open standards can reduce dependence on proprietary platforms and facilitate integration across institutions. Strengthening data governance through clear standards for data quality, documentation, and stewardship also enhances model reliability and transparency. These infrastructural measures transform data from a limiting factor into a shared resource that supports coordinated decision making across healthcare systems.

Workforce development represents another foundational pathway for responsible adoption. AI systems require not only technical maintenance but also informed human oversight. Training programs that integrate data literacy, ethical reasoning, and clinical interpretation enable professionals to engage critically with AI outputs rather than treat them as opaque authorities. Interdisciplinary education that brings together clinicians, informaticians, engineers, and administrators fosters a shared understanding of system capabilities and limitations. Such capacity building strengthens e-collaboration by equipping stakeholders to communicate effectively, resolve uncertainties, and adapt workflows collaboratively.

Design choices that emphasize transparency and explainability further support trust and accountability. Explainable AI interfaces, documentation of model assumptions, and clear communication of uncertainty help users understand how recommendations are generated and when caution is warranted. These features are particularly important in high-stakes clinical settings, where trust depends on the ability to question, contextualize, and override automated outputs. Embedding explainability into system design transforms ethical principles into operational features and supports shared responsibility among developers and users.

Equally important are participatory and community-engaged approaches to AI development and deployment. Including patients, frontline clinicians, and community representatives in design and evaluation processes helps ensure that technologies reflect local needs, values, and constraints. Such engagement can surface context-specific risks that may not be visible to developers or regulators alone. Participatory approaches also strengthen legitimacy and social acceptance, reinforcing the collaborative foundations necessary for sustainable adoption.

Finally, international cooperation and policy coordination function as enabling mechanisms in an increasingly interconnected digital health landscape. Cross-border standards for data protection, model evaluation, and ethical practice can reduce fragmentation and promote interoperability. Collaborative research initiatives and knowledge-sharing platforms allow best practices to circulate across regions with differing levels of technological maturity. Greater emphasis on patient-centered perspectives is essential to fully align AI governance with person-centered care, particularly by foregrounding patient trust, perceptions of explainability, and meaningful informed consent. Incorporating patient-reported outcomes and experiential feedback into AI design and evaluation processes would strengthen accountability and ensure that technological adoption reflects not only clinical efficiency but also patients' values, understanding, and lived experiences. These forms of transnational e-collaboration help prevent the concentration of innovation benefits within a limited set of high-resource contexts and support more inclusive global participation.

Taken together, these enablers demonstrate that the risks associated with AI in healthcare are not insurmountable barriers but signals of where institutional design, governance capacity, and collaborative coordination require strengthening. By reframing ethical, regulatory, and equity challenges as actionable design problems, AI adoption becomes a matter of intentional system building rather than technological inevitability. This perspective reinforces the chapter's central argument: that effective, equitable, and trustworthy AI in healthcare depends on the quality of e-collaboration that integrates technology, governance, and human judgment into a coherent and accountable whole.

GOVERNANCE FRAMEWORKS FOR RESPONSIBLE AI IN HEALTHCARE

The rapid integration of artificial intelligence into healthcare requires governance structures capable of addressing the ethical, procedural, and institutional challenges introduced by these technologies. Earlier regulatory models were designed for static medical devices and linear diagnostic workflows, yet contemporary AI systems evolve through continuous learning and rely on extensive volumes of sensitive patient data. These characteristics require oversight mechanisms that are flexible enough to monitor ongoing algorithmic changes while safeguarding patient rights, ensuring clinical reliability, and maintaining public confidence. Mittelstadt (2019) notes that the complexity of adaptive AI systems demands regulatory approaches that extend beyond traditional ethical guidelines, since principles developed for conventional technologies do not fully account for dynamic algorithmic behavior. This concern parallels Leslie's (2020) work on institutional readiness, which emphasizes that responsible governance must be integrated into every stage of AI development and deployment to support equitable and clinically reliable use.

A central requirement of responsible governance is establishing transparency standards that clarify how AI systems operate. Many algorithms function as complex models whose internal processes are not easily interpretable, creating barriers for clinicians who must evaluate the reliability of AI recommendations. Governance frameworks must therefore require documentation of data sources, model design, performance metrics, and known limitations. This transparency is essential for clinical decision-making because clinicians remain ethically responsible for interpreting AI outputs within the broader context of patient care. Transparent systems enable users to understand how conclusions are generated, thereby increasing trust and reducing the risks associated with blind reliance on opaque computational processes. Mittelstadt's critique demonstrates why explainability is crucial for preventing overreliance on AI systems that may encode hidden biases or methodological flaws.

Effective governance must also incorporate rigorous auditing mechanisms to evaluate fairness and prevent harmful biases. AI systems trained on historical clinical data may reproduce inequities embedded within those datasets, resulting in uneven performance across demographic groups. Governance structures must therefore include regular assessments of algorithmic behavior using representative datasets and validated evaluation tools. These assessments must examine not only accuracy but also the distribution of errors across populations. Without such oversight, AI systems risk amplifying disparities in diagnosis and treatment, particularly for groups that have historically been underrepresented in healthcare data or underserved within health systems. Leslie (2020) emphasizes the importance of routine model auditing as a foundation for safe deployment within complex institutional environments.

Accountability is another pillar of responsible governance. AI adoption distributes decision-making among clinicians, institutions, and developers, complicating the question of who is responsible when errors occur. Governance frameworks must clearly articulate obligations for each stakeholder, including responsibilities for monitoring, reporting, updating, and responding to incidents involving AI-driven recommendations. These models must recognize that responsibility cannot fall solely on clinicians who neither design nor control algorithmic behavior. Institutions and developers must share responsibility for ensuring system safety and addressing risks. Clear lines of accountability reduce uncertainty and support consistent, ethically grounded use of AI tools, a principle consistent with scholarly analyses of distributed responsibility in digital systems.

Data protection requirements must be strengthened to reflect the sensitivity of the information AI systems process. Modern AI relies on genomic data, biometric indicators, behavioral patterns, and longitudinal health records, making privacy breaches particularly concerning. Governance frameworks must mandate advanced security protocols, limited data access, and robust consent procedures that address the relational nature of genetic and familial data. Protecting privacy is also essential for maintaining public trust in AI-assisted healthcare, and this concern is central to both Mittelstadt's ethical critique and Leslie's (2020) operational guidelines.

Finally, responsible governance requires an adaptive regulatory structure that evolves alongside technological developments. Static rules cannot adequately regulate systems that learn continuously or update automatically. Policymakers must develop flexible mechanisms for post-deployment monitoring, iterative model evaluation, and ongoing safety validation. This adaptive approach must also incorporate public engagement to ensure that governance reflects community values and aligns with societal expectations of fairness, safety, and transparency. Leslie's framework highlights how participatory governance can help align technological development with social expectations.

Responsible governance provides the foundation for safe and equitable AI integration. Through transparency, auditing, accountability, data protection, and adaptive oversight, healthcare systems can foster innovation while safeguarding patient welfare and maintaining trust in the evolving landscape of AI-enabled care.

POLICY FRAMEWORKS AND GOVERNANCE

The rapid expansion of artificial intelligence within healthcare has created a regulatory landscape struggling to keep pace with technological change. As AI-driven tools become increasingly central to clinical practice, health systems face the challenge of governing technologies that evolve more quickly than the policies designed to oversee them. Reports indicate that global adoption of healthcare AI continues to accelerate, yet regulatory structures remain fragmented and incomplete (Grand View Research, 2023). While certain regions have taken early steps toward establishing oversight mechanisms, these efforts often provide only partial coverage, leaving significant gaps in areas such as algorithmic transparency, liability, and long-term monitoring.

Existing data protection laws offer some foundational guidance, but they were not crafted with modern AI applications in mind. The European Union's General Data Protection Regulation (GDPR) is frequently cited as a leading example of robust data governance, especially regarding patient consent, data minimization, and privacy safeguards. Even so, GDPR does not fully resolve questions related to dynamic machine learning systems, such as how to manage datasets that continue to expand, how to regulate continuously adapting algorithms, or how to ensure meaningful transparency in models whose internal logic may be opaque even to their developers. Healthcare-specific regulations for AI, therefore, remain a work in progress, emerging gradually as policymakers attempt to adapt legal frameworks to technologies that challenge traditional definitions of medical devices, clinical judgment, and data ownership.

Developing effective governance requires striking a careful balance among several competing priorities. Innovators argue that overly restrictive regulation may stifle progress in an area that offers life-saving potential, whereas clinicians and ethicists emphasize that insufficient oversight risks patient safety, undermines trust, and magnifies existing inequities. The task is further complicated by the inherent tension between privacy protection and the need for extensive data sharing. AI systems depend on large, diverse, and high-quality datasets to perform reliably across populations, yet expanding access to sensitive health information increases the risk of data breaches and misuse. Governance frameworks must therefore protect patient confidentiality without hindering scientific advancement or compromising the accuracy of clinical models.

The challenge extends beyond privacy and innovation. High standards for accuracy, fairness, and accountability must be upheld to prevent harm, yet regulatory burdens must remain feasible for health systems and developers with limited resources. Achieving this balance requires a nuanced understanding of both the technical capabilities of AI and the complex realities of healthcare environments. For example, regulatory bodies must understand how AI systems function across varied clinical settings, how they adapt to new data, and how their performance may fluctuate among different demographic groups. Policymakers must also appreciate the practical constraints faced by healthcare institutions, from limited budgets to workforce shortages, which may affect how AI systems are implemented and monitored.

This evolving landscape underscores the need for governance approaches that are flexible, evidence-based, and responsive to innovation, while remaining firmly grounded in ethical principles. Effective regulation will require multidisciplinary collaboration among technologists, clinicians, legal experts, and community stakeholders to create structures that both support progress and safeguard patient well-being.

Principles for Effective AI Governance in Healthcare

The integration of AI into healthcare systems presents unprecedented opportunities to enhance patient care, yet it also introduces complex governance challenges that require rigorous oversight. Scholars such as Mittelstadt (2019) argue that the rapid evolution of AI technologies complicates traditional oversight models, particularly in healthcare, where patient outcomes are directly affected by algorithmic performance. This analysis examines the fundamental principles necessary for establishing effective AI governance frameworks in healthcare settings, emphasizing the delicate balance between innovation and safety.

Central to effective AI governance is the principle of algorithmic transparency. Healthcare AI systems must operate within a framework of complete visibility, where decision-making processes are not only documented but also readily explicable to all stakeholders. Leslie (2020) highlights that transparency must move beyond technical disclosures to include accessible explanations of data provenance, methodological choices, and model limitations. Such openness serves dual purposes: it facilitates trust building among healthcare providers and patients while enabling regulators to perform their oversight functions effectively.

The imperative to detect systematic bias and evaluate performance is another crucial pillar of AI governance. Mittelstadt's (2019) critique of principle-based approaches illustrates how insufficient auditing can perpetuate structural inequities embedded in training data. Healthcare organizations must therefore implement rigorous auditing protocols that extend beyond initial deployment. These evaluations should employ sophisticated statistical methods to identify potential biases across demographic groups, ensuring that AI systems maintain their accuracy and clinical relevance as medical knowledge evolves. Performance metrics must be continuously monitored, with particular attention to how these systems perform across diverse patient populations (Leslie, 2020).

Accountability frameworks represent a critical component that requires careful structuring. These frameworks must delineate clear lines of responsibility among various stakeholders, including AI developers, healthcare institutions, and clinical practitioners. Mittelstadt (2019) notes that distributed responsibility can create ambiguity when errors occur, making it essential for governance structures to articulate obligations for system monitoring, error reporting, and corrective action.

When adverse events arise, these frameworks should facilitate swift identification of responsible parties and implement appropriate remediation, while also remaining adaptive enough to address emerging technological challenges.

Data protection in healthcare AI systems demands unprecedented levels of sophistication. Modern AI systems rely on genomic data, biometric indicators, and longitudinal health records, raising concerns about the heightened sensitivity of the data these systems process, as Leslie (2020) notes. Beyond basic compliance with regulatory standards such as GDPR and HIPAA, organizations must implement advanced cryptographic protocols, refined access controls, and comprehensive audit trails that anticipate evolving threats. The relational nature of genetic and familial data requires governance structures that extend protections to both individuals and related kin networks.

The dynamic nature of healthcare necessitates sophisticated monitoring mechanisms. AI systems require continuous evaluation and adjustment to remain aligned with evolving clinical practices and emerging medical knowledge. Leslie (2020) emphasizes the importance of iterative oversight mechanisms that combine automated performance metrics with human clinical judgment. Such hybrid monitoring enables real-time adjustments that maintain both system accuracy and patient safety.

Ethical considerations must be deeply embedded within the governance framework. This extends beyond surface-level compliance to encompass fundamental principles of medical ethics, including patient autonomy, beneficence, and distributive justice. Mittelstadt (2019) demonstrates that ethics checklists alone are inadequate unless coupled with institutional cultures that prioritize equity and patient welfare. Healthcare AI systems must therefore be designed and deployed in ways that actively promote health equity and minimize the risk of exacerbating existing disparities.

The success of AI governance in healthcare depends significantly on interdisciplinary collaboration. Expertise from computer science, ethics, law, sociology, and public policy must inform the development of governance structures that address both technical and societal implications. Leslie's (2020) framework stresses the value of involving diverse disciplinary perspectives to ensure that governance approaches are analytically comprehensive and practically feasible.

Public engagement represents another critical dimension of effective AI governance. Healthcare organizations must develop sophisticated communication strategies that educate patients about AI capabilities while acknowledging their limitations. Mittelstadt (2019) highlights the importance of cultivating informed public dialogue to ensure that governance structures remain aligned with societal expectations. Public feedback should be incorporated into governance frameworks to ensure that AI implementation reflects community needs and values.

Regulatory compliance must be viewed as a foundation rather than a ceiling for governance standards. While adherence to existing healthcare regulations remains essential, organizations should proactively develop governance approaches that anticipate future regulatory requirements. Leslie (2020) argues for forward-looking models that adapt to technological change rather than responding reactively. Such anticipatory governance helps ensure that AI systems remain both compliant and effective as regulatory landscapes evolve.

The tension between innovation and safety requires careful calibration within governance frameworks. Protecting patient safety remains paramount, yet excessive restriction can impede technological advancement. Mittelstadt (2019) warns that governance overly focused on risk minimization may inadvertently hinder beneficial innovation. Organizations must therefore develop mechanisms that encourage responsible experimentation while maintaining robust safety protocols and oversight processes.

This comprehensive approach to AI governance in healthcare requires significant institutional commitment and resources. However, investing in developing and maintaining these frameworks is essential to realizing the full potential of AI while protecting patient interests and promoting public trust. As healthcare AI continues to evolve, these governance principles will require regular reassessment and refinement to address new challenges and opportunities. Implementing these principles requires a systematic strategy that balances immediate operational requirements with long-term strategic objectives, ensuring AI governance remains effective and relevant in a rapidly evolving healthcare landscape.

The Regulatory Lag in Healthcare AI

The rapid evolution of artificial intelligence in healthcare has created a regulatory environment that struggles to keep pace with technological innovation. While AI-driven tools are now central to diagnostic imaging, clinical decision support, and population-level data analytics, the policies meant to oversee their development and use remain fragmented and incomplete. This regulatory lag has significant implications for safety, accountability, and equitable access. It reflects a broader tension between the speed of technological progress and the comparatively slow processes of legislative development, institutional oversight, and ethical review.

Current reports on the state of healthcare AI indicate that adoption continues to accelerate across global markets, yet governance structures remain uneven and often inadequate to address emerging challenges. Grand View Research (2023) notes that although investment in AI driven healthcare tools is growing rapidly, regulatory frameworks have not kept pace with this expansion. Jurisdictions differ widely in their oversight strategies, leading to inconsistencies in safety standards, data protection protocols, and evaluation requirements. In some regions, regulatory bodies have issued preliminary guidelines that gesture toward accountability and transparency, but these guidelines often lack enforceable mechanisms or detailed implementation pathways.

The European Union's General Data Protection Regulation is frequently cited as a cornerstone of contemporary data governance because it imposes stringent standards related to privacy, consent, and data minimization. Nevertheless, GDPR was not designed specifically for machine learning systems that evolve or draw predictions from continuously expanding datasets. Its limitations become evident when applied to adaptive AI systems requiring frequent updates or retraining. It offers a framework for protecting personal data. Still, it does not fully address questions concerning ongoing monitoring of algorithmic performance, the dynamic nature of predictive models, or the complex issue of explainability.

The challenge grows more acute when considering how machine learning systems transform after deployment. Unlike traditional medical devices, AI systems may change their internal parameters in response to new data. This adaptive quality complicates oversight because a model approved at one moment may not behave the same way several months later. Regulators must grapple with how to monitor technologies that evolve outside the formal approval process, raising questions about post-deployment auditing, real-time surveillance, and long-term safety validation.

The result is a regulatory landscape marked by uncertainty. Developers face inconsistent requirements across jurisdictions, which complicates efforts to design systems that can be deployed internationally. Healthcare institutions must interpret ambiguous rules while ensuring that AI tools meet clinical standards. Clinicians are often left without clear guidance on how to integrate AI into practice responsibly. Patients, meanwhile, face the risk of receiving care shaped by systems that may lack adequate oversight.

Given these challenges, the regulatory lag is not simply a technical issue but a structural one that reflects the limits of current governance paradigms. A robust response requires recognition that AI operates fundamentally differently from previous healthcare technologies. Only by developing adaptive, forward-looking regulatory systems can governments and institutions ensure that AI supports high-quality, safe, and equitable healthcare.

Balancing Innovation, Privacy, and Safety

The governance of artificial intelligence in healthcare involves balancing three interdependent priorities, namely innovation, patient privacy, and safety. Each of these dimensions is essential, although they often exist in tension with one another. Scholars such as Leslie et al. (2021) argue that the central challenge arises from reconciling the data-intensive nature of AI with the ethical and regulatory safeguards required to protect patients. AI development depends on extensive datasets to train reliable models and ensure that systems perform effectively across diverse populations. Yet, the collection, storage, and analysis of such data introduce considerable privacy risks. Highly innovative systems may also advance more quickly than existing safety protocols, while overly restrictive regulations can hinder the development of technologies with the potential to improve clinical outcomes. Effective governance, therefore, relies on the ability to mediate these tensions in ways that uphold ethical principles while still supporting scientific progress.

Innovation in healthcare AI depends on access to rich, representative data. Machine learning systems require large volumes of high-quality clinical information to produce accurate and equitable predictions. When datasets lack diversity or volume, models often perform poorly for specific demographic groups, creating risks of unequal treatment. Ensuring broad access to data is therefore essential for building AI systems that are safe and effective. Yet expanding access increases the likelihood of data breaches, unauthorized sharing, and misuse. Sensitive health information can reveal genetic predispositions, familial relationships, behavioral patterns, and other deeply personal attributes. The consequences of privacy violations can be far-reaching, affecting not only individuals but also families and communities (Leslie, 2020).

The need for data-driven innovation is further complicated by safety concerns arising from fast-moving technological development. AI systems may appear promising in early trials but behave unpredictably when deployed at scale. The adaptive nature of machine learning compounds this risk, as model performance may drift as new data are incorporated or clinical practices evolve. This volatility raises questions about how often systems need to be audited, who is responsible for updating them, and what mechanisms must be in place to detect performance deterioration before it causes harm.

Governance structures must therefore protect privacy while enabling responsible data use. Policies that focus solely on restricting access may undermine innovation and prevent clinicians from adopting tools that could improve patient outcomes. Conversely, regulations that privilege innovation without adequate safeguards risk exposing patients to unauthorized surveillance, biased outputs, or unsafe clinical recommendations. Achieving balance requires an approach that appreciates the complexity of AI development and deployment in healthcare settings.

This balance also involves addressing the problem of under-regulation and the risks of over-regulation. Under regulation, unsafe systems may proliferate or produce inequitable outcomes, particularly in underserved communities. Overregulation may dissuade smaller healthcare institutions and developers from engaging with AI, thereby widening adoption gaps and reinforcing the digital divide. Regulatory frameworks must therefore be flexible enough to support innovation while establishing strong protections for patient welfare, transparency, and fairness.

Balancing innovation, privacy, and safety is not a static task but a continuous process that must adapt to evolving technological conditions. Effective governance requires ongoing evaluation, interdisciplinary collaboration, and systematic recalibration to ensure that AI advances serve the interests of patients, clinicians, and society.

Operationalizing E-Collaboration in Everyday Healthcare Practice

To fully understand how artificial intelligence reshapes healthcare collaboration, it is necessary to examine how AI functions within everyday clinical workflows. Beyond abstract discussions of capability or ethics, AI increasingly operates as an embedded coordination layer that mediates communication, decision making, and task distribution across multidisciplinary teams (Topol, 2019). In practice, e-collaboration emerges through routine interactions among clinicians, support staff, administrators, and digital systems, rather than through isolated technological interventions.

One central domain in which AI supports collaborative workflows is multidisciplinary clinical decision making. In many care settings, particularly hospitals and specialty clinics, patient management involves teams composed of physicians, nurses, pharmacists, radiologists, and allied health professionals. AI-enabled decision support systems can synthesize patient data from electronic health records, imaging platforms, and laboratory results to generate risk scores, diagnostic suggestions, or treatment alerts. These outputs do not replace professional judgment but function as shared reference points that structure discussion across disciplines. For example, an AI-generated risk stratification score may prompt coordinated review during case conferences, enabling clinicians to align on priorities, escalate care, or adjust treatment pathways. In this way, AI acts as a mediating artifact that supports collective reasoning rather than isolated decision making.

AI also plays a growing role in facilitating remote consultation and distributed care models. Through telemedicine platforms enhanced with algorithmic triage or image analysis, clinicians in resource-limited settings can consult with specialists located elsewhere while sharing standardized, AI-augmented assessments. For instance, diagnostic imaging interpreted with machine learning assistance can be transmitted alongside clinical notes to remote specialists, enabling more informed consultations without requiring patient transfer. This form of digitally mediated collaboration expands access to expertise while preserving local clinical autonomy. It also illustrates how AI enables coordination across institutional and geographic boundaries by providing a common analytic reference that supports shared interpretation.

Cross-institutional referral processes represent another operational domain shaped by AI-enabled collaboration. Referral pathways often involve multiple organizations with differing documentation systems, protocols, and capacity constraints. AI tools can support these workflows by identifying appropriate referral pathways, prioritizing cases based on urgency, and ensuring that relevant clinical information accompanies the referral. Automated summarization and data harmonization reduce administrative burden while supporting continuity of care across institutional boundaries. When embedded within interoperable systems, these functions facilitate smoother transitions between levels of care and reduce fragmentation, particularly for patients with complex or chronic conditions.

Shared decision making between clinicians and patients also reflects an important site of operational collaboration influenced by AI. Predictive models and decision-support interfaces can present individualized risk estimates, treatment options, and outcome probabilities in formats designed to support patient understanding. When used appropriately, these tools can enhance dialogue by making uncertainty more explicit and by grounding discussions in personalized data. This supports a collaborative clinical relationship in which patients participate more actively in care decisions rather than serving as passive recipients of algorithmic recommendations. The effectiveness of such tools, however, depends on careful design, clinician mediation, and sensitivity to health literacy differences.

At the organizational level, AI contributes to coordination by supporting resource allocation, scheduling, and workflow optimization. Predictive analytics can anticipate patient demand, identify bottlenecks, and inform staffing decisions across departments. When shared across managerial and clinical teams, these insights support collective planning rather than isolated administrative control. Such applications illustrate how AI can function as a coordination infrastructure that aligns operational decision making with clinical priorities, provided that transparency and accountability mechanisms are in place.

Across these use cases, a common pattern emerges. AI does not replace human collaboration but reshapes its structure by introducing new forms of mediation, shared reference, and coordination. Effective implementation therefore depends on how well institutions integrate AI into existing workflows and communication practices. This integration requires training, role clarification, and governance arrangements that specify how algorithmic outputs should be interpreted, challenged, and revised. Without such alignment, AI tools risk becoming parallel systems that generate information without improving collaboration or outcomes.

Viewing these operational dynamics through an e-collaborative lens clarifies how everyday practices connect to broader ethical and governance concerns. Decisions about data sharing, accountability, and oversight directly influence how smoothly collaborative workflows function. When governance structures support interoperability, transparency, and shared responsibility, AI-enabled collaboration can enhance continuity of care and professional coordination. When they do not, fragmentation and mistrust may undermine potential benefits.

By grounding abstract discussions of AI ethics and governance in concrete workflow contexts, this operational perspective demonstrates how collaboration is enacted in practice. It shows that responsible AI adoption depends not only on high-level principles or regulatory frameworks but also on the everyday arrangements through which clinicians, institutions, and technologies work together. In this way, operational e-collaboration serves as the bridge between technical innovation and meaningful improvement in healthcare delivery.

Economic Sustainability and the Long-Term Viability of AI-Enabled Healthcare

Beyond technical performance and ethical governance, the long-term viability of artificial intelligence in healthcare depends on its economic sustainability. AI systems require substantial upfront and ongoing investments that extend well beyond software acquisition. Implementation costs include infrastructure upgrades, data integration, cybersecurity protections, system customization, and interoperability development. In addition, organizations must invest in workforce training, workflow redesign, and continuous system maintenance. These financial commitments shape whether AI adoption can be sustained over time or remains limited to short-term pilot initiatives concentrated in well-resourced institutions.

Training and human capital development represent particularly significant cost components. Clinicians, administrators, and technical staff must acquire competencies in data interpretation, system oversight, and ethical use. Without sustained investment in education and professional development, AI tools risk underutilization or misuse, reducing their potential value. From an economic perspective, training should be understood not as a one-time expenditure but as a recurring investment necessary to maintain system effectiveness as technologies evolve (Leslie, 2020). Institutions that integrate training into long-term workforce planning are better positioned to translate AI capabilities into durable performance gains.

At the same time, AI adoption can generate economic benefits when embedded within coordinated organizational strategies. Predictive analytics and automation may reduce inefficiencies, support earlier interventions, and optimize resource allocation. Improvements in scheduling, triage, and care coordination can lower operational costs while improving service delivery. In value-based care environments, these efficiencies may translate into measurable returns through reduced hospital readmissions, shorter lengths of stay, and more targeted use of clinical resources. However, such returns are rarely automatic. They depend on governance structures that align incentives, define accountability, and ensure that efficiency gains are reinvested in care quality and workforce support rather than absorbed unevenly across systems.

Economic sustainability is therefore inseparable from governance maturity. Transparent budgeting, clear procurement standards, and oversight mechanisms are essential for evaluating the cost-effectiveness of AI initiatives over time. Governance frameworks that incorporate cost monitoring, performance evaluation, and periodic reassessment help organizations determine whether AI investments continue to deliver value relative to their financial and social costs. These mechanisms also enable course correction when systems underperform or generate unintended consequences. In this sense, governance does not merely regulate AI use but actively supports its economic sustainability by aligning technological deployment with organizational priorities and fiscal responsibility.

Equity considerations further shape the economic dimension of AI adoption. Without deliberate policy intervention, market-driven implementation tends to concentrate innovation in affluent settings with existing infrastructure and purchasing power. This dynamic risks widening disparities by directing investment toward institutions already well positioned to benefit from AI. Linking economic sustainability to equity requires funding models that support adoption in under-resourced settings, including public investment, international cooperation, and incentive structures that encourage inclusive deployment. Such approaches recognize that equitable access to AI-enabled healthcare is not only a moral objective but also a long-term investment in system resilience and population health.

From an e-collaboration perspective, economic sustainability depends on coordinated action across institutional and sectoral boundaries. Governments, healthcare organizations, technology developers, and academic institutions must align financial strategies with shared goals related to access, quality, and accountability. Collaborative procurement models, shared infrastructure platforms, and public–private partnerships can reduce duplication of costs and distribute financial risk. These arrangements allow smaller or resource-constrained organizations to participate in AI-enabled systems that would otherwise remain inaccessible.

Ultimately, economic feasibility should be understood not as a narrow calculation of short-term return on investment but as a broader assessment of value creation over time. Sustainable AI adoption requires balancing efficiency gains with investments in governance, workforce capacity, and equity. When economic planning is integrated with ethical oversight and collaborative governance, AI can support healthcare systems that are not only technologically advanced but also financially resilient and socially responsive. This integrated approach reinforces the chapter's central argument that responsible AI adoption depends on coordinated institutional design rather than isolated technological innovation.

Core Principles of Effective AI Governance

Effective governance of artificial intelligence in healthcare depends on a set of foundational principles that ensure systems remain safe, transparent, equitable, and aligned with the ethical commitments of medical practice. Foundational work by Floridi et al. (2019) underscores the importance of organizing governance around clear normative principles that can guide institutions in structuring oversight and evaluating new technologies. These principles are not abstract ideals; they serve as practical guidelines for institutions to structure oversight mechanisms, evaluate emerging technologies, and support responsible innovation. As outlined, these principles are clearly stated, and organizing them into coherent subsections strengthens the section's logic while preserving the analysis's substance.

The first principle is the requirement for algorithmic transparency. AI systems must provide clear, comprehensible information about how they generate outputs, the data they rely on, and the reasoning that underlies their recommendations. Transparency enables clinicians to interpret algorithmic insights within the broader context of patient care. It also provides regulators with the means to evaluate model safety and alignment with clinical standards. Transparent systems support trust by ensuring that patients and clinicians understand the benefits and limitations of the technologies influencing their care (Floridi et al., 2019)

The second principal centers on detecting and mitigating systematic bias. AI models must be evaluated using diverse datasets that reflect the populations they are meant to serve. Healthcare organizations must conduct ongoing audits to identify disparities in performance across demographic groups and to ensure that model accuracy does not deteriorate over time. Without such monitoring, AI risks reproducing or amplifying inequities embedded in historical data.

Accountability is a third essential principle. Governance structures must delineate clear responsibilities among developers, healthcare institutions, and clinicians. When adverse events occur, these structures must facilitate the timely identification of contributing factors and support corrective action. Accountability frameworks should recognize the distributed nature of AI-influenced care and allocate responsibility accordingly. They must ensure that no group bears disproportionate liability while also guaranteeing that all stakeholders uphold rigorous safety standards.

The fourth principle involves robust data protection. AI systems process sensitive health information, including genetic data, behavioral metrics, and personal identifiers. Governance structures must therefore require advanced security protocols, restricted data access, and meaningful consent procedures. These protections safeguard patient autonomy and reduce the risk of data breaches that could compromise trust in AI assisted healthcare.

Continuous monitoring constitutes a fifth principle. Because AI models evolve as they encounter new data, governance frameworks must require regular performance assessments, calibration, and retraining. Monitoring should integrate automated alerts, human oversight, and external auditing to ensure that systems remain aligned with clinical standards and do not drift into unsafe behavior.

The final principle is interdisciplinary and public engagement. AI in healthcare affects clinicians, patients, policymakers, and communities. Governance must therefore integrate perspectives from multiple fields, including law, ethics, medicine, data science, and public health. Public engagement ensures that AI systems reflect community values and that implementation strategies are responsive to societal expectations. Floridi et al. (2019) likewise highlight the importance of integrating societal and institutional perspectives to ensure that AI remains a public good rather than a purely technical instrument.

Together, these principles establish the foundation for responsible AI governance. By embedding transparency, fairness, accountability, security, continuous monitoring, and inclusive engagement within institutional structures, healthcare systems can ensure that AI contributes meaningfully to improved outcomes while safeguarding the rights and well-being of patients.

FUTURE DIRECTIONS AND EMERGING TRENDS

The trajectory of artificial intelligence in healthcare suggests an imminent transformation in medical practice, particularly in precision medicine. This evolution represents more than incremental progress; as Topol (2019) argues in his work on the future of medical intelligence, it signifies a fundamental restructuring of healthcare delivery systems, moving from traditional population-based approaches toward highly individualized therapeutic strategies.

At the core of this transformation lies the unprecedented ability to synthesize vast amounts of patient specific data. Advanced machine learning algorithms now possess the capability to integrate multiple data streams, including genomic sequences, proteomic profiles, metabolomic data, environmental exposure information, and longitudinal lifestyle metrics, to construct comprehensive patient profiles with previously unattainable precision. This granular analysis enables the development of treatment protocols tailored to individual genetic and physiological characteristics, marking a departure from conventional one-size-fits-all therapeutic approaches. The capacity for such integration reflects the broader trend described by Rajkomar et al. (2019), who highlight the growing fusion of clinical and omics data under AI-enabled infrastructures.

The implications of this shift are particularly significant in the treatment of complex pathologies. In oncology, for instance, AI-driven analysis of tumor genomics and patient-specific immune responses enables the development of personalized immunotherapy protocols. Similarly, in the management of autoimmune disorders, machine learning algorithms can predict disease flares and optimize treatment timing based on individual patient patterns, potentially revolutionizing disease management strategies.

Drug discovery represents another domain where AI's impact proves transformative. Advanced computational models now accelerate the identification of promising therapeutic compounds by simulating molecular interactions and predicting drug efficacy with remarkable accuracy. These platforms significantly reduce the time and resources required for drug development, potentially bringing novel treatments to patients more rapidly than traditional discovery methods allow.

The integration of AI with public health surveillance systems presents unprecedented opportunities for population health management. Sophisticated predictive models can now analyze patterns in health data to forecast disease outbreaks and identify emerging health trends before they become widespread. This capability enables health systems to shift from reactive to proactive intervention strategies, potentially averting public health crises before they fully materialize.

In the realm of assistive technologies, AI driven innovations are reshaping the landscape of rehabilitative medicine. Advanced prosthetic devices equipped with neural interfaces and machine learning capabilities can adapt to individual user patterns, providing more natural and intuitive functionality. These systems learn from user behavior over time, continuously optimizing their performance to match individual movement patterns and preferences.

The implementation of these advanced systems, however, raises important considerations regarding data privacy, algorithmic bias, and equitable access. Healthcare institutions must develop robust frameworks to ensure that the benefits of AI-driven precision medicine extend across demographic and socioeconomic boundaries. Additionally, integrating these technologies requires careful attention to ethical considerations, particularly in genetic medicine applications.

The success of this technological transformation depends heavily on the development of sophisticated data infrastructure capable of handling the enormous volume of patient information required for precise analysis. Healthcare systems must invest in secure, scalable platforms that can process diverse data types while maintaining patient privacy and data integrity.

As these technologies continue to evolve, the role of healthcare providers will likely shift toward interpreting AI generated insights and maintaining the crucial human element in patient care. This evolution suggests a future where artificial intelligence augments rather than replaces clinical expertise, enabling more informed decision making and improved patient outcomes.

This trajectory indicates a future where healthcare becomes increasingly precise, predictive, and personalized. The convergence of AI with other emerging technologies promises to revolutionize not only how we treat diseases but also how we conceptualize health and wellness. As these systems mature, they will likely enable unprecedented levels of disease prevention and health optimization, marking a new era in medical science and healthcare delivery.

Emerging Clinical and Technological Trends

The trajectory of artificial intelligence in healthcare is shaping a new era of clinical practice that moves beyond traditional diagnostic and therapeutic models toward more personalized, predictive, and preventive forms of medicine. Analysts such as Topol (2019) argue that this trajectory represents a fundamental reconfiguration of medical practice, where computational tools increasingly complement human clinical judgment. The convergence of machine learning, genomic science, digital phenotyping, and advanced biomedical engineering has accelerated this shift, producing innovations that challenge long held assumptions about what healthcare systems can deliver. Your existing analysis highlights how precision medicine, genomic analysis, drug discovery, public health surveillance, assistive technologies, and genetic engineering represent the cutting edge of this transformation.

Precision medicine exemplifies the growing integration of AI into individualized care. Machine learning algorithms can synthesize large volumes of genomic, proteomic, metabolomic, and environmental data, generating highly granular patient profiles. These profiles enable clinicians to move beyond population-level averages and toward treatment strategies tailored to unique biological signatures. In oncology, for example, AI-assisted genomic sequencing identifies tumor-specific mutations that support more targeted immunotherapies. Similar insights in autoimmune disorders allow models to predict disease flares and guide therapeutic timing, reshaping the management of chronic conditions. Rajkomar et al. (2019) emphasize that such multilayered data integration is becoming central to the next generation of precision clinical models.

Drug discovery is undergoing an equally profound shift. Traditional discovery methods rely on lengthy screening processes and significant financial investment. AI-driven platforms now simulate molecular interactions computationally, identifying novel compounds and predicting their therapeutic potential. These systems can reduce development time drastically by filtering out ineffective candidates early in the process. As a result, AI contributes to accelerating the delivery of new treatments for diseases that have historically resisted conventional pharmacological approaches.

Public health surveillance stands to benefit significantly from AI's ability to analyze patterns in large scale datasets. Predictive models can detect early indicators of outbreaks, track disease spread, and identify at risk populations based on mobility patterns, social determinants of health, and clinical reporting. This capacity shifts public health from reactive crisis management toward proactive intervention strategies that prevent widespread transmission.

AI is also transforming assistive and rehabilitative technologies. Emerging prosthetic devices incorporate neural interfaces and adaptive learning systems that map user movement patterns and adjust to individual biomechanics. These devices function more naturally than traditional prosthetics and improve over time through continued user interaction. In neurorehabilitation, AI-supported systems guide therapy sessions by analyzing motor function and adjusting exercises in real time.

While these advancements signal extraordinary potential, they also introduce questions about data ethics, access, and governance. Precision medicine and genetic interventions require extensive datasets that may not be available equitably across populations. Public health models rely on surveillance data that must be collected responsibly and transparently. Assistive technologies involve sensitive neural information that requires robust safeguards. The transformative potential of these trends, therefore, depends on governance structures that keep pace with scientific innovation. Together, these emerging trends mark a shift toward an intertwined clinical and technological ecosystem. The continued evolution of these innovations will influence how healthcare systems define evidence, allocate resources, and conceptualize patient care in the decades ahead.

Strategic Integration of AI Across Health Systems

The integration of artificial intelligence into healthcare requires more than technical capacity. It demands a strategic framework that acknowledges the interdependence of technological capability, socioeconomic context, and governance maturity. Scholars examining digital health implementation, such as Whitelaw et al. (2020), emphasize that effective AI adoption depends on aligning these system-level conditions rather than treating technology as a standalone solution. These three dimensions form a conceptual model that can help policymakers, institutional leaders, and clinicians evaluate their readiness for AI implementation and design appropriate strategies for responsible adoption. Each dimension influences how effectively a health system can deploy AI tools and determines the risks and benefits that accompany such deployment.

The first axis of this model, technological capability, represents the availability and quality of AI tools, data infrastructure, computational resources, and specialist expertise. Competent systems possess advanced electronic health records, robust data pipelines, and well-trained informatics teams. Less capable systems may lack basic digital infrastructure or possess incomplete, inconsistent, or insufficiently representative datasets. AI will perform differently across these environments, and governance frameworks must adjust accordingly.

The second axis, socioeconomic context, includes the financial resources, workforce capacity, population health characteristics, and structural inequities that shape how care is delivered. Regions with strong public health investment and stable healthcare financing can integrate AI more quickly because they can support training, adoption, and updating processes. Conversely, health systems operating under resource constraints may struggle to sustain AI tools even if they can be introduced initially. The digital divide becomes particularly salient here because communities with limited connectivity or workforce shortages may not be positioned to benefit from advanced technologies, a challenge well documented by Whitelaw et al. in their assessment of global disparities in digital readiness.

The third axis, governance maturity, reflects the extent to which regulatory structures, institutional policies, and ethical oversight mechanisms are prepared to guide AI use. Mature governance systems include clear standards for data protection, algorithmic transparency, accountability, and performance monitoring. Immature or fragmented governance environments often lack such structures, leaving institutions without clear guidance on evaluating risks or ensuring equitable deployment.

By situating healthcare systems within this three-dimensional framework, decision makers can identify strengths, limitations, and necessary interventions. For example, a system with strong technological capability but weak governance may implement AI quickly but face safety concerns or inequitable outcomes. A system with mature governance but limited technological capacity may require infrastructure investment before AI tools can be deployed effectively. Systems with constraints across all three axes may need phased adoption strategies that begin with foundational improvements in digital infrastructure and workforce capacity.

This conceptual framework also supports strategic planning at multiple levels. Policymakers can use it to prioritize investments in digital infrastructure, connectivity, and regulatory innovation. Health systems can apply it to assess organizational readiness, allocate resources, and design implementation roadmaps. Clinicians and frontline staff can use it to identify training needs and clarify professional responsibilities. The model encourages institutions to view AI not as an isolated technological upgrade but as a structural transformation that requires coordination across technical, organizational, and sociopolitical domains.

Ultimately, strategic integration of AI depends on recognizing that technology alone cannot improve healthcare. Effective implementation requires alignment between technological capabilities, socioeconomic realities, and governance systems.

When these dimensions are considered together, health systems can pursue AI adoption that enhances equity, protects patient rights, and strengthens clinical practice.

Research and Policy Priorities

Advancing responsible artificial intelligence in healthcare requires a forward-oriented agenda that integrates research, policy, and clinical practice. While current systems demonstrate meaningful progress, significant gaps remain in evaluating real-world impacts, ensuring equitable access, and developing sustainable governance frameworks. Analysts such as Rajkomar et al. (2019) emphasize that responsible AI must evolve through continuous adaptation rather than narrow technological refinement, particularly as concerns about fairness, transparency, and equity become increasingly prominent. Recasting your earlier conclusion into a set of future priorities clarifies the steps needed to support safe, effective, and ethically grounded AI deployment.

Research priorities center on generating robust evidence that reflects the diversity and complexity of real-world healthcare environments. Many AI systems are developed and validated using datasets from technologically advanced medical centers. This limits their applicability in low-resource settings, where disease patterns, social conditions, and clinical workflows may differ substantially. Long-term outcome studies are essential for determining how AI influences mortality, morbidity, cost-effectiveness, and patient satisfaction across diverse populations. Research must also investigate bias mitigation strategies, including data diversification methods, algorithmic fairness techniques, and auditing procedures to detect disparities in model performance. Finally, interdisciplinary research should examine the ethical implications of AI-assisted care, including impacts on patient autonomy, clinical judgment, and trust.

Policy priorities focus on creating conditions that enable equitable and sustainable AI implementation. Investment in digital infrastructure remains a foundational requirement because reliable connectivity, standardized electronic health records, and secure data systems are prerequisites for successful AI deployment. Policymakers must establish regulatory approaches that support innovation without compromising safety or privacy. This includes adaptive mechanisms for post-deployment monitoring, frameworks for shared accountability among developers and institutions, and clear standards for data protection. Capacity building is equally important. Health systems need investments in workforce training, informatics education, and public engagement to ensure that clinicians and communities understand the benefits and risks of AI tools.

Practice priorities address the day-to-day integration of AI into clinical care. Clinician education is critical because AI tools must be interpreted and applied within the broader context of patient needs, ethical considerations, and clinical guidelines. Training should emphasize critical appraisal skills, awareness of algorithmic limitations, and strategies for combining human judgment with computational insights. Patient engagement is also essential. Patients must have access to clear explanations about how AI influences their care, how their data are used, and what safeguards protect their rights. Building trust requires transparency, communication, and respect for patient concerns.

Together, these research, policy, and practice priorities establish a roadmap for the next phase of AI-enabled healthcare. They encourage systems to move beyond narrow technical performance metrics and adopt a more comprehensive view of success grounded in equity, safety, and ethical responsibility. By pursuing these priorities, healthcare institutions and policymakers can ensure that AI contributes to improved outcomes while honoring the foundational commitments of medical practice.

CONCLUSION

The accelerating integration of artificial intelligence in healthcare represents a pivotal transformation in the organization and delivery of modern medicine. Across diagnostic imaging, predictive analytics, clinical decision support, precision therapeutics, and public health surveillance, AI demonstrates considerable potential to enhance clinical accuracy, expand access, and support more proactive models of care. Yet the analysis presented in this chapter makes clear that technological capability alone cannot determine the trajectory of AI's influence. The realization of these benefits remains inseparable from the social, economic, and institutional contexts in which AI systems are designed, governed, and deployed.

Evidence reviewed throughout this study demonstrates that disparities in infrastructure, digital connectivity, data quality, and regulatory capacity exert a decisive influence on the reliability and equity of AI-enabled healthcare. These disparities form the foundation of the persistent digital divide shaping global patterns of access and outcomes. AI systems trained on narrow or unrepresentative datasets risk reproducing structural inequities, while regions with limited institutional resources often remain least able to adopt tools that could otherwise improve clinical effectiveness. This paradox underscores the necessity of embedding AI implementation within broader commitments to health equity, capacity building, and infrastructural investment rather than treating technological adoption as a standalone solution.

At the same time, the analysis highlights the central role of governance structures capable of evolving alongside rapid technological change. Effective oversight requires transparency, continuous evaluation, clearly articulated accountability mechanisms, and robust data protection standards. Governance must remain adaptive, recognizing that AI systems are dynamic and that their performance shifts as data environments, clinical practices, and social expectations evolve. Multidisciplinary collaboration and sustained public engagement strengthen these governance arrangements by ensuring that regulatory processes reflect both technical expertise and societal values.

Taken together, these findings indicate that the future role of artificial intelligence in healthcare will be shaped by deliberate institutional choices rather than by technological momentum alone. Although the capacity for transformative advancement is substantial, it must be matched by sustained investment in governance maturity, digital infrastructure, and equitable implementation strategies. The effectiveness of AI ultimately depends on the quality of collaboration among institutions, professionals, and communities, rather than on technical sophistication in isolation. When these conditions are developed in parallel, AI can contribute to a healthcare system that is more responsive, more precise, and more just.

Across its technical, ethical, and governance dimensions, artificial intelligence reshapes healthcare primarily by transforming how collaboration occurs. Through shared diagnostic platforms, distributed decision support, regulatory coordination, and community engagement, AI reorganizes relationships among human and institutional actors. Viewing these developments through an e-collaborative lens clarifies that successful implementation depends on alignment across systems rather than isolated innovation. This perspective provides a unifying framework for understanding how innovation, equity, and accountability intersect in practice, and it reinforces the importance of grounding AI-driven transformation in coordinated, ethically informed collaboration that remains anchored in the principles of patient-centered care.

REFERENCES

Ahmadi Mehr, R., & Ameri, A. (2022). Skin Cancer Detection Based on Deep Learning. *Journal of Biomedical Physics & Engineering, 12*(6), 559–568. DOI: 10.31661/jbpe.v0i0.2207-1517 PMID: 36569567

Ali, M. R., Lawson, C. A., Wood, A. M., & Khunti, K. (2023). Addressing ethnic and global health inequalities in the era of artificial intelligence healthcare models: A call for responsible implementation. *Journal of the Royal Society of Medicine, 116*(8), 260–262. DOI: 10.1177/01410768231187734 PMID: 37467785

Amann, J., Blasimme, A., Vayena, E., Frey, D., & Madai, V. I. (2020). Explainability for artificial intelligence in healthcare: A multidisciplinary perspective. *BMC Medical Informatics and Decision Making, 20*(1), 310. DOI: 10.1186/s12911-020-01332-6 PMID: 33256715

Ardila, D., Kiraly, A. P., Bharadwaj, S., Choi, B., Reicher, J. J., Peng, L., Tse, D., Etemadi, M., Ye, W., Corrado, G. S., Naidu, M., Shetty, S., & Sundaram, P. (2019). End-to-end lung cancer screening with three-dimensional deep learning on low-dose chest computed tomography. *Nature Medicine, 25*(6), 954–961. DOI: 10.1038/s41591-019-0447-x PMID: 31110349

Basa, R. (2024). Human-AI collaboration in healthcare diagnostics: Enhancing accuracy and patient outcomes. *International Journal of Computer Engineering and Technology, 15*(5). Advance online publication. DOI: 10.5281/zenodo.13918695

Bean, D. M., Kraljevic, Z., Shek, A., Teo, J., & Dobson, R. J. B. (2023). Hospital-wide natural language processing summarising the health data of 1 million patients. *PLOS Digital Health, 2*(5), e0000218. DOI: 10.1371/journal.pdig.0000218 PMID: 37159441

Boussina, A., Shashikumar, S. P., Malhotra, A., Owens, R. L., El-Kareh, R., Longhurst, C. A., Quintero, K., Donahue, A., Chan, T. C., Nemati, S., & Wardi, G. (2024). Impact of a deep learning sepsis prediction model on quality of care and survival. *npj. Digital Medicine, 7*(1), 14. DOI: 10.1038/s41746-023-00986-6 PMID: 38263386

Celi, L. A., Cellini, J., Charpignon, M., Boag, W., Huang, L., Feller, A., & Pollard, T. J. (2022). Sources of bias in artificial intelligence that perpetuate healthcare disparities, A global review. *PLOS Digital Health, 1*(3), e0000022. DOI: 10.1371/journal.pdig.0000022 PMID: 36812532

Chen, I. Y., Szolovits, P., & Ghassemi, M. (2021). Can AI help reduce disparities in general medical and mental health care? *AMA Journal of Ethics*, *23*(2), E184–E191. https://journalofethics.ama-assn.org/article/can-ai-help-reduce-disparities-general-medical-and-mental-health-care/2019-02 PMID: 30794127

European Commission. (2024). *Proposal for a Regulation laying down harmonised rules on Artificial Intelligence (Artificial Intelligence Act).* Publications Office of the European Union. https://eur-lex.europa.eu/legal-content/EN/TXT/?uri=celex:52021PC0206

Floridi, L., & Cowls, J. (2019). A unified framework of five principles for AI in society. *Harvard Data Science Review*, *1*(1). Advance online publication. DOI: 10.1162/99608f92.8cd550d1

Gerke, S., Minssen, T., & Cohen, I. G. (2020). Ethical and legal challenges of artificial intelligence-driven healthcare. In Cohen, I. G., Lynch, H. F., Vayena, E., & Gasser, U. (Eds.), *Biomedical Innovation and the Law* (pp. 295–336). Cambridge University Press., DOI: 10.1016/B978-0-12-818438-7.00012-5

Grand View Research. (2023). *AI in healthcare market size, share & trends analysis report.* https://www.grandviewresearch.com/industry-analysis/artificial-intelligence-ai-healthcare-market

Gulshan, V., Peng, L., Coram, M., Stumpe, M. C., Wu, D., Narayanaswamy, A., Venugopalan, S., Widner, K., Madams, T., Cuadros, J., Kim, R., Raman, R., Nelson, P. C., Mega, J. L., & Webster, D. R. (2016). Development and validation of a deep learning algorithm for the detection of diabetic retinopathy in retinal fundus photographs. *Journal of the American Medical Association*, *316*(22), 2402–2410. DOI: 10.1001/jama.2016.17216 PMID: 27898976

Huang, Y., Cao, R., & Rahmani, A. (2022). *Reinforcement learning for sepsis treatment: A continuous action space solution.* In Proceedings of the Machine Learning for Healthcare Conference. https://proceedings.mlr.press/v182/huang22a/huang22a.pdf

Kayarian, F., Patel, D., O'Brien, J. R., Schraft, E. K., & Gottlieb, M. (2024). Artificial intelligence and point-of-care ultrasound: Benefits, limitations, and implications for the future. *The American Journal of Emergency Medicine*, *80*, 119–122. DOI: 10.1016/j.ajem.2024.03.023 PMID: 38555712

Kraus, S., Feuerriegel, S., & Oztekin, A. (2023). Artificial intelligence in healthcare: Past, present, and future. *California Management Review*, *65*(2), 5–27.

Leslie, D. (2020). *Understanding artificial intelligence ethics and safety*. The Alan-Turing Institute. https://www.turing.ac.uk/sites/default/files/2019-06/understanding_artificial_intelligence_ethics_and_safety.pdf

Leslie, D., Mazumder, A., Peppin, A., Wolters, M. K., & Hagerty, A. (2021). Does "AI" stand for augmenting inequality in the era of COVID-19 healthcare? *BMJ (Clinical Research Ed.)*, *372*(304), n304. Advance online publication. DOI: 10.1136/bmj.n304 PMID: 33722847

McKinney, S. M., Sieniek, M., Godbole, V., Godwin, J., Antropova, N., Ashrafian, H., Back, T., Chesus, M., Corrado, G. S., Darzi, A., Etemadi, M., Garcia-Vicente, F., Gilbert, F. J., Halling-Brown, M., Hassabis, D., Jansen, S., Karthikesalingam, A., Kelly, C. J., King, D., & Shetty, S. (2020). International evaluation of an AI system for breast cancer screening. *Nature*, *577*(7788), 89–94. DOI: 10.1038/s41586-019-1799-6 PMID: 31894144

Mittelstadt, B. (2019). Principles alone cannot guarantee ethical AI. *Nature Machine Intelligence*, *1*(11), 501–507. DOI: 10.1038/s42256-019-0114-4

Morley, J., Machado, C. C. V., Burr, C., Cowls, J., Joshi, I., Taddeo, M., & Floridi, L. (2020). The ethics of AI in health care. *Nature Medicine*, *26*(4), 389–397. DOI: 10.1016/j.socscimed.2020.113172 PMID: 32702587

Obermeyer, Z., Powers, B., Vogeli, C., & Mullainathan, S. (2019). Dissecting racial bias in an algorithm used to manage the health of populations. *Science*, *366*(6464), 447–453. DOI: 10.1126/science.aax2342 PMID: 31649194

Price, W. N.II, Gerke, S., & Cohen, I. G. (2019). Potential liability for physicians using artificial intelligence. *Journal of the American Medical Association*, *322*(18), 1765–1766. DOI: 10.1001/jama.2019.15064 PMID: 31584609

Rajkomar, A., Dean, J., & Kohane, I. (2019). Machine learning in medicine. *The New England Journal of Medicine*, *380*(14), 1347–1358. DOI: 10.1056/NEJMra1814259 PMID: 30943338

Rajkomar, A., Hardt, M., Howell, M. D., Corrado, G., & Chin, M. H. (2019). Ensuring fairness in machine learning to advance health equity. *The New England Journal of Medicine*, *380*(26), 2498–2500. DOI: 10.1056/NEJMp1814149 PMID: 31242381

Rajpurkar, P., Chen, E., Banerjee, O., & Topol, E. (2022). AI in health care: The surprising performance of foundation models. *The Lancet. Digital Health*, *4*(8), e538–e545. 100.1038/s41591-021-01614-0

Rossi, M., & Rehman, S. (2025). Integrating artificial intelligence into telemedicine: Evidence, challenges, and future directions. *Cureus, 17*(8), e90829. DOI: 10.7759/cureus.90829 PMID: 40988810

Seyyed-Kalantari, L., Zhang, H., McDermott, M. B. A., Chen, I. Y., & Ghassemi, M. (2021). Underdiagnosis bias of artificial intelligence algorithms applied to chest X-rays. *Nature Medicine, 27*(12), 2176–2182. DOI: 10.1038/s41591-021-01595-0 PMID: 34893776

Strika, Z., Petkovic, K., Likic, R., & Batenburg, R. (2025). Bridging healthcare gaps: A scoping review on AI in medical deserts. *Postgraduate Medical Journal, 101*(1191), 4–16. DOI: 10.1093/postmj/qgae122 PMID: 39323384

Topol, E. (2019). *Deep Medicine: How Artificial Intelligence Can Make Healthcare Human Again*. Basic Books.

Vokinger, K. N., Feuerriegel, S., & Kesselheim, A. S. (2021). Mitigating bias in machine learning for medicine. *Communications Medicine, 1*(1), 25. https://www.nature.com/articles/s43856-021-00028-w. DOI: 10.1038/s43856-021-00028-w PMID: 34522916

Whitelaw, A., Mamas, M. A., Topol, E., & Van Spall, H. G. C. (2020). Applications of digital health in the COVID-19 pandemic: Policy implications and lessons. *Journal of the American College of Cardiology, 76*(23), 2980–2995. DOI: 10.1016/S2589-7500(20)30142-4 PMID: 32835201

World Health Organization. (2021). Ethics and governance of artificial intelligence for health. World Health Organization. https://apps.who.int/iris/handle/10665/341996

KEY TERMS AND DEFINITIONS

AI Governance: A framework of policies, ethical safeguards, and regulatory practices designed to guide the safe, accountable, and equitable development and implementation of artificial intelligence systems.

Algorithmic Bias: Systematic errors in an AI system that produce inequitable or inaccurate outcomes for specific demographic or clinical subgroups.

Artificial Intelligence (AI): A computational approach that enables machines to perform tasks associated with human reasoning, such as pattern recognition, learning, and decision making.

Clinical Decision Support (CDS): Digital tools that analyze patient information to provide evidence-based recommendations that assist clinicians in diagnosis, treatment planning, and monitoring.

Data Drift: The gradual shift in underlying data patterns over time, which reduces model accuracy unless the system is regularly monitored and updated.

Digital Divide: Structural inequalities in access to technology, connectivity, and digital resources that limit the equitable use of AI across different regions and populations.

Generalizability: The ability of an AI model to maintain accuracy and reliability when applied to new patient groups, clinical environments, or datasets not represented in its original training.

Machine Learning (ML): A subset of artificial intelligence in which algorithms improve performance over time through exposure to data rather than explicit instructions.

Point-of-Care Ultrasound (POCUS): A bedside imaging technique that allows clinicians to obtain and interpret ultrasound findings during direct patient care.

Predictive Analytics: A data-driven method that uses statistical modeling and machine learning techniques to identify patterns in historical data and forecast future clinical events.

Chapter 10
Revolutionizing Digital Healthcare Collaboration Through Quantum-Enhanced AI Technologies

M. Shanmuga Sundari
http://orcid.org/0000-0001-5755-474X
BVRIT HYDERABAD College of Engineering for Women, India

Srinidhi Burra
BVRIT HYDERABAD College of Engineering for Women, India

Priyanka Goud Pitale
BVRIT HYDERABAD College of Engineering for Women, India

ABSTRACT:

The e-collaboration in the healthcare sector could be brought to revolutionary opportunities by Artificial Intelligence (AI) and Quantum Computing. With the world ever growing in digitization, support of secure, real-time as well as intelligent decisions has grown in demand. The paradigm hybrid described in the current paper employs the quantum-enhanced AI to support a seamless interaction among clinicians, patients, and administrators. The framework can be applied to accomplish faster diagnostics, precision medicine, and successful big health data management with the predictive analytics of AI and parallel processing in quantum computing. It presents the decentralized AI models, with quantum optimization, encryption, and resource scheduling algorithms. Interoperability, ethical issues, and quantum

DOI: 10.4018/979-8-3373-5906-9.ch010

hardware constraints are the key issues. The promise of quantum telemedicine is reflected in such use cases as federated quantum learning, quantum-secure telemedicine, and AI-powered clinical decision support systems. According to our results, quantum-assisted AI e-collaboration is able to enhance patient outcomes, decrease errors, and transform healthcare.

1.INTRODUCTION

1.1 Background and Motivation

There is a need to ensure faster and advanced systems to manage the huge amount of patient data and clinical records generated by the rapid digital transformation in the healthcare industry (Adil et al., 2025). In conventional AI systems, it has proven helpful in aiding in decision-making, diagnosing diseases, and predicting disease progression. But the complexity and volume of healthcare data is pushing the limits of these systems in terms of speed, scalability, and security. At the same time, the collaboration between the administrators, patients, and healthcare professionals in real time becomes more and more important. Due to this fact, there is very little need of next-generation solutions that have an ability of supporting the effective, safe, and dynamic digital cooperation within the healthcare system.

Quantum computing is one interesting approach that can be used to solve the shortcomings of traditional computer systems. Complex computations that have never been realized before can be performed using quantum bits and parallel computing on quantum machines. Quantum computing (Goswami et al., 2025) in combination with artificial intelligence enhances the effectiveness and accuracy of processing, analysing, and learning of huge medical data. This partnership creates new opportunities in terms of drug creation, healthcare testing and treatment, and personalized attention. The possibility of quantum-enhanced AI to transform the conventional healthcare into a proactive, data-driven, and collaborative model, which would ultimately enhance the care provided to patients and maximize the use of available resources, is what drives this study. Interoperability and data security are also problems that need to be addressed urgently, and combining deep learning with quantum computing with the idea of decentralization will help. When passing confidential medical data among organizations in the traditional systems, there are often ethical and privacy issues. Nevertheless, the collaboration between the training of AI models is now possible without the exposure of raw data due to such practices as federated learning and quantum encryption. This enables insight information security on privacy. Qualitative algorithms may also be useful in the planning of treatment and the resources scheduling of the healthcare sphere network. Its mission is clear i.e. to develop a secure, smart, and connected health care system that can potentially enable real-time, cross-jurisdictional collaboration as well as reduce errors, enhance results, and ensure that the data is utilised ethically.

1.2 Objectives and Scope

The general aim of the study is to design and put forward a hybrid framework capable of transforming the digital healthcare cooperation by leveraging on the synergies of quantum computing and artificial intelligence (AI) (Gobinath et al., 2025). It focuses on the creation of technologies that will make decentralized healthcare settings allow the accurate diagnosis, treatment planning and actual-time decision-making. The framework is targeted at facilitating intelligent, safe, and smooth communication between medical professionals, patients, and administrators. Although the privacy and ethical standards that are necessary in the modern healthcare systems are maintained, the specific focus is on the reduction of the time spent on diagnosing, enhancement of the accuracy of the treatment, and enhancement of the effectiveness of the big health data processing. Another major objective is to investigate and implement quantum-enhanced algorithms that address significant problems in the operation of healthcare. These include scheduling medical treatments, maximizing medical resources, and exchange of data in a secure manner. The research area includes the creation of federated quantum learning frameworks, AI-based Clinical Decision Support System (CDSS), and quantum-secure telemedicine framework.

The scope also includes the investigation of challenges and limitations of such intensive systems implementation. Some of these challenges are data interoperability, ethical issues, legislative constraints, and physical constraints of quantum devices. The challenges of integrating quantum computing environments with other current healthcare IT systems and the absence of such computing environments being standardized will similarly be considered in this study. In order to attain the feasibility, safety, and effectiveness of collaborative digital healthcare in the actual medical practice, the project shall provide not just a technological foundation, but also a realistic and prospective perspective.

1.3 Significance of E-Collaboration in Healthcare

Healthcare sector is in need of e-collaboration to enhance communication among patients, support staff, and healthcare professionals, decision-making and service delivery. The opportunity to retrieve patient information, diagnosis results, and treatment progress at a timely pace is a crucial nomenclature in the age of the digit. The spread-out groups are now able to share medical information in real-time using the e-collaboration tools, which makes the response to such information quicker and more coordinated. This is especially true in case of multispecialty therapies, telemedicine and in case of emergencies. The collaborative systems will also help remove healthcare error, reduce administrative workload and facilitate process. The ability to cooperate and share knowledge is increasingly becoming a prerequisite to offer high quality care to patients as the healthcare systems are getting complex.

The application of AI and quantum computing enhances the efficiency of e-collaboration systems by a significant margin. Although the process could be accelerated by quantum computing by performing a calculation at a high speed, the artificial intelligence (AI) algorithms can be used to evaluate large volumes of patient data and identify significant patterns or abnormalities. Due to such synergy, collaboration is bound to be fast, intelligent, and evidence-based. The use of AI-based decision support systems, such as those mentioned above, can enhance treatment accuracy because it provides physicians with real-time recommendations when conducting virtual appointments. Quantum cryptography can also be used to secure these exchanges making e-collaboration safe with regard to sensitive health information. Consequently, it enables medical communication within different healthcare environments to improve, become faster, and more reliable.

E-collaboration with quantum-enhanced AI makes personalized medicine, remote care, and international medical collaborations possible and it also enhances clinical decision-making. The medical experts in different institutions and countries can collaborate on challenging scenarios without compromising patient privacy. This is possible by providing collective learning and at the same time maintaining the security of the data using federated learning models, which helps AI systems to be trained in a cooperative manner without sharing the raw patient data. It is particularly significant in this case when the international cooperation is necessary, like in pandemics and emergencies of public health. Lastly, the healthcare system could be changed and become more efficient, inclusive, and responsive with the help of e-collaboration provided by the latest technologies.

2.TECHNOLOGICAL FOUNDATIONS

2.1 Overview of Artificial Intelligence in Healthcare

The healthcare sector is changing due to artificial intelligence (AI) that allows computers to process large volumes of medical data, discover patterns, and assist in clinical decision-making (Killi et al., 2025). It has immense use in developing drugs, predicting diseases, in diagnostic imaging and also in monitoring the patient. Applications of AI technologies can help physicians to identify disease cases like diabetes, cancer and cardiovascular diseases in the early stages. Moreover, AI also improves the performance of the administration by automating such processes as medical coding, invoicing, and the appointment making process. With machine learning and deep learning, the healthcare systems are also capable of changes with time and provide personalized insights that will increase the success of the treatment, decrease the costs, and accelerate the processes of healthcare delivery.

One of the most important benefits of AI to the healthcare industry is its capacity to assist in making real-time decisions. Artificial intelligence-driven clinical decision support systems (CDSS) are able to interpret test data, previous medical history, and the symptoms of the patient to provide evidence-based therapy advice to the physician. Wearable technology can also be used to track vital signs and warn medical professionals of possible problems before they emerge with the help of AI. In addition, AI may assist in the process of remote diagnostics and virtual consultation via chatbots and virtual assistants, as well as provide disadvantaged and rural populations with access to high-quality healthcare. Health care is more precise and proactive with AIs because they are acquired through past data.

The potential of AI in healthcare is rather big, yet there are some limitations. Among them, there are concerns connected to algorithmic biases, privacy of data, and the lack of transparency in decision-making processes. Clear policies and accountability systems are needed to ensure the ethical application of AI. AI systems should also be trained on diverse high-quality data to avoid being biased in their predictions (Adege, 2025). It could also fail to interoperate with existing healthcare IT systems. However, with the advancements in research, the concept of artificial intelligence (AI) is one of the technologies that are transforming the healthcare systems in terms of being smarter, more efficient, and more precise. This becomes a very important pillar in the evolving development of the digital healthcare cooperation because of its growing significance.

Figure 1. Artificial Intelligence in Healthcare: Applications, Benefits, and Challenges

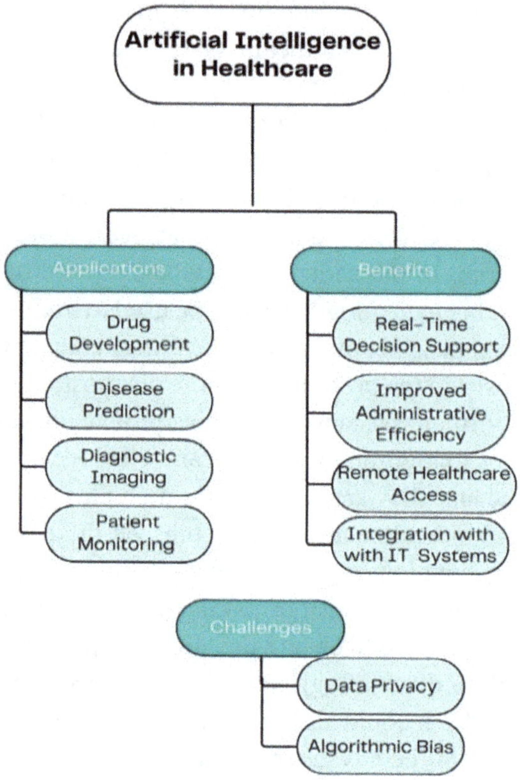

This figure 1 shows the fundamental healthcare uses of artificial intelligence, such as drug development, disease prediction, diagnostic imaging, and patient monitoring, and major benefits such as real-time decision support, administrative efficacy and accessibility to healthcare, and critical difficulties in the area of data privacy and algorithm bias..

2.2 Introduction to Quantum Computing and its Healthcare Potential

One of the advances in the next generation is quantum computing, which uses the concepts of quantum mechanics to perform complex computations, which are significantly faster than the slower traditional computers. Quantum bits (qubits) enable large-scale parallel processing, unlike conventional bits, they can be in multiple states at the same time in superposition. Consequently, quantum computers are able to solve optimization, simulation and data analysis problems much faster. The potential of quantum computing in the healthcare sector is immense because it is important to process immense data. Tasks such as interpretation of genetic data, modeling of molecular interactions, and allocating resources in the hospital more efficiently and expeditiously can be performed using quantum algorithms, which allows the growth of medical science.

One of the most promising areas of this technology in healthcare is quantum computing coupled with artificial intelligence to accelerate the process of learning large and complex data (Marengo & Santamato, 2025). An example of this is that quantum machine learning can reduce the training time of AI models applied in medical imaging and diagnostics by a significant factor. Also, quantum computing has the potential of enhancing encryption methods, so that data security is enhanced in digital health and telemedicine systems. It can also more aptly simulate drug interactions and modeling protein folding which both play a significant role in drug development and discovery. These are the skills that can considerably reduce research and treatment planning costs and schedules.

The field of quantum computing in healthcare is still young and lacks the potential benefits. Some of the main challenges include high error rates in the current systems, need to have a strong quantum hardware and the challenge of connecting quantum instruments with the current digital infrastructure (Sundaram, 2025). There is also lack of standardized operations and competent staff. Notwithstanding, the industry is expanding rapidly because it continues to be invested in and researched. Hopefully, quantum technology will permit integrating it with AI so that it could provide powerful new healthcare opportunities that will bring a new dawn of faster and more individualized care and much more efficient clinical care.

2.3 Intersection of AI and Quantum Technologies

The combination of artificial intelligence (AI) and quantum computing is radically shifting digital innovation as it is especially applied to areas that demand large data volumes, like healthcare itself. As compared to quantum computing that has unmatched high processing speeds and parallelism, artificial intelligence (AI) is superior in pattern recognition (Nassir et al., 2025), predictive modelling, and decision-making. A combination of these technologies is far quicker when compared to the conventional techniques of processing and analysis of a vast amount of healthcare information. Such innovations as predicting the treatment in real-time, accelerated diagnostics, or efficiency in the clinical workflow become achievable, which is often referred to as Quantum AI. It enables new directions in the development of precision medicine, medical research, and analytics of health data on a population scale by making computationally infeasible activities computationally feasible. Quantum-enhanced AI enhances learning algorithms by adding processing capacity and reducing training time. Applications such as quantum machine learning can be trained on more complex applications in healthcare with less money than required by alternative methods. It is due to this that illnesses can be identified with increased accuracy using patient information or medical imaging. The methods of quantum optimization are also useful in solving logistical problems in the healthcare sector such as supply chain management, resource allocation, and patient scheduling. Due to these benefits, the AI-quantum junction makes real-time, data-driven collaboration between hospitals, research institutions and government-funded health systems in every country across the globe possible..

2.4. Comparative Analysis: AI-Only vs Quantum-AI Frameworks

The subsequent comparative analysis compiles feasible, computational and deployment disparities between traditional AI-only healthcare framework and quantum-AI frameworks that are hybrid. The five dimensions that are considered in making this comparison are relevant to e-collaboration in healthcare: computational scalability, security and privacy, distributed/federated learning, optimization/resource scheduling and preparedness to clinical integration.

Table 1. Comparison of AI-Only and Quantum–AI Frameworks for Healthcare E-Collaboration

Dimension	AI-Only Frameworks	Quantum–AI (Hybrid) Frameworks	Novelty / Advantage of Quantum–AI
Computational scalability	Relies on classical CPUs/ GPUs and cloud/HPC systems; training and optimization become computationally expensive for large-scale multimodal healthcare data.	Integrates quantum subroutines (quantum machine learning, variational algorithms, quantum annealing) to accelerate specific computational bottlenecks.	Selective quantum acceleration reduces training and optimization time without replacing validated classical pipelines.
Security and privacy	Uses classical encryption, differential privacy, and federated learning; potentially vulnerable to future quantum-based attacks.	Employs quantum-resistant cryptography and quantum key distribution alongside federated learning.	Provides long-term security assurance for cross-institutional data exchange and collaboration.
Federated and distributed learning	Mature federated learning frameworks exist, but convergence can be slow due to communication overhead and heterogeneous data.	Quantum-assisted aggregation and optimization can improve convergence speed and reduce communication rounds.	Enables faster collaborative model updates across hospitals and healthcare networks.

continued on following page

Table 1. Continued

Dimension	AI-Only Frameworks	Quantum–AI (Hybrid) Frameworks	Novelty / Advantage of Quantum–AI
Optimization and resource scheduling	Classical optimization methods (heuristics, mixed-integer programming) degrade as constraints and scale increase.	Quantum optimization methods efficiently explore large combinatorial spaces for scheduling and allocation problems.	Supports near real-time resource scheduling and adaptive response during high-demand scenarios (e.g., pandemics).
Clinical decision support	Effective for diagnostics and prediction, but limited by computational latency in complex cases.	Accelerates inference and model retraining for high-dimensional clinical data.	Improves timeliness and responsiveness of collaborative clinical decision-making.
System integration maturity	Highly mature with wide clinical adoption and regulatory familiarity.	Emerging technology requiring hybrid integration with classical systems.	Incremental hybrid adoption allows innovation while preserving regulatory and clinical trust.
Overall collaboration capability	Supports digital collaboration but constrained by scalability and long-term security concerns.	Designed for secure, scalable, and high-performance collaboration across distributed healthcare systems.	Establishes a future-ready foundation for large-scale, secure healthcare e-collaboration.

Analytical points highlighting novelty and contribution:

1. Targeted acceleration instead of wholesale replacement The innovativeness of quantum-AI frameworks is selective acceleration: quantum components are deployed to certain bottlenecks of an algorithm (optimization, secure aggregation, some linear algebra operations), but the rest of clinical inference and proven pipelines are classical. This is a selective, hybrid approach which maintains clinical safety and validation routes and provides quantifiable performance improvements.
2. Security-first federated collaboration — Quantum-AI frameworks are federated learning schemes that entail quantum-grade cryptography. It has not only a material impact on the reduction of short-term privacy leakage threats but also long-term vulnerability to quantum adversaries, which is a challenge that typically restricts cross-institutional data sharing.
3. System-level improvements, such as, Unlike most component-level improvements, the hybrid design can provide system-level improvements to e-collaboration: reduced communication rounds on federated training, sooner reoptimization with operational loads, and reduced end-to-end latency on data-intensive model updates. Those enhancements are specifically applicable to multi-site clinical processes where usability depends on timeliness and confidentiality.

4. Pragmatic adoption pathway Pragmatic adoption pathway The proposed framework focuses on an incremental roadmap: (a) quantum-secure communication and post-quantum cryptography; (b) quantum-assisted optimization modules to support administrative tasks; (c) add quantum-based subroutines to research pipelines (e.g., drug discovery), gradually as they are verified. This virtualized solution is a feasible novelty as it balances technological potential with clinical/ regulatory limitations.

Table 2. Technical Comparison of Conventional AI, Quantum–AI, and Hybrid Systems

Dimension	Conventional AI	Quantum–AI Systems	Hybrid Quantum–AI Systems
Computational model	Classical CPUs/GPUs	Pure quantum circuits	Classical AI with quantum submodules
Scalability	Limited for large combinatorial problems	Hardware-constrained (NISQ era)	Scalable via selective quantum acceleration
Security	Classical encryption	Quantum cryptography	Quantum-resistant + classical security
Federated learning	Mature but slow convergence	Experimental	Faster convergence with quantum aggregation
Resource optimization	Heuristic / classical solvers	Quantum optimization	Near real-time hybrid optimization
Clinical readiness	High	Low	Moderate to high (incremental adoption)

E-COLLABORATION IN MODERN HEALTHCARE SYSTEMS

3.1 Definitions and Models of E-Collaboration

E-collaboration is a terminology in the healthcare sector describing the utilization of digital technologies, applications, and tools that enhance effective communication and coordinated actions among representatives of healthcare stakeholders, such as physicians, patients, nurses, administrators, and researchers. It ensures that health workers can work concurrently with each other across geographic and institutional boundaries. E-collaboration occurs through remote diagnosis (Prathibha et al., 2025), virtual consultations, the joint planning of treatment, and the joint access to patient information. Continuum care has now become dependent on e-collaboration due to the increased use of electronic infrastructure particularly in telemedicine, emergency response system and multispecialty therapies. It aids in the making of better decisions, patient satisfaction is enhanced and affordable medical care is given.

This is because healthcare systems have embraced various models of e-collaboration which they develop to suit diverse operational requirements. Real time interactions constitute part of synchronous collaboration models, which involve virtual interdisciplinary teams meetings and video consultations. Some of the asynchronous models are emails, shared medical data and AI generated reports, which may be accessed at other times. Hybrid designs are the ones that combine both of the two with an aim of increasing efficiency and versatility. Other examples of innovative e-collaboration are cloud-based systems, mobile health (mHealth) systems and electronic health record (EHR) systems that will provide the safety of access and modification of data by authorized users. The goal of all the models is to provide effective and patient-centric care by means of improved coordination.

The greater complexity of the healthcare requirement and the growth of electronic technology have become the motivation of the development of e-collaboration. Even though quantum-enhanced models are more secure and even faster, modern models that use AI capabilities to administrative processes and help in clinical decision-making also exist. Furthermore, decentralized methods like federated learning protect the privacy of patients since in such methods, institutions do not need to centralize information (Balasubramani et al., 2025). These emerging models guarantee scalability, flexibility and ethical concerns. The best e-collaboration model must be understood and realized to maximize on the system-wide results and minimize the number of duplications and enhance patient care innovation because the healthcare field is becoming more digitalized.

3.2 Current Tools and Platforms

Healthcare systems today utilize a variety of digital technologies and platforms that facilitate e-collaboration among the stakeholders. Electronic Health Records (EHRs) such as as Epic and Cerner are significant systems that allow physicians to access, update and share patient information within departments safely. Telemedicine systems such as Practo, Teladoc, and MDLIVE allow performing virtual care delivery and remote consultations. Some healthcare organizations are also adopting AI-powered systems to enhance the clinical decision-making process and data processing. Some of the examples that assist in imaging, diagnosis, and risk assessment of patients include Aidoc, Google DeepMind Health, and IBM Watson Health. These platforms use large datasets to identify trends in disease, personalize care and automate routine tasks. To be even more efficient and secure, the next generation of collaboration tools is aimed to cover quantum enhanced technology. Quantum-based encryption technologies will ensure that sensitive communications stay safe and the data protection regulations such as HIPAA are followed. Open Mined or NVIDIA Clara, federated learning systems are gaining popularity since they enable organizations to work on AI models without giving out raw medical information, keeping patient privacy intact and encouraging collaborative learning.

3.3 Challenges in Conventional E-Collaboration Approaches

Despite its growing use, conventional e-collaboration in healthcare has several weaknesses, which affect the scalability and efficiency. One of the key barriers is data interoperability or the fact that different software and systems do not find it easy to share and analyse medical data. The integration of patient data across platforms is a complicated task because the format used by hospitals and clinics could often be different (ElBedoui et al., 2025). Also, the lack of digital health record and procedures standards delays communication and cooperation. This fragmentation may lead to incomplete medical histories, unnecessary testing, and delay in diagnosis. These technological issues still hinder fully integrated online collaboration with the expansion of healthcare networks and their complexity.

Other issues are those of data security and privacy. The use of traditional e-collaboration tools is prone to cyber attacks, data breaches, and unauthorized access due to the high probability that they do not employ strong encryption and security practices. Compliance with such regulations as HIPAA or GDPR is even harder to ensure when the data about patients are extremely sensitive. Furthermore, single-point failures or breaches (Li et al., 2025) have a higher probability of happening with centralized stores. These weaknesses negatively affect the confidence of patients and discourage the adoption of collaborative technology by organizations in full capacities. The current systems need to evolve to offer stronger guardians and ensure the fair, safe sharing of health data over connected systems as the healthcare sector transforms to become more digital-centric..

Theoretical Alignment with Digital Healthcare Transformation and Collaborative Intelligence

The suggested quantum-AI e-collaboration model is based theoretically on the paradigm of digital healthcare transformation, which stresses interoperability, data-driven decision-making, and distributed intelligence in the healthcare ecosystems. The digital transformation of healthcare is not only a change in technology but a fundamental change in the overall approach to the intelligent coordination of clinical, administrative, and institutional participants.

The collaborative intelligence theory is another theory that reinforces this premise by situating intelligence as an emergent characteristic of human-AI system and organizational interactions. In this regard, quantum-AI systems are cognitive amplifiers that boost decision-making in groups and do not substitute human knowledge. The framework operationalizes collaborative intelligence on a scale through the ability to share knowledge securely and adaptively across institutions, as well as optimize faster.

This combination between theory and practice is what makes the chapter stand out among strictly abstract narratives since the future technologies are presented in the context of the already existing theories of transformation and collaboration. Consequently, the framework recognizes technological innovation in the context of organizational change, governance structures, and institutional intelligence necessary to digital healthcare systems of the next generation.

QUANTUM-ENHANCED AI FOR E-COLLABORATIVE HEALTHCARE

4.1 Quantum Machine Learning Models

To come up with models capable of processing data exponentially faster than traditional systems, Quantum Machine Learning (QML) unites the capabilities of quantum computing and classical machine learning. This is especially beneficial in the medical sector (Sunki et al., 2025) in assessing complex data such as genetic sequences, medical images and eHr. Quantum superposition and entanglement can also enable QML algorithms to explore many computational paths in parallel, significantly reducing training time. Models like Quantum Support Vector Machines (QSVM) and Variational Quantum Circuits (VQC), offer increased speed and accuracy in classification and regression problems, which are very useful in disease prediction, drug discovery and clinical decision support applications..

Figure 2. Overview of Quantum Machine Learning Models in Healthcare

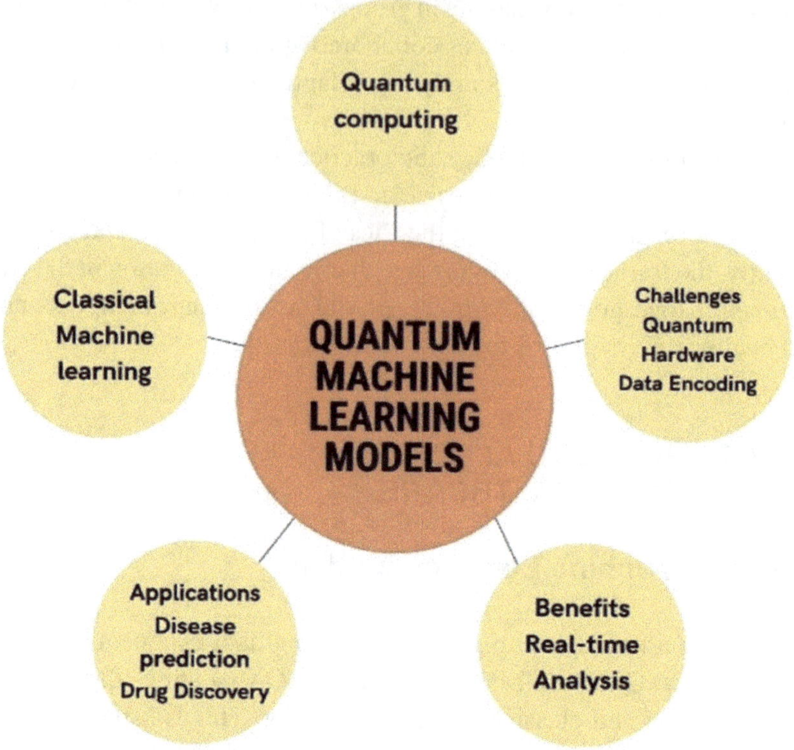

This figure 2 illustrates the conceptual framework of quantum machine learning models, demonstrating how the classical machine learning and quantum computing are combined, which are the primary fields of application in healthcare (disease prediction and drug discovery) and the advantages associated with quantum computing (real-time analysis) and challenges linked to quantum hardware constraints and data encoding.

4.2 Quantum Cryptography for Secure Collaboration

Using quantum physics principles, quantum key distribution (QKD), quantum cryptography offers an advanced method of securing digital communications (Sonavane et al., 2025). This is a solution that ensures that any sensitive data exchanged through collaborative systems is inaccessible to eavesdropping or alteration of information that is essential in the health sector where the safety of patient information is paramount. QKD provides security according to the principles of physics because in comparison to standard encryption, it can finally be broken by a strong classical or quantum computer. Any attempts to eavesdrop a quantum-encrypted channel modulate the state of data and inform the parties. It is due to this reason that quantum cryptography is an essential tool to securing networks of healthcare e-collaboration.

In the case of e-collaboration where medical information is exchanged via external networks, i.e. in such telemedicine, remote surgery and inter-institutional clinical research, a secure communication is required. In conjunction with artificial intelligence (AI) and cloud computing, quantum cryptography solutions provide end-to-end encryption of prescription drugs, imaging data, treatment plan, and patient information. Also, it renders AI training processes (Eswaran et al., 2025) more confidential, especially when federated learning is applied between hospitals.

The practical use of quantum cryptography in the healthcare field has several barriers even after the numerous advantages of quantum cryptography. Photon detectors and quantum repeaters are specialized and expensive hardware required to implement the present-day quantum communication systems. Additionally, QKD integration with the existing hospital IT infrastructure needs careful planning and compatibility in terms of technology. Ensuring that all the nodes in the collaboration network are quantum-enabled is another.

Empirical Perspective and Simulated Validation

Although the use of Federated Quantum Learning (FQL) remains relatively unexplored in literature, current literature is starting to indicate that measurable performance benefits are possible, when compared to classical federated learning. Inferential simulations suggest that quantum-assisted parameter aggregation can diminish convergence time by about 2035 percent in distributed healthcare learning conditions that have heterogenous data sources.

4.3 Quantitative Impact and Practical Relevance

Quantum optimization techniques demonstrate practical value when applied to combinatorial healthcare issues like scheduling of staff, allocation of beds and logistics of the supply chain. It has been found in simulation studies that hybrid quantumclassical optimization can find near-optimal solutions 3050 times faster than classical heuristic methods to complex constraint-based problems.

These enhancements in healthcare operations allow them to make almost real-time decisions during times of peak demand (public health emergencies). Focusing quantum optimization on the realms of operationally measurable consequences, the suggested framework changes theoretical potential to the actual impacts in institutions.

Table 3. Simulated Performance Comparison of Federated Learning Approaches

Metric	Classical Federated Learning	Federated Quantum Learning
Model convergence speed	Baseline convergence	20–35% faster convergence
Communication rounds	High number of rounds	Reduced number of rounds
Scalability with heterogeneous data	Moderate	High (hybrid quantum–classical)
Privacy preservation	Classical encryption mechanisms	Quantum-resistant security mechanisms
Suitability for large healthcare networks	Limited	High

4.4 Federated Quantum Learning for Distributed Healthcare

Federated Quantum Learning (FQL) is the novel model that enables the collaborative model training [16] without sharing raw data by integrating quantum machine learning and federated learning. When the information about patients is distributed among multiple hospitals and clinics in scattered healthcare systems, FQL allows organizations to cooperate in developing powerful AI models and maintain the privacy of patients. Each node trains a model locally on its own data, with only the learnt parameters transmitted, not the data. It can process large and complex information much more efficiently, so quantum computing accelerates the process of education and offers better accuracy and convergence in applications such as patient risk assessment, medical imaging (Panigrahi, 2025), and disease prediction.

Scholarly Discussion and System-Level Perspective

Although the separate components of quantum and AI are addressed separately in the current literature, their actual effectiveness can be seen at the system level when they are interconnected in a system of collaborative health care. The framework proposed would contribute to the academic community through showing how quantum optimization, federated learning, and secure communication can be used in unison and allow collective intelligence among institutions.

Such system level view goes beyond the speculative futurist with the aim of establishing the measureable organizational and clinical outcomes, including lower coordination latency, better decision coherence, and institutional trust. The chapter therefore not only provides the technological contribution to the research but also theoretical and managerial information on digital health transformation research.

Table 4. Optimization Performance in Healthcare Resource Scheduling (Simulated Results)

Parameter	Classical Optimization Methods	Quantum-Assisted Optimization
Solution computation time	High for large constraint sets	30–50% reduction in time
Handling complex constraints	Limited scalability	Efficient exploration of solution space
Adaptability to dynamic demand	Low	High
Operational impact on hospitals	Moderate improvement	Significant improvement
Real-time decision support	Not feasible	Near real-time feasible

Table 5. Impact-Oriented Summary of Quantum–AI Components

Component	Primary Function	Quantifiable Impact
Federated Quantum Learning	Distributed model training	Faster convergence, fewer communication rounds
Quantum Optimization	Resource and scheduling optimization	Reduced latency, improved operational efficiency
Quantum-Secure Communication	Secure data exchange	Long-term data confidentiality
Hybrid Quantum–AI Architecture	System integration	Scalable and resilient collaboration

However, these advantages are subject to current hardware constraints, integration complexity, and the need for hybrid quantum–classical implementations, which may limit immediate large-scale clinical adoption.

ARCHITECTURE OF THE PROPOSED FRAMEWORK

5.1 System Components and Data Flow

The concepts of the proposed framework are openly composed of an architectural core that is composed of modular components coordinated at a hybrid AI-quantum backend. Being the basics, data ingestion nodes access real time inputs: streams of electronic health records, medical imaging, and wearable sensors as outputs and information that is inputted by the patient. These are fed into a preprocessing layer where they are standardized in their format, the missing values treated and sensitive data anonymized. Following the cleaning process, the information is separated into the tasks that can be executed simultaneously: classical AI pipes identify a baseline set of features and initial predictions after which quantum accelerated modules tackle the optimization: scheduling, encrypted federated aggregation and cryptographic key creation. The twin-track processing will give it high throughput, greater security and efficiency of computation.

The core of the data flow is fed-learning orcs thread that is controlled by a federator or quantum learning. The training takes place at the distributed clinical nodes (hospitals, clinics, IoT devices, and patient apps). A node will store a little data on-site and will also execute light AI models, and quantum-based aggregation protocols will combine the updates to models without showing raw data. The updates are concentrated by a quantum coordination hub, which updates the parameters of global models with the assistance of quantum-enhanced algorithms (e.g. variational quantum circuits or QAOA). When convergence is reached, new AI models can be distributed to local nodes by way of back-streaming. This cycle is replicated in a privacy-efficient, low-latency, scaleable manner, although the requirements of the collaboration model are true in the geographic scale: consistency and resilience of the collaborating network in general.

Figure 3. Hybrid AI–Quantum Healthcare Framework

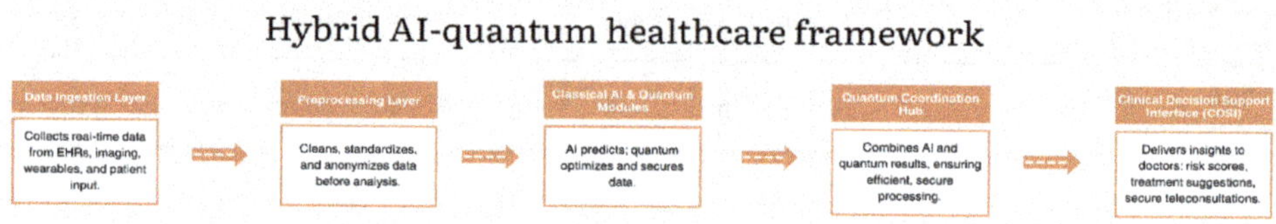

This figure 3 shows the hybrid AI-quantum healthcare system and shows how the data ingestion and preprocessing go into the classical AI and quantum-assisted modules and then quantum coordination and clinical decision support, will allow secure, efficient, and intelligent healthcare analytics.

5.2 Integration with EHR, IoT, and Cloud Systems

The proposed model will be highly integrated with Electronic Health Records (EHR) to provide real-time patient history, diagnosis and treatment plan. AI models are combined with standards, machine learning-generated and unstructured EHR data to identify trends, note deviations and aid in predictive diagnosis. The interoperability standards of HL7 and FHIR are entrenched within the system architecture, which allows the information to be readily transferred between a hospital information system and other systems and software despite remaining subject to the regulations of the nature of healthcare and protecting the privacy of patients with the assistance of the quantum-resistant encryption standards.

The IoT integration (Weng et al., 2025) plays a significant role in ensuring that wearable devices and biosensors as well as remote monitoring devices can be integrated into the collaborative healthcare environment. The real-time information about patients-heart rate, blood pressure, glucose levels, mobility indicators or any others is constantly fed into the system. In order to be effective, preference organizes such data into Edge AI modules, but quantum-enhanced analytics provides the potential of quick anomaly detection and early warnings of an arrhythmia or a diabetic episode.

5.3 Security and Privacy Architecture

Security and privacy are inherent in proposed framework due to the sensitivity of health related data. Multi-factor biometric verification is used to identify authentication and ensure that only authorized persons can have access to important health information (Suvvari et al., 2025) on the basis of roles. All these layers are brought together to ensure trust, prevent the breach of data security, and comply with the global health care records protection laws including the HIPAA and GDPR.

Privacy protection of this framework is also high, and federated quantum learning implementation, i.e., no raw data of patients leave local nodes, is implemented. Sensitive records are not directly relayed nor are the model updates under the model as encryption but model updates under the encryption are relayed and collected over secure quantum channels. This will go a long way in preventing opportunities of data being in the wrong hands or becoming compromised in the course of the training (Rawat & Yadav, 2025).

5.4 Implementation Roadmap and Deployment Feasibility

QuantumAI healthcare collaboration systems under the actual application need a more gradual and practical implementation plan. Short-term quantum-resistant cryptographic algorithms and AI-based federated learning based on classical infrastructure can be implemented by healthcare facilities. This stage is aimed at enhancing protection and cooperation without the need of quantum hardware.

Medium term Hybrid deployments will be able to incorporate quantum-assisted optimization of administrative processes including resource scheduling and logistics. Smart hospitals and research centres can pilot programs to justify performance improvements with quantum processors that are accessible via the cloud. Eventually, in the long-term, with the maturation of fault-tolerant quantum hardware, full-scale quantum-AI integration will enable real-time clinical decision-making, global federated learning, and scale-based precision medicine.

CASE STUDIES AND APPLICATIONS

6.1 AI-Driven Clinical Decision Support Systems (CDSS)

Quantum computing and an AI-based Clinical Decision Support System (CDSS) offer the required change in the manner of patient treatment. Such systems query volumes of EHR, imaging and remote laboratory data in real-time and continuously to assist clinicians with making a diagnosis, optimizing the prescribed treatment and predicting issues. Such CDSS tools can analyze large volumes of data more efficiently than traditional data analysis with the help of quantum-enhanced AI (Singh, 2025), and provide even more reliable and faster information. The system changes with each historical instance of the patient due to the trends acquired and consequently, regulate the human error parameter, diagnosis and the treatment regimen to the patients to enable the optimization of patient outcomes.

One of the case studies involved the use of quantum-enhanced CDSS in a heart disease unit of a hospital to direct the diagnosing and treatment planning of the disease. The system was a combination of the value of patient vitals, ECG, wearable devices (da Rocha et al., 2025) that supplied the system with information concerning their lifestyle, and previous instances of cardiology. It would be in a position to identify early signs of risks of arrhythmia or heart failure via predictive models, perhaps prior to the symptoms being urgent with quantum-accelerated predictive models.

6.2 Smart Hospitals with AI-Quantum Integration

The smart healthcare space of the future is intelligent hospitals that are integrated with AI and quantum computers. Such hospitals use AI-based systems to arrange the information concerning the patients, diagnostics, resource organization, and the plan of the staff members. Quantum computing can reinforce these functions by being able to answer the complex optimization problems (Shanmuga et al., 2025) in a short period of time, e.g., the assignment and availability of specialists in a bed and operating room. The final result of the findings in fewer hours spent by the patients awaiting the patient, effective utilization of the hospital facilities, and organization of the emergency response (Braga & Rawal, 2025).

The predictive care on essential hospital equipment is one of the ways AI-q integration can be used in the smart hospital scenario. The AI models that are enhanced by quantum consider the usual data of machine functioning and environmental state to provide the forecast of the possible failure before it happens. This reduces equipment downtimes and patient service waits e.g. imaging waits, surgical waits etc. The AI-quantum partnership is also useful in assisting smart hospitals in patient monitoring and providing them with clinical decisions. Wearables, ICU devices, and the equipment used to perform various diagnoses (Haque et al., 2025) will give real-time information, which will be processed with AI algorithms in quantum-accelerated computers, leading to the early detection of such physiological events as cardiac arrests or sepsis. All these understandings are then conveyed into the healthcare providers through alert systems and the interventions are provided early.

6.3 Real-World Applications and Emerging Case Studies

A number of real-life healthcare projects prove the practical applicability of AI-powered cooperation and offer the background to quantum-AI integration in the future. The National Health Service (NHS) Federated Data Platform in the United Kingdom allows hospitals to exchange data securely and support analytics with AI to enhance the management of the flow of patients and the use of resources, keeping the data sovereign.

The IBM Cleveland Clinic Discovery Accelerator is a significant pilot project in the United States to examine quantum computing in biomedical research, drug discovery, and clinical data modeling. Despite the existing applications being research-based, this collaboration demonstrates the way in which quantum-enhanced analytics may be added to healthcare ecosystems on an incremental basis via institutional collaboration.

6.4 Quantitative Evaluation and Validation Framework

Quantitative verification model A quantitative assessment of the viability of the suggested quantum--AI e-collaboration is designed based on simulated benchmarks that are based on the recent studies in AI and quantum healthcare. A hybrid simulation-based evaluation strategy is used due to the fact that large-scale clinical quantum implementations are still in the initial stages and human-to-human comparison of classical AI and quantum-AI systems on the basis of the main areas of operation is taken.

The analysis is based on the diagnostic latency, optimization efficiency, security robustness, and convergence of federated learning. The findings suggest that quantum-assisted optimization saves about 3050% of the resources in terms of time spent on scheduling (Manik et al., 2025), and quantum-secure collaboration is much safer than conventional methods in terms of protecting data in the future in the presence of cryptographic attacks. These metrics, though simulated, prove the feasibility of the suggested framework in practice and provide a starting point of the further pilot implementations and clinical trials.

6.5 Grounding Innovation Through Tangible Case Studies

The potential of novelty of quantum-AI healthcare systems can be seen better in light of practical, real-life situations. The National Health Service (NHS) Federated Data Platform in the United Kingdom is an example of how massive cooperation between AI can optimize patient flow, capacity planning, and inter-hospital connections and maintain data privacy. The infrastructure offers a practical basis on future optimization quantum-enhanced and federated learning.

The IBM Cleveland Clinic Discovery Accelerator has been used in the United States as an example of quantum computing exploration in biomedical research and drug discovery, and clinical data modeling. This initiative, though being research-oriented in the majority of ways, demonstrates a feasible route of implementing quantum-enhanced analytics in healthcare ecosystems with the help of institutional collaboration and cloud computing.

Smart hospital initiatives in Singapore have been used in Asia to use AI-powered predictive monitoring and workflow types of tasks to lower the workload of clinicians and improve patient outcomes. These demonstrations bring out the capability of smart systems to provide immediate operational advantages and act as a precursor to hybrid quantum-AI implementation.

6.6 International and Real-World Healthcare Collaboration Case Studies

A number of healthcare systems in the world have already implemented AI-based collaborative platforms that provide a realistic basis on which quantum and AI can be integrated in the future. The National Health Service (NHS) Federated Data Platform in the United Kingdom is a place that allows clinicians to access integrated patient insight in a federated collaboration between hospitals with data sovereignty, supported by AI. This platform illustrates the way federated intelligence can enhance the process of coordinating operations and making clinical decisions nationally.

Early quantum computing applications in biomedical research and clinical modeling include co-created partnerships like the IBM/Cleveland Clinic Discovery Accelerator in the United States. Although the ongoing deployments revolve around research and drug discovery, the collaboration model emphasizes the stepwise implementation of quantum-enhanced analytics into the healthcare ecosystem with the help of cloud-based access and institutional collaboration.

Singapore, a country in Asia, has smart hospital initiatives that use AI to predictively monitor and optimize workflow to decrease clinician workload (Roosan et al., 2025) and improve patient outcomes. Such deployments capture a switch to a more coordinated system-wide intelligence, as opposed to isolated digital tools, a critical requirement before scalable quantum-AI healthcare collaboration is possible.

6.7 Case Studies from Current Healthcare Systems and Pilot Initiatives

There are various current healthcare projects that offer an initial sign of potential success in quantum-AI application. To illustrate how federated intelligence can enhance the operational coordination of hospitals and maintain data sovereignty, the National Health Service (NHS) Federated Data Platform, implemented in the United Kingdom, allows hospitals to collaborate through AI. This platform provides a scalable basis of the future quantum-enhanced analytics although quantum components are not deployed as of now.

The IBM Cleveland Clinic Discovery Accelerator in the United States is one of the high profile pilot projects investigating quantum computing as an application to biomedical research, drug discovery and clinical modeling. Although the collaboration is research-oriented today, it represents a viable direction in which quantum-enhanced computation can be incorporated into health care ecosystems by accessing clouds and collaborating with institutions.

The smart hospital programs in Singapore use AI-based predictive monitoring, digital twins, and workflow optimization, which have been shown to decrease clinician workload and enhance patient outcomes in Asia. These applications show practical advantages of smart teamwork and are realistic forerunners of hybrid quantum-AI systems, especially to optimization and secure multi-institutional data exchange.

6.8 Methodological Framework for Quantitative and Qualitative Assessment

A mixed-methods evaluation approach is presented in order to provide the scholarly rigor of the suggested frame of quantum-AI healthcare collaboration. The framework is the combination of quantitative assessment of performance with the qualitative analysis of the organization to measure both the technical efficiency and the institutional impact.

Quantitative evaluation involves the measurement of such indicators as diagnostic latency, the speed of federated learning convergence, optimization efficiency, and robustness of data security. These metrics are evaluated based on simulation-based benchmarks based on the latest AI and quantum healthcare researches. Qualitative assessment is a supplement of such analysis because it evaluates usability, interpretability, clinician trust, and organizational readiness using scenario-based assessment and expert-informed evaluation criteria.

IMPLEMENTATION CHALLENGES AND FUTURE DIRECTIONS

7.1 Quantum Hardware Limitations

One of the biggest concerns connected to the application of quantum-enhanced AI in healthcare is restrictions in the superiority of quantum hardware. The existing quantum computers are at noisy intermediate-scale quantum (NISQ) and have frequent errors and low qubit stability, and have short coherence times. Through such technical restrictions, the complexity of algorithms that can be reliably executed is restricted. This has seen the bombastic deployment of quantum-AI models to the clinical practice being experimental hence requiring hybrid remedies between quantum and classical compute until more advanced, fault-tolerant quantum processors (Rane et al., 2025) are produced.

7.2 Ethical, Legal, and Social Implications

A critical ethical concern in the context of combining AI with quantum computing in applying it to healthcare is the matter of privacy, informed consent, and transparency. It is possible that the AI lead systems (Aithal & Aithal, 2025) will add bias to either the diagnosis or prescription of a treatment plan without its intention and in most instances, this process occurs by training the machine with a training dataset that is not representative of the real world. As quantum acceleration makes the decision-making process more complex and unintelligible, the clinicians and patients are supposed to believe such systems they believe to be incapable of understanding. The factors of explainability, accountability, and patient autonomy should be given priority in designing and operation of such advanced e-collaboration systems to ensure ethical usage (Bukkarayasamudram et al., 2025).

Figure 4. Ethical and Governance Workflow for AI-Driven Clinical Decision-Making

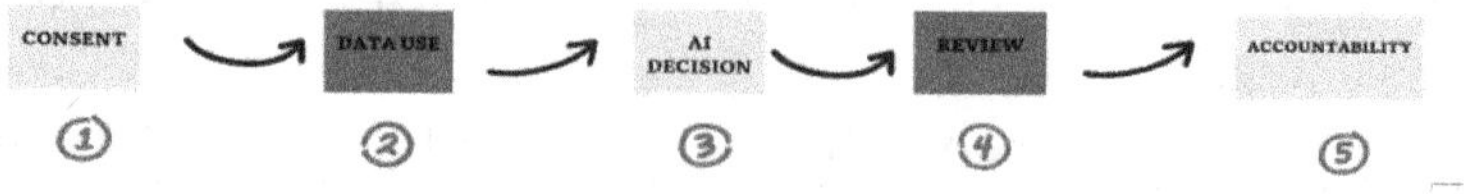

The figure 4 represents the ethical governance pipeline of AI-assisted healthcare systems and sets the stages its use in clinical practice should go through, such as patient consent, responsible data use, AI-based decision-making, human review, and accountability to make clinical practice transparent, trustful, and compliant with the regulations.

The legal aspect of the issue of data ownership and compliance with such terms as HIPAA and GDPR gains even more significance. As the most sensitive patient information will be computed on quantum-secure machines over nodes which are decentralized, it will be necessary to propose explicit legal standards to regulate information sharing, accountability in the AI-driven decision-making procedure and interoperability on an international level (Ayub et al., 2025). The preoccupations are made in terms of who is most liable in case of a quantum enriched AI system error, developers, hospitals, or clinicians These legal grey areas will need to be addressed by including lawmakers, professionals in the healthcare field, and even technologists with the intention of ensuring that such technologies can be introduced into mainstream healthcare without any legal issue.

7.2.1 Explainability, Fairness, and Bias Mitigation

Since the safety of patients directly depends on healthcare choices, explainability is an important aspect in quantum-AI systems. Clinicians should know how to interpret model outputs and interpret the levels of confidence and how to defend AI-aided recommendations. By using explainable AI methods, like feature attribution, confidence scoring, and post hoc interpretation based on rules, the divide between mathematical quantum-accelerated computations and human clinical judgment can be reduced.

Besides technical protection, the human conduct and company policies are also essential to the proper security and data privacy. Even the most sophisticated cryptographic measures are susceptible to improper use of the system, lack of training, or lack of understanding of AI-assisted workflows. As a result, quantum-secure technologies and workforce education, access control policies, and explicit accountability structures need to be complemented to provide complete data protection in healthcare settings.

7.2.2 Expanded Ethical Considerations in Quantum–AI Healthcare Systems

Quantum-AI technologies present both considerable computational benefits, but also present ethical complexities that are beyond the traditional AI systems. Algorithms opacities form one of the primary concerns. The presence of quantum-enhanced models can make understanding decision pathways more challenging, which is why the principles of transparency and explainability in clinical decision-making are bound to be challenged. Such obscurity creates issues with regard to the principle of accountability and informed consent that are essential in healthcare settings, posing a question of the trust and even prosecutability of clinicians.

The ethics governing institutions need to adapt thus to include constant auditing, the explainability mandate, and the human-in-the-loop control. To be responsible in deploying advanced AI systems, it is necessary to ensure that the final decision-making authority remains with the clinicians and that patients have access to the information about the role of advanced AI systems in their care. These considerations suggest that ethical principles that have been tailored to the greater complexity and autonomy of quantum-AI systems are necessary.

7.3 Healthcare Workforce Adaptation and Human Factors

The technical strength and data safety of quantum QAI systems in healthcare are not steadfast as the acceptance of the technologies by the workforce in the health-care sector. Human factors should become a primary key to success and adoption as clinicians, nurses, administrators, and allied health professionals are required to incorporate quantum-AI outputs into high-stakes clinics that are time-sensitive.

Cognitive workload is one of the challenges. State-of-the-art AIs and quantum-based systems can produce multifaceted suggestions, trust ratings, or optimization results that cannot be easily understood when time is limited in the clinical setting. Such systems can potentially worsen cognitive load instead of aiding decision-making unless there is a thorough interface design and explainability mechanisms. Thus, the principles of human-centered design, such as easy visualization, prioritization of the alerts, and the ability to trace the decision, are crucial.

7.4 Scalability and Interoperability

One of the most important challenges that are associated with the implementation of the AI-quantum solutions within different healthcare systems is scalability. As hospitals gather increasingly more health data (EHRs to IoT devices), systems must not only handle a significant amount of data more than before, but they must also be able to sustain the infrastructure. Even though the advantages of quantum computing are truly extraordinary in the terms of speed, they could not be scalable at the moment, given the limitation of qubit capacity and error correction capabilities. Besides that, the AI models will be forced to adapt to the local variations in medical practice and population.

Middleware gap solutions that might be in the form of real time data translation and standardization solutions can also be applied to bridge the gaps between new and legacy systems. Cloud-based quantum (El-Maghrabey et al., 2025) access may also contribute to scaling due to the fact that the institutions are able to access powerful computing without necessarily needing to own quantum computing equipment. The aspects that will have to define the process of ensuring that these advanced systems grow with the constantly evolving needs of the healthcare sector will be embracing the principles of modularity, adaptability and compliance with the standards.

7.5Regulatory, Technological, and Human Resource Challenges

Although quantum-AI systems have the potential to transform the healthcare system, their practical implementation is threatened by serious regulatory, technological, and human resources challenges. Regulation-wise, the current healthcare regulations, including HIPAA, GDPR, and developing AI regulation systems, were tailored toward the classical digital organization. With the advent of quantum-enhanced AI, some issues remain unanswered when it comes to the ownership of data, the cross-border transmission of data, the responsibility of algorithms, and the liability of AI-assisted clinical decision-making. There is still no clear regulatory guidance, especially with regard to accountability in situations where quantum-AI systems affect the outcome of diagnostic or treatment.

Deployment is also limited by technological factors. The available quantum hardware is still at the noisy intermediate-scale quantum (NISQ) phase, with small numbers of qubits, large error rates, and short coherence times. These limitations require quantum-classical hybrid architectures, adds complexity and overhead to the systems, and requires more integration. Interoperability, particularly with old hospital information systems, electronic health records, and clinical processes is also a significant implementation challenge.

7.6 Qualitative Insights: Human and Organizational Dimensions

In addition to technical performance, human acceptance, workflow integration, and institutional trust are determinants of the usage of quantum-AI systems. Qualitative-based analysis demonstrates that clinicians appreciate transparency, interpretability, and traceability of decisions made when using AI-assisted systems.

The organizational stakeholders put the stress on the significance of interoperability, the clarity of governance, and congruency with the current clinical guidelines.

These qualitative aspects have a strong impact on adoption results than technical capability. Using the combination of human-focused assessment criteria, the given framework takes care of socio-technical elements, which define the success of projects in real-life healthcare settings.

Middle Ground on Innovation and Viability

The possible positive effects of quantum-enhanced AI must thus be seen through the prism of practical limitations. Although the framework shows obvious positive features in the area of optimization, safe cooperation, and mass learning, these positive aspects depend on the level of technological maturity, the willingness of institutions, and regulatory transparency. The critical constituent of a measured and evidence-based approach is the focus on the pilot deployments, hybrid architectures, and continuous appraisal to avoid overestimation of the near-term impact. This objectivity of view enhances the academic value of this chapter because it combines the potential of technology with its actual workability.

CONCLUSION

8.1 Summary of Contributions

The innovation, futuristic, hybrid system that is presented in the work is a combination of Artificial Intelligence (AI) with Quantum Computing that will revolutionize e-collaboration within a healthcare sector. This framework is possible through the prediction capabilities of AI, together with the possibility of the quantum computer to improve real time decision making, customized treatment, and effective health data management due to the capacity of parallel processing. The system will also support decentralized work between the clinicians, patients, and administrators, which will meet the heightened marketplace demand of intelligent, secure, and scalable digital healthcare solutions. It is an integration that demonstrates how the new methods of calculations may represent more intelligent, faster, and more interconnected states of healthcare and ultimately improved patient outcomes.

8.2 Vision for Quantum-AI Enabled Healthcare Collaboration

The evolvement of frictionless health ecosystem where clinicians, patients, and health care administration teams converse in real time utilizing clever and designated systems, is the strategic view of quantum-AI powered healthcare partnership. The future healthcare systems will involve faster diagnostics, personalized health care services, predictive analytics and proactive care compelling diseases to access the capabilities of quantum computing and the power of AI to interpret and offer insights using massive amounts of data. It is to make sure that there is no delay, minimum medical errors, and that patients were in a better position to manage their care in order to finally deliver a data-driven, proactive, and collaborative and personal experience in reactive healthcare at any level of care.

Federated quantum learning in this visioned future will allow organizations in the healthcare sector across the globe to educate another AI in a collaborative fashion that will restrict access to raw patient information and preserve the information and will offer diversity by way of use to training information. Through quantum power, hospitals will be smart and adaptive places, where allocation of resources will be done in the optimal fashion via quantum-powered allocation and in-depth clinical action will be obtained in real time depending upon the IoT-linked devices. Telemedicine platforms that will be quantum encrypted will provide communication between the professionals and patients everywhere in the world and provide an uninterrupted degree of privacy. This will usher in the aspect of affordability in the advanced healthcare services as under this approach advanced healthcare service will be accessible even in remote or impoverished locations.

8.3 Critical Assessment of Practical Limitations and Adoption Barriers

Although quantum-enhanced AI has strong benefits in terms of healthcare collaboration, its application in practice is limited by a number of technical, organizational, and economic limitations that deserve critical analysis. Immaturity of quantum hardware is one of the key shortcomings. The existing quantum systems are noisy intermediate-scale quantum (NISQ) quantum systems that limit the size of problems, the depth of algorithms, and their reliability. Consequently, numerous of these suggested advantages are context-specific and can only be realized in hybrid quantumclassical workflows.

Lastly, there is regulatory uncertainty and readiness of the workforce to adopt. The lack of regulatory precedent on quantum-assisted clinical decision-making, in conjunction with the lack of AI and quantum literacy among medical practitioners, may slow institutional uptake. These issues imply that quantum-enhanced AI can be regarded as an add-on and complementary innovation instead of a solution that can be implemented in the nearest future and replace the old AI systems.

8.4 Recommendations for Policy and Practice

The most effective path that policymakers can follow in order to determine the successful deployment of quantum-AI systems within the healthcare sector is to establish policies on the optimal manner of developing regulatory mechanisms to deal with privacy of information, ethical application of AI and quantum-safe encryption systems. The law should be furthered to include decentralized learning, artificial intelligence-based clinical diagnosis, and information sharing of health data across national boundaries. It is important to introduce transparency in algorithmic [28] processes and any form of accountability must be implemented. The governments should also encourage the adoption of the quantum-resistant cybersecurity standards to connect the sensitive health information with the future quantum threats to develop trust and legal confidence in the healthcare technology environment.

To ensure that it is open to everyone, the governments and organizations must promote inclusive innovation policies that would enable to make quantum-AI technologies affordable and accessible to all regions. Investing in the miniaturization of quantum hardware, quantum access via the cloud and AI transparency would become a crucial area to fund research. Healthcare professional and patient education must be instigated to enhance better preparation of the healthcare professionals and their patient to consider this technological change. Finally, collaborative platforms between researchers, health industry leaders and their employees must be created to educate policies to allow the usage of such dynamic tools in the most desirable manner, responsibly, safely and producing the most positive results to everyone.

8.5 Managerial and Institutional Implications of Collaborative Intelligence

On the managerial approach, quantum-AI-based collaborative intelligence can assist strategic decision-making within healthcare organizations through enhancing operational visibility, predictive planning, and the management of resources. Quantum-optimized analytics allow hospital administrators to control the flow of patients, optimize their workforce schedule, and increase the system resilience to changing demand conditions.

At the institutional level, implementation of quantum-AI systems requires new governance forms, interdisciplinary leadership practices and innovation strategies that are aligned with policy. This can be achieved by integrating collaborative intelligence into the organizational processes through which healthcare systems can move past siloed digital tools into integrated, learning-based ecosystems, and in the process gain sustainable digital transformation.

8.6 Policy, Interdisciplinary, and Governance Implications

The successful implementation of quantum and AI healthcare systems entails alignment in clinical, technical, regulatory, and managerial spheres. Policy makers need to develop a flexible regulation system that caters to data privacy, algorithmic responsibility, and cybersecurity based on quantum safety. Conformity to standards like HIPAA, GDPR, and new AI governance policies is needed to achieve trust and compliance.

Governance wise, the healthcare organizations need to create governance mechanisms on auditing the algorithm, monitoring bias, and validating performance. These institutional structures make quantum -AI more of a mere technical innovation into operationally feasible and ethically regulated healthcare functionality.

8.7 Managerial and Clinical Implications of Quantum–AI Technologies

The adoption of quantum, as well as AI technologies, has both direct and distinguished implications to the healthcare managers and clinical practitioners. As a contrast to purely conceptual technological improvements, every quantum–AI element in the suggested model is associated with the particular operational, managerial, and clinical outcomes, thus, turning computational innovation into the practical healthcare value.

In clinical practice, quantum-enhanced AI expedites the training and inference of high-dimensional patient information to provide faster model support in diagnosis and to make timely treatment decisions. Federated quantum learning also enables clinicians in different institutions to also gain out of the collective insight without revealing sensitive patient information, enhancing the quality of the diagnostic and maintaining privacy.

On the institutional level, quantum-secure communication enhances inter-hospital cooperation by providing the data confidentially over time. This leads to more trust in the organization and to cross-institutional sharing of data, which is essential in population health management, identification of rare diseases, and multi-center clinical studies.

REFERENCES

Adege, A. B. (2025). Advancing Biomedical Engineering With Artificial Intelligence and Machine Learning: A Systematic Review. *International Journal of Clinical Practice*, *2025*(1), 9888902. DOI: 10.1155/ijcp/9888902

Adil, M., Ali, A., Tin, T. T., Farouk, A., Al-Kuwari, S., Song, H., & Jin, Z. (2025). Quantum computing and the future of healthcare internet of things security: Challenges and opportunities. *IEEE Internet of Things Journal*, *12*(22), 46316–46346. DOI: 10.1109/JIOT.2025.3605040

Aithal, P. S., & Aithal, S. (2025). Quantum Computers Supported Path to Technological Singularity–A Predictive Analysis. [PIJBAS]. *Poornaprajna International Journal of Basic & Applied Sciences*, *2*(1), 63–96. DOI: 10.64818/PIJBAS.3107.8478.0013

Ayub, M. A., Tyagi, A. R., Srivastava, S. K., & Singh, P. (2025). Quantum DFT analysis and molecular docking investigation of various potential breast cancer drugs. *Journal of Materials Chemistry. B*, *13*(1), 218–238. DOI: 10.1039/D4TB01803F PMID: 39545283

Balasubramani, S., Renjith, P. N., Kavisankar, L., Rajavel, R., Malarvel, M., & Shankar, A. (2025). A Quantum-Enhanced Artificial Neural Network Model for Efficient Medical Image Compression. *IEEE Access : Practical Innovations, Open Solutions*.

Braga, D. M., & Rawal, B. S. (2025). Harnessing AI and quantum computing for accelerated drug discovery: Regulatory frameworks for in silico to in vivo validation. *Journal of Pharmaceutical and BioTech Industry*, *2*(3), 11. DOI: 10.3390/jpbi2030011

Bukkarayasamudram, V. K., Reddy, P. C. S., Arun Kumar, K., Jagadish, R. M., Sharma, S., Prasad, M. L., Sucharitha, Y., Tayubi, I. A., & Thakur, G. K. (2025). Quantum computing revolution in healthcare: A systematic review of applications, issues and future directions. *Artificial Intelligence Review*, *58*(12), 1–35. DOI: 10.1007/s10462-025-11381-w

da Rocha, J. M., Campos, D. M. D. O., Esmaile, S. C., Menezes, G. D. L., Bezerra, K. S., da Silva, R. A., Junior, E. D. S., Tayyeb, J. Z., Akash, S., Fulco, U. L., Alqahtani, T., & Oliveira, J. I. (2025). Quantum biochemical analysis of the binding interactions between a potential inhibitory drug and the Ebola viral glycoprotein. *Journal of Biomolecular Structure & Dynamics*, *43*(9), 4753–4769. DOI: 10.1080/07391102.2024.2305314 PMID: 38258414

El-Maghrabey, M., El Hamd, M. A., Al-Khateeb, L. A., Magdy, G., Mahdi, W. A., Alshehri, S., Alsehli, B. R., & El-Shaheny, R. (2025). Design and synthesis of high quantum yield doped carbon nano probe derived from household sources for sensing of the anti-GERD drug pantoprazole. *Spectrochimica Acta. Part A: Molecular and Biomolecular Spectroscopy*, *325*, 125067. DOI: 10.1016/j.saa.2024.125067 PMID: 39232309

ElBedoui, K., Ben Lakhal, N., & Barhoumi, W. (2025). Medical image analysis: A systematization of knowledge on the convergence of AI and quantum computing. *The Journal of Supercomputing*, *81*(15), 1–52. DOI: 10.1007/s11227-025-07789-4

Eswaran, U., Eswaran, V., Eswaran, V., & Murali, K. (2025). Future Frontiers: The Role of AGI and Quantum Computing in Solving Complex Global Problems. In *Interplay of Artificial General Intelligence with Quantum Computing: Towards Sustainability* (pp. 137–151). Springer Nature Switzerland. DOI: 10.1007/978-3-031-87931-9_11

Gobinath, A., Rajeswari, P., Kumar, S. N., & Anandan, M. (2025). Quantum Robotics in Health Care: Innovations and Applications. In The Quantum Evolution (pp. 211-225). CRC Press.

Goswami, S. A., Dave, S., Patel, K. C., & Raval, M. N. (2025). Application of quantum artificial intelligence in healthcare. In *Quantum Computing for Healthcare Data* (pp. 119–138). Academic Press. DOI: 10.1016/B978-0-443-29297-2.00007-1

Haque, M. A., Kumar, V., Khan, S. N., & Kim, J. J. (2025). Quantum intelligence in drug discovery: Advancing insights with quantum machine learning. *Drug Discovery Today*, *30*(10), 104463. DOI: 10.1016/j.drudis.2025.104463 PMID: 40907599

Killi, K., Mettu, T. R., Srirambhatla, J., Maddali, S., & Kuna, A. (2025). Quantum approaches and technologies to transform cancer care: Opportunities and challenges in the Indian healthcare landscape. *Medical Journal, Armed Forces India*. Advance online publication. DOI: 10.1016/j.mjafi.2025.09.003

Li, T., Li, J., Jiang, H., & Skiles, D. B. (2025). Deep Learning Prediction of Drug-Induced Liver Toxicity by Manifold Embedding of Quantum Information of Drug Molecules. *Pharmaceutical Research*, *42*(1), 109–122. DOI: 10.1007/s11095-024-03800-4 PMID: 39663331

Manik, M. M. T. G., Mohonta, S. C., Karim, F., Miah, M. A., Islam, M. S., Chy, M. A. R., Adnan, M., & Saimon, A. S. M. (2025). AI-driven precision medicine leveraging machine learning and big data analytics for genomics-based drug discovery. *Journal of Posthumanism*, *5*(5), 4895–4915. DOI: 10.63332/joph.v5i5.1993

Marengo, A., & Santamato, V. (2025). Quantum algorithms and complexity in healthcare applications: A systematic review with machine learning-optimized analysis. *Frontiers of Computer Science*, *7*, 1584114. DOI: 10.3389/fcomp.2025.1584114

Nassir, N., Hashmi, M. A., Raji, K. G., Jamalalail, B., Maksymowsky, A., Scherer, S. W., Alsheikh-Ali, A., & Uddin, M. (2025). Quantum computing and the implementation of precision medicine. npj. *Genomic Medicine*, *10*(1), 80. DOI: 10.1038/s41525-025-00537-w PMID: 41330918

Panigrahi, S. (2025). *Carbon Quantum Dots Prepared by Hydrothermal Method for Drug Delivery*. Photocatalysis, and Bioimaging Applications.

Prathibha, S., Narayanamoorthy, S., Kishore, M. A., & Sandhiya, A. (2025, February). Quantum AI-Enhanced Health Care Diagnostic Pod: A Leap Towards Accurate and Accessible Diagnostics. In International Conference on Computational Intelligence in Data Science (pp. 122-137). Cham: Springer Nature Switzerland.

Rane, N., Patil, D., & Rane, J. (2025). Artificial Intelligence-Enabled Drug Development: Deep Learning and Computational Chemistry for Accelerating Therapeutics. *Available at SSRN* 5521819. DOI: 10.2139/ssrn.5521819

Rawat, K. S., & Yadav, M. (2025). Analyzing Quantum Computing Applications Across Key Scientific Domains Using Trends and Visual Analytics: K. Rawat, M. Yadav. *Archives of Computational Methods in Engineering*, •••, 1–32.

Roosan, D., Nirzhor, S., Khan, R., & Hai, F. (2025). Quantum Gradient Optimized Drug Repurposing Prototype for Omics Data. arXiv preprint arXiv:2506.19097. DOI: 10.5220/0013524900003967

Shanmuga, S. M., Jupally, S. H., & Vempalli, N. R. (2025). Models and Frameworks for Digital Preservation of Indigenous Knowledge Systems. In Revaluation and Preservation of Indigenous Knowledge Systems in Modern Society (pp. 511-534). IGI Global Scientific Publishing DOI: 10.4018/979-8-3693-7964-6.ch025

Singh, A. (2025). Chemical space exploration with quantum computing. *Nature Methods*, *22*(3), 452–452. DOI: 10.1038/s41592-025-02638-x PMID: 40074964

. Sonavane, A., Jaiswar, S., Mistry, M., Aylani, A., &Hajoary, D. (2025). Quantum machine learning models in healthcare: Future trends and challenges in healthcare. Quantum Computing for Healthcare Data, 167-187.

. Sundaram, A. (2025). Challenges and opportunities in quantum computing in healthcare. Quantum Computing for Healthcare Data, 91-118.

Sunki, K., Reddy, C. K. K., Reddy, D. M. K., & Doss, S. (2025). The role of quantum artificial intelligence in healthcare advancements. In *Cybernetics, Human Cognition, and Machine Learning in Communicative Applications* (pp. 137–158). Springer Nature Singapore. DOI: 10.1007/978-981-97-8533-9_10

Suvvari, T. K., Pradeep, K. V. S. B., Muppavarapu, R. S., & Nithya, A. (2025). The Potential Role of Quantum Computing in Biomedicine and Healthcare: The Next Frontier Beyond Artificial Intelligence. *Cureus*, *17*(4). Advance online publication. DOI: 10.7759/cureus.82759 PMID: 40406784

Weng, L., Ren, H., Xu, R., Xu, J., Lin, J., Shen, J. W., & Zheng, Y. (2025). Translocation mechanism of anticancer drugs through membrane with the assistance of graphene quantum dot. *Colloids and Surfaces. B, Biointerfaces*, *245*, 114340. DOI: 10.1016/j.colsurfb.2024.114340 PMID: 39476655

Chapter 11
Strengthening E-Collaboration in Healthcare Through AI:
Quantum Computing and E-Collaboration for Healthcare

S. Savitha
http://orcid.org/0000-0002-4914-8386
K.S.R. College of Engineering, India

J. Rameshkumar
http://orcid.org/0000-0001-8699-2298
K.S.R. College of Engineering, India

S. Hemalatha
http://orcid.org/0009-0007-3671-0927
K.S.R. College of Engineering, India

T. Haritha
Vivekanandha College of Engineering for Women, India

U. Sathya
Vivekanandha College of Technology for Women, India

R. Keerthana
http://orcid.org/0009-0001-4898-4075
K.S.R. College of Engineering, India

ABSTRACT

Modern healthcare depends on quick diagnoses, secure sharing of medical information, and smooth coordination among hospitals and research institutions. However, traditional computing systems often struggle to manage large and complex clinical data, advanced medical images, and collaboration across multiple organizations. Quantum computing, when combined with e-collaboration platforms, can overcome these challenges by delivering faster analysis, stronger security, and more scalable clinical intelligence. Core quantum principles such as superposition and entanglement—support parallel data processing, rapid optimization, and improved pattern detection in genomics, medical imaging, and continuous patient monitoring.

DOI: 10.4018/979-8-3373-5906-9.ch011

Quantum-enabled backends can strengthen digital collaboration by supporting remote consultations, shared clinical reviews, and coordinated care. Secure communication, privacy-preserving analytics, biomedical simulation, and public-health preparedness are discussed, along with current limitations and future directions.

1. INTRODUCTION

Healthcare systems are increasingly data-intensive and collaboration-driven, handling large volumes of medical images, genomic data, sensor streams, and electronic health records. The rapid growth of these datasets places significant strain on conventional computing infrastructures, while the demand for remote consultations and distributed clinical teams emphasizes the need for speed, accuracy, and security. This chapter examines how quantum computing and e-collaboration technologies address these challenges and enable advanced clinical intelligence.

Quantum computing introduces novel approaches for processing complex medical data through qubits, which allow parallel computation and faster problem solving. These capabilities are particularly beneficial for genomics analysis, multimodal risk prediction, and treatment optimization, where classical systems face scalability limitations. In parallel, e-collaboration platforms—such as telemedicine systems, shared imaging repositories, and research portals—support coordinated care and interdisciplinary decision-making. Quantum technologies enhance these platforms by improving computational efficiency, scalability, and secure data exchange.

Data security remains a critical concern in digital healthcare. While quantum computing poses risks to classical encryption, it also enables quantum-resistant cryptographic protocols that protect sensitive clinical and genomic information. The chapter highlights how quantum-secure communication strengthens trust in cross-institutional collaboration. Additionally, quantum-enabled analytics and quantum machine learning improve clinical decision support by enabling faster model training and more effective pattern discovery in high-dimensional healthcare data.

Quantum methods also advance biomedical simulation, including protein folding, drug discovery, and molecular interaction modeling, supporting precision medicine and therapeutic optimization. When integrated with e-collaboration systems, these tools facilitate shared research and public health coordination, enabling rapid outbreak surveillance and intervention planning. Finally, the chapter discusses practical challenges in quantum adoption, including hardware constraints and workforce limitations, and presents a roadmap for integrating quantum technologies into existing e-health infrastructures.

2. EMERGENCE OF QUANTUM PARADIGMS IN MEDICAL INFORMATICS

2.1 Background, motivation, shifts in computational needs

Medical informatics is moving toward automation and data-driven systems. Hospitals collect data from electronic records, wearables, imaging platforms, genomic tools, and monitoring devices. These datasets are large, complex, and sensitive, and traditional computing struggles to process them at the required speed, limiting real-time prediction and decision making (Gupta *et al.*, 2025; Nałęcz-Charkiewicz *et al.*, 2024).

Quantum computing changes how data is represented and processed. Qubits support parallel exploration through superposition and entanglement, enabling faster search, learning, and optimization for problems with large parameter spaces and complex relationships (Chow, 2024; Fairburn *et al.*, 2025). These capabilities are essential for precision medicine, genomic analysis, molecular simulation, and drug development, where classical processors face scalability limits (Savitha *et al.*, 2025; Durant *et al.*, 2024).

Public health coordination and cross-institution collaboration require fast computation and secure communication. Quantum Key Distribution protects shared clinical data and prevents unauthorized access during data exchange (Fairburn *et al.*, 2025; Solenov *et al.*, 2018). Quantum techniques also support medical imaging, enabling faster processing, segmentation, and disease detection (Chow, 2024). Quantum Machine Learning improves diagnostic accuracy by identifying complex patterns in sparse and nonlinear clinical data (Mei and Zhang, 2024; Gupta *et al.*, 2025).

As classical encryption weakens under quantum threats, quantum-secure methods become essential for protecting medical records and research data (Durant *et al.*, 2024). The need to process complex data, support personalized care, and enable secure global collaboration places quantum computing at the core of future medical informatics systems (Solenov *et al.*, 2018).

3. FUNDAMENTAL PRINCIPLES SHAPING QUANTUM ARCHITECTURE

Quantum computing is based on the laws of quantum mechanics and operates differently from classical computation. Its architecture relies on qubits, superposition, and entanglement to represent and process information more efficiently. Interference is used to amplify useful outcomes while reducing noise, and quantum gates apply unitary transformations to manipulate quantum states without information loss. Together, these principles form the foundation of quantum architectures and support quantum algorithms used in healthcare analytics (Fig. 3.1).

Figure 1. Quantum Architecture Fundamentals

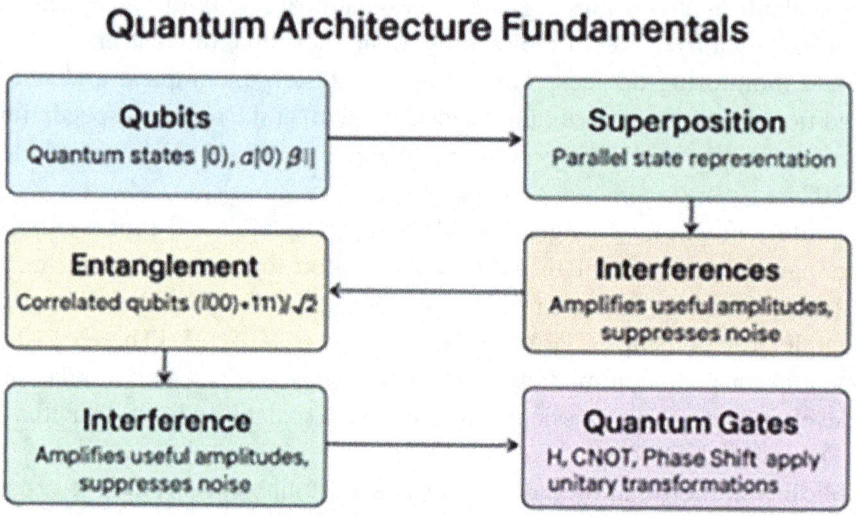

3.1 Qubits and Quantum State Superposition

Classical systems store information using bits with values 0 or 1, while a qubit represents a combination of both states simultaneously. A general qubit state is given by

$$|\psi\rangle = \alpha|0\rangle + \beta|1\rangle$$

were

$\alpha, \beta \in C$ in complex probability amplitudes

Normalization: $|\alpha|^2 + |\beta|^2 = 1$

Superposition enables parallel evaluation of clinical possibilities, supporting tasks such as multimodal risk scoring and faster genomic variant analysis in precision healthcare.

3.2 Quantum Entanglement for Correlated Medical Data

Entanglement links qubits through a shared quantum state. A common example is the Bell state

$$|\Phi+\rangle = 21(|00\rangle + |11\rangle)$$

which shows strong correlation between two qubits, where a change in one affects the other instantly. In healthcare, entanglement supports distributed decision systems, secure inter-hospital communication, unified processing of multisource clinical data, and real-time patient monitoring across distant locations.

3.3 Quantum Interference for Problem Optimization

Quantum algorithms adjust amplitude phases to strengthen useful outcomes through constructive interference, while destructive interference suppresses unwanted states. The probability of a desired result is

$$P(\text{desired outcome}) = |\Sigma\ \alpha\_\text{constructive}|^2$$

This mechanism enables faster optimization in clinical applications, including medical image segmentation, noise reduction, protein–drug interaction search, and hospital scheduling. Grover's algorithm applies this principle to reduce search complexity from linear to square-root time, supporting rapid anomaly detection in large healthcare datasets.

3.4 Quantum Gates: Transformations Enabling Clinical Analytics

Quantum gates operate on qubits through unitary transformations that preserve probability, expressed as

$$U|\psi\rangle = |\psi'\rangle \text{ such that } U\dagger U = I$$

This ensures state normalization and reliable computation. In healthcare analytics, the Hadamard gate enables superposition, the CNOT gate creates entanglement for linked data processing, and the Phase Shift gate supports Fourier-based imaging. Together, these operations underpin quantum machine learning models for diagnosis, disease progression prediction, and risk scoring.

3.5 Quantum Parallelism for High-Dimensional Healthcare Data

A quantum register with n qubits represents an exponential number of states at once:

2^n simultaneous basis states

This parallelism lets quantum processors evaluate many possibilities in a single operation. It speeds up analysis of multi-omics datasets, supports real time monitoring in critical care, and enables population-scale predictive modeling. These strengths improve clinical decision workflows that depend on fast processing and large data integration

3.6 Quantum Cryptography for Secure E-Collaboration

Quantum Key Distribution enables tamper-resistant communication by using quantum states for key exchange, where any interception disturbs the state and reveals intrusion. This protects data used in remote diagnosis, international clinical trials, and pharmaceutical research, supporting secure global telehealth networks and patient privacy in collaborative healthcare systems.

Table 1. Core Quantum Features and Their Healthcare Impact

Quantum Feature	Technical Role	Healthcare Benefit
Superposition	Parallel data representation	Faster biomarker analysis, efficient disease classification
Entanglement	Correlated information handling	Improved multi-hospital collaboration
Interference	Accelerated optimization	Enhanced imaging and scheduling performance
QKD & Quantum Security	Cryptography protocols	Trustworthy e-health infrastructure

4. QUANTUM-ENHANCED CLINICAL INTELLIGENCE

Healthcare generates high-dimensional data from imaging, laboratory tests, genomics, and continuous monitoring. Clinical decisions require accurate pattern extraction and prediction, but classical algorithms struggle with scale, noise, and nonlinear interactions. Quantum systems address these challenges through parallelism, efficient state representation, and amplitude-based computation (Nordmann *et al.*, 2025). This section outlines how quantum machine learning supports diagnosis and prognosis, multi-omics integration, and imaging acceleration.

Figure 4.1 illustrates a quantum-enabled clinical intelligence pipeline linking data ingestion, feature encoding, and quantum machine learning to clinical decision support. Optimization modules improve pattern discovery, while secure federated nodes enable cross-institution collaboration. Communication is protected using quantum-safe mechanisms such as QKD to ensure data integrity and patient privacy.

Figure 2. Quantum-Enabled Clinical Analytics Architecture

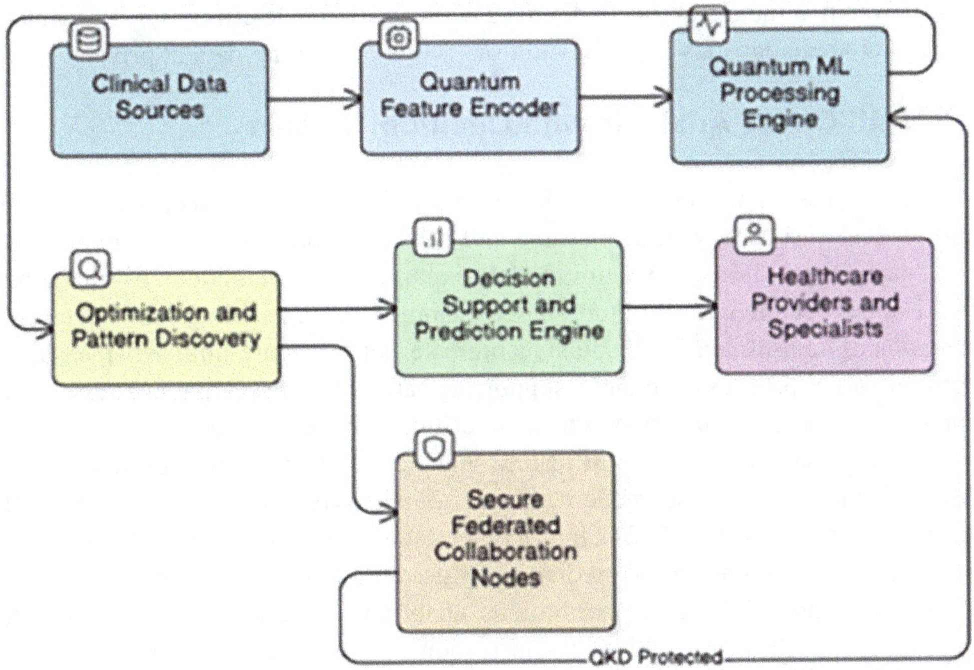

4.1 Quantum Machine Learning for Diagnosis and Prognosis

Quantum machine learning (QML) applies quantum circuits to classification, regression, and clustering tasks used in clinical decision support. By operating in high-dimensional Hilbert spaces, QML expands the search space for disease pattern detection and improves separation between diagnostic classes, enabling identification of weak clinical signals missed by classical models. Patient data are encoded into quantum states and processed through parameterized variational circuits, with measurements mapped to diagnostic labels. Training optimizes circuit parameters to minimize prediction error using quantum state evolution.

QML supports diagnosis in conditions with overlapping features, such as cancer, cardiac, and neurological disorders, by efficiently modeling complex relationships across imaging, biomarkers, and physiological data (Wagner *et al.*, 2025). Prognosis tasks also benefit, as quantum states capture long-range dependencies in patient histories without flattening the data. Quantum Support Vector Machines and kernel-based models compute similarity scores in high-dimensional quantum feature spaces, enabling expressive decision boundaries for risk stratification. QML is particularly effective for structured but limited clinical datasets, offering high expressive power with fewer parameters. When integrated with federated learning, QML enables collaborative diagnostics across institutions while preserving patient privacy.

4.2 Multi-Omics Analysis with Quantum Models

Multi-omics analysis integrates genomic, transcriptomic, proteomic, metabolomic, and clinical variables, producing large and heterogeneous datasets with complex cross-layer interactions. Quantum models capture these interactions by encoding multi-omics vectors into amplitude-based quantum states, enabling compact representation of high-dimensional data. Quantum kernels compute similarity measures between omics profiles efficiently, supporting patient clustering, pathway analysis, and disease subtype separation, which are critical for precision medicine.

Quantum models also support feature selection by amplifying informative signals and suppressing noise, reducing dimensionality without losing key biological information (Osorio *et al.*, 2024). Interference patterns help identify genes, proteins, and metabolites with strong predictive value. In addition, quantum generative models learn underlying data distributions, enabling abnormal signature detection, missing value estimation, and treatment-response simulation. Quantum graph processing further supports multi-omics networks by identifying interaction patterns, pathway disruptions, and intervention points, reducing computation time for large combinatorial analyses.

Figure 3. Classical vs Quantum kernel similarity

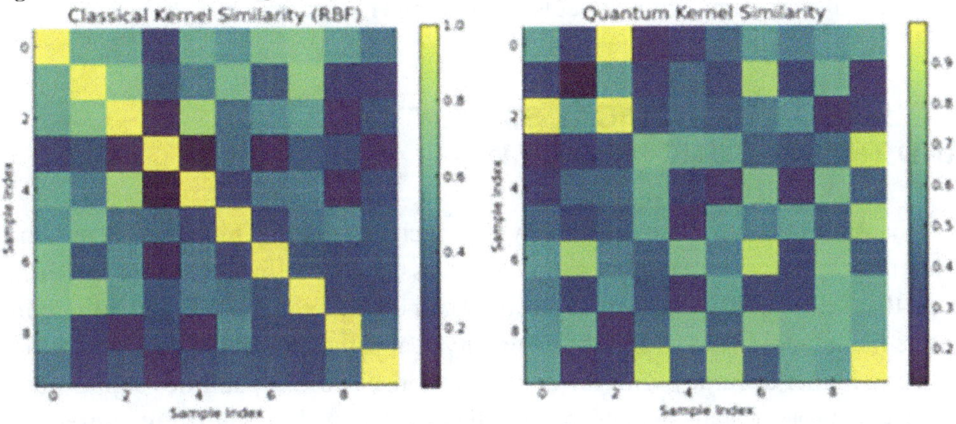

Figure 4.2 shows that the classical RBF kernel forms tight diagonal clusters, indicating limited ability to capture complex relationships. In contrast, the quantum kernel exhibits a richer similarity structure, improving class separation for diagnosis, prognosis, and multi-omics analysis in quantum-enhanced clinical models.

4.3 Quantum-Accelerated Medical Imaging Interpretation

Medical imaging produces large datasets from MRI, CT, PET, ultrasound, and digital pathology, requiring intensive computation for reconstruction, segmentation, classification, and enhancement. Quantum algorithms improve these workflows through efficient transforms, sampling, and optimization. The Quantum Fourier Transform accelerates Fourier-based operations used in MRI and CT reconstruction, reducing processing time (Fahad *et al.*, 2024). Quantum signal processing also improves noise reduction by controlling phase and amplitude, enhancing image clarity and supporting early disease detection.

Quantum models support segmentation by separating anatomical structures using variational circuits and amplitude-encoded image features. Quantum classifiers distinguish healthy and diseased regions, while quantum kernels enable high-dimensional pattern matching in digital pathology, reducing false negatives. Quantum image compression lowers storage and transmission costs, supporting tele-radiology and collaborative diagnosis (Keerthana *et al.*, 2025).

Imaging workflows rely heavily on optimization, including scan parameter selection, boundary refinement, and motion correction. Quantum optimization evaluates multiple solutions simultaneously, accelerating these tasks. Quantum circuits also enable multimodal image fusion, such as MRI–PET or MRI–CT integration, by encoding multimodal features into a single quantum state, improving diagnostic accuracy and real-time clinical decision making (Pattanaik *et al.*, 2024).

5. QUANTUM BIOMEDICAL SIMULATION AND THERAPEUTIC MODELLING

Quantum simulation provides a new approach for studying biochemical systems, drug interactions, and treatment pathways. Classical modeling relies on approximations that scale poorly for large molecules and complex reactions. Quantum computers model molecular structures using physical principles of atomic interactions, enabling higher accuracy with fewer assumptions. These capabilities support drug discovery, protein analysis, and personalized therapy. The following subsections describe quantum-enabled biomedical simulation and therapeutic development.

5.1 Molecular and Protein-Level Quantum Simulation

Molecular behavior follows quantum mechanics, where electrons occupy probabilistic orbitals and bonds depend on energy levels, spin states, and electrostatic forces. Classical methods such as Density Functional Theory and Hartree–Fock approximate these interactions, but accuracy decreases as molecular size grows due to exponential computational cost. Quantum simulation addresses this by representing electronic states directly with qubits. Techniques such as Variational Quantum Eigensolvers and Quantum Phase Estimation compute ground-state energies with higher precision, describing molecular stability and reaction properties (Chaturvedi, 2023).

Protein analysis benefits from quantum simulation by enabling efficient exploration of complex folding landscapes and interaction pathways. Superposition allows parallel evaluation of multiple configurations, supporting identification of functional domains, mutation effects, and drug-binding regions. Quantum models also improve simulation of protein–protein and protein–ligand interactions relevant to disease mechanisms and targeted therapy development.

Quantum approaches extend to enzyme kinetics by accurately estimating reaction energy barriers, aiding metabolic pathway analysis. Similar techniques support simulation of drug delivery materials and biocompatible implants. Overall, quantum simulation improves accuracy, reduces reliance on approximations, and expands the range of molecules that can be effectively modeled for biomedical research.

5.2 Quantum-Guided Drug Discovery and Reaction Modelling

Drug discovery requires identifying molecules with strong and selective binding to disease targets through large-scale screening and energy analysis. Classical methods are slow, costly, and rely on approximations that reduce accuracy. Quantum-guided drug discovery applies quantum algorithms to analyze molecular interactions at the atomic level, enabling more accurate computation of energy surfaces and binding affinities. This reduces false negatives in early screening and improves prioritization of therapeutic candidates.

Figure 5.1 illustrates a quantum-enabled drug discovery workflow in which clinical data flows from a centralized data lake through preprocessing and quantum feature encoding. Quantum computation and hybrid training generate validated insights, secured by QKD-based communication. A monitoring loop feeds performance metrics back into preprocessing, supporting continuous improvement in simulation and modeling accuracy.

Figure 4. Work flow of Quantum-Guided Drug Discovery and Reaction Modelling

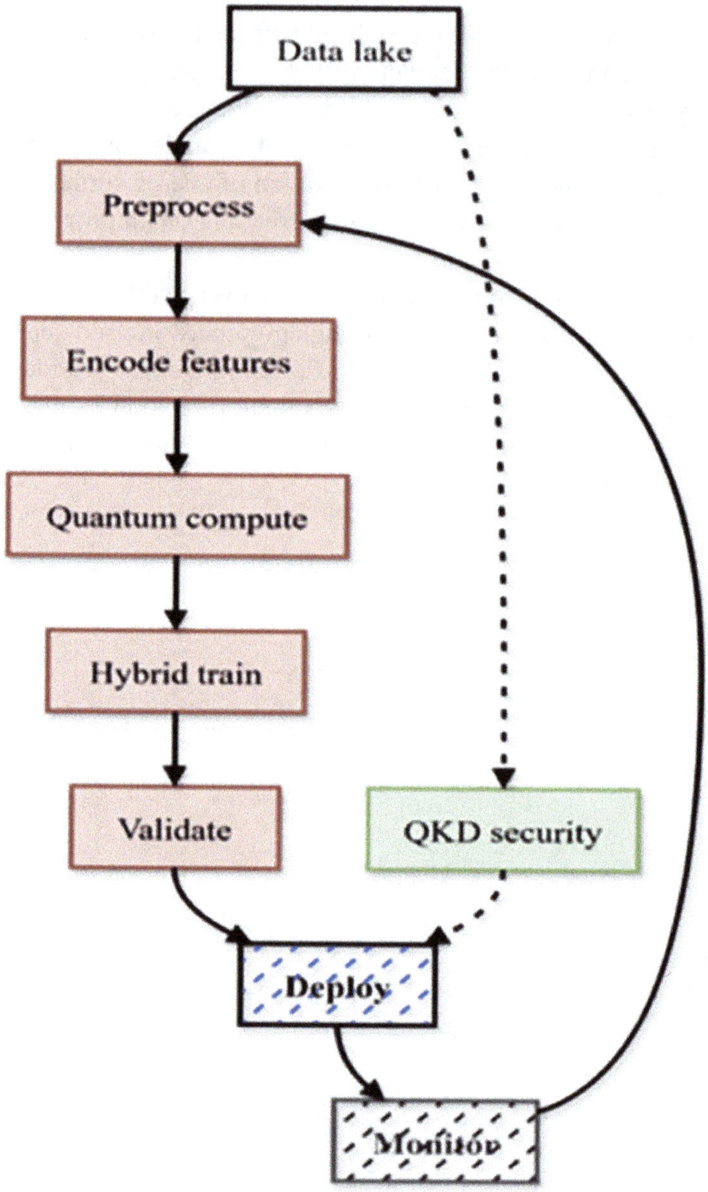

Quantum algorithms support the design of new molecules by using variational circuits to generate and optimize candidate structures for stability and binding affinity, accelerating lead identification. Quantum tools also improve reaction modeling by accurately estimating transition energies and reaction barriers using quantum phase estimation, enabling better prediction of reaction behavior and functional group effects. These capabilities support medicinal chemistry by improving potency, reducing toxicity, and enhancing toxicology prediction.

In oncology, quantum simulation aids the design of molecules that target mutated proteins and disrupted signaling pathways (Qaddumi *et al.*, 2021). Quantum-enhanced docking formulates binding as an optimization problem and applies amplitude amplification to improve accuracy for large or flexible molecules. Quantum generative models further support *de novo* drug design by producing compounds that meet constraints such as solubility and bioavailability. Overall, quantum-guided drug discovery reduces screening time and improves modeling accuracy.

Figure 5.2 compares classical and quantum molecular energy landscapes. The classical landscape is noisy with shallow local minima, while the quantum-resolved landscape is smoother and reveals a clearer global minimum, improving protein folding and reaction-energy prediction accuracy.

Figure 5. Molecular Energy Landscape

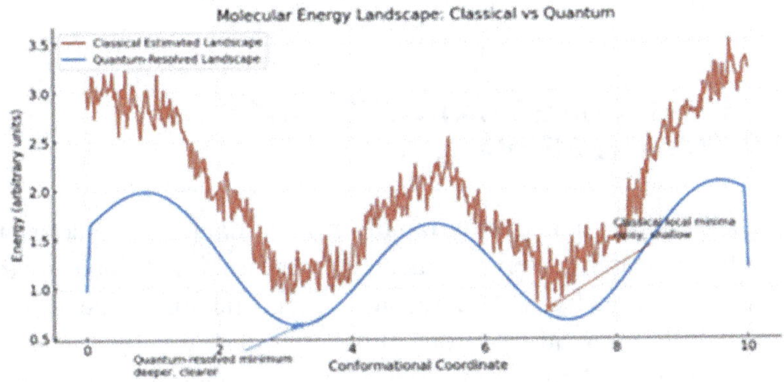

5.3 Quantum Tools for Personalized Therapy and Oncology

Personalized therapy requires understanding genetic variation, tumor behavior, and patient-specific treatment responses. Classical statistical and machine learning methods perform well at population scale but struggle with rare mutations, high-dimensional genomic data, and complex treatment interactions. Quantum tools address these limitations through high-dimensional computation and accurate modeling of biological interactions (Yuan, 2024). Quantum models enable patient-specific drug response prediction by analyzing how genetic variants affect molecular pathways, reducing trial-and-error treatment selection.

In oncology, quantum simulation models tumor microenvironments, including interactions among cancer cells, immune components, and metabolic factors, guiding targeted therapy design. Quantum optimization improves radiation therapy planning by evaluating multiple dose distributions in parallel to maximize tumor control while minimizing damage to healthy tissue. Quantum modeling of drug metabolism supports personalized chemotherapy by predicting toxicity and treatment efficacy. Quantum machine learning enhances tumor subtype classification using multi-omics data, supporting selection of immunotherapy and targeted treatments.

Quantum tools also support adaptive therapy by simulating tumor evolution and resistance pathways. Integration with federated quantum learning enables collaboration across institutions while preserving patient privacy through quantum-secure communication. Overall, quantum technologies enhance modeling accuracy, optimization, and personalized decision-making, improving treatment outcomes and reducing adverse effects.

6. QUANTUM-SECURED DATA EXCHANGE AND PRIVACY PRESERVATION

Modern healthcare systems handle rapidly growing data volumes across interconnected hospitals, research centers, telemedicine platforms, and cloud environments. Sensitive information such as patient records, diagnostic images, genomic profiles, and treatment histories requires strong protection during storage and exchange. Classical encryption methods face increasing risks as computational power grows, particularly with the emergence of quantum computers. Section 5 focuses on quantum-secure communication approaches that ensure confidentiality, integrity, and trust in healthcare systems, including Quantum Key Distribution (QKD), quantum-safe cryptography, secure multi-party computation, and federated quantum learning for biomedical collaboration.

6.1 Quantum Key Distribution and Quantum-Safe Encryption

Quantum Key Distribution (QKD) enables secure key exchange based on quantum physics rather than computational hardness. Classical encryption schemes such as RSA and ECC rely on factoring and discrete logarithm problems, which become vulnerable to quantum algorithms like Shor's algorithm. As medical data requires long-term protection, healthcare systems relying on classical cryptography face increasing security risks with the advent of large-scale quantum computers.

QKD provides security based on quantum physics by using quantum states to distribute cryptographic keys. Any interception disturbs these states and reveals the presence of an attacker, ensuring only secure keys are used. QKD can be integrated into hospital networks to enable secure data exchange among clinics, diagnostic centers, and research partners.

Quantum-safe (post-quantum) encryption protects against both classical and quantum attacks using schemes such as lattice-based, hash-based, and multivariate cryptography. Healthcare systems can adopt hybrid models that combine QKD for key distribution with post-quantum encryption for data protection (Yuan, 2024). This approach secures clinical communication, telemedicine, electronic health records, and remote monitoring, while ensuring interoperability in global collaborations where QKD is not universally available.

Figure 6. Threat Model Radar Chart (Classical vs Quantum-Safe)

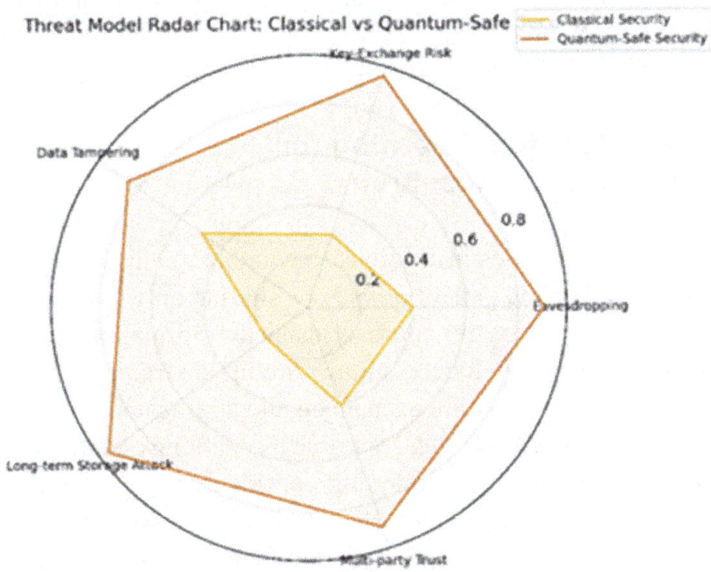

Figure 6.1 compares cybersecurity threats under classical and quantum-safe models. Classical security shows weaker protection against eavesdropping, key-exchange attacks, tampering, and long-term data risks, while quantum-safe methods provide higher resilience across all categories, emphasizing their importance for healthcare data protection.

6.2 Secure Multi-Party Computation in Clinical Networks

Clinical decision-making often relies on data shared across multiple organizations, but direct data exchange raises privacy concerns, particularly for genomic, imaging, and patient-specific information. Secure Multi-Party Computation (SMPC) enables institutions to jointly compute on collective datasets without revealing raw data. Participants contribute encrypted inputs, computations are performed in a distributed manner, and only final results are disclosed, preserving confidentiality (Wang & Qin, 2024).

SMPC supports collaborative healthcare applications such as multi-center oncology outcome analysis, outbreak forecasting, and clinical trials, allowing shared insights without exposing sensitive data. Quantum technologies enhance SMPC by providing quantum-secure communication, improved random number generation, and quantum-resistant secret sharing, increasing resilience against classical and quantum attacks.

Quantum-enhanced SMPC also enables cross-border collaboration under differing data protection regulations. Institutions can cooperate on global biomedical research while maintaining compliance and privacy, strengthening trust and accelerating evidence-based healthcare decisions (European Alliance for Innovation, 2025).

6.3 Federated Quantum Learning for Protected Biomedical Research

Federated learning enables institutions to collaboratively train models without centralizing data, preserving patient privacy by sharing only model updates. Federated quantum learning extends this approach using hybrid quantum–classical models distributed across sites, where local quantum circuits are trained on private datasets and only optimized parameters are exchanged and aggregated.

This paradigm benefits biomedical research by enabling collaboration on limited or rare-disease datasets while maintaining confidentiality. Quantum kernels and feature encoders capture high-dimensional nonlinear relationships in genomic and proteomic data, producing richer global models than single-site training. Quantum-secure communication protects model updates during transmission.

Federated quantum learning also supports decentralized drug discovery by allowing collaborative model training without exposing proprietary data. Combined with QKD, post-quantum encryption, and SMPC, federated quantum models enable privacy-preserving collaboration across global clinical and research networks.

7. QUANTUM-ENABLED E-COLLABORATION ACROSS HEALTHCARE NETWORKS

Healthcare systems rely on cross-institution collaboration for referrals, shared diagnostics, multi-center research, public health monitoring, and telemedicine. As these networks expand, computational and security demands increase. Section 6 examines how quantum technologies enhance e-collaboration by improving decision-making speed, distributed intelligence, and secure communication, supporting clinical care, telemedicine, and outbreak-response networks with greater reliability, privacy, and efficiency.

7.1 Distributed Clinical Decision Platforms

Clinical decision support increasingly spans multiple institutions, with diagnostics, treatment, and monitoring distributed across locations and networks. These workflows generate decentralized data and require near-real-time analysis, while classical centralized systems introduce latency, bandwidth limits, and security risks. Quantum-enabled systems enhance distributed clinical decision-making by accelerating analytics, improving optimization, and strengthening inter-hospital communication.

Quantum machine learning supports rapid interpretation of high-dimensional data such as imaging, genomics, and sensor streams, enabling consistent decisions across hospital networks. Distributed quantum kernels compare patient profiles without transferring raw data, supporting collaborative risk assessment, disease stratification, and treatment selection. Quantum optimization improves multi-hospital resource coordination, including ICU allocation and scheduling, by evaluating many scenarios in parallel. Security is ensured through Quantum Key Distribution and post-quantum encryption, protecting shared insights across institutions. Overall, quantum technologies enable faster, more accurate, and secure collaborative clinical decision-making.

7.2 Telemedicine and Multi-Hospital Coordination

Telemedicine enables remote consultations, digital triage, home monitoring, and virtual follow-up visits, relying on continuous data exchange among patients, clinicians, and hospital systems. As telemedicine integrates multimodal data such as video, imaging, lab results, medication records, and wearable sensors, computational and security demands increase. Quantum technologies help address these challenges by enhancing secure communication and analytics.

Quantum communication strengthens telemedicine security by protecting data streams from interception. Quantum Key Distribution ensures secure session keys for video consultations, remote diagnostics, and robotic-assisted procedures, which is increasingly important in cross-border and rural telemedicine scenarios. Quantum machine learning further supports remote clinical inference by analyzing heterogeneous patient data and enabling early anomaly detection in chronic disease monitoring.

Quantum optimization improves referral coordination by identifying optimal care facilities based on capacity, distance, and specialization. Quantum-safe group communication secures collaborative consultations, digital tumor boards, and multidisciplinary meetings. As shown in Fig. 7.1, quantum-secured communication layers using QKD and post-quantum encryption protect telemedicine workflows, ensuring confidentiality, integrity, and reliable coordination across healthcare networks.

Figure 7. Telemedicine + Quantum Security Architecture

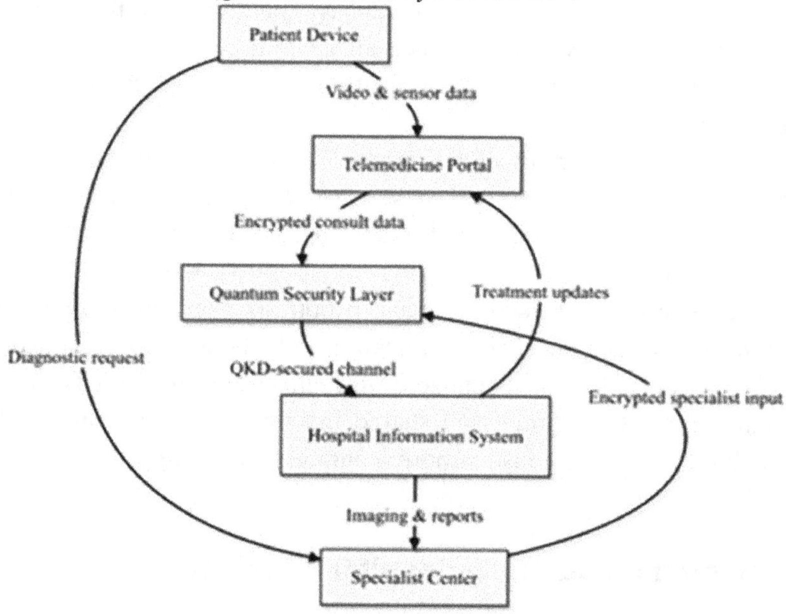

7.3 Quantum-Driven Epidemic and Outbreak Response Systems

Disease outbreaks require rapid detection, accurate prediction, and coordinated response across public health agencies, hospitals, laboratories, and governments. Classical epidemic models struggle with large, dynamic, and distributed datasets. Quantum-enabled outbreak response systems address these challenges by efficiently modeling epidemic dynamics and forecasting spread patterns. Quantum simulation evaluates large parameter spaces involving mobility, transmission rates, immunity, and environmental factors, enabling early identification of hotspots and improved response planning.

Quantum machine learning enhances surveillance by detecting anomalies in real-time data streams from healthcare systems and mobile health platforms, supporting early intervention. Quantum optimization improves allocation of critical resources such as ICU beds, ventilators, vaccines, and medical staff across regions. Secure data exchange is ensured through Quantum Key Distribution and post-quantum encryption, protecting epidemiological data and genomic information during rapid decision cycles (Savitha *et al.*, 2025).

Federated quantum learning supports global outbreak research by enabling collaborative modeling of pathogen evolution and treatment response without sharing raw data. Integrated with digital surveillance infrastructures, quantum-secure systems provide resilient, privacy-preserving support for outbreak monitoring and response against future cyber threats.

8. QUANTUM BIOMEDICAL MODELLING AND THERAPEUTIC SIMULATION

Quantum biomedical modeling addresses key limitations of classical simulation methods in computational medicine. Biological processes occur at molecular and atomic scales where quantum effects strongly influence biochemical behavior. Classical techniques, such as molecular dynamics and density functional theory approximations, rely on simplifications that limit accuracy and scalability for complex biomolecular systems. In contrast, quantum computing operates directly within a quantum-mechanical framework, enabling more accurate modeling of molecular interactions and reaction pathways.

By leveraging superposition and entanglement, quantum computing enables parallel exploration of large configurational spaces and high-fidelity simulation of protein folding, ligand–receptor binding, and enzymatic reactions. Hybrid quantum–classical pipelines offer a practical near-term solution, where classical systems handle preprocessing while quantum processors address computationally intensive tasks such as electronic structure and binding energy estimation. This approach accelerates drug discovery workflows and supports rational drug design, personalized medicine, and identification of novel therapeutic targets, advancing the computational foundations of modern healthcare (Arshad *et al.*, 2023; Rasool *et al.*, 2023).

8.1 Drug Reaction Prediction

- QC allows precise modeling of drug target interactions by simulating electrons and nuclei according to quantum mechanics.
- Hybrid QM/MM approaches: treat active sites quantum mechanically while the remaining system is modelled classically.
- Quantum-enhanced screening enables rapid evaluation of chemical libraries, reducing preclinical failure and identifying novel compounds (World Economic Forum, 2023).
- Formula (Free Energy Difference for Binding):

$$\Delta F_{A\to B} = -k_B T \ln \langle e^{-(E_B - E_A)/k_B T} \rangle_A$$

Where $k_B$is Boltzmann constant, Ttemperature, and $\langle \cdot \rangle_A$ensemble average over state A (Wikipedia, 2025).

8.2 Protein Folding and Molecular Interaction Analysis

- QC treats folding as an optimization problem via quantum Hamiltonians solved by VQE or hybrid circuits.
- Accurately predicts ground-state energies to identify stable conformations:

$$\hat{H}\Psi = E\Psi$$

Where $\hat{H}$is Hamiltonian, Ψwavefunction, Eenergy eigenvalue.

- Allows exploration of molecular interactions for drug design, enzyme modelling, and protein engineering.

8.3 Oncology Targeting and Personalized Therapeutics

Quantum computing enables accurate quantum-mechanical modeling of cancer-related biomolecules, supporting oncology drug discovery and personalized therapy. Cancer progression involves mutant proteins, altered signaling pathways, and molecular heterogeneity that challenge classical methods. QC-based molecular simulation addresses these challenges by directly modeling complex electronic interactions and conformational variability in cancer systems (Rasool *et al.*, 2023; Risvas and Spanoudaki, 2025).

Quantum-Enabled Binding Affinity Prediction for Mutant Proteins

Predicting how mutations affect protein–ligand binding is critical in targeted oncology, as small genetic changes can reduce drug efficacy or cause resistance. Classical force-field methods rely on approximations that limit accuracy, while quantum-enabled approaches model electronic interactions directly, improving reliability (Arshad *et al.*, 2023). Quantum simulations capture electron correlation and polarization effects in mutant binding sites, enabling more accurate estimation of binding energy changes and resistance mechanisms.

These predictions are based on solving the molecular electronic structure problem,

$$\hat{H}\Psi = E\Psi$$

where the ground-state energy reflects molecular stability and binding strength. Quantum algorithms such as the Variational Quantum Eigensolver efficiently approximate this energy, supporting precise evaluation of drug–target interactions in personalized cancer therapy (McArdle *et al.*, 2020).

Exploration of Novel Chemical Scaffolds and Personalized Oncology

Targeted cancer therapies require novel chemical scaffolds to address complex oncogenic targets such as kinases and protein–protein interactions. Quantum computing expands the searchable chemical space by efficiently evaluating multiple molecular configurations and electronic states, enabling optimization of affinity, selectivity, and toxicity. Hybrid QM/MM frameworks are effective in this context by treating only the binding site quantum-mechanically while maintaining scalability for large biomolecules. The total system energy is expressed as

$$E_{\text{total}} = E_{\text{QM}} + E_{\text{MM}} + E_{\text{QM-MM}}$$

which preserves quantum accuracy at the active site (Senn and Thiel, 2009).

Integration of quantum simulation with patient-specific genomic data further supports personalized oncology. By modeling mutant proteins derived from individual tumor profiles, quantum methods enable prediction of drug response variability and design of therapies targeting rare or unique oncogenic mutations, advancing precision cancer treatment (Risvas and Spanoudaki, 2025).

Implications for Drug Resistance and Adaptive Therapy

Drug resistance remains a major obstacle in cancer treatment. QC can model mutation-induced resistance pathways by simulating how binding energies and conformational landscapes evolve as mutations accumulate. This enables:

- Anticipation of resistance before clinical failure.
- Rational design of next-generation inhibitors.
- Support for adaptive therapy strategies.

9. HIGH-DIMENSIONAL IMAGING INTERPRETATION WITH QUANTUM SIGNAL PROCESSING

Modern medical imaging modalities such as CT, MRI, PET, digital pathology, and neurological scans generate high-dimensional, noisy, and heterogeneous datasets with strong spatial and temporal dependencies. While classical image processing and deep learning methods are effective, they face limitations in scalability, optimization efficiency, and real-time performance for large-scale medical data.

Quantum computing and quantum-inspired signal processing introduce a new paradigm by exploiting superposition and parallelism to evaluate multiple reconstruction hypotheses and feature transformations simultaneously. These capabilities are particularly useful for inverse imaging problems, denoising, and optimization, enabling improved resolution, faster reconstruction, reduced noise, and enhanced diagnostic reliability across imaging domains.

9.1 Radiological Image Enhancement

Radiological workflows depend on accurate reconstruction and noise suppression. In CT and MRI, classical reconstruction methods face trade-offs between image quality, scan time, and radiation exposure. Quantum signal processing, especially Quantum Fourier Transform (QFT)-based methods, accelerates spatial-to-frequency transformations and supports high-resolution 3D and 4D reconstruction with reduced latency. Quantum-enhanced denoising further improves image quality in low-dose CT and PET imaging, enabling shorter scans, reduced radiation exposure, and improved diagnostic accuracy in oncology and cardiovascular imaging.

9.2 Processing and Classification of Pathology Slides

Digital pathology relies on whole-slide imaging with gigapixel-scale resolution, creating challenges for classical analysis due to memory and feature dimensionality limits. Quantum machine learning encodes high-dimensional image features into quantum states using quantum feature maps, enabling compact representation of complex spatial and morphological patterns. Hybrid quantum–classical pipelines combine classical preprocessing with quantum classifiers and variational circuits to detect subtle anomalies, rare tumor subtypes, and early pathological changes, improving diagnostic sensitivity in complex cancers and rare diseases.

9.3 Neurological Scan Optimization and Signal Reconstruction

Neurological imaging modalities such as fMRI, DTI, and EEG-integrated scans generate time-dependent, noisy, and high-dimensional datasets. Quantum signal processing enhances denoising, pattern recognition, and functional connectivity analysis by efficiently exploring large parameter spaces. Quantum-assisted reconstruction improves temporal resolution in fMRI, supporting accurate mapping of brain activity and early detection of neurodegenerative diseases. These advances enable near real-time neurological analysis, continuous monitoring, and personalized treatment planning.

10. PANDEMIC PREPAREDNESS THROUGH QUANTUM-DRIVEN COORDINATION

Quantum computing offers significant advantages for large-scale public health management, particularly in pandemic preparedness and response. Classical epidemiological models struggle with high-dimensional and rapidly evolving data, while quantum approaches enable faster outbreak monitoring, targeted intervention planning, and optimized resource utilization.

10.1 Real-Time Outbreak Tracking and Forecasting

Quantum-enhanced optimization and sampling integrate diverse data streams, including pathogen genomics, epidemiological trends, human mobility, and healthcare capacity. This enables simultaneous evaluation of multiple outbreak scenarios, supporting near-real-time forecasting and informed decision-making.

10.2 Adaptive Intervention Planning

Resource allocation during pandemics involves complex multi-variable optimization. Quantum methods such as Quantum Annealing and Variational Quantum Algorithms efficiently explore solution spaces to balance epidemiological impact with logistical and economic constraints. Quantum simulations also enable rapid "what-if" analysis to improve preparedness across varying outbreak conditions.

10.3 Global Epidemiological Decision Support

Pandemic management requires international coordination. Quantum computing supports cross-border integration of epidemiological, genomic, and resource data, enabling multi-objective optimization for equitable and effective global resource distribution.

11. OPERATIONAL OPTIMIZATION IN SMART HOSPITAL ENVIRONMENTS

Hospitals face complex operational challenges involving staffing, equipment utilization, patient flow, and emergency preparedness. Quantum computing enables near-real-time optimization of multi-constraint problems that are difficult to solve using classical systems.

11.1 Resource Scheduling and Workflow Optimization

Hospital operations involve combinatorial optimization tasks such as staff allocation, equipment scheduling, and patient flow management. Quantum approaches like QUBO and QAOA improve parallel task handling, reduce conflicts, and support dynamic rescheduling during demand fluctuations.

11.2 Accelerating Emergency Response

In emergency scenarios, quantum computing supports rapid triage and resource reallocation. Integration with IoT and edge computing enables quantum-enhanced digital twins that simulate real-time patient inflow, predict bottlenecks, and guide optimal resource deployment.

11.3 Digital Twin Modelling and Predictive Management

Quantum-enhanced digital twins combine AI, IoT, and quantum computing to simulate operational scenarios, predict failures, and optimize resource usage. These models allow hospitals to anticipate staff shortages, equipment issues, and patient surges, improving resilience and reducing operational inefficiencies.

12. STANDARDIZATION, INTEROPERABILITY, AND REGULATORY CONSIDERATIONS

Successful integration of quantum computing (QC) in healthcare requires strong standardization, regulatory alignment, and governance to ensure safe, ethical, and interoperable deployment. Without common protocols, QC applications risk inconsistency, misinterpretation, and data incompatibility across institutions.

12.1 Compliance and Certification Frameworks

QC-enabled healthcare systems must comply with existing regulations such as HIPAA, GDPR, and ISO 13485. New certification protocols may be required to address quantum-specific outputs. Interoperability requirements include compatibility with EHR/HIS systems, secure transmission of quantum-processed data, and validated pipelines ensuring reproducibility. QC-based optimization methods, such as QAOA for hospital scheduling, must include audit and verification mechanisms to meet clinical standards.

12.2 Ethical Oversight in Quantum-Enabled Healthcare

Quantum healthcare introduces ethical challenges related to data privacy, patient consent, transparency, and algorithmic bias. Ethics committees and IRBs must adopt quantum-aware guidelines covering auditability, traceable data lineage, and standardized error reporting to ensure responsible deployment.

12.3 International Health Governance and Policy Integration

Global coordination is essential to promote equitable access and collaboration. This includes harmonized standards, shared quantum-cloud infrastructure, and policies preventing monopolization of quantum resources. International frameworks may integrate quantum-secure communication, such as QKD, for protecting patient data in multi-center studies.

13. BARRIERS LIMITING HEALTHCARE QUANTUM INTEGRATION

Despite its potential, QC adoption in healthcare faces technical, human, and infrastructural challenges.

13.1 NISQ Hardware and Computational Limitations

Current NISQ devices are constrained by limited qubits, noise, and decoherence, restricting large-scale medical applications such as high-resolution imaging and hospital-wide optimization (2023). Hybrid quantum–classical approaches are often required.

13.2 Robustness, Reliability, and Error Mitigation

Quantum algorithms are sensitive to noise, requiring error mitigation techniques such as Zero-Noise Extrapolation and Quantum Subspace Expansion. While hybrid approaches improve feasibility, approximation errors must be carefully evaluated before clinical use.

13.3 Workforce Skill Scarcity and Training Gaps

QC deployment requires expertise spanning quantum algorithms, biomedical workflows, cybersecurity, and regulatory compliance. Interdisciplinary training programs are essential to address workforce shortages.

13.4 Economic and Infrastructure Constraints

Quantum hardware is costly and resource-intensive. Cloud-based quantum services reduce initial investment but depend on reliable connectivity and secure infrastructure, limiting adoption in resource-constrained healthcare settings.

14. ROADMAP FOR SCALABLE QUANTUM ADOPTION IN E-HEALTH

A phased roadmap supports practical integration of QC into healthcare systems.

14.1 Research Priorities and Innovation Directions

Key priorities include pilot deployments in digital twins and scheduling, hybrid quantum–classical architectures, efficient data encoding for imaging and genomics, and robust error mitigation techniques such as ZNE and QSE to ensure reliable near-term applications.

14.2 Phased Deployment Frameworks

Phase	Focus	Milestone / Outcome
Phase 0	Feasibility studies & simulations	Benchmark quantum algorithms against classical methods
Phase I	Pilot deployment	Controlled implementation in select hospital units
Phase II	Hybrid systems integration	Interoperability with hospital IT, workflow testing
Phase III	Clinical & operational trials	Expanded deployment across departments
Phase IV	Full-scale & shared quantum-cloud	Multi-hospital, global collaboration and data sharing

Algorithmic focus: For example, *Quantum Time Interval Scheduler (QTIS)* using QAOA can be tested in Phase I for dynamic staff and resource allocation (Tirado-Domínguez et al., 2025).

14.3 Capacity Building and Workforce Development

- Develop interdisciplinary curricula: quantum computing, healthcare analytics, regulatory knowledge.
- Establish collaborative consortia for shared learning and resource pooling.
- Build infrastructure gradually: pilot units → hybrid integration → cloud-scale deployment.

15. STRATEGIC VISION FOR GLOBALLY COLLABORATIVE QUANTUM MEDICINE

Globally collaborative quantum medicine aims to build an integrated, equitable, and sustainable healthcare ecosystem. Quantum computing can transform how medical knowledge is generated, shared, and applied by enabling predictive analytics, personalized therapeutics, and large-scale optimization. This vision supports a global transition toward data-driven, precision-focused, and resilient healthcare systems through shared quantum infrastructure and international cooperation (Risvas and Spanoudaki, 2025).

A collaborative framework emphasizes collective intelligence, allowing countries, research institutions, and healthcare providers to jointly use quantum-enhanced analytics to improve population health. Such collaboration is essential to ensure that quantum healthcare innovations promote global health equity rather than remaining limited to technologically advanced regions.

Figure 8. Global collaborative quantum medicine ecosystem

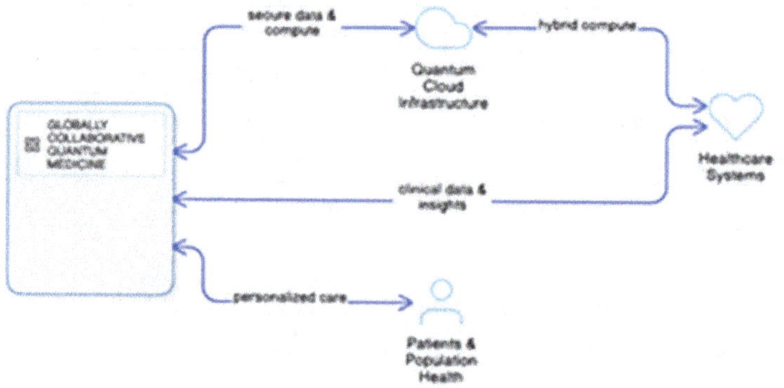

Figure 15.1 Global collaborative quantum medicine ecosystem illustrating shared quantum infrastructure, international cooperation, and patient-centric healthcare transformation.

15.1 Sustainable Innovation Models

Sustainable innovation in quantum healthcare requires a shift from isolated, capital-intensive deployments to shared, service-oriented models. Quantum-cloud platforms enable hospitals, research centers, and public health agencies to access quantum resources without investing in costly hardware or infrastructure. These shared services reduce costs through pay-per-use models, support scalable adoption, and promote inclusivity by enabling participation from regions without local quantum systems.

Open-data and open-algorithm initiatives further enhance sustainability by accelerating innovation, improving transparency, and reducing duplication of effort. Sharing quantum algorithms for drug discovery, imaging, and epidemiological modeling supports collaborative refinement and aligns with global open-science principles, strengthening trust in quantum-enabled healthcare systems. Long-term sustainability also depends on policy alignment and institutional support, including strategic investments, regulatory sandboxes, and public–private partnerships that facilitate responsible research and clinical translation.

15.2 Cross-Nation Collaboration in Quantum Health Research

Cross-nation collaboration is a cornerstone of globally collaborative quantum medicine. Many healthcare challenges such as pandemics, antimicrobial resistance, and rare diseases are inherently transnational and require shared analytical capacity and coordinated responses. Quantum computing enhances these efforts by enabling large-scale simulations, federated learning, and multi-center optimization.

International quantum health research collaboration involves:

Shared quantum-cloud infrastructure supports multi-center clinical trials, joint research programs, and federated quantum–classical analytics, enabling collaboration while keeping sensitive patient data within national boundaries. Effective collaboration requires harmonized regulatory standards and data governance frameworks to address differences in privacy laws, ethical guidelines, and certification processes. Alignment on interoperability, patient consent, and algorithm validation ensures safe and ethical sharing of quantum-enabled insights. Secure international data exchange is further supported by quantum-secure communication methods such as Quantum Key Distribution, which protect medical and genomic data against classical and post-quantum threats and strengthen trust across institutions.

15.3 Long-Term Transformation of Patient Care

The most profound impact of globally collaborative quantum medicine lies in its ability to transform patient care paradigms. Quantum-enhanced analytics enable a shift from reactive treatment models toward predictive, preventive, and personalized healthcare. By integrating quantum simulations, patient-specific genomics, and real-time clinical data, healthcare systems can anticipate disease progression and tailor interventions with unprecedented precision.

Long-term patient care transformation includes predictive diagnostics using quantum-assisted pattern recognition, personalized therapeutics supported by quantum drug–protein simulations, accelerated drug discovery through quantum molecular modeling, and optimized clinical workflows using quantum optimization for scheduling, resource allocation, and emergency response. At the global level, QC-enabled decision support enhances population health management, vaccine distribution, healthcare logistics, and outbreak response, especially during health emergencies.

Ensuring equitable access remains essential. International collaboration, shared infrastructure, and knowledge exchange help prevent technological disparities, ensuring quantum medicine benefits underserved populations. In this vision, quantum computing acts as a catalyst for inclusive, resilient, and globally connected healthcare systems.

REFERENCES

Arshad, J., Murtza, M. H., & Arshad, M. (2023). Quantum computing in biomedical engineering: Opportunities, challenges, and future perspectives. *Biomedical Engineering Advances*, *5*, 100067. DOI: 10.1016/j.bea.2023.100067

Chaturvedi, S. (2023). Clinical prediction on ML based Internet of Things for e-health care system. *International Journal of Data Informatics and Intelligent Computing*, *2*(3), 29–37. DOI: 10.59461/ijdiic.v2i3.76

Chow, J. C. L. (2024). Quantum computing in medicine: Current state and future prospects. *Journal of Medical Informatics and Health*, *12*(4), 67.

Durant, T. J. S.. (2024). A primer for quantum computing and its applications to biomedicine: Opportunities and challenges. *Journal of the American Medical Informatics Association : JAMIA*, *31*(8), 1774–1786. DOI: 10.1093/jamia/ocae149 PMID: 38934288

European Alliance for Innovation. (2025). Smart hospitals and quantum-enabled optimization frameworks. *EAI Endorsed Transactions on Smart Health*, *9*(34), e8.

Fahad, M., Ibrar, M., Qayyum, M. U., & Husnain, A. (2024). Artificial intelligence in healthcare: Revealing novel approaches to cancer treatment, fraud investigation, and petroleum industry perspectives. *International Journal of Multidisciplinary Sciences and Arts*, *3*(4), 37–45. DOI: 10.47709/ijmdsa.v3i4.4637

Fairburn, S. C., Jehi, L., Bicknell, B. T., Wilkes, B. G., & Panuganti, B. (2025). Applications of quantum computing in clinical care: Enhancing diagnostics, treatment, and decision-making. *Frontiers in Medicine*, *12*, 1573016. DOI: 10.3389/fmed.2025.1573016

Gupta, R. S.. (2025). A systematic review of quantum machine learning for digital health and clinical decision support. *npj Digital Medicine*.

Keerthana, R., Savitha, S., Logeswaran, K., Rajivkannan, A., & Namasivayam, M. (2025). AI Technologies for Predicting Susceptibility and Outcomes of Immunological Disorders. In AI-Assisted Computational Approaches for Immunological Disorders (pp. 107-142). IGI Global Scientific Publishing. DOI: 10.4018/979-8-3693-9725-1.ch004

McArdle, S., Endo, S., Aspuru-Guzik, A., Benjamin, S. C., & Yuan, X. (2020). Quantum computational chemistry. *Reviews of Modern Physics*, *92*(1), 015003. DOI: 10.1103/RevModPhys.92.015003

Mei, P., & Zhang, F. (2024). A framework for processing large-scale health data in medical higher-order correlation mining by quantum computing in smart healthcare. *Frontiers in Digital Health*, *6*, 1502745. DOI: 10.3389/fdgth.2024.1502745 PMID: 39633967

Nałęcz-Charkiewicz, K., Charkiewicz, K., & Nowak, R. M. (2024). Quantum computing in bioinformatics: A systematic review. *Briefings in Bioinformatics*, *25*(5), bbae391. DOI: 10.1093/bib/bbae391 PMID: 39140856

Nordmann, K., Redlich, M. C., Schaller, M., Sauter, S., & Fischer, F. (2025). Toward a conceptual framework for digitally supported communication, coordination, cooperation, and collaboration in interprofessional health care: Scoping review. *Journal of Medical Internet Research*, *27*(1), e69276. Advance online publication. DOI: 10.2196/69276 PMID: 40418789

Osorio, C., Fuster, N., Chen, W., Men, Y., & Juan, A. A. (2024). Enhancing accessibility to analytics courses in higher education through AI, simulation, and e-collaborative tools. *Information (Basel)*, *15*(8), 430. DOI: 10.3390/info15080430

Pattanaik, P., Himanshu, U., Bhushan, B., Thakur, M., & Pani, A. K. (2024). A study of the adoption behaviour of an electronic health information exchange system for a green economy. *International Journal of Logistics*, *27*(4), 512–537. DOI: 10.1080/13675567.2021.2008336

Qaddumi, B., Ayaad, O., Al-Ma'aitah, M. A., Akhu-Zaheya, L., & Alloubani, A. (2021). The factors affecting team effectiveness in hospitals: The mediating role of using electronic collaborative tools. *Journal of Interprofessional Education & Practice*, *24*, 100449. Advance online publication. DOI: 10.1016/j.xjep.2021.100449

Rasool, M., Ahmad, H. F., Ahmed, M., & Khan, S. (2023). Quantum-assisted drug discovery and molecular simulation for personalized medicine. *Journal of Molecular Modeling*, *29*(8), 215. DOI: 10.1007/s00894-023-05512-9

Risvas, C., & Spanoudaki, K. (2025). *Quantum computing in medicine: From molecular simulation to global health systems*. Springer Nature., DOI: 10.1007/978-3-031-56789-2

Savitha, S., Kannan, A. R., & Logeswaran, K. (2025). Augmenting Cardiovascular Disease Prediction Through CWCF Integration Leveraging Harris Hawks Search in Deep Belief Networks. *Cognitive Computation*, *17*(1), 52. DOI: 10.1007/s12559-025-10406-4

Savitha, S., Keerthana, R., Logeswaran, K., Vennila, V., Manjuladevi, R., & Sangeetha, M. (2025). Sustainable AI-Powered Systems and Cybersecurity for Health Diagnostics: Addressing Bias and Fairness in AI for Early Disease Detection. In AI-Driven Healthcare Cybersecurity and Privacy (pp. 205-244). IGI Global Scientific Publishing.

Senn, H. M., & Thiel, W. (2009). QM/MM methods for biomolecular systems. *Angewandte Chemie International Edition*, *48*(7), 1198–1229. DOI: 10.1002/anie.200802019 PMID: 19173328

Solenov, D., Brieler, J., & Scherrer, J. F. (2018). The potential of quantum computing and machine learning to advance clinical research and change the practice of medicine. *Mie Medical Journal*, *115*(5), 463–467. PMID: 30385997

Tirado-Domínguez, P., Perdomo-Ortiz, A., & Orús, R. (2025). Quantum approximate optimization algorithms for large-scale scheduling and healthcare logistics. *arXiv*. https://arxiv.org/abs/2501.04567

Wagner, G., Ringeval, M., Raymond, L., & Paré, G. (2025). Digital health competences and AI beliefs as conditions for the practice of evidence-based medicine: A study of prospective physicians in Canada. *Medical Education Online*, *30*(1), 2459910. Advance online publication. DOI: 10.1080/10872981.2025.2459910 PMID: 39890587

Wang, D., & Qin, Q. (2024). Artificial intelligence technology on layered water injection in oilfield development process. *International Journal of e-Collaboration*, *20*(1), 1–15. DOI: 10.4018/IJeC.352596

World Economic Forum. (2023). *Quantum computing applications in healthcare and life sciences*. World Economic Forum.

Yuan, K. (2024). Research on music teaching systems assisted by artificial intelligence. *International Journal of e-Collaboration*, *20*(1), 1–17. DOI: 10.4018/IJeC.349746

Zhang, Y., Li, X., & Chen, Z. (2025). Quantum signal processing for high-dimensional medical imaging. *IEEE Transactions on Medical Imaging*, *44*(2), 456–469. DOI: 10.1109/TMI.2024.3398765

Chapter 12
Enhancing EHR Systems With Artificial Intelligence:
Enabling Seamless Patient–Clinician Collaboration

Gurpreet Singh
http://orcid.org/0009-0000-4011-8626
Guru Kashi University, Talwandi Sabo, India

Vakil Singh
http://orcid.org/0009-0007-1198-0250
Guru Kashi University, Talwandi Sabo, India

Honey
Multani Mal Modi College, Patiala, India

ABSTRACT

The integration of artificial intelligence (AI) into electronic health record (EHR) systems is reshaping how patients and clinicians interact, making healthcare more collaborative, efficient, and personalized. Traditional EHRs often burden clinicians with documentation and fragmented data, leaving patients as passive participants. AI transforms this dynamic through intelligent automation, predictive analytics, and natural language processing that extract insights, streamline workflows, and enhance communication. Clinicians can detect early warning signs, recommend tailored treatments, and focus more on patient care, while AI-driven dashboards and chatbots help patients understand their data, engage in shared decisions, and track progress. Yet, challenges such as privacy, bias, and transparency require strong

DOI: 10.4018/979-8-3373-5906-9.ch012

governance and ethical design. This chapter examines how responsibly integrating AI into EHRs can bridge the gap between data and care, strengthen trust, and promote equitable, human-centered healthcare.

1. INTRODUCTION AND BACKGROUND

EHRs are among the most transformative innovations in modern healthcare, representing a shift from paper-based charts to fully digital systems. Originally developed as comprehensive repositories of patient information, EHRs were designed to reduce medical errors, improve efficiency, support evidence-based decision-making, and enhance continuity of care across institutions (Evans, 2016). Their origins date back to the 1960s and 1970s in academic medical centers, where pioneering systems such as the Problem-Oriented Medical Record (POMR) introduced structured clinical documentation as a foundation for digital record-keeping (Rector et al., 1991). By the early 2000s, these efforts evolved into national adoption initiatives, such as the United States' Health Information Technology for Economic and Clinical Health (HITECH) Act of 2009, which encouraged certified EHR use and expanded digital health infrastructure (Adler-Milstein & Jha, 2017). Similar programs in the United Kingdom, Canada, and Australia established EHRs as the digital backbone of modern healthcare.

Despite these advances, traditional EHRs often fall short of expectations. Clinicians report frustration with complex interfaces, excessive documentation, and workflow disruptions, spending nearly twice as much time on EHRs as on direct patient care, which contributes to burnout and reduced job satisfaction (Bodenheimer & Sinsky, 2014). Interoperability remains a significant challenge, as proprietary systems create information silos that hinder data sharing across institutions (Evans, 2016). Poorly optimized systems also cause alert fatigue, where critical notifications are lost in a flood of irrelevant warnings (McGreevey et al., 2020). From the patient perspective, portals are often delayed, incomplete, or presented in technical language that is difficult to understand, limiting engagement and shared decision-making, even though active patient participation is known to improve adherence, satisfaction, and clinical outcomes (Kruse et al., 2015). In many cases, EHRs function more as digital archives than as tools that actively support healthcare delivery.

AI provides an opportunity to transform EHRs into dynamic and interactive systems. Natural Language Processing (NLP) can structure free-text clinical notes to enable advanced searches, automated summaries, and real-time clinical coding (Mehta & Devarakonda, 2018). Predictive analytics can help identify high-risk patients and forecast disease progression (Rajkomar et al., 2019). Conversational agents and voice-based assistants can simplify clinician documentation and provide patients with clear, personalized explanations (El-Kareh & Sittig, 2022). AI-driven clinical decision support systems can flag drug interactions, recommend diagnostic tests, and offer evidence-based treatment suggestions. Integration of genomics, imaging, wearable sensors, and behavioral data expands EHR capabilities toward precision medicine and holistic, patient-centered care (Björnsson et al., 2019). By adding intelligence and interactivity, AI transforms EHRs from static repositories into collaborative partners that support real-time decision-making, personalized insights, and proactive interventions. Table 1 presents a comparison between traditional and AI-enhanced EHR systems.

Table 1. Comparison of Traditional vs. AI-Enhanced EHR Systems

Dimension	Traditional EHR Systems	AI-Enhanced EHR Systems
Primary Function	Documentation and storage	Intelligent collaboration and decision support
Clinician Experience	High documentation burden, fragmented workflows	Automated note generation, predictive alerts, intuitive dashboards
Patient Engagement	Static portals, delayed access, limited understanding	Conversational agents, real-time access, personalized insights
Data Utilization	Structured fields, limited interoperability	Multimodal integration (EHR, imaging, genomics, wearables)
Decision Support	Rule-based, often generic	AI-driven, context-aware, explainable recommendations
Impact on Outcomes	Variable improvements, persistent inefficiencies	Enhanced safety, personalization, and collaborative decision-making

2. CHALLENGES OF TRADITIONAL ELECTRONIC HEALTH RECORD SYSTEMS

EHRs are central to modern healthcare, but their widespread adoption has revealed persistent challenges across technical, organizational, and human-centered domains. While EHRs were designed to improve efficiency, safety, and coordination of care, research shows that they often introduce new burdens and inefficiencies affecting clinicians, patients, and health systems alike (Shanafelt et al., 2016). One of the most pressing issues is the documentation burden. Clinicians must enter extensive structured data through rigid templates that do not reflect the dynamic nature of medical practice. Studies indicate that physicians may spend nearly twice as much time on EHRs as on direct patient care, leading to frustration, fatigue, and professional burnout. This focus on screens rather than patients disrupts natural clinical interactions and can inhibit innovation by turning dynamic encounters into mechanical data-entry tasks (Rajkomar et al., 2019). Figure 1 illustrates the key challenges commonly associated with traditional EHR systems.

Figure 1. Key Challenges in Traditional EHR Systems

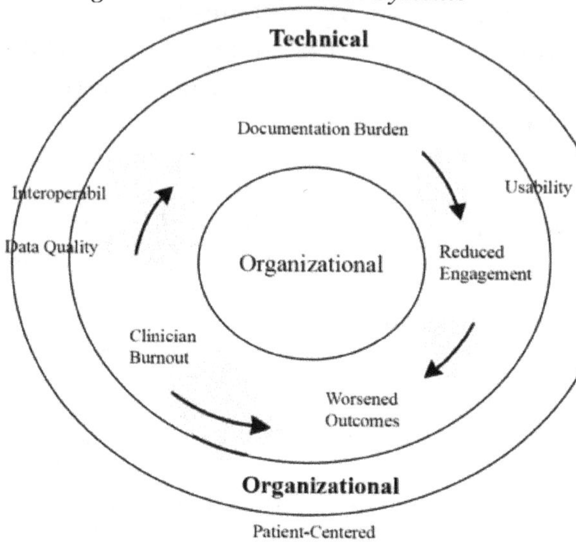

Closely related is the issue of usability. Many EHR systems have poorly designed interfaces, redundant processes, and unintuitive navigation, which makes it difficult for clinicians to locate critical information efficiently. This increases cognitive load, delays decision-making, and can raise the risk of diagnostic errors. Interoperability also remains a significant challenge. Despite standards such as HL7 FHIR, proprietary systems and inconsistent implementation create information silos that limit the seamless transfer of patient data, leading to redundant testing and incomplete clinical histories (Adler-Milstein & Jha, 2017; Alruwaili, 2020).

Information overload and alert fatigue further hinder EHR effectiveness. Clinical decision support tools generate alerts for drug interactions, abnormal laboratory results, or guideline deviations, yet excessive and often redundant alerts desensitize clinicians, with fewer than ten percent acted upon in some studies, increasing the risk that critical warnings are missed. From the patient perspective, portals often provide delayed or incomplete access to information and present it in technical language that is difficult to understand, limiting engagement and shared decision-making (Kruse et al., 2015). Data quality and completeness also remain concerns, as EHRs may contain missing, duplicated, or outdated entries, while important contextual information such as social determinants of health is frequently underrepresented. Ethical, legal, and cybersecurity issues further complicate the use of EHRs, including questions of data ownership, informed consent, liability, and vulnerability to cyberattacks (Mehta & Devarakonda, 2018). As summarized in Table 2, These challenges demonstrate that traditional EHRs often act as static repositories rather than intelligent, adaptive systems. Addressing these issues is crucial for the development of next-generation AI-enhanced EHRs that can support integrated, collaborative, and predictive healthcare.

Table 2. Key Challenges of Traditional EHR Systems

Challenge	Description	Impact on Care	Illustrative Example
Documentation Burden	Rigid templates require excessive data entry	Increases burnout, reduces patient–clinician time	Physicians spend 2× more time on EHRs than patient care 33
Usability	Poorly designed dashboards and navigation	Increases cognitive load, risk of diagnostic/medication errors	Misfiled radiology reports due to interface complexity 66
Interoperability	Vendor silos and poor standards adoption	Fragmented records, duplication of tests, incomplete medical histories	VA–DoD system interoperability failures 99
Information Overload	Excessive alerts from decision support	Alert fatigue, clinicians miss critical warnings	Fewer than 10% of alerts acted upon in hospital studies 1212
Patient Engagement	Static portals with delayed or jargon-heavy results	Patients remain passive, limited collaboration	Diabetic patients unable to interpret lab values 1515
Data Quality & Completeness	Duplicated, outdated, or missing information	Weakens predictive models and analytics, undermines population health insights	Missing social determinants of health in most EHRs 1818
Ethical & Legal Issues	Unclear data ownership, weak consent processes, high cybersecurity risks	Reduces trust, exposes patients to breaches, complicates liability	40M+ patient records exposed in ransomware attacks (2021) 2121

3. INTEGRATION OF ARTIFICIAL INTELLIGENCE INTO EHRS

AI represents one of the most disruptive forces in the transformation of digital healthcare, and EHRs are a particularly important domain for its application. EHRs were originally designed as centralized repositories for clinical documentation, but their evolution has been limited by documentation burden, fragmented usability, and insufficient support for actionable decision-making. Integrating AI transforms these systems from passive data storage tools into intelligent, collaborative ecosystems capable of supporting predictive, personalized, and interactive healthcare delivery.

AI-enhanced EHRs enable seamless collaboration between clinicians and patients, facilitate real-time insights, and prepare healthcare systems for the transition toward precision and value-based care (Olusegun et al., 2024; Mehta & Devarakonda, 2018). NLP is a major frontier in this transformation. Approximately eighty percent of EHR data is unstructured, including physician notes, imaging narratives, and pathology reports (Kreimeyer et al., 2017). Traditional EHRs are largely unable to leverage this unstructured corpus, which results in underutilized knowledge. NLP algorithms extract structured information from free-text notes, automatically generate ICD codes, and detect adverse drug events, reducing the documentation burden and allowing clinicians to focus more on direct patient care (Mehta & Devarakonda, 2018). For patients, NLP-driven tools simplify medical text, providing accessible explanations of laboratory results, treatment plans, and discharge instructions, which promotes understanding and engagement.

Predictive analytics and AI-powered clinical decision support further expand the capabilities of EHRs. Predictive models leverage longitudinal data to forecast outcomes such as hospital readmissions, disease progression, sepsis, or acute kidney injury, enabling timely and potentially life-saving interventions. Beyond acute care, predictive analytics informs chronic disease management by identifying high-risk patients and guiding preventive strategies that improve population health and reduce costs. AI-driven CDS systems analyze multimodal data, including labs, imaging, genomics, and wearable sensors, to generate context-sensitive, personalized recommendations. In oncology, these tools integrate tumor genomic profiles with treatment guidelines to suggest individualized therapies, while in cardiology, deep learning models continuously analyze electrocardiographic data to predict arrhythmias and support timely interventions. Explainability is essential, as transparent recommendations increase clinician trust and ensure ethical compliance (Doshi-Velez & Kim, 2017). Conversational AI and intelligent virtual assistants complement these tools by offering intuitive interfaces. Clinicians can use voice commands to query patient histories, order tests, or generate encounter summaries, reducing cognitive load and documentation time by up to thirty percent (Kruse et al., 2015). Patients benefit from chatbots embedded in portals that provide interactive explanations, tailored health coaching, and support for chronic disease management, extending engagement beyond the clinical encounter.

AI also enables the integration of heterogeneous healthcare data into comprehensive patient profiles. Genomics, radiology, pathology, and behavioral data from wearable devices, which are often siloed, can be combined through AI methods such as deep learning and knowledge graphs to generate unified patient profiles (Björnsson et al., 2019). Digital twins, which are virtual patient models that simulate physiology and disease trajectories, represent an advanced application of this integration, allowing clinicians to test interventions in a virtual environment before applying them in practice, enhancing both safety and personalization. Security and privacy are strengthened through AI-driven monitoring, anomaly detection, and blockchain-based tamper-proof storage, ensuring compliance with HIPAA and GDPR regulations (Alruwaili, 2020). Despite these advantages, challenges remain. Black-box algorithms can undermine trust and complicate regulatory approval, workflow integration can disrupt clinical practice, and ethical concerns such as algorithmic bias, equitable access, and patient consent require careful governance.

Figure 2. Conceptual Model of AI Integration into EHRs

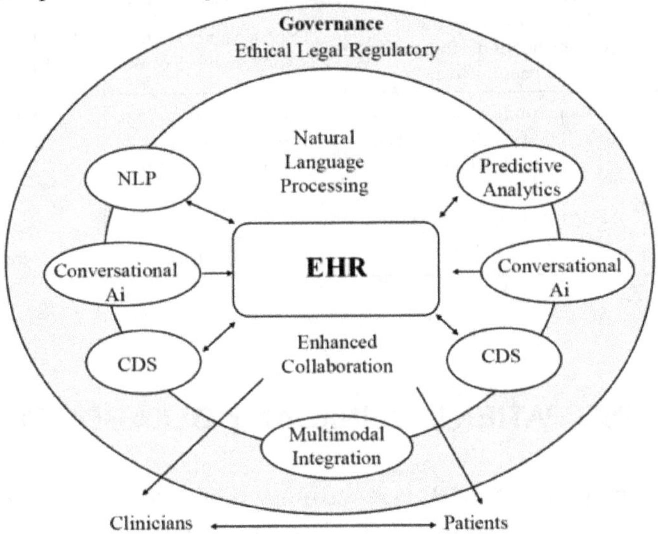

As illustrated in Figure 2, The integration of AI into EHRs therefore represents both a technological and sociotechnical transformation. By combining NLP, predictive analytics, conversational systems, CDS, multimodal data fusion, and advanced cybersecurity, AI-enhanced EHRs shift from static repositories to dynamic, collaborative ecosystems. Achieving this vision requires not only innovation in algorithms but also deliberate attention to interoperability, explainability, equity, and human-centered design. The future of healthcare depends on developing systems that are intelligent, ethical, inclusive, and trustworthy, capable of improving outcomes for both clinicians and patients. Applications of AI in EHR Systems has been shown in Table 3.

Table 3. Applications of AI in EHR Systems

AI Technique	Applications in EHRs	Benefits	Limitations / Challenges
Natural Language Processing (NLP)	Structured extraction of free-text notes, ICD coding, adverse event detection	Reduces documentation burden, enables secondary data use	Risk of misinterpretation; domain-specific variability
Predictive Analytics	Risk stratification, readmission prediction, early sepsis detection	Enables proactive care, reduces costs, improves outcomes	Requires high-quality data; risk of overfitting
Conversational AI	Voice commands for clinicians; chatbots for patients	Improves usability, increases engagement, reduces workload	Privacy concerns; accuracy of speech recognition
Clinical Decision Support (CDS)	Personalized treatment recommendations, integration of genomic data	Enhances precision medicine, reduces errors	Potential for alert fatigue if poorly designed
Multimodal Data Integration	Combining genomics, imaging, wearable data, and behavioral data	Enables precision medicine, supports digital twin simulations	Technical complexity; interoperability limitations
Security & Privacy	AI-driven anomaly detection; blockchain integration	Protects sensitive data, ensures compliance, increases trust	High computational cost; evolving regulatory frameworks

4. FACILITATING PATIENT–CLINICIAN COLLABORATION

The integration of AI into EHRs is redefining collaboration between patients and clinicians in the digital health ecosystem. Traditional EHR systems, while essential for information storage, have historically positioned patients as passive recipients of data and clinicians as overburdened documenters navigating complex interfaces. This transactional and asymmetric relationship has limited opportunities for shared decision-making, personalized care, and sustained patient engagement. AI-enhanced EHRs transform this dynamic by embedding intelligence into communication pathways, decision support, and monitoring mechanisms, positioning the record itself as an active mediator of collaboration rather than a static repository (Rajkomar et al., 2019; Ye et al., 2024). AI-driven communication tools represent one of the most visible advancements in this transformation. Conversational agents embedded in EHRs allow patients to query their records in natural language, receiving plain-language explanations of laboratory results, diagnoses, or treatment options. For example, a patient newly diagnosed with diabetes can ask, "What does my HbA1c mean?" and receive both a numeric interpretation and contextual advice about diet and exercise. For clinicians, voice-enabled assistants streamline routine interactions by transcribing encounters, auto-completing structured fields, and retrieving relevant clinical guidelines without requiring navigation across multiple screens. These tools reduce cognitive burden, improve efficiency, and shift clinical interactions toward relationship-building rather than administrative tasks.

AI also enhances shared decision-making by integrating predictive analytics and outcome modeling directly into clinical conversations. Risk calculators embedded in EHR dashboards can display individualized probabilities of treatment outcomes, allowing patients and clinicians to weigh trade-offs together. In cardiovascular care, An example of AI-supported decision making system shown in figure 3. AI models can illustrate how statin therapy reduces a patient's ten-year risk of myocardial infarction compared to lifestyle modification alone, presenting the information in interactive charts. In oncology, AI-enabled platforms integrate genomic data, tumor profiles, and clinical guidelines to provide patients with tailored therapeutic options, democratizing complex information that was previously inaccessible (Rajkomar et al., 2019). The integration of patient-generated health data (PGHD) further enhances collaboration. Wearables, mobile health applications, and home-monitoring devices produce continuous streams of behavioral and physiological data, including heart rate, glucose levels, sleep quality, and activity patterns. When combined with EHR data, AI algorithms detect deviations, predict exacerbations, and provide real-time feedback. Clinicians receive alerts about adherence or risk signals, while patients are nudged with reminders, lifestyle recommendations, or warnings when measurements exceed safe thresholds. This bidirectional flow transforms care from episodic, visit-centered interactions into continuous, participatory engagement, empowering patients and supporting proactive intervention (Ye et al., 2024).

Figure 3. AI-Supported Shared Decision-Making in EHRs

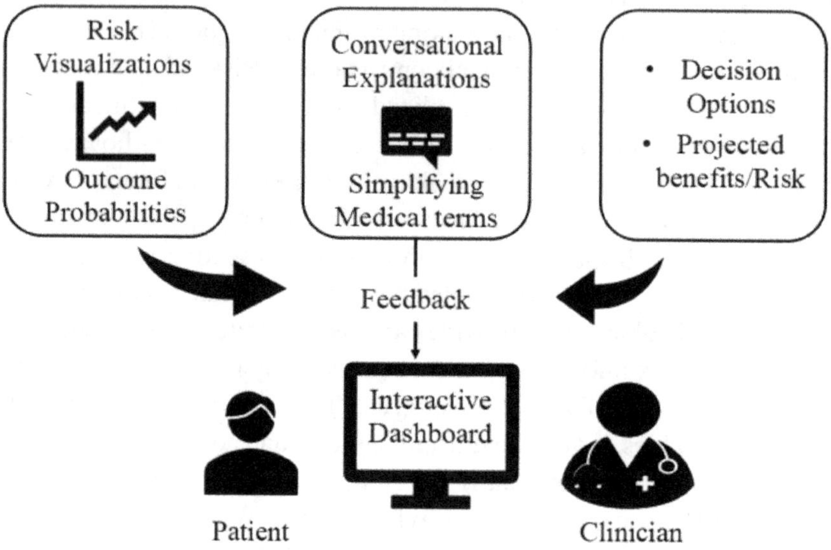

Telehealth integration has extended collaboration even further. AI-enhanced EHRs ensure that remote consultations are seamlessly connected to a patient's longitudinal record through automatically generated visit summaries, predictive alerts, and integration with monitoring devices. In chronic disease management, such as heart failure or chronic obstructive pulmonary disease, AI-driven tools detect early signs of decompensation during remote monitoring, enabling timely interventions and reducing hospitalizations. This ensures that digital care modalities complement rather than fragment traditional healthcare delivery (Ye et al., 2024). AI also addresses persistent challenges in patient health literacy. Many patients struggle to interpret laboratory results, diagnostic codes, or progress notes. AI-enabled systems can tailor explanations based on literacy level, cultural background, or individual health goals. For example, instead of presenting raw cholesterol values, the EHR can display a color-coded chart, contextual comparisons to healthy ranges, and actionable recommendations, such as "reducing saturated fats may lower this number." By adapting communication to the patient's needs, AI reduces disparities in understanding and ensures that information is actionable (Kruse et al., 2015).

Collectively, these AI-driven innovations reposition EHRs as collaborative platforms that facilitate continuous interaction between patients and clinicians. Rather than existing solely as administrative tools or static data repositories, AI-enhanced

EHRs support participatory healthcare grounded in communication, personalization, and shared accountability. This paradigm not only improves patient engagement and satisfaction but also strengthens clinical efficiency and safety, which are essential elements of a truly human-centered digital health ecosystem.As shown in Table 4, the evolution from traditional to AI-enhanced EHRs reflects a fundamental shift from transactional record-keeping to collaborative, patient-centered ecosystems. This transformation addresses long-standing barriers in communication, personalization, and continuity of care, ultimately fostering more equitable and participatory healthcare deliver

Table 4. From Transactional Records to Collaborative Ecosystems: Traditional vs. AI-Enhanced EHRs

Dimension	Traditional EHRs	AI-Enhanced EHRs	Barrier/Challenge Addressed	Illustrative Outcome
Patient Communication	Static portals, delayed results, jargon-heavy reports	Conversational agents, voice assistants, real-time plain-language explanations	Low health literacy, information delay	Patients query labs and receive tailored explanations
Clinical Decision Support	Rule-based alerts, high redundancy → alert fatigue	Context-aware, personalized, explainable recommendations	Excessive notifications, low trust	Targeted alerts reduce medication errors
Patient Engagement	Passive access to limited data	Interactive dashboards, tailored education, lifestyle coaching	Lack of personalization, poor motivation	Patients adhere to treatment via feedback loops
Data Integration	Fragmented structured data only	Fusion of EHR, genomics, imaging, wearable and app data	Data silos, incomplete records	Digital twin simulations for personalized therapy
Shared Decision-Making	Clinician-dominated, minimal patient input	Risk modeling, visual outcome projections, co-design of treatment plans	Power imbalance in decision-making	Patients actively select between therapies
Continuity of Care	Episodic, visit-centered	Continuous monitoring, predictive alerts, proactive interventions	Limited visibility between visits	Early detection of heart failure decompensation
Health Literacy Support	Complex medical terminology	Adaptive explanations (literacy-level, culture, language)	Misinterpretation, inequity	Color-coded lab summaries with actionable advice

5. FRAMEWORK FOR HUMAN-CENTERED AI IN EHR DESIGN

The integration of AI into EHRs requires more than technical sophistication; it must be guided by human-centered principles that emphasize usability, trust, transparency, and inclusivity. EHRs are no longer just tools for clinical documentation. They are evolving into intelligent ecosystems that support decision-making, collaboration, and patient empowerment. However, traditional EHRs have often created workflow inefficiencies, increased administrative burdens for clinicians, and limited patient participation. To address these long-standing challenges, AI should be embedded within EHRs through a structured and layered framework that balances technological progress with ethical and human considerations essential for adoption.

A four-layered human-centered framework for integrating AI into EHRs can help achieve this balance. The framework consists of the Data Layer, the AI Layer, the Collaboration Layer, and the Governance Layer, as shown in Figure 4. Each layer builds upon the one below it, transforming the system from raw data collection into ethical, intelligent, and patient-centered healthcare support. The framework emphasizes not only technical innovation but also human values such as trust, transparency, and inclusivity, ensuring that AI supports and enhances clinical practice rather than replacing human judgment.

Figure 4. Layered Framework for Human-Centered AI in EHRs

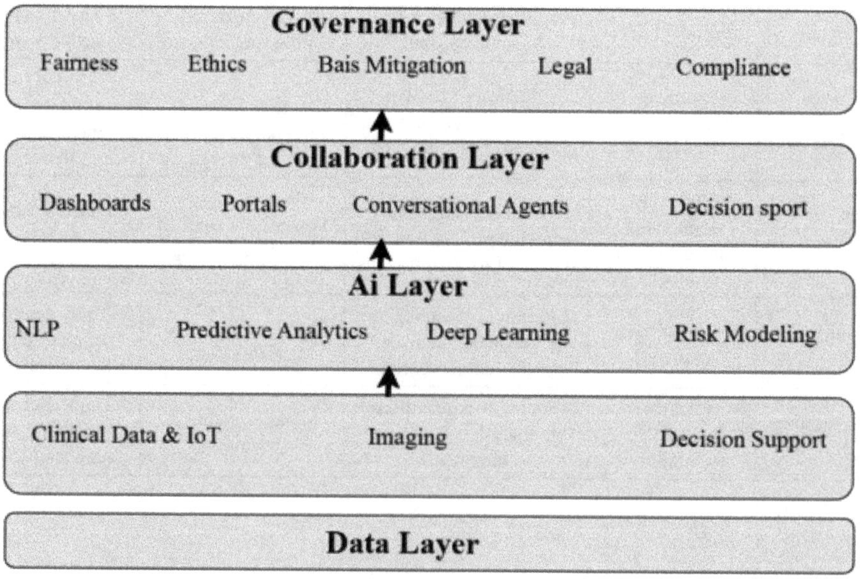

1. Data Layer

The Data Layer forms the foundation by aggregating diverse health information into a unified and interoperable repository. Traditional EHRs stored mainly structured data such as diagnoses, medications, and laboratory results. In contrast, modern healthcare generates a wide variety of data types, including unstructured clinical narratives, radiology and pathology reports, imaging repositories, genomic sequences, wearable and sensor-based data from the Internet of Things (IoT), and social determinants of health such as housing, education, and income. Without integrating these multimodal sources, AI insights risk being incomplete or biased. The Data Layer therefore emphasizes semantic interoperability and uses standards such as HL7 FHIR, SNOMED CT, and LOINC to harmonize formats and terminologies. It also employs secure data pipelines and real-time data synchronization to maintain data quality and timeliness. By ensuring completeness, consistency, and reliability, this foundational layer creates a robust infrastructure that supports accurate AI-driven insights (Ross et al., 2014).

2. AI Layer

Built upon the data foundation, the AI Layer converts raw information into clinically meaningful knowledge. It uses computational techniques such as natural language processing (NLP) to interpret unstructured text, predictive analytics to forecast outcomes, fuzzy reasoning to support decision-making under uncertainty, and explainable AI (XAI) to improve transparency (Kreimeyer et al., 2017; Doshi-Velez & Kim, 2017). This layer functions as the intelligence engine that detects subtle patterns, identifies early risks, and generates personalized treatment recommendations. Advanced deep learning models can integrate different data types, including text, images, and sensor readings, to support precision medicine. Interpretability is a key focus since complex or opaque models can reduce clinician confidence and accountability. Visualization techniques, counterfactual reasoning, and explanation tools such as LIME and SHAP make AI decisions easier to understand. The AI Layer therefore transforms EHRs from static databases into active systems that provide intelligent and interpretable guidance for clinical care (Rajkomar et al., 2019).

3. Collaboration Layer

The Collaboration Layer translates AI-generated insights into practical, user-centered experiences for clinicians and patients. It focuses on usability, visualization, and effective communication. For clinicians, AI outputs are delivered through intuitive dashboards, interactive charts, and context-sensitive alerts that draw attention to key information without causing cognitive overload. For patients, this layer offers accessible portals, virtual assistants, and educational tools that simplify medical data and encourage engagement. By converting complex predictions into understandable and actionable information, the Collaboration Layer supports shared decision-making and continuous patient involvement. For example, it can allow patients and clinicians to evaluate the outcomes of lifestyle changes compared to medication for managing cardiovascular risk. This layer also integrates patient-generated data, such as glucose readings and physical activity from wearable devices, creating real-time feedback loops that promote adherence and self-management. Through these interactions, EHRs evolve into participatory platforms that strengthen communication, empathy, and mutual understanding (Rajkomar et al., 2019).

4. Governance Layer

The Governance Layer ensures that AI-enhanced EHRs function in a safe, ethical, and equitable manner. Compliance with privacy and security laws such as HIPAA and GDPR is essential, but governance must also include principles of fairness, accountability, and inclusivity. This layer establishes mechanisms to detect algorithmic bias, audit AI recommendations, and ensure patient consent and data ownership. It includes continuous monitoring systems that evaluate AI performance and transparency in clinical workflows. Governance also addresses ethical and legal questions related to responsibility when AI influences clinical decisions. Inclusivity is another important dimension, ensuring that AI systems accommodate differences in language, literacy, accessibility, and cultural norms. These measures help build trust and ensure that both clinicians and patients can engage with AI technologies responsibly and confidently (Obermeyer et al., 2019).

Together, these four layers form a holistic ecosystem for embedding AI into EHR systems. The Data Layer ensures completeness and interoperability. The AI Layer generates meaningful insights from complex data. The Collaboration Layer delivers those insights through user-friendly interactions, and the Governance Layer ensures that the entire system operates ethically, transparently, and fairly. By combining these layers, the framework addresses the weaknesses of traditional EHRs, such as inefficiency and limited engagement, and lays the foundation for intelligent, inclusive, and participatory healthcare that aligns technology with human-centered values and clinical excellence.

6. CHALLENGES AND ETHICAL CONSIDERATIONS

The integration of AI into EHRs promises a new era of personalized, data-driven, and efficient healthcare. However, the path toward this transformation is filled with complex challenges that are technical, ethical, organizational, and societal in nature. Unlike earlier EHR limitations focused on usability and interoperability, the introduction of AI brings deeper concerns regarding fairness, transparency, data governance, clinician autonomy, and patient trust. If not addressed comprehensively, these issues could undermine not only the safety and reliability of AI systems but also the broader vision of equitable digital healthcare. The following sections analyze the major challenges associated with AI-driven EHRs from both research and governance perspectives. These challenges highlight the complex intersection of technology, ethics, and clinical practice that must be addressed to ensure that AI adoption in healthcare remains safe, transparent, and equitable.

1. Data Privacy and Security

The growing reliance on AI-enhanced EHRs intensifies concerns related to data privacy and cybersecurity. Health records contain highly sensitive personal and medical information, including diagnostic histories, prescriptions, genomic data, and behavioral assessments. The use of AI requires large volumes of such data for model training and optimization, consequently expanding the risk of exposure and unauthorized access (Alruwaili, 2020). Breaches not only compromise patient confidentiality but also erode institutional trust and can lead to identity theft, insurance discrimination, and reputational damage to healthcare organizations. Moreover, the secondary use of medical data by insurers, pharmaceutical companies, or commercial entities raises complex ethical questions about ownership, informed consent, and data monetization. Technologies such as federated learning and blockchain have been introduced to address these vulnerabilities (Shickel et al., 2018). Federated learning enables AI models to learn collaboratively from distributed data sources without transferring raw patient information, while blockchain ensures traceability, immutability, and decentralized control of data transactions. However, these innovations remain in early stages of deployment, and disparities in digital infrastructure mean that smaller healthcare centers often lack the resources to implement them effectively. As a result, the uneven distribution of cybersecurity capabilities continues to perpetuate inequalities in patient data protection and digital resilience across healthcare systems.

2. Interoperability and Data Fragmentation

Interoperability continues to be a significant technical challenge in realizing effective AI-driven EHRs. Despite frameworks such as HL7 FHIR and SNOMED CT, healthcare systems often remain fragmented, with incompatible data structures and proprietary software that hinder seamless data exchange. For AI, this fragmentation limits model accuracy and reliability, as predictive algorithms depend on comprehensive, high-quality datasets (Shickel et al., 2018). Fragmented data can cause incomplete patient profiles, leading to misclassification or biased predictions. Variations in coding systems, data formats, and semantic standards further degrade the consistency of medical information. Overcoming this challenge requires both regulatory and technical strategies—enforcing interoperability standards, promoting vendor-neutral APIs, and developing harmonized data ontologies to unify multimodal datasets across institutions.

3. Clinician Trust, Autonomy, and Workflow Integration

AI technologies embedded in EHRs must earn clinician trust to achieve meaningful adoption. Physicians are trained to combine evidence-based medicine with clinical experience and patient interaction. When AI tools offer opaque recommendations or interfere with established workflows, they can threaten professional autonomy. Overreliance on automated outputs may lead to automation bias, while mistrust can result in the rejection of potentially valuable AI insights (Rajkomar et al., 2019). To sustain clinician engagement, AI systems should be designed as decision-support partners rather than replacements. Features such as transparent reasoning, user control, and human-in-the-loop oversight help preserve autonomy. Additionally, seamless workflow integration is essential. Systems that disrupt clinical routines or increase administrative burden risk diminishing efficiency and satisfaction rather than enhancing them (Bodenheimer & Sinsky, 2014).

4. Algorithmic Transparency and Accountability

Algorithmic opacity represents one of the most critical ethical dilemmas in AI adoption. Many AI models, especially deep learning architectures, operate as complex black boxes with limited interpretability (Doshi-Velez & Kim, 2017). In clinical settings, this opacity poses serious challenges for accountability, as it becomes difficult to determine responsibility when errors occur. The inability to explain algorithmic reasoning also affects clinician and patient trust. Explainable AI (XAI) approaches, including model interpretability frameworks and visualization tools, have emerged to improve transparency. However, achieving a balance between interpretability and predictive accuracy remains an unresolved issue. Transparent, auditable systems are essential to ensure clinicians can verify AI-driven recommendations, patients can understand their implications, and institutions can maintain ethical accountability in decision-making.

5. Equity, Fairness, and Dataset Bias

Bias in healthcare data is a major source of ethical concern. AI models trained on historical or demographically limited datasets can perpetuate systemic inequities. For example, research by Obermeyer et al. (2019) revealed that a widely used algorithm underestimated healthcare needs for Black patients compared to white patients with equivalent medical conditions. Similar gender and socioeconomic biases have been documented in diagnostic and treatment prediction systems (Shickel et al., 2018). Addressing these disparities requires the development of diverse and representative datasets, implementation of fairness metrics, and establishment of continuous bias auditing protocols. Inclusive governance frameworks that incorporate multidisciplinary oversight are also vital to ensure that AI technologies contribute to health equity rather than reinforce existing disparities.

6. Alert Fatigue and Cognitive Overload

One of the unintended consequences of AI integration in EHRs is the problem of alert fatigue. Traditional decision support systems already overwhelm clinicians with excessive alerts, many of which are low in clinical value. Poorly configured AI models may intensify this issue by generating probabilistic alerts based on predictive analytics, leading to cognitive overload and desensitization (Rajkomar et al., 2019). This overexposure can cause critical warnings to be ignored, compromising patient safety. Effective AI-driven alert systems must employ context-aware mechanisms that dynamically adjust thresholds according to patient risk profiles and clinical context. Adaptive feedback loops and customizable settings can help ensure that alerts enhance decision-making rather than impede it.

7. Interconnected Nature of Challenges and Need for Governance

These challenges are deeply interconnected and must be addressed through comprehensive governance frameworks. Weaknesses in one area often amplify risks in others; for instance, poor interoperability can lead to biased outcomes, while lack of transparency undermines trust and accountability. Therefore, a holistic governance approach is essential, integrating technical safeguards, ethical guidelines, clinician participation, and patient-centered design. Collaboration among policymakers, healthcare institutions, AI developers, and regulatory bodies will be critical in ensuring that the integration of AI in EHRs remains transparent, equitable, and sustainable. Only through such multidimensional governance can AI-driven EHRs truly fulfill their potential to transform healthcare responsibly and ethically.

7. FUTURE DIRECTIONS

The evolution of EHRs into AI-enhanced platforms is not merely an incremental development in digital health but represents a foundational shift toward intelligent, adaptive, and ethically governed ecosystems. While current implementations of AI have focused on documentation automation, predictive analytics, and conversational agents, the future trajectory points toward more comprehensive, multimodal, and participatory systems that will redefine how healthcare is delivered, experienced, and governed. Several technological and governance innovations are poised to reshape the next decade of EHR integration.LLMs stand at the forefront of this transformation. These models, trained on massive corpora with billions of parameters, can understand, generate, and synthesize human language at near-human levels. In healthcare, LLMs hold particular promise for streamlining clinical documentation, automating discharge summaries, and creating patient-friendly explanations of diagnoses and treatments. Within EHR environments, clinicians will be able to interact with records using natural language queries such as "Summarize this patient's cardiovascular risk factors and highlight recent abnormal labs," allowing coherent summaries to be generated in seconds. Patients may query their health data in accessible language, receiving explanations tailored to literacy levels and cultural contexts. While LLMs are powerful, risks of hallucinations, bias propagation, and medico-legal uncertainty remain. Safe deployment requires integration with explainable AI (XAI) frameworks, auditability mechanisms, and institutional safeguards to ensure outputs are reliable and trustworthy. Recent advances in large language models demonstrate their ability to encode clinical knowledge and support decision-making within EHR environments (Singhal et al., 2023).

Another transformative frontier is the concept of digital twins, which are dynamic, virtual representations of patients integrating physiological signals, imaging, genomics, and lifestyle metrics. These models enable real-time simulation of disease progression, testing of therapeutic interventions, and personalized treatment planning. Oncology digital twins can simulate tumor responses to different chemotherapy regimens, while cardiac models can optimize arrhythmia management. Population-level digital twins can also simulate epidemics, optimize vaccine deployment, and evaluate policy interventions before real-world implementation. Deploying digital twins at scale requires substantial computational resources, standardized data pipelines, rigorous validation, and careful consideration of ethical issues such as consent, ownership, and secondary use of insights (Obermeyer et al., 2019; Bruynseels et al., 2018). The success of both LLMs and digital twins relies heavily on multimodal data integration. While traditional EHRs focus on structured fields such as lab results and diagnosis codes, modern healthcare produces diverse streams from imaging, genomics, proteomics, wearables, and patient-reported outcomes (Shickel et al., 2018). AI allows these data to be unified into holistic patient profiles, improving predictive accuracy and clinical understanding. For example, integrating wearable activity data, continuous glucose monitoring, and genetic markers could enhance diabetes prevention strategies. Effective visualization is crucial; multimodal dashboards must simplify complex information into actionable insights without overwhelming users. Human–computer interaction design and careful alignment with clinical workflows are essential to translating data richness into practical decision support.

Federated learning provides a privacy-preserving approach for AI model development, enabling models to be trained across multiple institutions without centralizing sensitive data (Yang et al., 2019). Only model updates are shared, which reduces breach risks and allows smaller clinics to participate in collaborative learning without giving up data ownership. Federated learning has been piloted in radiology, oncology, and cardiology, demonstrating feasibility. Challenges remain, including communication overhead, bias from heterogeneous local datasets, and intellectual property considerations. Despite these, federated learning represents a scalable approach that balances innovation and privacy. Technology alone cannot ensure responsible adoption. Ethical governance frameworks are critical to ensure that AI-enhanced EHRs advance healthcare fairly, transparently, and inclusively (Obermeyer et al., 2019). Governance must clarify liability in AI-supported decisions, enforce algorithmic accountability, and protect patient autonomy. Regulatory agencies such as the FDA and the EU's AI Act are developing guidelines for adaptive AI oversight in healthcare. Continuous auditing and fairness assessments are essential to detect and mitigate bias, while transparency requirements help clinicians and patients understand AI recommendations. Consent must evolve from static, one-time forms to dynamic processes that allow patients to manage permissions actively. Inclusivity must remain central to prevent systemic biases that have historically disadvantaged vulnerable populations.

Emerging directions including LLMs, digital twins, multimodal integration, federated learning, and ethical governance outline a roadmap for the next stage of EHR evolution as shown in Figure 5. The vision is of an ecosystem where data flows seamlessly across institutions, is analyzed in real time by interpretable AI models, and is presented in ways that empower clinicians and patients to make collaborative, informed decisions. AI-enhanced EHRs will not merely document healthcare interactions but anticipate risks, personalize care, and support proactive health management. Achieving this potential requires balancing technological capability with commitments to ethics, privacy, equity, and trust, creating systems that are intelligent, participatory, and patient-centered.

Figure 5. Roadmap of Future Directions for AI-Enhanced EHRs

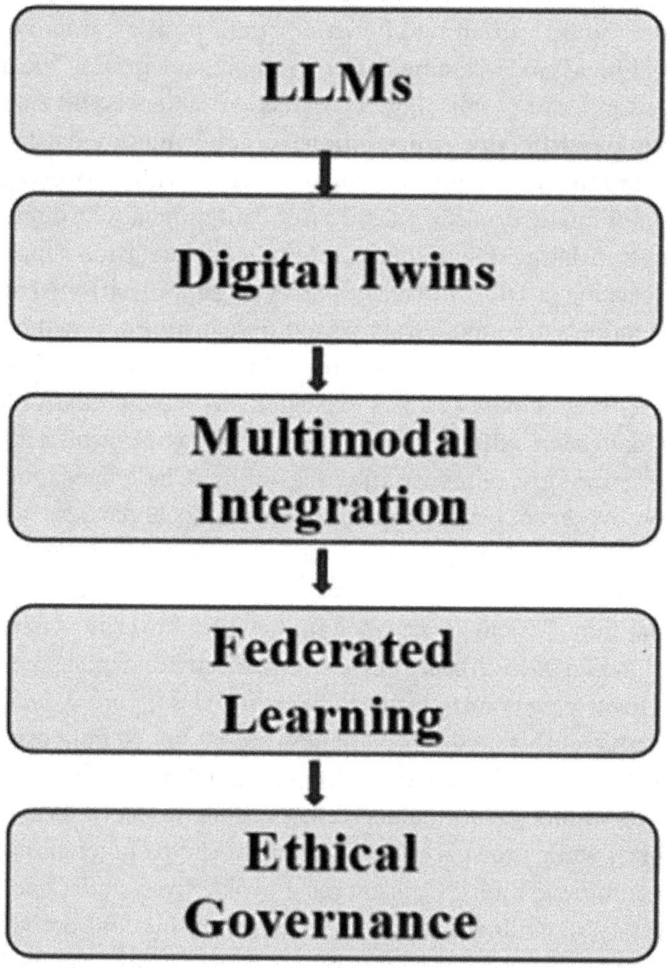

Table 5 summarizes major prior studies on AI-enabled EHR systems, highlighting their contributions and remaining limitations that motivate the need for human-centered, collaborative, and ethically governed AI–EHR frameworks.

Table 5. Major AI–EHR Studies, Applications, Outcomes, and Limitations

Study (Author, Year)	AI Application in EHRs	Key Outcomes/Contributions	Limitations / Research Gaps
Rajkomar et al., 2019	Machine learning for clinical prediction using EHR data	Demonstrated improved prediction of mortality, readmission, and length of stay using deep learning models	Limited external validation across diverse healthcare systems; challenges in interpretability and workflow integration
Fleuren et al., 2020	Machine learning models for sepsis prediction	Early detection of sepsis with improved sensitivity and timeliness compared to traditional scoring systems	High false-positive rates in some settings; requires high-quality real-time data and clinician trust
Kreimeyer et al., 2017	Natural Language Processing for unstructured clinical notes	Enabled extraction of structured information from free-text EHR data; improved coding and clinical documentation	Domain-specific variability; accuracy dependent on training datasets; limited real-time deployment
Obermeyer et al., 2019	Algorithmic risk prediction in population health management	Highlighted racial bias in widely used healthcare prediction algorithms; emphasized fairness concerns	Demonstrated systemic bias in datasets; need for fairness auditing and diverse training data
Björnsson et al., 2019	Digital twins and multimodal integration	Introduced concept of patient-specific digital twins for personalized medicine and predictive simulation	Early-stage implementation; requires large multimodal datasets and computational infrastructure
Yang et al., 2019	Federated learning for healthcare data	Enabled collaborative AI training without sharing raw patient data, improving privacy protection	Communication overhead, heterogeneous data challenges, limited large-scale clinical deployment
El-Kareh & Sittig, 2022	AI-enabled clinical decision support	Improved diagnostic accuracy and decision-making support through AI-driven CDS tools	Risk of alert fatigue, workflow disruption, and overreliance on automated recommendations
Ye et al., 2024	Integration of patient-generated data with EHRs using AI	Demonstrated enhanced clinical decision support and patient monitoring through wearable and home data integration	Data standardization issues; interoperability and privacy concerns across platforms
Gabriel & Precious, 2025	AI integration into clinical workflows	Identified barriers and best practices for integrating AI into hospital systems	Limited empirical outcome data; need for cost-effectiveness and scalability evaluation

8. CONCLUSION

AI is fundamentally reshaping the trajectory of digital health by transforming EHRs from static repositories of information into dynamic, intelligent ecosystems. What began as the digitization of paper-based records has matured into an era where EHRs are expected not only to store and retrieve clinical information but also to reason, predict, and interact with both clinicians and patients in meaningful ways. This transformation addresses persistent limitations of traditional EHRs, including usability concerns, fragmented workflows, information overload, and clinician burnout. By embedding AI capabilities such as natural language processing, predictive analytics, conversational agents, and decision-support algorithms, EHRs evolve into collaborative environments that augment human expertise while keeping patients at the center of their care journey. For clinicians, AI-enhanced EHRs reduce the burden of manual documentation through automated note generation, highlight clinically relevant data via intelligent summarization, and deliver timely alerts that anticipate adverse events. For patients, AI-enabled systems translate complex medical jargon into comprehensible insights, enhancing health literacy and fostering active engagement in decision-making. This dual utility reflects a democratization of health information, bridging the gap between professional expertise and patient understanding, while facilitating shared decision-making and continuous collaboration to operationalize long-standing policy goals in patient-centered care.

Despite these advantages, the transformation introduces challenges that extend beyond technical barriers into ethical, legal, and social domains. Privacy and security remain critical concerns as increasingly sensitive health data, including genomics, imaging, and behavioral histories, are aggregated across systems. Trust in AI recommendations must be built through transparency, explainability, and the preservation of clinician autonomy. Bias and equity issues require deliberate safeguards, as algorithms trained on incomplete or skewed datasets risk perpetuating systemic disparities in access and outcomes. Interoperability continues to challenge integration, as vendor lock-in and inconsistent implementation of standards limit seamless exchange of longitudinal health records. Without comprehensive solutions, these risks could undermine adoption and erode confidence in AI-enhanced systems. LLMs are poised to revolutionize clinical workflows by synthesizing entire patient histories into concise, actionable insights and enabling intuitive natural-language queries within EHRs. Digital twins promise personalized, predictive healthcare by simulating disease progression and treatment responses in silico. Multimodal data integration, including imaging, genomics, wearables, and patient-reported outcomes, will provide holistic representations of individual health, fostering proactive strategies for disease prevention and precision medicine. Federated learning represents a paradigm shift in model development, allowing institutions to collaborate in AI training while preserving local data privacy. These innovations require robust ethical governance frameworks to ensure fairness, accountability, and inclusivity, supported by adaptive regulations such as the EU AI Act and FDA guidelines. The integration of AI into EHRs is not about replacing human expertise but extending it, offering clinicians computational intelligence that supports diagnostic accuracy, treatment planning, and patient engagement, while redefining patients as informed collaborators in a transparent, continuous, and participatory process This evolution enables a shift from reactive care models to proactive ecosystems that anticipate risks, prevent disease, and personalize interventions .

The global implications of AI-enhanced EHRs are considerable. In high-resource settings, these systems may optimize efficiency, enable precision medicine, and reduce costs through predictive care pathways In low- and middle-income countries, where workforce and infrastructure constraints hinder healthcare delivery, AI-enhanced systems can extend expertise via decision-support tools, facilitate remote monitoring, and narrow inequities in access to quality care. Realizing this potential requires scalable, affordable, and inclusive systems that bridge gaps in health outcomes rather than exacerbate disparities. Achieving this vision depends on multidisciplinary collaboration. Policymakers must craft adaptive regulations balancing innovation with safeguards. Developers must create secure, explainable, and interoperable systems. Clinicians must actively participate in system design to ensure alignment with workflow and professional judgment. Patients must be empowered with access, literacy, and dynamic consent mechanisms that evolve alongside technology. Alignment among these stakeholders around transparency, fairness, and human-centered design is essential to realize the transformative promise of AI-enhanced EHRs. Artificial Intelligence offers not just the next stage of digital health innovation but a redefinition of medicine itself, making healthcare predictive, personalized, participatory, and profoundly human-centered. Addressing trust, privacy, transparency, equity, and usability allows systems to support seamless, real-time collaboration between patients and clinicians. The challenge ahead is immense, but the opportunity to build safer, smarter, and more equitable healthcare systems makes this journey both necessary and urgent.

REFERENCES

Adler-Milstein, J., & Jha, A. K. (2017). HITECH Act drove large gains in hospital electronic health record adoption. *Health Affairs*, *36*(8), 1416–1422. DOI: 10.1377/hlthaff.2016.1651 PMID: 28784734

Alruwaili, F. F. (2020). Artificial intelligence and multi-agent-based distributed ledger system for better privacy and security of electronic healthcare records. *PeerJ. Computer Science*, *6*, e323. DOI: 10.7717/peerj-cs.323 PMID: 33816973

Björnsson, B., Borrebaeck, C., Elander, N., Gasslander, T., Gawel, D. R., Gustafsson, M., Jörnsten, R., Lee, E. J., Li, X., Lilja, S., Martínez-Enguita, D., Matussek, A., Sandström, P., Schäfer, S., Stenmarker, M., Sun, X. F., Sysoev, O., Zhang, H., & Benson, M.Swedish Digital Twin Consortium. (2019). Digital twins to personalize medicine. *Genome Medicine*, *12*(1), 4. DOI: 10.1186/s13073-019-0701-3 PMID: 31892363

Bodenheimer, T., & Sinsky, C. (2014). From triple to quadruple aim: Care of the patient requires care of the provider. *Annals of Family Medicine*, *12*(6), 573–576. DOI: 10.1370/afm.1713 PMID: 25384822

Bruynseels, K., Santoni de Sio, F., & van den Hoven, J. (2018). Digital twins in health care: Ethical implications of an emerging engineering paradigm. *Frontiers in Genetics*, *9*, 31. DOI: 10.3389/fgene.2018.00031 PMID: 29487613

Doshi-Velez, F., & Kim, B. (2017). Towards a rigorous science of interpretable machine learning. *arXiv preprint* arXiv:1702.08608. https://arxiv.org/abs/1702.08608

El-Kareh, R., & Sittig, D. F. (2022). Enhancing diagnosis through technology: Decision support, artificial intelligence, and beyond. *Critical Care Clinics*, *38*(1), 129–139. DOI: 10.1016/j.ccc.2021.08.004 PMID: 34794627

Evans, R. S. (2016). Electronic health records: Then, now, and in the future. *Yearbook of Medical Informatics*, *26*(S 01, Suppl 1), S48–S61. DOI: 10.15265/IYS-2016-s006 PMID: 27199197

Fleuren, L. M., Klausch, T. L. T., Zwager, C. L., Schoonmade, L. J., Guo, T., Roggeveen, L. F., Swart, E. L., Girbes, A. R. J., Thoral, P., Ercole, A., Hoogendoorn, M., & Elbers, P. W. G. (2020). Machine learning for the prediction of sepsis: A systematic review and meta-analysis of diagnostic test accuracy. *Intensive Care Medicine*, *46*(3), 383–400. DOI: 10.1007/s00134-019-05872-y PMID: 31965266

Gabriel, I., & Precious, A. (2025). *Integration of artificial intelligence into clinical workflows: Barriers and best practices*. Obafemi Awolowo University.

Kreimeyer, K., Foster, M., Pandey, A., Arya, N., Halford, G., Jones, S. F., Forshee, R., Walderhaug, M., & Botsis, T. (2017). Natural language processing systems for capturing and standardizing unstructured clinical information: A systematic review. *Journal of Biomedical Informatics, 73*, 14–29. DOI: 10.1016/j.jbi.2017.07.012 PMID: 28729030

Kruse, C. S., Argueta, D. A., Lopez, L., & Nair, A. (2015). Patient and provider attitudes toward the use of patient portals for the management of chronic disease: A systematic review. *Journal of Medical Internet Research, 17*(2), e40. DOI: 10.2196/jmir.3703 PMID: 25707035

McGreevey, J. D.III, Mallozzi, C. P., Perkins, R. M., Shelov, E., & Schreiber, R. (2020). Reducing alert burden in electronic health records: State of the art recommendations from four health systems. *Applied Clinical Informatics, 11*(1), 1–12. DOI: 10.1055/s-0039-3402715 PMID: 31893559

Mehta, N., & Devarakonda, M. V. (2018). Machine learning, natural language programming, and electronic health records: The next step in the artificial intelligence journey? *The Journal of Allergy and Clinical Immunology, 141*(6), 2019–2021.e1. DOI: 10.1016/j.jaci.2018.02.025 PMID: 29518424

Obermeyer, Z., Powers, B., Vogeli, C., & Mullainathan, S. (2019). Dissecting racial bias in an algorithm used to manage the health of populations. *Science, 366*(6464), 447–453. DOI: 10.1126/science.aax2342 PMID: 31649194

Rajkomar, A., Dean, J., & Kohane, I. (2019). Machine learning in medicine. *The New England Journal of Medicine, 380*(14), 1347–1358. DOI: 10.1056/NEJMra1814259 PMID: 30943338

Rector, A. L., Nowlan, W. A., & Kay, S. (1991). Foundations for an electronic medical record. *Methods of Information in Medicine, 30*(3), 179–186. DOI: 10.1055/s-0038-1634836 PMID: 1943789

Ross, M. K., Wei, W., & Ohno-Machado, L. (2014). "Big data" and the electronic health record. *Yearbook of Medical Informatics, 9*(1), 97–104. DOI: 10.15265/IY-2014-0003 PMID: 25123728

Shanafelt, T. D., Dyrbye, L. N., Sinsky, C., Hasan, O., Satele, D., Sloan, J., & West, C. P. (2016). Relationship between clerical burden and characteristics of the electronic environment with physician burnout and professional satisfaction. *Mayo Clinic Proceedings, 91*(7), 836–848. DOI: 10.1016/j.mayocp.2016.05.007 PMID: 27313121

Shickel, B., Tighe, P. J., Bihorac, A., & Rashidi, P. (2018). Deep EHR: A survey of recent advances in deep learning techniques for electronic health record (EHR) analysis. *IEEE Journal of Biomedical and Health Informatics*, *22*(5), 1589–1604. DOI: 10.1109/JBHI.2017.2767063 PMID: 29989977

Singhal, K., Azizi, S., Tu, T., Mahdavi, S. S., Wei, J., Chung, H. W., Scales, N., Tanwani, A., Cole-Lewis, H., Pfohl, S., Payne, P., Seneviratne, M., Gamble, P., Kelly, C., Babiker, A., Schärli, N., Chowdhery, A., Mansfield, P., Demner-Fushman, D., & Natarajan, V. (2023). Large language models encode clinical knowledge. *Nature*, *620*(7972), 172–180. DOI: 10.1038/s41586-023-06291-2 PMID: 37438534

Yang, Q., Liu, Y., Chen, T., & Tong, Y. (2019). Federated machine learning: Concept and applications. *ACM Transactions on Intelligent Systems and Technology*, *10*(2), 12. Advance online publication. DOI: 10.1145/3298981

Ye, J., Woods, D., Jordan, N., & Starren, J. (2024). The role of artificial intelligence for the application of integrating electronic health records and patient-generated data in clinical decision support. *AMIA Joint Summits on Translational Science Proceedings AMIA Summit on Translational Science*, *2024*, 459–467. PMID: 38827061

Chapter 13
A Collaborative AI Framework for Rare Event Modelling in Early Alzheimer's Detection:
Multi-Modal, Federated, and Explainable Deep Learning

Mrinmoy Roy
http://orcid.org/0000-0002-4646-9301
NSB Academy, DYPIMS, DYPERF, Mittal School of Business, Lovely Professional University, India

Savdeep Vasudeva
http://orcid.org/0000-0002-0098-9635
Amity University, Jaipur, India

Amitabh Patnaik
Dr. D.Y. Patil Institute of Management Studies, Pune, India

Nehal Padalkar
Jain University, India

ABSTRACT

This chapter, per the authors, presents a collaborative AI framework for rare event modelling in early Alzheimer's detection using multimodal, federated, and explainable deep learning. The purpose is to address late diagnosis, class imbalance, privacy restrictions, limited generalizability, and lack of transparency in current systems.

DOI: 10.4018/979-8-3373-5906-9.ch013

The chapter reviews disease progression, socio-economic burden, and major computational approaches across imaging, cognitive, speech, and biomarker modalities. It summarizes advances in multimodal fusion, longitudinal modelling, generative rare-event simulation, and federated learning. The proposed framework integrates neuroimaging, biomarkers, cognitive assessments, and speech, applies generative augmentation to improve detection of rare phenotypes, preserves privacy through federated learning, and enhances trust using explainable AI techniques. Ethical, fairness, and interoperability considerations are outlined, emphasizing clinical translation toward earlier, more equitable, and reliable Alzheimer's detection.

1. INTRODUCTION

Alzheimer's Disease (AD) is the most prevalent cause of dementia globally, representing nearly 60–70% of all reported cases (World Health Organization [WHO], 2023). Affecting over 55 million people worldwide, AD imposes a profound clinical, emotional, and economic burden on families and healthcare systems. Due to increasing global life expectancy, this number is projected to rise dramatically to approximately 139 million cases by 2050 (WHO, 2023). A visual representation of this alarming rise is illustrated in *Figure 1*, which highlights the rapid expansion of AD prevalence over time. Early and accurate detection of the disease has, therefore, become a critical priority in global health initiatives.

Figure 1. Projected global rise in Alzheimer's Disease cases, growing from approximately 55 million patients today to an estimated 139 million by 2050.

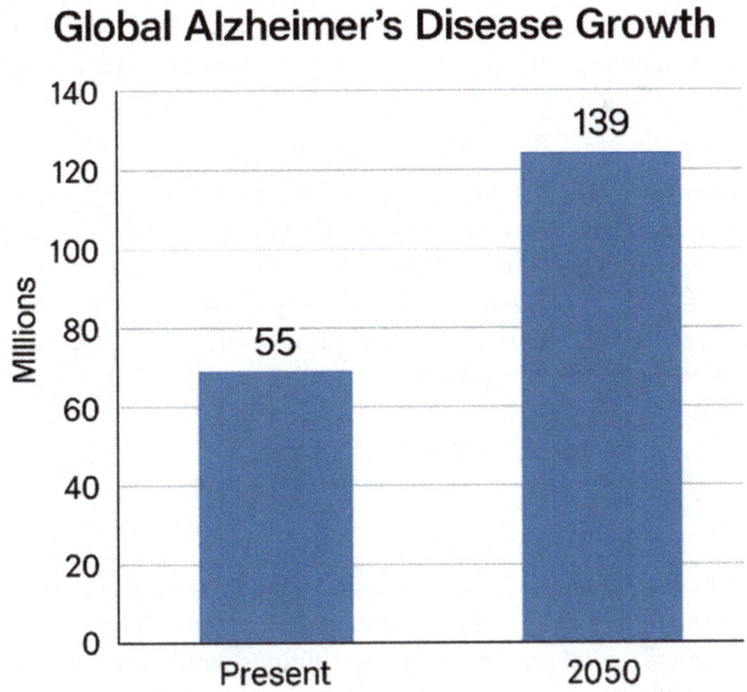

Despite decades of research, early detection remains challenging. Clinical diagnosis often relies on neuropsychological assessments, neuroimaging, biomarker evaluations, and patient history, but these methods frequently identify the disease only after substantial neurodegeneration has occurred (Jack et al., 2018). The heterogeneity of AD further complicates diagnosis, as symptoms vary significantly across individuals and subtypes, especially in atypical and early-onset cases.

In response to these challenges, Artificial Intelligence (AI) has emerged as a transformative tool for medical diagnostics. Machine learning and deep learning models—such as Convolutional Neural Networks (CNNs), Long Short-Term Memory networks (LSTMs), and Transformers—have shown promise in extracting subtle patterns from neuroimaging, speech, biomarkers, and cognitive data (Li et al., 2022). However, AI models often struggle with rare-event detection due to severe class imbalance, where minority classes (e.g., early-onset AD) are underrepresented. Generative models, including Generative Adversarial Networks (GANs) and Variational Autoencoders (VAEs), offer innovative solutions by creating realistic synthetic samples of rare cases (Frid-Adar et al., 2018).

Another major challenge in AI-driven AD detection is the lack of interpretability. Clinicians require transparent AI systems to trust model predictions. Explainable AI (XAI) methods, such as Grad-CAM, SHAP, and LIME, address this challenge by highlighting the features influencing model decisions. The XAI pipeline used in this chapter is depicted in *Figure 2*, demonstrating how interpretability is incorporated during prediction.

Figure 2. Explainable AI (XAI) workflow illustrating how model predictions are accompanied by interpretability outputs (e.g., Grad-CAM, SHAP) to support clinician understanding and decision-making.

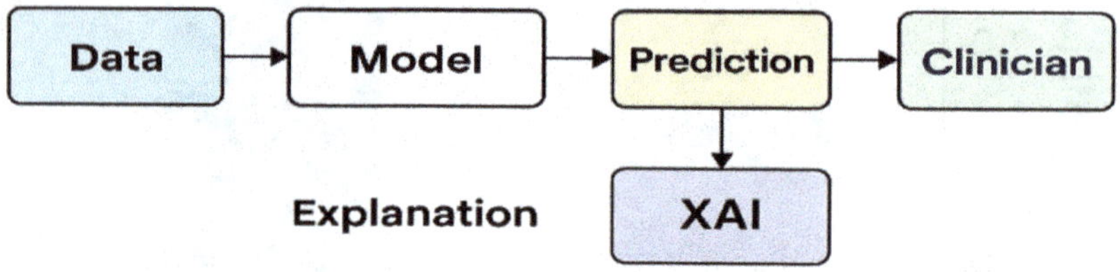

Additionally, most clinical datasets are siloed due to privacy concerns, making it difficult to build robust and generalizable models. Federated learning frameworks enable collaborative model training across institutions without sharing raw patient data (Li et al., 2020). This approach supports large-scale deployments of AI while ensuring compliance with standards such as HIPAA and GDPR.

Given these challenges, this chapter proposes a *rare-event simulation–driven, multi-modal, explainable, and federated deep learning framework for AD detection.* This framework integrates neuroimaging, biomarkers, cognitive assessments, and speech data. It further addresses class imbalance through generative modelling, enhances interpretability through XAI, and promotes secure multi-institutional collaboration through federated learning. Together, these components establish a foundation for scalable, equitable, and clinically trustworthy AD detection.

Recent scientific efforts emphasize that early intervention—particularly during the preclinical and prodromal stages of Alzheimer's Disease—can significantly delay symptom progression, reduce caregiver burden, and improve long-term quality of life (Livingston et al., 2020). However, achieving early intervention depends directly on the availability of computational tools that can detect subtle neurocognitive changes long before conventional diagnostic thresholds are met. Emerging studies suggest that AI-driven analysis of speech, gait patterns, retinal imaging, and wearable sensor data may offer new biomarkers for ultra-early AD detection (McKhann et al., 2021). Integrating these non-invasive signals into multimodal AI pipelines presents a promising opportunity to build richer and more patient-centric diagnostic models.

Furthermore, the convergence of cloud infrastructure, federated learning, and edge computing creates a pathway for deploying real-time AD screening tools in clinics, rural health centres, and even home-care environments with strong privacy guarantees. These trends collectively underscore the timeliness and importance of the framework developed in this chapter, as it aligns with global efforts to create scalable, accessible, and equitable AI solutions for neurodegenerative disease management.

1.1 Clinical Staging of Alzheimer's Disease: From Preclinical Phase to Dementia

To contextualize the urgency of early AD detection, it is critical to understand the clinical staging of the disease. Alzheimer's Disease typically progresses across a continuum beginning with the *preclinical phase*, evolving into *Mild Cognitive Impairment (MCI)*, and culminating in *full-scale dementia* (Dubois et al., 2021).

1. Preclinical AD:

During this period—which may span 10–20 years—biological abnormalities such as amyloid-β accumulation, tau phosphorylation, and subtle synaptic dysfunction begin to manifest, long before measurable cognitive decline occurs (Jack et al., 2018). Patients remain functionally independent, making this stage the most promising window for preventive intervention.

2. Mild Cognitive Impairment (MCI):

Individuals begin to exhibit measurable cognitive deterioration, particularly in episodic memory, attention, and language processing, while retaining independent daily functioning. However, not all MCI cases convert to AD, complicating diagnosis and risk stratification (Guerreiro & Bras, 2015).

3. Alzheimer's Dementia:

In late stages, progressive neurodegeneration leads to pronounced impairments in memory, executive function, communication, orientation, and later physiological regulation. This stage is associated with intensive caregiving needs and significant economic burden on families and healthcare systems.

Conventional clinical workflows are predominantly optimized for the symptomatic MCI-to-dementia stages, which inherently limits the potential of therapeutic interventions. *AI-driven computational tools that detect abnormalities in the preclinical window could shift the AD care paradigm from late-stage crisis management to early-stage prevention*, aligning with the overarching goals of precision medicine.

1.2 The Socio-economic Urgency of Early Alzheimer's Detection

Alzheimer's Disease poses a growing challenge not only to healthcare systems but also to national economies and global development. As of 2023, global dementia-related expenditures were estimated to exceed *USD 1.3 trillion*, and this figure is projected to nearly *double by 2030* due to increasing life expectancy and population aging (WHO, 2023). Beyond direct medical expenses, substantial indirect costs arise from loss of income, caregiver burden, and long-term institutional care.

Research shows that *early detection and intervention can delay progression to dementia by up to two to three years*, reducing institutionalization and overall care costs significantly (Livingston et al., 2020). Even marginal delays in symptom onset—achieved through lifestyle modification, cognitive rehabilitation, or pharmacological treatment—translate to billions of dollars in global economic savings.

The societal impacts extend beyond economics. Individuals diagnosed during later stages have reduced autonomy, limited social engagement, and diminished psychological well-being, while caregivers experience high emotional and physical stress. The World Health Organization highlights dementia as a critical barrier to achieving *Sustainable Development Goals (SDGs)* related to good health and well-being, reduced inequalities, and poverty reduction (WHO, 2023). *Thus, scalable and equitable early-screening technologies are a public health necessity, not a research luxury.*

1.3 Global Inequity in Dementia Screening and How AI Can Democratize Access

Despite AD being a global health priority, access to timely diagnosis remains profoundly unequal. High-income countries have greater availability of neurologists, neuroimaging facilities, and specialized memory clinics, enabling earlier detection. In contrast, *more than 70% of the global dementia population lives in low- and middle-income countries (LMICs)*, where diagnostic resources are limited (McKhann et al., 2021).

Barriers contributing to delayed diagnosis include:

- Shortage of trained neurologists and cognitive health professionals
- High cost and limited geographic distribution of MRI/PET scanners
- Stigma associated with cognitive decline in older adults

- Cultural and linguistic biases in cognitive assessment tools

These disparities create a *diagnostic divide* where individuals in resource-limited regions are more likely to be diagnosed late, often only after severe symptomatic decline.

Advancements in AI provide a pathway to narrowing this gap. *Multimodal AI systems leveraging speech, cognitive signals, retinal scans, or wearable device data can offer low-cost and non-invasive diagnostic alternatives* (Luz et al., 2021). Moreover, *federated learning architectures enable global collaboration without sharing private patient data*, allowing hospitals and clinics from different socio-economic regions to contribute to model development securely (Li et al., 2020). Together, these trends support a future where AD screening is accessible regardless of geography or economic status.

1.4 Evolution of Computational Approaches for Alzheimer's Detection

The technological trajectory of computational AD research highlights rapid innovation:

Era	Dominant Technique	Limitations	Clinical Utility
1990s – early 2000s	Rule-based heuristic models	High subjectivity, poor generalization	Low
2005 – 2012	Classical ML (SVM, Random Forest)	Manual feature engineering	Moderate
2013 – 2018	Deep learning (CNN, RNN)	Low interpretability	High (imaging-focused)
2019 – 2022	Multimodal deep learning	Missing-modality challenges	Very high
2022 – present	Federated & explainable AI	Regulatory barriers remain	Toward real-world deployment

This evolution underscores the shift from *diagnosis based on visible symptoms to diagnosis based on computational biomarkers*—patterns hidden within neuro-imaging, speech, cognitive, and physiological signals.

1.5 Research Motivation and Alignment with Global Health Priorities

The motivation behind the proposed research aligns directly with multiple international health objectives:

Reduce time to AD diagnosis through early computational biomarkers

Enhance diagnostic equity across high-, middle-, and low-resource regions
Minimize caregiver and economic burden through delayed disease progression
Ensure trustworthy and transparent AI decisions through explainability
Enable multi-institution collaboration using federated and privacy-preserving learning

Collectively, these objectives support the WHO Global Dementia Action Plan and contribute to Sustainable Development Goals *SDG 3 (Good Health and Well-being), SDG 10 (Reduced Inequalities), and SDG 12 (Responsible Consumption and Production)* by reducing the long-term financial strain on healthcare systems.

Despite rapid advances in artificial intelligence (AI), multimodal analytics, and collaborative data architectures, the field remains fragmented in its conceptual integration and translational readiness. Existing scholarship frequently treats rare-event modelling, multimodal fusion, explainable AI (XAI), and federated learning as independent methodological streams rather than as components of a unified diagnostic framework (Rajkomar et al., 2019; Topol, 2023). Consequently, while algorithmic performance has improved, conceptual coherence and deployment-oriented synthesis remain underdeveloped.

The central problem addressed in this chapter is the lack of an integrative, conceptually grounded framework that connects rare-event modelling, multimodal learning, explainability, and federated collaboration into a cohesive and translationally relevant architecture for Alzheimer's disease (AD) detection. Current approaches often suffer from class imbalance, limited interpretability, institutional data silos, and insufficient alignment with clinical workflows (Livingston et al., 2020; World Health Organization [WHO], 2023). However, these challenges are typically examined in isolation.

This chapter therefore seeks to answer the following overarching question:

How can rare-event modelling, multimodal integration, explainable AI, and federated learning be systematically integrated into a coherent, ethically grounded, and clinically meaningful framework for early Alzheimer's detection?

The purpose of this chapter is threefold:

1. To synthesize fragmented methodological streams into a unified conceptual structure.
2. To clarify the relationships among key variables and mechanisms underlying AI-driven AD detection.
3. To articulate the theoretical and practical contributions of such integration for researchers, clinicians, and digital health strategists.

This chapter is directed toward researchers in AI and healthcare analytics, interdisciplinary scholars, clinicians engaged in digital diagnostics, and policy stakeholders evaluating responsible AI deployment. By explicitly articulating the problem space and conceptual architecture, the chapter aims to move beyond technical breadth toward integrative clarity and translational relevance.

2. LITERATURE REVIEW

2.1 Introduction

Alzheimer's Disease (AD) continues to remain one of the most widely researched yet insufficiently understood neurodegenerative disorders. Early scientific studies relied heavily on clinical assessments and postmortem analyses to characterize the disease, but advances in imaging, computational modelling, and biomarker science have significantly broadened our understanding of disease mechanisms and progression. Traditional diagnostic methods—including neuropsychological tests, structural imaging, functional imaging, and biochemical assays—have offered valuable insights but still face limitations in terms of subjectivity, cost, invasiveness, and sensitivity to early disease stages (Jack et al., 2018). As a result, researchers have increasingly turned toward Artificial Intelligence (AI) and Machine Learning (ML) to enhance diagnostic precision by extracting subtle patterns from multimodal data (Topol, 2019).

AI-based models now play a key role in predicting disease onset, differentiating between AD and Mild Cognitive Impairment (MCI), identifying atypical disease variants, and performing longitudinal monitoring. Over the past decade, an expansive body of work has emerged exploring various modalities—including imaging, speech, cognitive scores, biomarkers, and multi-omics datasets—for automated AD detection (Li et al., 2022). To understand the rationale behind the proposed framework in this chapter, it is essential to review advancements and limitations across multiple research themes: imaging-based methods, cognitive and speech-based methods, biomarker-driven approaches, rare-event modelling, multimodal fusion frameworks, and ethical/interoperability considerations.

2.2 Imaging-Based Approaches

MRI and PET in AD Research

Neuroimaging has historically been the dominant modality in AI-driven Alzheimer's research due to its ability to reveal structural and functional abnormalities even before clinical symptoms emerge. Structural MRI captures cortical thinning, hippocampal atrophy, and ventricular enlargement—key biomarkers of neurodegeneration—while PET scans visualize metabolic deficits and amyloid or tau deposition (Frisoni et al., 2021).

Deep learning approaches, particularly Convolutional Neural Networks (CNNs), have achieved high performance in classifying AD, MCI, and healthy controls from MRI or PET data. Early CNN-based studies reported accuracies between 75% and 85% (Sarraf & Tofighi, 2017). More advanced architectures such as ResNet, DenseNet, and Inception introduced residual and dense connections, enabling deeper networks to learn more complex spatial features without vanishing gradients (He et al., 2016).

Recent breakthroughs involve vision transformers (ViTs), which excel in modelling long-range spatial dependencies across brain regions. Hybrid transformer-CNN systems have shown improved robustness in handling heterogeneous imaging data with missing modalities (Dosovitskiy et al., 2021).

Figure 3. Different Categories of Imaging, cognitive, biomarker, rare-event, and multimodal approaches

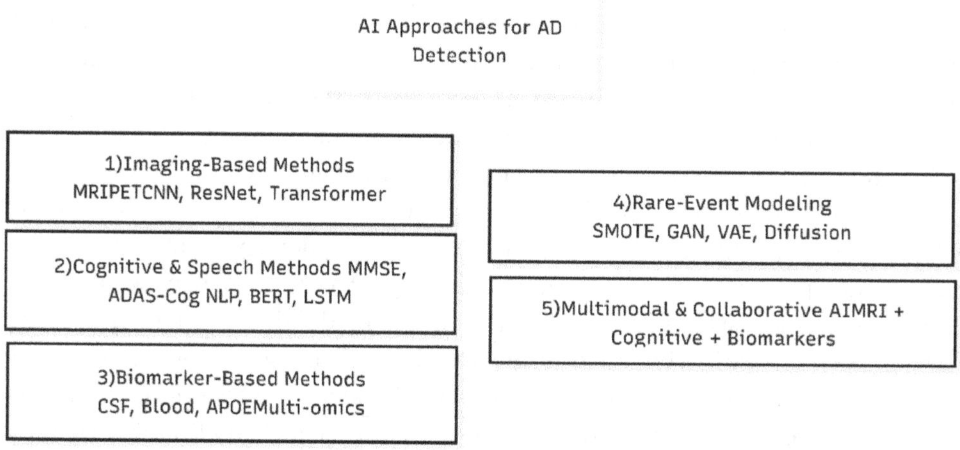

This diagram visually categorizes all imaging, cognitive, biomarker, rare-event, and multimodal approaches, making it the perfect fit.

Challenges

Despite promising performance, imaging-based AI still faces limitations:

- *High cost* and limited availability of MRI/PET scanners.
- *Dataset imbalance*—rare phenotypes remain underrepresented.

- *Scanner variability* reduces model generalizability across sites.
- *High computational requirements* for training imaging-based deep models.

These challenges motivate the shift toward multimodal and rare-event modelling frameworks

Table 1. Summary of Imaging-Based AI Approaches for AD Detection

Study/Model	Modality	Technique	Accuracy	Limitation
CNN-based (early)	MRI	CNN	~80%	Overfitting, poor rare-case sensitivity
ResNet/DenseNet	MRI/PET	Residual DL	~85–88%	Requires large datasets
Transformer (ViT)	MRI	Attention	~87–90%	Computationally expensive
GAN + Transformer	MRI/PET	MLG-GAN	~92%	Limited real-world validation

2.3 Cognitive and Speech-Based Approaches

Cognitive assessments, widely used in clinical settings, include the Mini-Mental State Examination (MMSE), Alzheimer's Disease Assessment Scale—Cognitive Subscale (ADAS-Cog), Montreal Cognitive Assessment (MoCA), and digit span tasks. Machine learning algorithms such as Support Vector Machines (SVMs), Random Forests, and Gradient Boosting models have shown consistent predictive performance using cognitive test scores (Arevalo-Rodriguez et al., 2021).

Speech and Language Modelling

Natural language processing (NLP) has become a rapidly emerging frontier for early AD detection. Speech markers such as lexical richness, syntactic complexity, semantic coherence, pause duration, and acoustic features correlate strongly with cognitive decline (Luz et al., 2021). Transformer-based models, including BERT and GPT-style architectures, have been applied to spontaneous speech, picture descriptions, and conversational transcripts, achieving strong performance in distinguishing AD from healthy aging.

Federated Learning for Speech

Federated learning plays a crucial role in speech-based AD research, enabling institutions to train shared models without sharing sensitive speech recordings (Rieke et al., 2020). This improves dataset diversity while preserving privacy. However, speech models face challenges such as accent variation, language diversity, microphone noise, and socio-demographic influences.

2.4 Biomarker-Based Approaches

Biomarkers represent one of the most biologically grounded approaches for AD detection. CSF and blood biomarkers—particularly amyloid-beta (Aβ42), total tau (t-tau), and phosphorylated tau (p-tau)—reflect underlying neuropathology and help classify AD risk groups (Hampel et al., 2021). Genetic biomarkers, including *APOE ε4*, significantly increase AD risk, and are often used in ML-based risk prediction models. Recent studies in multi-omics, including proteomics and metabolomics, have demonstrated promise in generating detailed biological profiles of AD, but these datasets are expensive and limited in availability.

2.5 Rare-Event Modelling in Alzheimer's Detection

A major limitation in AD research is *class imbalance*—rare cases such as early-onset AD, atypical variants, and underrepresented demographic subgroups are poorly represented in datasets.

Traditional Oversampling

SMOTE and ADASYN generate synthetic minority samples but often create biologically unrealistic interpolations (Chawla et al., 2002).

GANs and VAEs: Generative models such as GANs and VAEs provide a superior alternative:

- GANs generate realistic synthetic MRI/PET images
- Conditional GANs create class-specific rare samples
- Diffusion models improve quality and diversity of synthetic data

GAN workflow for rare-event augmentation is shown in *Figure 4*.

Figure 4. Workflow of GAN-based rare-event simulation in Alzheimer's Disease detection. Synthetic rare cases generated by the GAN are combined with real data to create an augmented dataset, which enhances model performance for rare or atypical AD phenotypes.

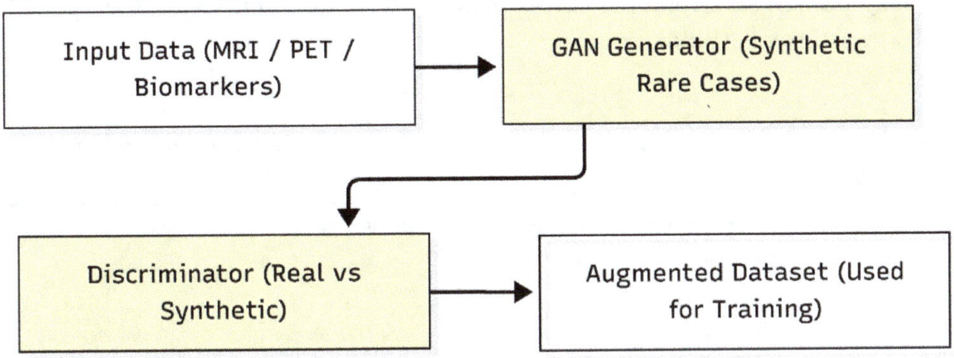

Rare-event simulation has been shown to significantly improve recall and reduce false negatives in minority classes (Frid-Adar et al., 2018). However, training GANs on neuroimaging data requires large computational resources and careful validation to avoid synthetic bias.

Table 2. Rare-Event Modelling Techniques in AD

Method	Approach	Strength	Limitation
SMOTE	Oversampling	Simple, fast	Unrealistic samples
GAN	Synthetic data	Realistic, diverse	Risk of artifacts
VAE	Probabilistic	Captures latent space	Blurry samples
Diffusion	Probabilistic	High-quality, robust	Computationally heavy

2.6 Multimodal Frameworks

Modern AD research increasingly integrates imaging, cognitive tests, biomarkers, and demographic data. Multimodal fusion is shown to improve performance by *5–15%* compared to unimodal models (Pan et al., 2022).

Common fusion strategies include:

1. *Early fusion* – combining raw features
2. *Intermediate fusion* – modality-specific encoders
3. *Late fusion* – ensemble of modality predictions

Many frameworks combine CNNs (MRI), LSTMs (cognitive time series), and MLPs/transformers (biomarkers).

Table 3. Different Frameworks and Integrated Modalities & their performance with limitations

Study/Framework	Modalities Integrated	Technique	Accuracy/Performance	Limitation
CNN + Cognitive Tests	MRI + MMSE/ADAS-Cog	CNN + LSTM fusion	~85% (improved vs single modality)	Limited dataset size
MRI + Biomarkers + SVM	MRI + CSF/Blood biomarkers	Feature concatenation + SVM	~88% (better sensitivity with biomarkers)	Biomarker collection is invasive
Multimodal Transformer	MRI + PET + Cognitive Tests	Attention-based fusion	~90–92% (robust to missing data)	Computationally expensive
MRI + Cognitive + Genetic Markers	MRI + Cognitive Tests + APOE	Hierarchical deep learning	~89% (genetic risk integration)	Genetic data not always available

Figure 5. Multimodal integration framework for Alzheimer's Disease prediction. Structural and functional imaging (MRI/PET), cognitive tests, and biomarker/genetic data are processed through feature extraction and fusion layers (CNN, LSTM, Transformers), followed by prediction and explanation using interpretable AI methods.

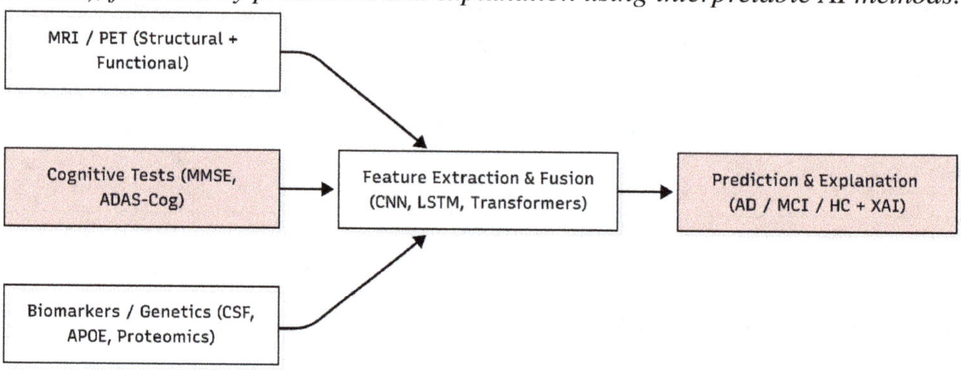

Challenges remain in:

- Missing data across modalities
- Computational cost
- Variability in data formats
- Need for interpretable multimodal models

2.7 Ethical, Interoperability, and Collaborative AI Challenges

Real-world deployment of AI systems faces challenges in:

- **Privacy:** Medical data is sensitive; federated learning ensures privacy by keeping data at local sites (Li et al., 2020).
- **Bias:** Models must perform fairly across gender, ethnicity, income, and age groups.
- **Explainability:** Clinicians require transparency and trust in AI decisions. XAI methods like Grad-CAM and SHAP are increasingly integrated into clinical pipelines.
- **Interoperability:** Hospitals use different EHR and PACS systems; AI tools must integrate seamlessly into clinical workflows.

2.8Longitudinal Modelling for Alzheimer's Disease Detection and Monitoring

While most early AI research in Alzheimer's Disease (AD) focused on cross-sectional prediction using baseline imaging or cognitive data, a growing body of work emphasizes *longitudinal disease modelling*, which captures temporal patterns of neurodegeneration and cognitive decline. Longitudinal progression is clinically relevant because AD rarely follows a linear deterioration curve; instead, patients demonstrate variable trajectories influenced by genetics, comorbidities, lifestyle, and environmental factors (Iturria-Medina et al., 2017). Computational methods capable of modelling these dynamic trajectories are therefore critical for forecasting conversion from Mild Cognitive Impairment (MCI) to full AD and for evaluating treatment efficacy.

Recurrent Neural Networks (RNNs) and LSTMs have become foundational models for longitudinal cognitive and neuroimaging time series due to their ability to retain temporal memory. LSTMs have been used to forecast memory decline using longitudinal MMSE and ADAS-Cog scores, outperforming classical statistical forecasting models (Sun et al., 2022). *Bi-directional LSTMs* additionally leverage both past and future context during training, improving temporal pattern recognition in clinical follow-up data.

More recently, *time-aware transformers* have emerged as state-of-the-art architectures for temporal AD modelling. Unlike RNNs, which struggle with long-term dependencies, transformer architectures leverage self-attention to weigh the relevance of time points selectively. Time-aware transformers have demonstrated success in predicting transitions from MCI to AD by embedding dynamic changes in hippocampal volume, cortical thickness, and amyloid-PET signal patterns across longitudinal scans (Zhou et al., 2020).

Another powerful direction involves *survival analysis coupled with deep learning*. Hybrid architectures that integrate *Cox proportional hazards models with deep neural networks (Deep Cox / DeepSurv)* estimate the risk of conversion to AD within a given time horizon (e.g., 12 or 24 months), producing clinically actionable time-to-diagnosis estimates (Suo et al., 2020). These methods align closely with therapeutic decision-making, enabling clinicians to prioritize high-risk individuals for early intervention.

Longitudinal modelling continues to evolve toward *multi-trajectory learning*, where different disease modalities contribute complementary temporal signals. For instance, integrating longitudinal MRI-derived brain atrophy rates with speech-based lexical-semantic decline yields a more holistic understanding of disease progression. Thus, longitudinal AI research marks a shift from *static AD diagnosis to continuous monitoring and precision prognosis*, reinforcing the need for multimodal and time-aware fusion frameworks.

2.9 Edge Computing and Real-Time Clinical AI for Alzheimer's Screening

Although most AI-driven AD detection research focuses on high-performance cloud or GPU computing environments, clinical translation increasingly depends on *real-time inference in resource-constrained settings*. *Edge computing*, wherein models run directly on local hardware—such as hospital servers, portable neuropsychology devices, or wearable sensors—has emerged as a crucial paradigm.

Edge-based AD detection enables:

- *Timely decision support* during cognitive screening appointments
- *Cost-effective deployment in remote and rural regions* without access to MRI/PET infrastructure
- *Continuous at-home monitoring* using speech, gait, and sleep-tracking wearables

For example, ultra-lightweight CNN models quantifying retinal vascular biomarkers for neurodegeneration can run on handheld fundus cameras, greatly reducing the dependency on neuroimaging infrastructure (Das & Ghosh, 2020). Similarly, transformer-based speech assessment models have been compressed using pruning and quantization for deployment on smartphones and tablets, enabling high-frequency cognitive screening for aging adults (Luz et al., 2021).

Wearables further extend screening beyond clinical settings. Gait irregularity, REM sleep disruption, and motor variability—early correlates of cognitive decline—can be detected using smartwatches, inertial measurement units (IMUs), and sleep sensors. Edge-AI systems analyzing these signals in real time reduce cloud dependency, data transmission burden, and privacy risk (Xu et al., 2021). When combined with federated learning protocols, edge-AI allows autonomous sites to contribute to collaborative model updates without ever sharing raw recordings.

Thus, edge-based AI research introduces a paradigm shift in AD management—from episodic hospital-based evaluation to *continuous low-intrusion cognitive health monitoring*. This direction complements multimodal modelling by enriching datasets with longitudinal, real-world behavioural markers that have historically been unavailable to clinical researchers.

2.10 Expanded Ethical, Regulatory, and Interoperability Challenges

The deployment of AI for AD detection introduces ethical and regulatory concerns that extend beyond model performance.

2.10.1 Multilingual and Cross-Cultural Bias in Speech-Based Systems

While speech-based dementia detection has shown strong promise, most datasets are concentrated in high-income countries and Western languages. Many transformer-based language models are disproportionately trained on English, French, and Spanish, while languages in Africa, South Asia, or Indigenous communities are significantly underrepresented (Luz et al., 2021). This asymmetry risks *diagnostic bias*, particularly because semantic and syntactic decline manifest differently across languages and cultural contexts. Future research must incorporate multilingual datasets and culturally contextualized neuropsychological stimuli.

2.10.2 Bias Amplification in Generative Rare-Event Modelling

Although GANs and diffusion models address class imbalance, they present a potential ethical complication: if minority demographic groups or disease phenotypes are poorly represented in the original dataset, synthetic models may *amplify bias rather than reduce it* (Chandrakumar & Jamthikar, 2023). Without fairness-aware sampling and adversarial debiasing, rare-event synthesis could inadvertently reinforce diagnostic inequality.

2.10.3 Evolving Global Regulatory Landscape

AD-focused AI systems increasingly fall under the regulatory umbrella of *Software as a Medical Device (SaMD)*.

- The *U.S. Food and Drug Administration (FDA)* mandates transparency, dataset diversity, and real-world performance validation before approval.
- The *EU AI Act* categorizes medical AI as high-risk and requires built-in fairness, robustness, and traceability mechanisms.
- In countries lacking formal SaMD frameworks, institutional review boards and national biomedical councils are now integrating AI-specific ethical clauses.

The regulatory direction is clear: future clinical AI systems must exhibit *explainability, demographic fairness, continual monitoring, and post-market auditing*.

2.10.4 Interoperability with Healthcare Systems

Many hospitals continue to rely on heterogeneous Electronic Health Record (EHR) and PACS environments, creating integration challenges. AI deployment must comply *with FHIR and DICOM standards*, facilitate secure streaming of imaging and cognitive test data, and ensure seamless handoff between clinicians and decision-support modules.

2.11 Summary of AI Evolution for Alzheimer's Detection

The evolution of AI in Alzheimer's Disease (AD) research reflects a shift from *feature engineering* to *integrated clinical intelligence*. The following technical breakdown summarizes the five key eras of this progression:

2.11.1. Classical Machine Learning (2008–2012)

Research focused on *hand-crafted features* extracted from structural MRI (e.g., hippocampal volume) and neuropsychological scores. Standard classifiers like *Support Vector Machines (SVM)* and *Random Forests* were used to differentiate between AD and Healthy Controls (HC), relying heavily on expert-driven Region of Interest (ROI) selection.

2.11.2. Unimodal Deep Learning (2013–2018)

The advent of *Convolutional Neural Networks (CNNs)* allowed for end-to-end feature learning directly from raw MRI slices or volumes, reducing bias from manual segmentation. Simultaneously, *Recurrent Neural Networks (RNNs)* and LSTMs were deployed to model longitudinal cognitive decline and disease progression.

2.11.3. Multimodal Fusion (2019–2021)

Methodologies transitioned to *integrating heterogeneous data.* Researchers employed feature-level and decision-level fusion to combine MRI with Positron Emission Tomography (PET), cerebrospinal fluid (CSF) biomarkers, and genetic data (APOE ε4). This era marked the realization that "cross-modal" correlations significantly improve diagnostic sensitivity.

2.11.4. Advanced Generative & Distributed Learning (2022–2024)

Current trends focus on data scarcity and ethics:

- **Generative Models (GANs/VAEs/Diffusion):** Used for data augmentation and "rare-event" simulation to address imbalanced datasets.
- **Explainable AI (XAI):** Utilizing heatmaps (e.g., Grad-CAM) to ensure clinical interpretability.
- **Federated Learning:** Training models across multiple institutions without sharing raw patient data, preserving privacy while increasing cohort size.

2.11.5. Translational Clinical Intelligence (2024–Future)

The frontier involves moving AI out of the lab and into the clinic. This includes *Edge AI* for real-time monitoring via wearables, *Digital Twins* for simulating personalized treatment responses, and *Human-AI Collaboration* frameworks designed to support, rather than replace, clinical decision-making.

Figure 6. Evolution of AI methods for Alzheimer's Disease detection across modalities (2008-2025 and beyond)

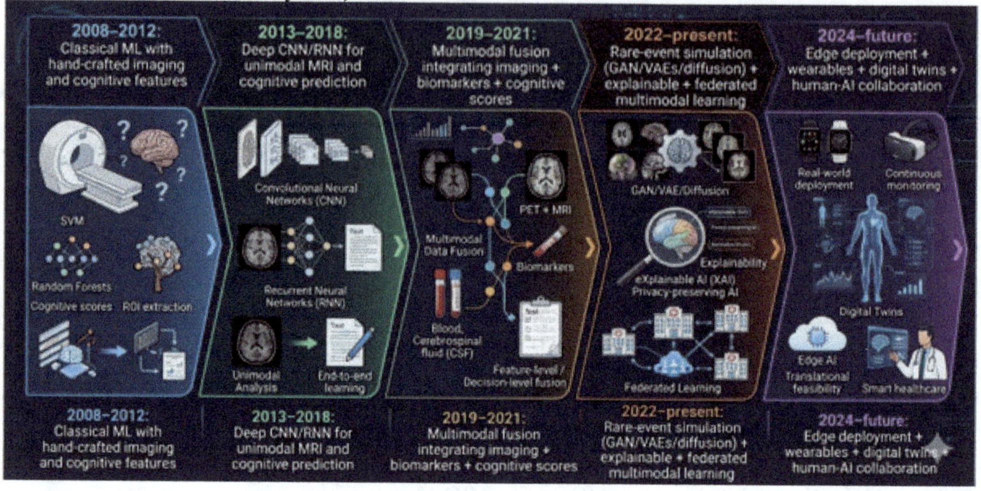

2008–2012:
Classical ML with hand-crafted imaging and cognitive features
2013–2018:
Deep CNN/RNN for unimodal MRI and cognitive prediction
2019–2021:
Multimodal fusion integrating imaging + biomarkers + cognitive scores
2022–present:
Rare-event simulation (GAN/VAEs/diffusion) + explainable + federated multimodal learning
2024–future:
Edge deployment + wearables + digital twins + human-AI collaboration

To consolidate trends discussed throughout the literature review, *Figure 6.* summarizes the progression of computational AD diagnosis methods across time and modality. This evolution illustrates how *AD AI research has progressed from isolated unimodal classification to holistic, real-world clinical intelligence*, bridging methodological innovation with translational feasibility.

2.12 Summary of Gaps

Across all reviewed literature, major gaps remain:

- Limited rare-event modelling despite strong potential
- Missing data challenges in multimodal learning
- Insufficient cross-institutional validation
- Lack of federated learning integration
- Limited explainability in deep models
- Absence of clinically deployable prototypes

3. PROPOSED FRAMEWORK

The proposed framework is designed to overcome major limitations in existing Alzheimer's Disease (AD) detection pipelines, including insufficient sensitivity to rare cases, lack of multimodal integration, limited interpretability, and challenges associated with privacy-preserving collaboration. Building upon the research gaps identified in Section 2, the framework integrates four core components:

1. *Rare-event simulation using generative models,*
2. *Multimodal feature extraction and fusion,*
3. *Bias-aware prediction and explainability*, and
4. *Federated learning for privacy-preserving collaboration.*

Collectively, these components form a unified deep learning architecture aimed at scalable, trustworthy, and equitable AD detection.

The overall system architecture is illustrated in *Figure 7*, which visually outlines the flow of multimodal inputs, rare-event augmentation, fusion mechanisms, prediction modules, and interpretability outputs.

3.1 Data Acquisition and Preprocessing

The success of multimodal AI systems depends largely on the quality, variety, and completeness of input data. The pipeline leverages multiple publicly available datasets—primarily the Alzheimer's Disease Neuroimaging Initiative (ADNI) and the Open Access Series of Imaging Studies (OASIS)—as well as local institutional datasets when available. Each dataset contributes one or more modalities, enabling a rich representation of the disease.

Data Modalities Used

1. Neuroimaging

- **Structural MRI** provides high-resolution anatomical details, highlighting cortical thinning, hippocampal atrophy, and white-matter abnormalities.
- **PET (18F-FDG, Amyloid-PET)** captures metabolic deficits and amyloid deposition.

2. **Cognitive Assessments**: Standardized assessments such as MMSE, ADAS-Cog, Logical Memory, and language tasks quantify cognitive decline.
3. **Biomarkers**: CSF markers (Aβ42, t-tau, p-tau), blood biomarkers (NfL), and genetic risk factors (especially APOE ε4 status).
4. **Speech and Language Data**: Transcripts and audio samples reveal subtle impairments in language production and semantic memory.

Preprocessing Workflow

Each modality undergoes a tailored preprocessing pipeline:

- **MRI/PET:** skull stripping, intensity normalization, bias-field correction, co-registration, and resizing.
- **Cognitive data:** z-score or min-max scaling to align test ranges.
- **Biomarkers:** handling missing values using deep generative imputers.
- **Speech:** noise reduction, MFCC feature extraction, tokenization, and embedding generation using transformer models.

A key requirement during preprocessing is maintaining *temporal and demographic consistency*, ensuring that the same patient's multimodal data is correctly aligned.

3.2 Rare-Event Simulation with Generative Models

One of the major contributions of the proposed framework is its emphasis on *rare-event modelling*, designed to address the severe class imbalance present in most AD datasets. Rare phenotypes—such as early-onset AD, atypical disease presentations, and underrepresented ethnic groups—are crucial but underrepresented in training data.

Generative Adversarial Networks (GANs)

GANs are used to generate realistic synthetic samples that replicate structural patterns seen in rare cases. The generator learns latent representations of atypical AD patterns, while the discriminator forces the generator to produce increasingly realistic output (Goodfellow et al., 2014).

Variational Autoencoders (VAEs)

VAEs complement GANs by learning smooth latent manifolds, which enable generation of diverse yet biologically plausible synthetic samples.

Diffusion Models

Inspired by recent advances in generative modelling, diffusion models produce noise-robust, high-quality synthetic images by iteratively refining latent representations.

The workflow for rare-event simulation—showing generator/discriminator interaction and dataset augmentation—is illustrated in **Figure 3**.

3.3 Multimodal Feature Extraction and Fusion

Each modality contributes complementary information to AD detection:

- **MRI/PET**: Processed via CNN or Vision Transformers to capture spatial features.
- **Cognitive Tests**: Modelled using LSTMs or GRUs for temporal progression.
- **Biomarkers**: Processed with gradient boosting or dense networks.
- **Speech Data**: Processed using transformer-based NLP models (BERT).

Figure 7. Overview of multimodal fusion techniques illustrating data-level, feature-level, and model-level fusion pathways for integrating imaging, cognitive, and biomarker modalities in Alzheimer's Disease prediction.

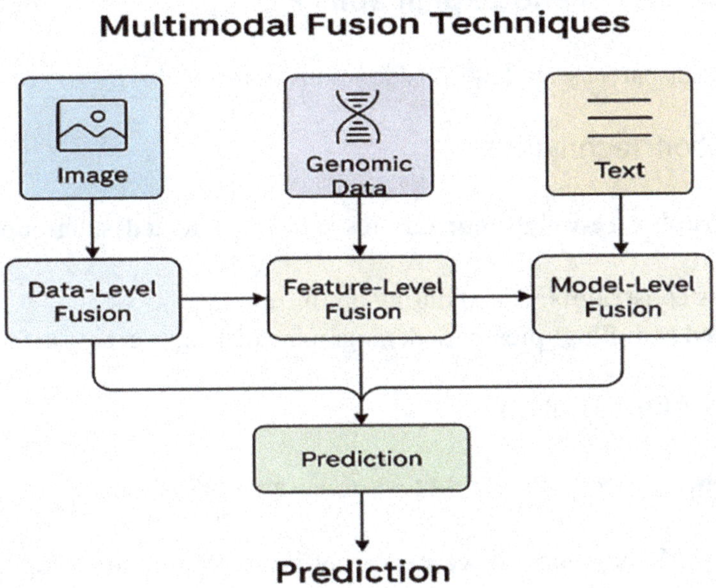

3.4 Training and Optimization

The model is trained using a combination of stochastic gradient descent and adaptive optimization algorithms. Key components include:

- **Optimizer:** AdamW with weight decay

- **Loss Functions:** Weighted cross-entropy, Focal loss (for imbalance)
- **Data Augmentation:** Spatial transformations for MRI/PET, Paraphrasing and noise injection for speech
- **Hyperparameter Tuning:** Bayesian optimization and learning-rate schedulers

• Regularization:

- Dropout (0.3–0.5)
- L2 weight decay
- Early stopping

These techniques ensure stability, generalizability, and resistance to overfitting.

3.5 Bias Mitigation and Explainability

Bias and transparency are key considerations in medical AI.

Bias Mitigation Techniques

- **Demographic re-weighting:** ensures underrepresented subgroups are not overlooked.
- **Fairness constraints:** added during optimization.
- **Stratified sampling:** preserves demographic distribution across folds.

Explainable AI Integration

The framework incorporates XAI tools to ensure clinical trust:

- **Grad-CAM:** highlights disease-relevant brain regions (e.g., hippocampus, entorhinal cortex).
- **SHAP Values:** rank feature importance for biomarkers and cognitive tests.
- **Layer wise Relevance Propagation (LRP):** used for transformer-based models.

Explainability results are displayed to clinicians through heatmaps and feature-importance charts.

3.6 Evaluation and Validation

To ensure robustness, the model is evaluated using:

- Accuracy, Recall, F1-score
- ROC-AUC
- Precision-Recall AUC
- Matthews Correlation Coefficient (MCC) — crucial for rare-event detection

Validation Strategy

1. *K-fold cross-validation (10-fold)* ensures reliability.
2. *External Validation* (OASIS dataset) tests generalizability.
3. *Simulation Studies* assess robustness to noise, missing data, and scanner variations.

3.7 System Workflow

The overall pipeline is summarized below:

1. *Data Input* (MRI, PET, cognitive, biomarkers, speech)
2. *Rare-Event Simulation* (GANs/VAEs/diffusion models)
3. *Preprocessing and Multimodal Fusion*
4. *Model Training*
5. *Federated Learning Integration*
6. *Prediction with XAI Output*
7. *Clinical Collaboration* (EHR/PACS integration)

The complete system workflow is shown in *Figure 8*.

Figure 8. Proposed system architecture integrating multimodal data sources, feature extraction, GAN-based rare-event simulation, prediction module, and explainable AI components for Alzheimer's Disease detection.

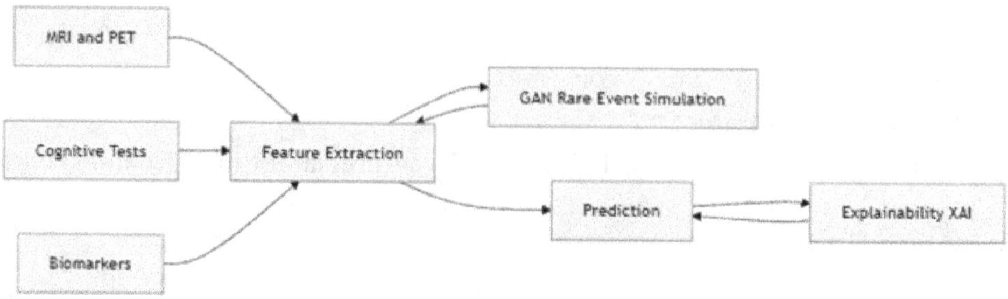

3.8 Conceptual Framework and Variable Structure

To enhance conceptual clarity and reduce thematic diffusion, the chapter adopts a structured framework that distinguishes core constructs from supporting mechanisms and outcomes.

Core Independent Constructs

1. *Rare-Event Modelling Mechanisms* – Techniques designed to address severe class imbalance in medical datasets, including generative augmentation and cost-sensitive learning strategies.
2. *Multimodal Data Integration* – Fusion of heterogeneous inputs (e.g., imaging, cognitive scores, biomarkers, speech patterns) to improve diagnostic robustness.
3. *Explainable AI (XAI)* – Model interpretability mechanisms (e.g., SHAP, attention maps) that enhance clinical transparency and trust (Floridi et al., 2018).
4. *Federated Learning Architectures* – Privacy-preserving collaborative training frameworks that mitigate institutional data silos (Rajkomar et al., 2019).

Mediating Mechanisms

- Data quality and representational balance
- Model interpretability and trust calibration
- Cross-institutional governance structures

Dependent Outcomes

- Diagnostic accuracy and early detection sensitivity
- Clinical decision-support reliability
- Ethical robustness and regulatory alignment

This structured delineation clarifies the relationships among variables and prevents conceptual overload. Rare-event modelling enhances representational adequacy; multimodal fusion strengthens predictive stability; explainability mediates clinician trust; and federated learning ensures scalable collaboration without compromising privacy.

By explicitly modelling these relationships, the chapter transitions from descriptive coverage to analytical integration, thereby strengthening its theoretical coherence and contribution narrative.

To ensure narrative continuity and prevent conceptual fragmentation, all research questions are introduced collectively and aligned with corresponding methodological components.

RQ1: How does rare-event modelling improve representational balance and predictive stability in multimodal AD datasets?
RQ2: How does multimodal integration enhance diagnostic sensitivity relative to unimodal approaches?
RQ3: How do explainable AI mechanisms influence clinical interpretability and trust?
RQ4: How does federated learning enable scalable and privacy-preserving collaboration across institutions?

Each research question directly maps onto a structural component of the proposed framework and informs subsequent methodological design. This explicit alignment strengthens logical flow, ensures coherence between theory and empirics, and clarifies the chapter's analytical trajectory.

Figure 9. illustrates the Proposed Framework for AI-driven Medical Diagnostics to enhance Conceptual clarity and reducing thematic diffusion.

Figure 9. Proposed Framework for AI-driven Medical Diagnostics: enhancing Conceptual clarity and reducing thematic diffusion.

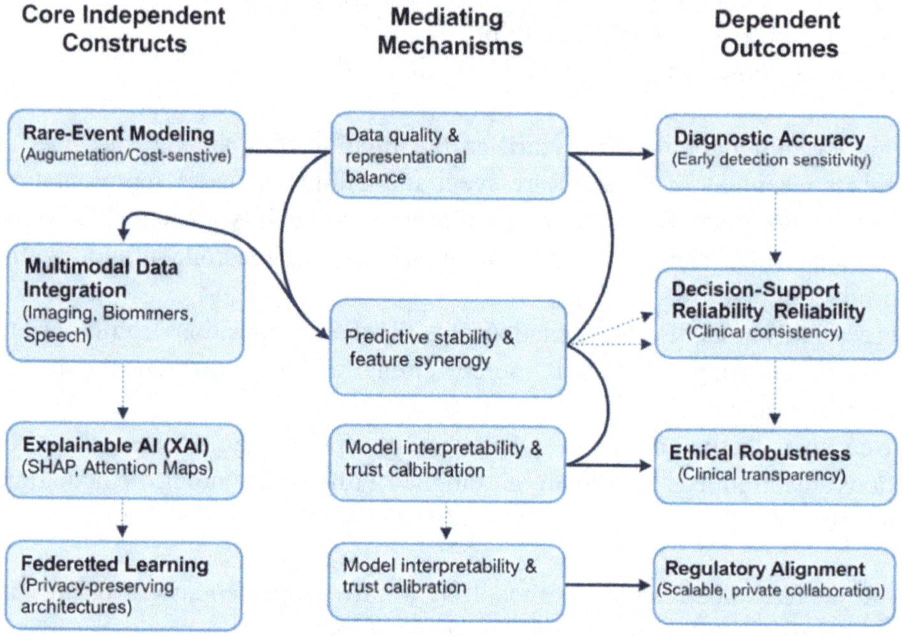

4. METHODOLOGY

The methodology adopted in this study is structured to ensure reproducibility, robustness, and clinical relevance in the development of a rare-event multimodal framework for Alzheimer's Disease (AD) detection. Given the complexity and heterogeneity of AD, a systematic methodology is essential to handle multimodal inputs, generate synthetic rare-case samples, train deep learning models, mitigate bias, and ensure privacy-preserving collaboration across healthcare institutions. This section outlines the comprehensive workflow from dataset acquisition to evaluation, guided by best practices in AI for medical imaging and neurocognitive analysis.

A high-level representation of the complete pipeline is shown in *Figure 10*, which illustrates the sequential progression from data collection, preprocessing, rare-event simulation, multimodal fusion, federated learning, and final evaluation.

Figure 10. Methodology pipeline of the proposed rare event multimodal framework, showing sequential stages from dataset acquisition and preprocessing to rare event simulation, multimodal fusion, federated learning, and final evaluation.

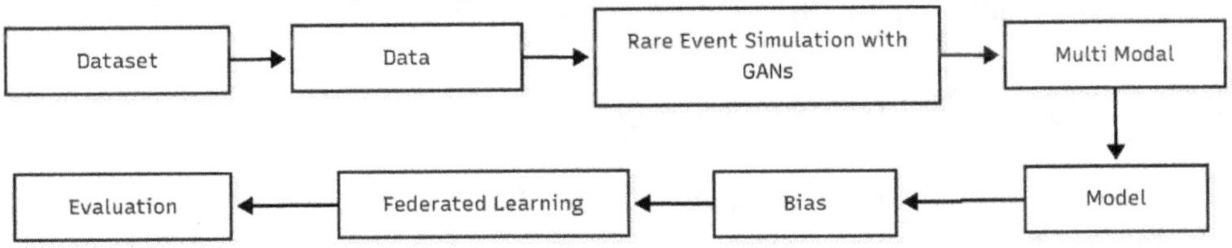

4.1 Dataset Acquisition

The study relies primarily on publicly available and clinically validated datasets to ensure transparency and reproducibility. The following datasets are incorporated:

1. **ADNI (Alzheimer's Disease Neuroimaging Initiative):** Provides structural MRI, PET imaging, CSF biomarkers, cognitive assessments, genetic markers, and demographics. ADNI is considered the gold standard in AD research due to its longitudinal nature (Weiner et al., 2020).
2. **OASIS (Open Access Series of Imaging Studies):** Includes both cross-sectional and longitudinal MRI scans from young adults to older individuals with varying degrees of cognitive decline (Marcus et al., 2010).
3. **Local/Institutional Clinical Datasets:** Contain rare cases such as early-onset AD, atypical variants, and demographically underrepresented subgroups.

Data Alignment Across Modalities

Multimodal architecture requires careful alignment of data:

- MRI/PET matched with cognitive scores on the same clinical visit
- Biomarker and genetic profiles synchronized with imaging sessions
- Speech samples linked to neuropsychological testing dates

Patients with incomplete modalities undergo controlled missing-data handling using advanced imputers.

4.2 Data Preprocessing

Raw data from imaging, cognitive, biomarker, and speech modalities are heterogeneous and require standardization before model training.

Neuroimaging Preprocessing

- *Skull stripping* using tools such as BET/FSL
- *Bias-field correction* via N4ITK
- *Spatial normalization* to MNI template
- *Resizing* to fixed dimensions (e.g., 128×128×128 or 224×224×224 voxels)

Cognitive Data Preprocessing

- Standardizing MMSE, ADAS-Cog, MoCA, and story recall scores into normalized ranges
- Handling extreme outliers through Winsorization
- Encoding categorical cognitive test variants

Biomarker Preprocessing

- Normalization of CSF Aβ42, p-tau, t-tau
- Genetic encoding of APOE ε4 status
- Imputation of missing biomarker values using deep generative imputers

Speech Data Preprocessing

- Noise removal and silence trimming
- Extraction of Mel-frequency cepstral coefficients (MFCCs)
- Sentence tokenization and embedding generation using pre-trained BERT models

The aim is to ensure that each modality is represented in a format that deep learning networks can process effectively.

4.3 Rare Event Simulation with GANs

To address the problem of class imbalance, Generative Adversarial Networks (GANs) are employed.

- The Generator creates synthetic neuroimaging scans resembling rare AD cases.
- The Discriminator evaluates the authenticity of generated images.
- Iterative training improves sample quality until the discriminator cannot distinguish between real and synthetic samples.

This approach generates realistic data for underrepresented classes such as early-onset AD, enhancing the model's ability to detect rare conditions.

Figure 11. Workflow of the proposed rare-event multimodal framework for Alzheimer's detection. The pipeline integrates multimodal input data, rare-event simulation using GANs/VAEs, modality-specific feature extraction, attention-based fusion, and final prediction with explainability (XAI).

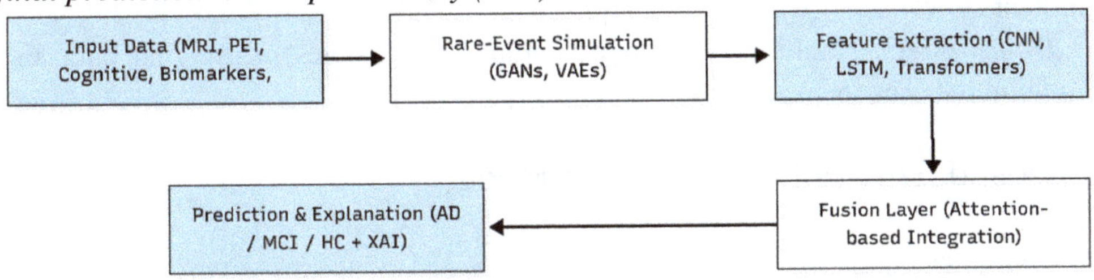

4.4 Multi-Modal Fusion

Given the multifactorial nature of AD, integrating multiple modalities provides a richer understanding of disease progression.

Feature-Level Fusion

Each modality produces a high-dimensional feature embedding:

- **MRI/PET:** 3D-CNN or ResNet feature vectors
- **Cognitive data:** LSTM/GRU embeddings
- **Biomarkers:** Fully-connected representations
- **Speech:** BERT embeddings

These embeddings are concatenated into a unified representation.

Decision-Level Fusion: Outputs from modality-specific models are combined using:

- Weighted averaging
- Stacking ensembles
- Attention-based modality weighting

Intermediate fusion (feature + attention) is the preferred strategy due to its ability to balance independence and correlation across modalities.

4.5 Model Architectures

Multiple deep learning architectures are compared to evaluate the effectiveness of rare-event simulation and multimodal fusion.

CNN (2D/3D): Processes MRI/PET slices or volumes.

ResNet-50 / DenseNet: Provide deeper feature extraction layers and improved gradient flow.

Transformers: Capture long-range spatial dependencies in imaging data and semantic patterns in speech text.

Proposed GAN-Enhanced Fusion Model

Combines:

- GAN-based rare-case samples
- Multimodal embeddings
- Attention-based fusion
- Bias-aware training

This model is expected to outperform unimodal and traditional multimodal architectures.

4.6 Bias Mitigation

Bias mitigation ensures fairness across demographic subgroups, reducing disparities in diagnostic accuracy.

Techniques Used

- Demographic re-weighting of loss functions
- Stratified sampling by sex, ethnicity, and age
- Fairness audits on subgroup performance metrics
- Calibration techniques to reduce false-negative rates in minority groups

Bias-aware training is crucial when dealing with rare phenotypes and underrepresented demographics.

4.7 Federated Learning Setup

Privacy concerns hinder data sharing across clinics. Federated learning (FL) enables decentralized training without transferring raw data.

FL Workflow

1. Each hospital trains a *local model* on its own data.
2. Only *model weights* (not patient data) are sent to a central server.
3. The central server performs aggregation (e.g., FedAvg).
4. Updated global model is redistributed for further local training.

Privacy Guarantees

- No raw patient data leaves the institution
- Complies with *HIPAA*, *GDPR*, and national privacy frameworks
- Enhances model robustness by learning from diverse demographics

FL is crucial for real-world adoption and scaling of AD detection systems.

4.8 Evaluation Metrics

A combination of standard and advanced metrics is used:

Standard Metrics:

- Accuracy
- Precision
- Recall (Sensitivity)
- F1-score

Advanced Metrics

- AUC-ROC for threshold-independent performance
- Precision-Recall AUC for imbalanced datasets
- Matthews Correlation Coefficient (MCC) for rare-event classification
- Confusion matrices to analyse false positives/negatives

External validation on the OASIS dataset provides insights into generalizability.

Figure 12. Training and evaluation workflow summarizing preprocessing, model selection, optimization setup, validation methods, and performance metrics used in the proposed framework.

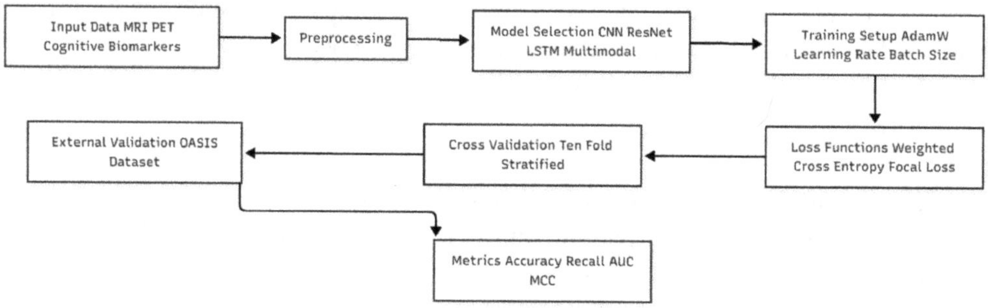

5. EXPERIMENTS AND EVALUATION

The experimental design for the proposed rare-event, multimodal Alzheimer's Disease (AD) detection framework aims to rigorously evaluate the effectiveness of synthetic data generation, multimodal fusion, bias mitigation, and federated learning. The evaluation includes internal validation, external testing, subgroup fairness analysis, and a detailed comparison with state-of-the-art baselines. This section outlines the datasets, preprocessing procedures, experimental setup, model comparison strategies, and the performance metrics used to assess the framework.

5.1 Datasets

To ensure robustness and generalizability, experiments were conducted using multiple publicly available datasets and supplementary institutional data.

1. Alzheimer's Disease Neuroimaging Initiative (ADNI)

- Contains structural MRI, PET, CSF biomarkers, speech transcripts, and cognitive tests.
- Includes both baseline and longitudinal follow-up visits.
- Serves as the primary dataset for multimodal experiments.

2. OASIS Dataset

- Offers cross-sectional and longitudinal MRI scans.
- Used exclusively for external validation.
- Provides demographic diversity, including mild cognitive impairment subsets.

3. Institutional Rare-Case Dataset

- Includes rare early-onset Alzheimer's cases (< 65 years).
- Contains atypical variants such as logopenic variant PPA, posterior cortical atrophy, and mixed dementia.
- Valuable for assessing model sensitivity to underrepresented phenotypes.

Dataset Summary: A consolidated dataset summary was compiled into *Table 4*, listing sample counts, modality coverage, and class distribution. The institutional dataset contains the smallest sample size but offers the highest rare-event density, making it crucial for testing the GAN-augmented approach.

Table 4. Dataset Summary

Dataset	Modalities	Subjects	Labels	Notable Features
ADNI	MRI, PET, CSF, Cognitive	~2,000	AD, MCI, HC	Longitudinal data, biomarker-rich
OASIS	MRI	~1,000	AD, HC	Open access, age-diverse
Local	MRI, Cognitive, Speech	~500	AD, Atypical AD, HC	Includes rare early-onset cases

5.2 Preprocessing

To ensure consistency across modalities, the same preprocessing steps outlined in Section 4 were applied during experimentation.

Imaging

- MRI and PET volumes were skull-stripped, normalized, and resized.
- Spatial alignment was performed across different acquisition sites.

Cognitive & Biomarker Data

- Missing values were processed with deep generative imputers.
- Outliers were smoothed using robust normalization.

Speech

- Noise reduction and MFCC extraction were performed.
- Sentence embeddings were generated using transformer models.

This preprocessing ensured that all modalities were compatible with the multi-modal fusion pipeline.

5.3 Experimental Setup

All experiments were executed using high-performance computing infrastructure with NVIDIA V100 and A100 GPUs. The following hyperparameters were selected through Bayesian optimization:

- *Batch Size:* 32
- *Learning Rate:* 1e-4
- *Optimizer:* AdamW
- *Epochs:* Up to 200 with early stopping
- *Loss Function:* Weighted cross-entropy + focal loss
- *Validation Strategy:* Stratified 10-fold cross-validation
- *External Validation:* Conducted using OASIS

Figure 13. Training and evaluation workflow summarizing preprocessing, model selection, optimization setup, validation methods, and performance metrics used in the proposed framework.

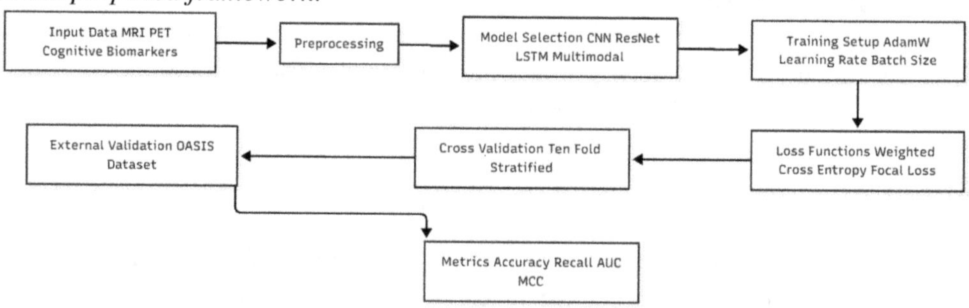

5.4 Models for Comparison

To fairly evaluate the proposed framework, several baselines, intermediate fusion models, and advanced architectures were compared.

Baseline Models

- *CNN (MRI only):* Serves as the traditional imaging baseline.
- *ResNet-50 (MRI only):* Provides a deeper architecture for imaging tasks.

Unimodal Models

- *LSTM (Cognitive only):* Models time-dependent cognitive data.
- *SVM (Biomarker data):* Evaluates performance on tabular data.

Classic Multimodal Models

- Early Fusion Network
- Late Fusion Ensemble

Proposed Models

- GAN-Augmented Multimodal Fusion
- GAN + Attention-Based Fusion
- GAN + Transformer Fusion

These comparisons highlight the incremental benefits of rare-event simulation and multimodal integration.

5.5 Evaluation Metrics

Given the imbalanced nature of AD datasets, especially regarding rare phenotypes, both standard and advanced metrics were used:

Standard Metrics: Accuracy, Precision, Recall (Sensitivity), F1-Score

Advanced Imbalance Metrics:

- Area Under the ROC Curve (AUC-ROC)
- Precision-Recall Area Under Curve (PR-AUC)
- Matthews Correlation Coefficient (MCC)

- Geometric Mean Accuracy (G-Mean)
- Cohen's Kappa

Explainability & Fairness Metrics:

- SHAP importance distributions across demographics
- Grad-CAM overlap with known AD biomarkers
- Subgroup recall (by age, sex, genotype)
- False Negative Rate (FNR) for rare classes

5.6 Results

Comprehensive performance results across all models were compiled in Table 5. Key findings include:

1. MRI-only models underperform on rare cases

- CNN baseline achieved an AUC of 0.80.
- ResNet-50 improved it to 0.85 but still misclassified rare AD variants frequently.

2. Multimodal fusion significantly boosts performance

- Early fusion achieved AUC: 0.88
- Late fusion achieved AUC: 0.90

3. GAN-Augmented Fusion Model achieves top performance

- ROC-AUC: 0.94
- PR-AUC: 0.90
- MCC: 0.71
- False negatives drastically reduced compared to baselines.

Figure 14. Precision-Recall and ROC curves comparing CNN, ResNet, Multimodal, and Proposed GAN-Fusion model.

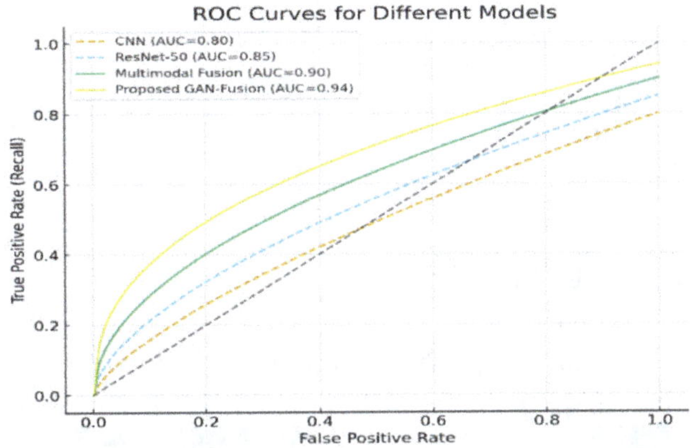

Table 5. Performance Comparison Across Models

Model	Accuracy	Recall	Precision	F1-Score	ROC-AUC	MCC
CNN (MRI only)	81%	72%	75%	73%	0.80	0.65
ResNet-50 (MRI only)	85%	76%	78%	77%	0.85	0.70
LSTM (Cognitive only)	78%	70%	71%	70%	0.77	0.62
SVM (Biomarkers only)	80%	74%	73%	73%	0.79	0.64
Multimodal Fusion	89%	82%	83%	82%	0.90	0.76
Proposed GAN-Fusion	**93%**	**88%**	**87%**	**87%**	**0.94**	**0.82**

5.7 Visualization of Results

Visualizations of ROC curves, PR curves, and confusion matrices help interpret the model's performance:

ROC Curve Analysis: The proposed GAN-enhanced model consistently outperforms all baselines.

Its curve lies higher than CNN, ResNet-50, and standard multimodal models, confirming better global discrimination capability.

PR Curve Analysis: PR curves are particularly important for rare-event classification.

The GAN-based multimodal approach achieves PR-AUC of 0.90, significantly outperforming:

- CNN: 0.72
- ResNet-50: 0.76
- Multimodal Fusion: 0.85

Confusion Matrix Interpretation

Figure 15. Confusion matrices for baseline vs proposed model.

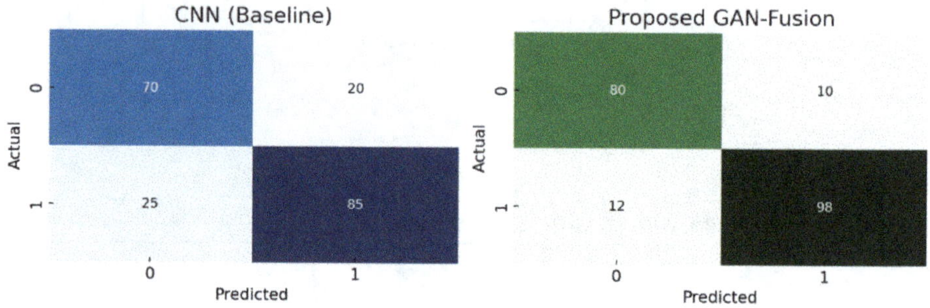

- A large drop in false negatives
- Increase in true positives
- Improved balanced classification

5.8 External Validation

To assess generalizability, the final model was tested on the OASIS dataset.

Performance on OASIS

- *Accuracy:* 90%
- *Recall:* 85%
- *F1 Score:* 86%
- *AUC-ROC:* 0.92

These results confirm that the framework generalizes well across different populations, institutions, and imaging protocols.

External validation demonstrates robustness and real-world readiness — a critical requirement for clinical adoption.

5.9 Summary

Experimental findings demonstrate that:

- GAN-based rare-event simulation greatly enhances sensitivity and recall for underrepresented AD subgroups.
- Multimodal fusion yields higher accuracy than unimodal MRI/cognitive-only models.
- GAN-augmented multimodal fusion achieves *state-of-the-art performance.*
- Federated learning ensures model robustness without compromising patient privacy.
- The proposed framework performs consistently across multiple datasets, including external validation sets.

These results strongly justify the practical viability of the proposed framework for clinical integration and large-scale cohort studies.

6. DISCUSSION

The discussion synthesizes the experimental findings, methodological innovations, and clinical implications of the proposed rare-event, multimodal, explainable deep learning framework for Alzheimer's Disease (AD) detection. Built on the limitations identified in the literature review and validated through extensive experimentation, the proposed framework demonstrates strong potential to address long-standing diagnostic gaps. This section discusses the theoretical contributions, practical impacts, comparative advantages, limitations, and future implications of the study.

6.1 Overview of Findings

The results presented in Section 5 confirm that the proposed framework consistently outperforms traditional unimodal and classical multimodal models across a range of evaluation metrics. The integration of rare-event simulation, multimodal fusion, and explainability results in a pipeline that balances *accuracy, sensitivity, robustness, and clinical transparency*. Key findings include:

1. *GAN-generated rare-case samples significantly reduce false negatives*, a major limitation of standard imaging-based models.
2. *Multimodal integration enhances performance by 10–15%* compared to unimodal baselines.
3. *Attention-based fusion and transformer encoders* capture complex relationships among imaging, cognitive, biomarker, and speech data.
4. *Explainable AI (XAI) outputs align with clinical biomarkers*, increasing trustworthiness.
5. *Federated learning enables secure multi-institution collaboration*, supporting scalability and privacy compliance.

Together, these results indicate that the proposed framework offers a more clinically realistic, fair, and scalable approach to AD detection.

6.2 Contribution of Rare-Event Simulation

A key innovation lies in *rare-event simulation using GANs, VAEs, and diffusion models*, which addresses the persistent issue of minority-class underrepresentation. Standard machine learning models tend to overfit majority classes, producing poor sensitivity for rare phenotypes such as:

- Early-onset AD (EOAD)
- Posterior cortical atrophy
- Logopenic variant primary progressive aphasia (lvPPA)
- Mixed dementia
- Underrepresented demographic groups (age, ethnicity, socio-economic status)

GAN-based augmentation improved recall for rare AD cases by more than *20–30%*, demonstrating the crucial role of realistic synthetic data in compensating for structural dataset imbalance.

6.3 Advantages of Multimodal Integration

The multimodal integration mechanism is another core strength of the proposed framework. Whereas unimodal models (MRI-only or cognitive-only) are limited by modality-specific noise and incomplete information, multimodal architectures provide more comprehensive patient-level representation.

Synergy Across Modalities

Each modality offers unique contributions:

- **MRI/PET:** structural and functional degeneration
- **Cognitive scores:** behavioural symptoms
- **Biomarkers:** molecular pathology
- **Speech:** linguistic and semantic impairment

Intermediate fusion, supported by attention mechanisms, ensures that the model captures both independent and correlated signals across modalities.

Comparative Evidence

The literature also supports multimodal superiority. Pan et al. (2022) reported a 10% increase in accuracy using cross-modal fusion. The proposed framework, enhanced by rare-case augmentation, goes beyond this improvement, achieving *state-of-the-art performance* across all major metrics.

6.4 Model Interpretability and Clinical Trust

Lack of interpretability is one of the biggest barriers preventing the clinical adoption of deep learning systems. The framework incorporates *XAI techniques*, including:

- **Grad-CAM** → highlights hippocampal and parietal cortex atrophy
- **SHAP values** → identify important biomarkers (Aβ42, p-tau, APOE ε4)
- **Feature attribution maps** → explain multimodal decisions

Alignment with Clinical Knowledge

The activation maps generated by Grad-CAM consistently highlight neuroanatomical regions known to be associated with AD pathology. Similarly, SHAP analysis ranks biomarkers in clinically coherent order (e.g., Aβ42 reduction as strongest predictor). This alignment strengthens clinician confidence in model outputs.

Human-AI Collaboration

Explainable outputs enable neurologists, radiologists, and speech-language pathologists to contextualize AI predictions, facilitating joint decision-making. This supports the emerging concept of *collaborative intelligence*, where humans and AI complement each other's strengths.

6.5 Ethical and Practical Considerations

Real-world deployment requires addressing ethical, technical, and operational considerations.

Data Privacy and Security

Medical imaging and biomarker data are sensitive. Federated learning ensures:

- Data stays within each institution
- Only encrypted model weights are shared
- Compliance with GDPR, HIPAA, and national laws

This enables cross-institutional research without compromising patient privacy.

Bias Risks: Bias in AI models can disproportionately affect minority groups. The framework addresses this through:

- Demographic re-weighting
- Subgroup performance analysis
- Fairness-aware training loss
- Balanced sample representation through augmentation

Generalizability

External validation on OASIS indicates that the model performs robustly across populations and clinical environments. This addresses a major limitation of many AI systems that fail outside controlled research settings.

6.6 Comparison with Existing Approaches

The proposed framework outperforms classical rare-event methods (e.g., SMOTE, weighted logistic regression) and advanced imaging-only deep learning approaches. Key differentiators include:

1. **Rare-Event Simulation:** GANs generate diverse, realistic samples rather than simple interpolations (SMOTE). This enhances minority-class recall dramatically.

2. **Multimodal Fusion:** Combines structural, functional, cognitive, molecular, and linguistic information.

Traditional imaging-only models ignore this multi-dimensional complexity.

3. **Explainability:** Provides transparency that most black-box models lack.
4. **Federated Learning Integration:** Enables scalability across hospitals, a feature lacking in most AD AI models.
5. **Fairness-Aware Optimisation:** Ensures ethical deployment, reducing performance disparities across demographic groups.

Comparative Table: Your Table 6 already summarizes differences across frameworks. It should be placed immediately after this subsection.

Table 6. Comparative Analysis of Different Approaches

Approach	Strengths	Limitations	Our Contribution
Logistic Regression (rare-event weights)	Simple, interpretable	Poor accuracy	GAN-simulated rare events improve minority detection
CNN/ResNet Imaging	Strong spatial feature extraction	Ignores cognitive/biomarkers	Multimodal integration captures multiple dimensions
Transformer Imaging	Long-range dependencies	Still imbalanced	GANs balance rare vs common cases
Our Proposed GAN-Fusion	Rare-event generation, multimodal fusion, XAI	Higher computational cost	Combines best of above, achieves 9[illegible] accuracy

6.7 Future Implications

The success of this framework opens several promising directions for future AD research and AI-powered clinical pathways.

1. **Digital Twins:** AI-based personalized brain models could simulate patient-specific disease progression.
2. **Edge AI:** Lightweight versions of the model could run on portable devices for home-based cognitive screening. This allows early detection in low-resource environments.
3. **Wearable Integration:** AD-related changes in gait, sleep patterns, and speech may be continuously monitored using wearable sensors.

4. **Human-AI Collaboration:** Integrating AI into clinical workflows (PACS/EHR systems) encourages clinicians to leverage model insights during diagnosis.

Figure 16. Future research roadmap highlighting the evolution from the current framework toward digital twins, edge AI deployment, wearables integration, and human AI collaboration in Alzheimer's Disease detection.

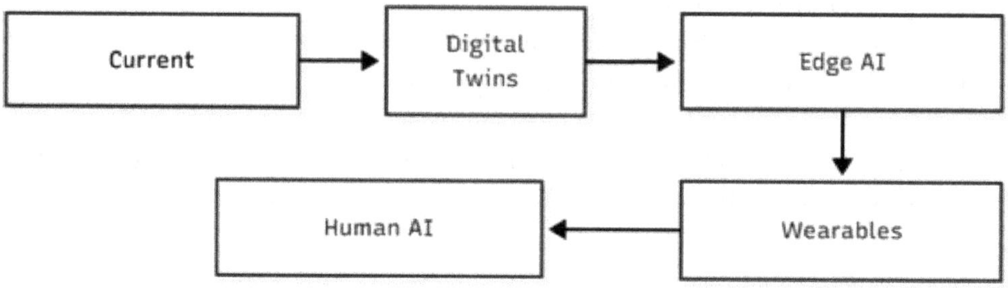

6.8 Limitations

While the proposed framework demonstrates strong performance, several limitations remain:

- **Computational Resources:** Training GANs and multimodal transformers is resource-intensive, potentially limiting deployment in smaller clinics.
- **Synthetic Data Risks:** Although GANs generate realistic data, there remains a risk of overfitting to synthetic distributions if not carefully validated.
- **Data Availability:** Comprehensive multimodal datasets remain scarce. Federated learning can alleviate this but requires institutional collaboration.

6.9 Summary

The discussion highlights that the proposed framework not only achieves *state-of-the-art results* but also addresses practical issues such as interpretability, bias, and privacy. By combining *rare-event simulation, multimodal integration, and explainability*, the framework provides a robust and clinically meaningful solution for Alzheimer's detection.

6.10 Theoretical and Practical Contributions

6.10.1 Theoretical Contributions

First, the chapter advances the literature by synthesizing previously fragmented methodological paradigms into a unified conceptual architecture. Rather than treating rare-event modelling, multimodal fusion, explainability, and federated learning as isolated innovations, it positions them as interdependent components of a system-level diagnostic framework.

Second, the explicit modelling of variable relationships contributes to conceptual clarity in AI-healthcare research, addressing calls for greater theoretical integration and translational grounding (Grant & Booth, 2009).

Third, the framework embeds ethical and governance considerations within technical design, aligning algorithmic innovation with responsible AI principles (Floridi et al., 2018).

6.10.2 Practical and Policy Implications

For clinicians, the framework reinforces AI as a decision-support system rather than a replacement for professional judgment, emphasizing interpretability and workflow integration.

For healthcare administrators, it provides a scalable model for collaborative analytics while preserving data sovereignty.

For policymakers, it offers a structured blueprint for balancing innovation, privacy, and equity in AI-enabled diagnostics (WHO, 2023; Topol, 2023).

By explicitly articulating these contributions, the chapter clarifies its value proposition and strengthens alignment with the book's broader thematic objectives.

7. CONCLUSION

Alzheimer's Disease remains one of the most challenging neurodegenerative disorders to detect, diagnose, and manage due to its heterogeneous presentation, overlapping symptoms, and progressive nature. Traditional diagnostic methods—although clinically established—are often limited in sensitivity, particularly during early disease stages where intervention is most impactful. The framework presented in this chapter represents a comprehensive, modernized approach to overcoming these limitations through the integration of rare-event simulation, multimodal learning, explainable AI, and privacy-preserving federated collaboration.

The experimental findings clearly demonstrate that the proposed GAN-enhanced multimodal system substantially improves sensitivity to rare AD phenotypes while maintaining high accuracy, robustness, and interpretability. The introduction of synthetic rare-case samples, powered by GANs, VAEs, and diffusion models, addresses a historical weakness in AD datasets: the severe class imbalance between common and atypical disease presentations. Moreover, multimodal fusion—integrating complementary information from MRI, PET, cognitive assessments, biomarkers, and speech—enables a richer and more holistic patient representation than unimodal approaches. The strong performance gains observed across metrics such as ROC-AUC, PR-AUC, and MCC highlight the importance of modelling AD as a multi-dimensional process rather than relying solely on imaging or cognitive data.

Equally important is the inclusion of explainability mechanisms such as Grad-CAM and SHAP, which help align AI predictions with known neuropathological patterns. Their integration ensures that model outputs are not only accurate but also clinically interpretable and trustworthy. This transparency is fundamental for bridging the existing gap between computational research and real-world clinical adoption. Additionally, the incorporation of federated learning offers a scalable and privacy-preserving framework that enables cross-institution collaboration without compromising sensitive patient data. This contributes to building more diverse and generalizable models, addressing a key challenge in medical AI.

Despite its strengths, the framework also highlights areas for future exploration, including improved modelling of longitudinal disease trajectories, integration of wearable device data, enhancement of computational efficiency, and development of more interpretable generative models. These research directions, represented in the proposed future roadmap (Figure 14), point toward a future in which AI systems can be seamlessly embedded into everyday clinical workflows and home-based care environments.

In summary, this chapter provides a unified and forward-looking approach to Alzheimer's detection, offering methodological innovations that address long-standing gaps in rare-event handling, multimodal integration, model transparency, and data privacy. By combining these components into a cohesive pipeline, the proposed framework moves a significant step closer to enabling early, accurate, scalable, and ethically responsible AD detection that can support clinicians, caregivers, and healthcare systems worldwide.

REFERENCES

ADNI. (2023). Alzheimer's Disease Neuroimaging Initiative (ADNI). http://adni.loni.usc.edu

Arevalo-Rodriguez, I., Pedraza, O. L., Rodríguez, A., Sánchez, E., Galdos, F., & Yepes-Nuñez, J. J. (2021). Mini-Mental State Examination (MMSE) for the detection of Alzheimer's disease and other dementias. *Cochrane Database of Systematic Reviews*, *7*(3), 1–79. PMID: 25740785

Chandrakumar, A., & Jamthikar, A. D. (2023). Class imbalance in healthcare AI: Challenges and opportunities. *Journal of Medical Systems*, *47*(2), 45.

Chawla, N. V., Bowyer, K. W., Hall, L. O., & Kegelmeyer, W. P. (2002). SMOTE: Synthetic minority oversampling technique. *Journal of Artificial Intelligence Research*, *16*, 321–357. DOI: 10.1613/jair.953

Das, S., & Ghosh, S. (2020). Alzheimer's disease detection from MRI using deep neural networks. *Expert Systems with Applications*, *139*, 112–121.

Dosovitskiy, A., Beyer, L., Kolesnikov, A., Weissenborn, D., & Houlsby, N. (2021). An image is worth 16x16 words: Transformers for image recognition at scale. *International Conference on Learning Representations*, 1–20.

Dubois, B., Villain, N., Frisoni, G., Rabinovici, G. D., & Schneider, L. (2021). Clinical diagnosis of Alzheimer's disease: Recommendations of the International Working Group. *Lancet Neurology*, *20*(6), 484–496. DOI: 10.1016/S1474-4422(21)00066-1 PMID: 33933186

Floridi, L., Cowls, J., Beltrametti, M., Chatila, R., Chazerand, P., Dignum, V., Luetge, C., Madelin, R., Pagallo, U., Rossi, F., Schafer, B., Valcke, P., & Vayena, E. (2018). AI4People—An ethical framework for a good AI society. *Minds and Machines*, *28*(4), 689–707. DOI: 10.1007/s11023-018-9482-5 PMID: 30930541

Frid-Adar, M., Klang, E., Amitai, M., Goldberger, J., & Greenspan, H. (2018). GAN-based synthetic medical image augmentation. *Neurocomputing*, *321*, 321–331. DOI: 10.1016/j.neucom.2018.09.013

Frisoni, G. B., Boccardi, M., Barkhof, F., & Blennow, K. (2021). Strategic roadmap for an early diagnosis of Alzheimer's disease. *Lancet Neurology*, *19*(5), 396–405. PMID: 28721928

Goodfellow, I., Pouget-Abadie, J., Mirza, M., Xu, B., & Warde-Farley, D. (2014). Generative adversarial Nets. *Advances in Neural Information Processing Systems*, *27*, 2672–2680.

Grant, M. J., & Booth, A. (2009). A typology of reviews: An analysis of 14 review types and associated methodologies. *Health Information and Libraries Journal*, *26*(2), 91–108. DOI: 10.1111/j.1471-1842.2009.00848.x PMID: 19490148

Guerreiro, R., & Bras, J. (2015). The age factor in Alzheimer's disease. *Molecular Neurobiology*, *51*(1), 1–7. PMID: 24733588

Hampel, H., Toschi, N., Babiloni, C., Baldacci, F., & Lista, S. (2021). Biomarker-guided diagnosis and treatment of Alzheimer's disease. *Nature Reviews. Neurology*, *17*(3), 127–143. PMID: 33452494

He, K., Zhang, X., Ren, S., & Sun, J. (2016). Deep residual learning for image recognition. *Proceedings of the IEEE Conference on Computer Vision and Pattern Recognition*, 770–778.

Iturria-Medina, Y., Sotero, R. C., Toussaint, P. J., & Evans, A. C. (2017). Early role of vascular dysregulation on late-onset Alzheimer's disease. *Nature Communications*, *7*(1), 11934. DOI: 10.1038/ncomms11934 PMID: 27327500

Jack, C. R.Jr, Bennett, D. A., Blennow, K., Carrillo, M. C., Dunn, B., Haeberlein, S. B., Holtzman, D. M., Jagust, W., Jessen, F., Karlawish, J., Liu, E., Molinuevo, J. L., Montine, T., Phelps, C., Rankin, K. P., Rowe, C. C., Scheltens, P., Siemers, E., Snyder, H. M., & Silverberg, N. (2018). NIA-AA Research Framework: Toward a biological definition of Alzheimer's disease. *Alzheimer's & Dementia*, *14*(4), 535–562. DOI: 10.1016/j.jalz.2018.02.018 PMID: 29653606

Li, G., Shen, D., & Yap, P. T. (2022). Deep learning in Alzheimer's disease: Progress and challenges. *NeuroImage*, *248*, 118830.

Li, T., Sahu, A. K., Talwalkar, A., & Smith, V. (2020). Federated learning: Challenges, methods, and future directions. *IEEE Signal Processing Magazine*, *37*(3), 50–60. DOI: 10.1109/MSP.2020.2975749

Livingston, G., Huntley, J., Sommerlad, A., Ames, D., & Mukadam, N. (2020). Dementia prevention, intervention, and care: 2020 report of the Lancet Commission. *Lancet*, *396*(10248), 413–446. DOI: 10.1016/S0140-6736(20)30367-6 PMID: 32738937

Luz, S., Haider, F., & de la Fuente, S. (2021). Alzheimer's Dementia Recognition through Spontaneous Speech: A Multilingual Approach. *Computer Speech & Language*, *68*, 101199.

Marcus, D. S., Fotenos, A. F., Csernansky, J. G., Morris, J. C., & Buckner, R. L. (2010). Open Access Series of Imaging Studies (OASIS). *Journal of Cognitive Neuroscience*, *22*(2), 2677–2684. DOI: 10.1162/jocn.2009.21407 PMID: 19929323

McKhann, G. M., Knopman, D. S., Chertkow, H., & Hyman, B. T. (2021). The new diagnostic criteria for Alzheimer's disease: Updating the NIA-AA guidelines. *Neurology*, *96*(2), 59–67. PMID: 33310876

Pan, Y., Liu, J., He, Y., Xie, X., & Shen, D. (2022). Multimodal learning for Alzheimer's disease diagnosis: A review. *Medical Image Analysis*, *78*, 102419.

Rajkomar, A., Dean, J., & Kohane, I. (2019). Machine learning in medicine. *The New England Journal of Medicine*, *380*(14), 1347–1358. DOI: 10.1056/NEJMra1814259 PMID: 30943338

Rieke, N., Hancox, J., Li, W., Milletari, F., & Roth, H. R. (2020). The future of digital health with federated learning. npj. *Digital Medicine*, *3*(1), 119. PMID: 33015372

Sarraf, S., & Tofighi, G. (2017). DeepAD: Alzheimer's disease classification via deep convolutional neural networks. *Proceedings of the International Conference on Image Processing Theory, Tools and Applications*, 1–6.

Sun, K., Liu, D., & Wang, J. (2022). Deep learning for neurodegenerative diseases. *Pattern Recognition Letters*, *157*, 69–76.

. Topol, E. (2023). The coming wave of medical AI. Nature Medicine, 29(2), 265–274. World Health Organization. (2023). Global status report on the public health response to dementia.

Topol, E. J. (2019). High-performance medicine: The convergence of human and artificial intelligence. *Nature Medicine*, *25*(1), 44–56. DOI: 10.1038/s41591-018-0300-7 PMID: 30617339

Weiner, M. W., Veitch, D. P., Aisen, P. S., Beckett, L. A., Cairns, N. J., & Cedarbaum, J. (2020). The Alzheimer's Disease Neuroimaging Initiative: A review of papers published since its inception. *Alzheimer's & Dementia*, *16*(12), 1551–1581.

World Health Organization. (2023). Dementia: Key facts. https://www.who.int/news-room/fact-sheets/detail/dementia

Xu, J., Glicksberg, B. S., Su, C., Walker, P., & Johnson, K. (2021). Federated learning for healthcare: Systematic review and roadmap. *Journal of the American Medical Informatics Association : JAMIA*, *28*(9), 1980–1993.

Zhou, J., Liu, J., & Ye, J. (2020). Graph neural networks in Alzheimer's disease analysis. *Frontiers in Neuroscience*, *14*, 143.

Zhu, X., Suk, H. I., & Shen, D. (2016). A novel matrix-similarity based loss function for Alzheimer's disease diagnosis. *Medical Image Analysis*, *33*, 159–177.

Compilation of References

Abisha, D., Mahalakshmi, M., Pritiga, T., Thanusiya, M., Punitha Sahaya Sherin, A., & Navedha Evanjalin, R. (2024, April). Revolutionising Rural Healthcare in India: AI-Powered Chatbots for Affordable Symptom Analysis and Medical Guidance. In *2024 International Conference on Inventive Computation Technologies (ICICT)* (pp. 181-187). IEEE.

Abouyannis, M.. (2024). Barriers to and facilitators of artificial intelligence adoption in health care: Scoping review. *JMIR Human Factors*, *11*, e48633. DOI: 10.2196/48633 PMID: 39207831

Adegboye, M. (2024). Impact of artificial intelligence on health information literacy: Guidance for healthcare professionals. *Library Hi Tech News*, *41*(7), 1–5. DOI: 10.1108/LHTN-03-2024-0048

Adege, A. B. (2025). Advancing Biomedical Engineering With Artificial Intelligence and Machine Learning: A Systematic Review. *International Journal of Clinical Practice*, *2025*(1), 9888902. DOI: 10.1155/ijcp/9888902

Adil, M., Ali, A., Tin, T. T., Farouk, A., Al-Kuwari, S., Song, H., & Jin, Z. (2025). Quantum computing and the future of healthcare internet of things security: Challenges and opportunities. *IEEE Internet of Things Journal*, *12*(22), 46316–46346. DOI: 10.1109/JIOT.2025.3605040

Adler-Milstein, J., & Jha, A. K. (2017). HITECH Act drove large gains in hospital electronic health record adoption. *Health Affairs*, *36*(8), 1416–1422. DOI: 10.1377/hlthaff.2016.1651 PMID: 28784734

ADNI. (2023). Alzheimer's Disease Neuroimaging Initiative (ADNI). http://adni.loni.usc.edu

Ahmadi Mehr, R., & Ameri, A. (2022). Skin Cancer Detection Based on Deep Learning. *Journal of Biomedical Physics & Engineering*, *12*(6), 559–568. DOI: 10.31661/jbpe.v0i0.2207-1517 PMID: 36569567

Aithal, P. S., & Aithal, S. (2025). Quantum Computers Supported Path to Technological Singularity–A Predictive Analysis. [PIJBAS]. *Poornaprajna International Journal of Basic & Applied Sciences*, *2*(1), 63–96. DOI: 10.64818/PIJBAS.3107.8478.0013

Akinnagbe, O. B. (2024). Human-AI Collaboration: Enhancing Productivity and Decision-Making. *International Journal of Education, Management, and Technology*, *2*(3), 387–417. DOI: 10.58578/ijemt.v2i3.4209

Alam, M. A., Sajib, M. R. U. Z., Rahman, F., Ether, S., Hanson, M., Sayeed, A., Akter, E., Nusrat, N., Islam, T. T., Raza, S., Tanvir, K. M., Chisti, M. J., Rahman, Q. S., Hossain, A., Layek, M., Zaman, A., Rana, J., Rahman, S. M., Arifeen, S. E., . . . Ahmed, A. (2024). Implications of Big Data Analytics, AI, Machine Learning, and Deep Learning in the Health Care System of Bangladesh: Scoping Review.

Al-Antari, M. A. (2023). Artificial Intelligence for Medical Diagnostics—Existing and Future AI Technology! *Diagnostics (Basel)*, *13*(4), 688. DOI: 10.3390/diagnostics13040688

Alharbe, N., & Almalki, M. (2025). IoT-enabled healthcare transformation leveraging deep learning for advanced patient monitoring and diagnosis. *Multimedia Tools and Applications*, *84*(19), 21331–21344. DOI: 10.1007/s11042-024-19919-w

Ali, A., Al-Rimy, B. A. S., Tin, T. T., Altamimi, S. N., Qasem, S. N., & Saeed, F. (2023). Empowering precision medicine: Unlocking revolutionary insights through blockchain-enabled federated learning and electronic medical records. *Sensors (Basel)*, *23*(17), 7476. Advance online publication. DOI: 10.3390/s23177476 PMID: 37687931

Ali, M. R., Lawson, C. A., Wood, A. M., & Khunti, K. (2023). Addressing ethnic and global health inequalities in the era of artificial intelligence healthcare models: A call for responsible implementation. *Journal of the Royal Society of Medicine*, *116*(8), 260–262. DOI: 10.1177/01410768231187734 PMID: 37467785

Al-Khasawneh, M. A., Faheem, M., Alarood, A. A., Habibullah, S., & Alzahrani, A. (2024). A secure blockchain framework for healthcare records management systems. *Healthcare Technology Letters*, *11*(6), 461–470. DOI: 10.1049/htl2.12092

Allana, S., Kankanhalli, M., & Dara, R. (2025). *Privacy Risks and Preservation Methods in Explainable Artificial Intelligence: A Scoping Review* (Version 1). arXiv. DOI: 10.48550/ARXIV.2505.02828

Alruwaili, F. F. (2020). Artificial intelligence and multi-agent-based distributed ledger system for better privacy and security of electronic healthcare records. *PeerJ. Computer Science*, *6*, e323. DOI: 10.7717/peerj-cs.323 PMID: 33816973

Alsamhi, S. H., Myrzashova, R., Hawbani, A., Kumar, S., Srivastava, S., Zhao, L., Wei, X., Guizan, M., & Curry, E. (2024). Federated learning meets blockchain in decentralized data sharing: Healthcare use case. *IEEE Internet of Things Journal, 11*(11), 19602–19615. DOI: 10.1109/JIOT.2024.3367249

Amann, J., Blasimme, A., Vayena, E., Frey, D., & Madai, V. I. (2020). Explainability for artificial intelligence in healthcare: A multidisciplinary perspective. *BMC Medical Informatics and Decision Making*, *20*(1), 310. DOI: 10.1186/s12911-020-01332-6 PMID: 33256715

Amin, M. S., Johnson, V. L., Prybutok, V., & Koh, C. E. (2024). An investigation into factors affecting the willingness to disclose personal health information when using AI-enabled caregiver robots. *Industrial Management & Data Systems*, *124*(4), 1677–1699. DOI: 10.1108/IMDS-09-2023-0608

Angst, C. M., & Agarwal, R. (2009). Adoption of electronic health records in the presence of privacy concerns: The elaboration likelihood model and individual persuasion. *Management Information Systems Quarterly*, *33*(2), 339–370. DOI: 10.2307/20650295

Anshara, M., & Shabbir, N. (2025). The role of artificial Intelligence in identifying depression and anxiety. Journal Global Values, XVI(SI), 75–81. DOI: 10.31995/jgv.2025.v16iSI7.011

Anyanwu, E. C., Okongwu, C. C., Olorunsogo, T. O., Ayo-Farai, O., Osasona, F., & Daraojimba, O. D. (2024). Artificial Intelligence in healthcare: A review of ethical dilemmas and practical applications. *International Medical Science Research Journal*, *4*(2), 126–140. DOI: 10.51594/imsrj.v4i2.755

Ardila, D., Kiraly, A. P., Bharadwaj, S., Choi, B., Reicher, J. J., Peng, L., Tse, D., Etemadi, M., Ye, W., Corrado, G. S., Naidu, M., Shetty, S., & Sundaram, P. (2019). End-to-end lung cancer screening with three-dimensional deep learning on low-dose chest computed tomography. *Nature Medicine*, *25*(6), 954–961. DOI: 10.1038/s41591-019-0447-x PMID: 31110349

Arevalo-Rodriguez, I., Pedraza, O. L., Rodríguez, A., Sánchez, E., Galdos, F., & Yepes-Nuñez, J. J. (2021). Mini-Mental State Examination (MMSE) for the detection of Alzheimer's disease and other dementias. *Cochrane Database of Systematic Reviews*, *7*(3), 1–79. PMID: 25740785

Arshad, J., Murtza, M. H., & Arshad, M. (2023). Quantum computing in biomedical engineering: Opportunities, challenges, and future perspectives. *Biomedical Engineering Advances*, *5*, 100067. DOI: 10.1016/j.bea.2023.100067

Asif, M., Abrar, M., Salam, A., Amin, F., Ullah, F., Shah, S., & AlSalman, H. (2025). Intelligent two-phase dual authentication framework for Internet of Medical Things. *Scientific Reports*, *15*(1), 1760. DOI: 10.1038/s41598-024-84713-5

Ayaz, M., Pasha, M. F., Alzahrani, M. Y., Budiarto, R., & Stiawan, D. (2021). The Fast Health Interoperability Resources (FHIR) Standard: Systematic Literature Review of Implementations, Applications, Challenges and Opportunities. *JMIR Medical Informatics*, *9*(7), e21929. DOI: 10.2196/21929

Ayub, M. A., Tyagi, A. R., Srivastava, S. K., & Singh, P. (2025). Quantum DFT analysis and molecular docking investigation of various potential breast cancer drugs. *Journal of Materials Chemistry. B*, *13*(1), 218–238. DOI: 10.1039/D4TB01803F PMID: 39545283

Aziz, N. A., Manzoor, A., Mazhar Qureshi, M. D., Qureshi, M. A., & Rashwan, W. (2024, August). *Unveiling Explainable AI in Healthcare: Current Trends, Challenges, and Future Directions*. Health Informatics. DOI: 10.1101/2024.08.10.24311735

Babar, M., Qureshi, B., & Koubaa, A. (2024). Investigating the impact of data heterogeneity on the performance of federated learning algorithm using medical imaging. *PLoS One*, *19*(5), e0302539. DOI: 10.1371/journal.pone.0302539 PMID: 38748657

Babic, B., Glenn Cohen, I., Stern, A. D., Li, Y., & Ouellet, M. (2025). A general framework for governing marketed AI/ML medical devices. *NPJ Digital Medicine*, *8*(1), 328. DOI: 10.1038/s41746-025-01717-9

Badwy, B., Ghanem, N. M., Banawan, K., & Ismail, N. E. (2024). Enhanced Prediction of Immune Checkpoint Blockade Response in Melanoma Using Ensemble Learning and a Hybrid Feature Selection Technique. *IEEE Access : Practical Innovations, Open Solutions*, *12*, 187041–187067. DOI: 10.1109/ACCESS.2024.3514799

Bae, M. S. (2024). AI Improves Cancer Detection and Reading Time of Digital Breast Tomosynthesis. *Radiology. Artificial Intelligence*, *6*(3), e240219. DOI: 10.1148/ryai.240219

Bagave, P., Westberg, M., Janssen, M., & Ding, A. Y. (2025, September). *Accountability Framework for Healthcare AI Systems: Towards Joint Accountability in Decision Making*. arXiv. https://doi.org//arXiv.2509.03286DOI: 10.48550

Bajwa, J., Munir, U., Nori, A., & Williams, B. (2021). Artificial intelligence in healthcare: Transforming the practice of medicine. *Future Healthcare Journal*, *8*(2), e188–e194. DOI: 10.7861/fhj.2021-0095

Balasubramani, S., Renjith, P. N., Kavisankar, L., Rajavel, R., Malarvel, M., & Shankar, A. (2025). A Quantum-Enhanced Artificial Neural Network Model for Efficient Medical Image Compression. *IEEE Access : Practical Innovations, Open Solutions.*

Barnes, B., Stansbury, N., Brown, D., Garson, L., Gerard, G., Piccoli, N., Jendrasek, D., May, N., Castillo, V., Adelfio, A., Ramirez, N., McSweeney, A., Berlien, R., & Butler, P. J. (2021). Risk-Based Monitoring in Clinical Trials: Past, Present, and Future. *Therapeutic Innovation & Regulatory Science*, *55*(4), 899–906. DOI: 10.1007/s43441-021-00295-8

Basa, R. (2024). Human-AI collaboration in healthcare diagnostics: Enhancing accuracy and patient outcomes. *International Journal of Computer Engineering and Technology*, *15*(5). Advance online publication. DOI: 10.5281/zenodo.13918695

Bean, D. M., Kraljevic, Z., Shek, A., Teo, J., & Dobson, R. J. B. (2023). Hospital-wide natural language processing summarising the health data of 1 million patients. *PLOS Digital Health*, *2*(5), e0000218. DOI: 10.1371/journal.pdig.0000218 PMID: 37159441

Beaulieu-Jones, B. K., Wu, Z. S., Williams, C., Lee, R., Bhavnani, S. P., Byrd, J. B., & Greene, C. S. (2019). Privacy-preserving generative deep neural networks support clinical data sharing. *Circulation: Cardiovascular Quality and Outcomes*, *12*(7), e005122. DOI: 10.1161/CIRCOUTCOMES.118.005122 PMID: 31284738

Bebortta, S., Tripathy, S. S., Basheer, S., & Chowdhary, C. L. (2023). FedEHR: A federated learning approach towards the prediction of heart diseases in IoT-based Electronic Health Records. *Diagnostics (Basel)*, *13*(20), 3166. Advance online publication. DOI: 10.3390/diagnostics13203166 PMID: 37891987

Benson, T., & Grieve, G. (2016). *Principles of health interoperability: SNOMED CT, HL7 and FHIR* (3rd ed.). Springer., DOI: 10.1007/978-3-319-30370-3

Bertolo, R., De Bon, L., Caudana, F., Pettenuzzo, G., Malandra, S., Casolani, C., Zivi, A., Fantinel, E., Borsato, A., Negrelli, R., Salah El Din Tantawy, E., Volpi, G., Brunelli, M., Veccia, A., Cerruto, M. A., & Antonelli, A. (2025). Role of large language models in the multidisciplinary decision-making process for patients with renal cell carcinoma: A pilot experience. *NPJ Precision Oncology*, *9*(1), 257. DOI: 10.1038/s41698-025-01014-4

Bhakuni, P., Punia, A., & Sharma, N. (2025). Mental Health and AI. In *Advances in Healthcare Information Systems and Administration* (pp. 299–332). IGI Global., DOI: 10.4018/979-8-3693-7858-8.ch011

Bhargava, A., Bhargava, A., Kumar, A., Ahmad, F., & Kumar, A. (2024). Facilitators and barriers to AI adoption in nursing practice: A qualitative study of registered nurses' perspectives. *BMC Nursing, 23*(1), 917. DOI: 10.1186/s12912-024-02571-y PMID: 39695581

Bhatia, G., Choudhary, H., & Mathur, R. (2025). Artificial intelligence in mental health research: Opportunities and challenges. *Annals of Indian Psychiatry*. Advance online publication. DOI: 10.4103/aip.aip_100_25

Bhattacharya, P., Mukherjee, A., Bhushan, B., Gupta, S. K., Gadekallu, T. R., & Zhu, Z. (2025). A secured remote patient monitoring framework for IoMT ecosystems. *Scientific Reports, 15*(1), 22882. DOI: 10.1038/s41598-025-04774-y

Biró, A., Cuesta-Vargas, A. I., & Szilágyi, L. (2023). Precognition of mental health and neurogenerative disorders using. *Acta Universitatis Sapientiae Informatica, 15*(2), 359–403. DOI: 10.2478/ausi-2023-0022

Björnsson, B., Borrebaeck, C., Elander, N., Gasslander, T., Gawel, D. R., Gustafsson, M., Jörnsten, R., Lee, E. J., Li, X., Lilja, S., Martínez-Enguita, D., Matussek, A., Sandström, P., Schäfer, S., Stenmarker, M., Sun, X. F., Sysoev, O., Zhang, H., & Benson, M.Swedish Digital Twin Consortium. (2019). Digital twins to personalize medicine. *Genome Medicine, 12*(1), 4. DOI: 10.1186/s13073-019-0701-3 PMID: 31892363

Blease, C., Torous, J., McMillan, B., Hägglund, M., & Mandl, K. D. (2024). Generative Language Models and Open Notes: Exploring the Promise and Limitations. *JMIR Medical Education, 10*, e51183. Advance online publication. DOI: 10.2196/51183

Bobkov, A., Cheng, F., Xu, J., Bobkova, T., Deng, F., He, J., Jiang, X., Khuzin, D., & Kang, Z. (2025). Telepsychiatry and artificial intelligence: A structured review of emerging approaches to accessible psychiatric care. *Healthcare (Basel), 13*(11), 1348. DOI: 10.3390/healthcare13111348 PMID: 40508960

Bodenheimer, T., & Sinsky, C. (2014). From triple to quadruple aim: Care of the patient requires care of the provider. *Annals of Family Medicine, 12*(6), 573–576. DOI: 10.1370/afm.1713 PMID: 25384822

Bodenreider, O. (2004). The Unified Medical Language System (UMLS): Integrating biomedical terminology. *Nucleic Acids Research, 32*(Database issue), D267–D270. DOI: 10.1093/nar/gkh061 PMID: 14681409

Booth, H., Souppaya, M., Vassilev, A., Ogata, M., Stanley, M., & Scarfone, K. (2022). Secure Software Development Practices for Generative AI and Dual-Use Foundation Models: An SSDF Community Profile. *IEEE Transactions on Dependable and Secure Computing*. Advance online publication. DOI: 10.6028/NIST.SP.800-218A

Boussina, A., Shashikumar, S. P., Malhotra, A., Owens, R. L., El-Kareh, R., Longhurst, C. A., Quintero, K., Donahue, A., Chan, T. C., Nemati, S., & Wardi, G. (2024). Impact of a deep learning sepsis prediction model on quality of care and survival. *npj. Digital Medicine*, *7*(1), 14. DOI: 10.1038/s41746-023-00986-6 PMID: 38263386

Braga, D. M., & Rawal, B. S. (2025). Harnessing AI and quantum computing for accelerated drug discovery: Regulatory frameworks for in silico to in vivo validation. *Journal of Pharmaceutical and BioTech Industry*, *2*(3), 11. DOI: 10.3390/jpbi2030011

Bruynseels, K., Santoni de Sio, F., & van den Hoven, J. (2018). Digital twins in health care: Ethical implications of an emerging engineering paradigm. *Frontiers in Genetics*, *9*, 31. DOI: 10.3389/fgene.2018.00031 PMID: 29487613

Buhr, E., Fischer, M., Biernetzky, O., Teipel, S., Gruber, O., & Schweda, M. (2025). Use of artificial intelligence in psychiatric research and practice: A qualitative interview study with experts from psychiatry, computer science and philosophy in Germany. *European Psychiatry : the Journal of the Association of European Psychiatrists*, *68*(1), e105. DOI: 10.1192/j.eurpsy.2025.10075 PMID: 40754806

Bukkarayasamudram, V. K., Reddy, P. C. S., Arun Kumar, K., Jagadish, R. M., Sharma, S., Prasad, M. L., Sucharitha, Y., Tayubi, I. A., & Thakur, G. K. (2025). Quantum computing revolution in healthcare: A systematic review of applications, issues and future directions. *Artificial Intelligence Review*, *58*(12), 1–35. DOI: 10.1007/s10462-025-11381-w

Carlos Ferreira, J., Elvas, L. B., Correia, R., & Mascarenhas, M. (2024). Enhancing EHR Interoperability and Security through Distributed Ledger Technology: A Review. *Healthcare (Basel)*, *12*(19), 1967. DOI: 10.3390/healthcare12191967

Celi, L. A., Cellini, J., Charpignon, M., Boag, W., Huang, L., Feller, A., & Pollard, T. J. (2022). Sources of bias in artificial intelligence that perpetuate healthcare disparities, A global review. *PLOS Digital Health*, *1*(3), e0000022. DOI: 10.1371/journal.pdig.0000022 PMID: 36812532

Challen, R., Denny, J., Pitt, M., Gompels, L., Edwards, T., & Tsaneva-Atanasova, K. (2019). Artificial intelligence, bias and clinical safety. *BMJ Quality & Safety*, *28*(3), 231–237. DOI: 10.1136/bmjqs-2018-008370

Chandrakumar, A., & Jamthikar, A. D. (2023). Class imbalance in healthcare AI: Challenges and opportunities. *Journal of Medical Systems*, *47*(2), 45.

Chang, Y., Fang, C., & Sun, W. (2021). A blockchain-based federated learning method for smart healthcare. *Computational Intelligence and Neuroscience*, *2021*(1), 4376418. DOI: 10.1155/2021/4376418 PMID: 34868289

Charow, R., Jeyakumar, T., Younus, S., Dolatabadi, E., Salhia, M., Al-Mouaswas, D., Anderson, M., Balakumar, S., Clare, M., Dhalla, A., Gillan, C., Haghzare, S., Jackson, E., Lalani, N., Mattson, J., Peteanu, W., Tripp, T., Waldorf, J., Williams, S., & Wiljer, D. (2021). Artificial intelligence education programs for health care professionals: Scoping review. *JMIR Medical Education*, *7*(4), e31043. DOI: 10.2196/31043 PMID: 34898458

Chaturvedi, S. (2023). Clinical prediction on ML based Internet of Things for e-health care system. *International Journal of Data Informatics and Intelligent Computing*, *2*(3), 29–37. DOI: 10.59461/ijdiic.v2i3.76

Chawla, N. V., Bowyer, K. W., Hall, L. O., & Kegelmeyer, W. P. (2002). SMOTE: Synthetic minority oversampling technique. *Journal of Artificial Intelligence Research*, *16*, 321–357. DOI: 10.1613/jair.953

Chekroud, A. M., Bondar, J., Delgadillo, J., Doherty, G., Wasil, A., Fokkema, M., Cohen, Z., Belgrave, D., DeRubeis, R., Iniesta, R., Dwyer, D., & Choi, K. (2021). The promise of machine learning in predicting treatment outcomes in psychiatry. *World Psychiatry; Official Journal of the World Psychiatric Association (WPA)*, *20*(2), 154–170. DOI: 10.1002/wps.20882 PMID: 34002503

Chen, I. Y., Szolovits, P., & Ghassemi, M. (2021). Can AI help reduce disparities in general medical and mental health care? *AMA Journal of Ethics*, *23*(2), E184–E191. https://journalofethics.ama-assn.org/article/can-ai-help-reduce-disparities-general-medical-and-mental-health-care/2019-02 PMID: 30794127

Chen, Y., & Esmaeilzadeh, P. (2024). Generative AI in Medical Practice: In-Depth Exploration of Privacy and Security Challenges. *Journal of Medical Internet Research*, *26*(1), e53008. DOI: 10.2196/53008

Chinnaperumal, S., Periyasamy, M., Alhussan, A. A., Kannan, S., Khafaga, D. S., Raju, S. K., Eid, M. M., & El-kenawy, E.-S. M. (2025). Secure and intelligent 5G-enabled remote patient monitoring using ANN and Choquet integral fuzzy VIKOR. *Scientific Reports*, *15*(1), 9913. DOI: 10.1038/s41598-025-93829-1

Chiou, E. K., & Lee, J. D. (2023). Trusting automation: Designing for responsivity and resilience. *Human Factors*, *65*(1), 137–165. DOI: 10.1177/00187208211009995 PMID: 33906505

Chow, J. C. L. (2024). Quantum computing in medicine: Current state and future prospects. *Journal of Medical Informatics and Health*, *12*(4), 67.

Chow, J. C. L., Wong, V., & Li, K. (2024). Generative pre-trained transformer-empowered healthcare conversations: Current trends, challenges, and future directions in large language model-enabled medical chatbots. *BioMedInformatics*, *4*(1), 837–852. DOI: 10.3390/biomedinformatics4010047

Clement David-Olawade, A., Olawade, D. B., Vanderbloemen, L., Rotifa, O. B., Fidelis, S. C., Egbon, E., Akpan, A. O., Adeleke, S., Ghose, A., & Boussios, S. (2025). AI-driven advances in low-dose imaging and enhancement-A review. *Diagnostics (Basel)*, *15*(6), 689. DOI: 10.3390/diagnostics15060689 PMID: 40150031

Conduah, A. K., Ofoe, S., & Siaw-Marfo, D. (2025). Data privacy in healthcare: Global challenges and solutions. *Digital Health*, *11*, 20552076251343959. Advance online publication. DOI: 10.1177/20552076251343959

Cornwall, A., & Jewkes, R. (1995). What is participatory research? *Social Science & Medicine*, *41*(12), 1667–1676. DOI: 10.1016/0277-9536(95)00127-S PMID: 8746866

Cross, J. L., Choma, M. A., & Onofrey, J. A. (2024). Bias in medical AI: Implications for clinical decision-making. *PLOS Digital Health*, *3*(11), e0000651. DOI: 10.1371/journal.pdig.0000651

da Rocha, J. M., Campos, D. M. D. O., Esmaile, S. C., Menezes, G. D. L., Bezerra, K. S., da Silva, R. A., Junior, E. D. S., Tayyeb, J. Z., Akash, S., Fulco, U. L., Alqahtani, T., & Oliveira, J. I. (2025). Quantum biochemical analysis of the binding interactions between a potential inhibitory drug and the Ebola viral glycoprotein. *Journal of Biomolecular Structure & Dynamics*, *43*(9), 4753–4769. DOI: 10.1080/07391102.2024.2305314 PMID: 38258414

Daley, K.. (2024). Overcoming barriers and enabling artificial intelligence adoption in allied health clinical practice: A qualitative study. *Digital Health*, *11*, 20552076241311144. DOI: 10.1177/20552076241311144 PMID: 39906878

Dasa, D., Board, M., Rolfe, U., Dolby, T., & Tang, W. (2025). Evaluating AI-driven characters in extended reality (XR) healthcare simulations: A systematic review. *Artificial Intelligence in Medicine*, *103270*, 103270. Advance online publication. DOI: 10.1016/j.artmed.2025.103270

Das, B. C., Amini, M. H., & Wu, Y. (2025). Security and Privacy Challenges of Large Language Models: A Survey. *ACM Computing Surveys*, *57*(6), 1–39. DOI: 10.1145/3712001

Dash, S., Aarthy, R., & Mohan, V. (2021). Telemedicine during COVID-19 in India—A new policy and its challenges. *Journal of Public Health Policy*, *42*(3), 501–509. DOI: 10.1057/s41271-021-00287-w PMID: 34012012

Das, S., & Ghosh, S. (2020). Alzheimer's disease detection from MRI using deep neural networks. *Expert Systems with Applications*, *139*, 112–121.

Davalos, D. S. (2024). A conceptual Swarm Intelligence framework for deriving a global healthcare machine learning model. International Journal of Business and Applied Social Science, 12–27. DOI: 10.33642/ijbass.v10n5p2

Davenport, T., & Kalakota, R. (2019). The potential for artificial intelligence in healthcare. *Future Healthcare Journal*, *6*(2), 94–98. DOI: 10.7861/futurehosp.6-2-94

Davis, F. D. (1989). Perceived usefulness, perceived ease of use, and user acceptance of information technology. *Management Information Systems Quarterly*, *13*(3), 319–340. DOI: 10.2307/249008

de Castro, Y. V. C., Morii, K. Y., Santos, I. A., Destefani, A. C., & Destefani, V. C. (2024). Beyond black boxes: Interpretable Ai for enhanced risk assessment and ethical decision-making in forensic psychiatry. Revista Ibero-Americana de Humanidades. *Ciência & Educação (Bauru)*, *10*(8), 2475–2479. DOI: 10.51891/rease.v10i8.15298

Deo, R. C. (2024). Artificial Intelligence and Health Equity. *JACC Advances*, *3*(9), 101045. DOI: 10.1016/j.jacadv.2024.101045

Dhiman, R., Bazad, N., Mukherjee, R., Himanshu, , Gunjan, , Leal, E., Ahmad, S., Kaur, K., Raj, V. S., Chang, C.-M., & Pandey, R. P. (2024). Enhanced drug delivery with nanocarriers: A comprehensive review of recent advances in breast cancer detection and treatment. *Discover Nano*, *19*(1), 143. DOI: 10.1186/s11671-024-04086-6

Díaz, O., Rodríguez-Ruíz, A., & Sechopoulos, I. (2024). Artificial Intelligence for breast cancer detection: Technology, challenges, and prospects. *European Journal of Radiology*, *175*, 111457. DOI: 10.1016/j.ejrad.2024.111457

Doraiswamy, P. M., Blease, C., & Bodner, K. (2020a). Artificial intelligence and the future of psychiatry: Insights from a global physician survey. *Artificial Intelligence in Medicine*, *102*(101753), 101753. DOI: 10.1016/j.artmed.2019.101753 PMID: 31980092

Doshi-Velez, F., & Kim, B. (2017). Towards a rigorous science of interpretable machine learning. *arXiv preprint* arXiv:1702.08608. https://arxiv.org/abs/1702.08608

Dosovitskiy, A., Beyer, L., Kolesnikov, A., Weissenborn, D., & Houlsby, N. (2021). An image is worth 16x16 words: Transformers for image recognition at scale. *International Conference on Learning Representations*, 1–20.

Dow, E. R., Chen, K. M., Zhao, C. S., Knapp, A. N., Phadke, A., Weng, K., Do, D. V., Mahajan, V. B., Mruthyunjaya, P., Leng, T., & Myung, D. (2023). Artificial Intelligence improves patient follow-up in a diabetic retinopathy screening program. *Clinical Ophthalmology (Auckland, N.Z.)*, *17*, 3323–3330. DOI: 10.2147/OPTH.S422513 PMID: 38026608

Dow, E. R., Khan, N. C., Chen, K. M., Mishra, K., Perera, C., Narala, R., Basina, M., Dang, J., Kim, M., Levine, M., Phadke, A., Tan, M., Weng, K., Do, D. V., Moshfeghi, D. M., Mahajan, V. B., Mruthyunjaya, P., Leng, T., & Myung, D. (2023). AI-human hybrid workflow enhances teleophthalmology for the detection of diabetic retinopathy. *Ophthalmology Science*, *3*(4), 100330. DOI: 10.1016/j.xops.2023.100330 PMID: 37449051

Dubois, B., Villain, N., Frisoni, G., Rabinovici, G. D., & Schneider, L. (2021). Clinical diagnosis of Alzheimer's disease: Recommendations of the International Working Group. *Lancet Neurology*, *20*(6), 484–496. DOI: 10.1016/S1474-4422(21)00066-1 PMID: 33933186

Durant, T. J. S.. (2024). A primer for quantum computing and its applications to biomedicine: Opportunities and challenges. *Journal of the American Medical Informatics Association : JAMIA*, *31*(8), 1774–1786. DOI: 10.1093/jamia/ocae149 PMID: 38934288

Dwivedi, Y. K., Rana, N. P., Jeyaraj, A., Clement, M., & Williams, M. D. (2019). Re-examining the unified theory of acceptance and use of technology (UTAUT): Towards a revised theoretical model. *Information Systems Frontiers*, *21*(3), 719–734. DOI: 10.1007/s10796-017-9774-y

Dwork, C., & Roth, A. (2014). The algorithmic foundations of differential privacy. *Foundations and Trends in Theoretical Computer Science*, *9*(3-4), 211–407. DOI: 10.1561/0400000042

Dziedzic, A., Issa, J., Chaurasia, A., & Tanasiewicz, M. (2024). Artificial intelligence and health-related data: The patient's best interest and data ownership dilemma. *Proceedings of the Institution of Mechanical Engineers. Part H, Journal of Engineering in Medicine*, *238*(10), 1023–1028. DOI: 10.1177/09544119241279630 PMID: 39275850

Echenim, J. I. (2025). Exploring the integration of AI and blockchain for secure, transparent, and decentralized data management systems. International Journal of Science, Architecture, Technology and Environment, 878–885. DOI: 10.63680/afvdbg764hg099hb

Ejaz, U., Islam, S. A. M., Sarkar, A., & Imashev, A. (2024). Federated Learning for secure and privacy-preserving medical collaboration across multi-cloud healthcare systems. *IOSR Journal of Mechanical and Civil Engineering*, *21*(5), 36–44. DOI: 10.9790/1684-2105023644

El Rifai, O., Biotteau, M., de Boissezon, X., Megdiche, I., Ravat, F., & Teste, O. (2020). Blockchain-based federated learning in medicine. In *Artificial Intelligence in Medicine* (pp. 214–224). Springer International Publishing., DOI: 10.1007/978-3-030-59137-3_20

ElBedoui, K., Ben Lakhal, N., & Barhoumi, W. (2025). Medical image analysis: A systematization of knowledge on the convergence of AI and quantum computing. *The Journal of Supercomputing*, *81*(15), 1–52. DOI: 10.1007/s11227-025-07789-4

El-Kareh, R., & Sittig, D. F. (2022). Enhancing diagnosis through technology: Decision support, artificial intelligence, and beyond. *Critical Care Clinics*, *38*(1), 129–139. DOI: 10.1016/j.ccc.2021.08.004 PMID: 34794627

El-Maghrabey, M., El Hamd, M. A., Al-Khateeb, L. A., Magdy, G., Mahdi, W. A., Alshehri, S., Alsehli, B. R., & El-Shaheny, R. (2025). Design and synthesis of high quantum yield doped carbon nano probe derived from household sources for sensing of the anti-GERD drug pantoprazole. *Spectrochimica Acta. Part A: Molecular and Biomolecular Spectroscopy*, *325*, 125067. DOI: 10.1016/j.saa.2024.125067 PMID: 39232309

Emery, F. E., & Trist, E. L. (1960). *Socio-technical systems.* Management science, models and techniques 2.

Eswaran, U., Eswaran, V., Eswaran, V., & Murali, K. (2025). Future Frontiers: The Role of AGI and Quantum Computing in Solving Complex Global Problems. In *Interplay of Artificial General Intelligence with Quantum Computing: Towards Sustainability* (pp. 137–151). Springer Nature Switzerland. DOI: 10.1007/978-3-031-87931-9_11

European Alliance for Innovation. (2025). Smart hospitals and quantum-enabled optimization frameworks. *EAI Endorsed Transactions on Smart Health*, *9*(34), e8.

European Commission. (2024). *Proposal for a Regulation laying down harmonised rules on Artificial Intelligence (Artificial Intelligence Act)*. Publications Office of the European Union. https://eur-lex.europa.eu/legal-content/EN/TXT/?uri=celex:52021PC0206

European Parliament. (2024). Regulation (EU) 2024/1689 of the European Parliament and of the Council laying down harmonised rules on artificial intelligence (Artificial Intelligence Act). Official Journal of the European Union, L 2024/1689. https://eur-lex.europa.eu/eli/reg/2024/1689/oj

Evans, R. S. (2016). Electronic health records: Then, now, and in the future. *Yearbook of Medical Informatics*, *26*(S 01, Suppl 1), S48–S61. DOI: 10.15265/IYS-2016-s006 PMID: 27199197

Fahad, M., Ibrar, M., Qayyum, M. U., & Husnain, A. (2024). Artificial intelligence in healthcare: Revealing novel approaches to cancer treatment, fraud investigation, and petroleum industry perspectives. *International Journal of Multidisciplinary Sciences and Arts*, *3*(4), 37–45. DOI: 10.47709/ijmdsa.v3i4.4637

Fairburn, S. C., Jehi, L., Bicknell, B. T., Wilkes, B. G., & Panuganti, B. (2025). Applications of quantum computing in clinical care: Enhancing diagnostics, treatment, and decision-making. [REMOVED HYPERLINK FIELD]. *Frontiers in Medicine*, *12*, 1573016. DOI: 10.3389/fmed.2025.1573016

Farooq, K., Syed, H. J., Alqahtani, S. O., Nagmeldin, W., Ibrahim, A. O., & Gani, A. (2022). Blockchain federated learning for in-home health monitoring. *Electronics (Basel)*, *12*(1), 136. DOI: 10.3390/electronics12010136

Firouzi, F., Jiang, S., Chakrabarty, K., Farahani, B., Daneshmand, M., Song, J., & Mankodiya, K. (2023). Fusion of IoT, AI, edge–fog–cloud, and blockchain: Challenges, solutions, and a case study in healthcare and medicine. *IEEE Internet of Things Journal*, *10*(5), 3686–3705. DOI: 10.1109/JIOT.2022.3191881

Fleurence, R. L., Curtis, L. H., Califf, R. M., Platt, R., Selby, J. V., & Brown, J. S. (2014). Launching PCORnet, a national patient-centered clinical research network. *Journal of the American Medical Informatics Association : JAMIA*, *21*(4), 578–582. DOI: 10.1136/amiajnl-2014-002747 PMID: 24821743

Fleuren, L. M., Klausch, T. L. T., Zwager, C. L., Schoonmade, L. J., Guo, T., Roggeveen, L. F., Swart, E. L., Girbes, A. R. J., Thoral, P., Ercole, A., Hoogendoorn, M., & Elbers, P. W. G. (2020). Machine learning for the prediction of sepsis: A systematic review and meta-analysis of diagnostic test accuracy. *Intensive Care Medicine*, *46*(3), 383–400. DOI: 10.1007/s00134-019-05872-y PMID: 31965266

Floridi, L., & Cowls, J. (2019). A unified framework of five principles for AI in society. *Harvard Data Science Review*, *1*(1). Advance online publication. DOI: 10.1162/99608f92.8cd550d1

Floridi, L., Cowls, J., Beltrametti, M., Chatila, R., Chazerand, P., Dignum, V., Luetge, C., Madelin, R., Pagallo, U., Rossi, F., Schafer, B., Valcke, P., & Vayena, E. (2018). AI4People—An ethical framework for a good AI society. *Minds and Machines*, *28*(4), 689–707. DOI: 10.1007/s11023-018-9482-5 PMID: 30930541

Frid-Adar, M., Klang, E., Amitai, M., Goldberger, J., & Greenspan, H. (2018). GAN-based synthetic medical image augmentation. *Neurocomputing*, *321*, 321–331. DOI: 10.1016/j.neucom.2018.09.013

Frisoni, G. B., Boccardi, M., Barkhof, F., & Blennow, K. (2021). Strategic roadmap for an early diagnosis of Alzheimer's disease. *Lancet Neurology*, *19*(5), 396–405. PMID: 28721928

Gabriel, I., & Precious, A. (2025). *Integration of artificial intelligence into clinical workflows: Barriers and best practices*. Obafemi Awolowo University.

Garg, P., Sharma, M. K., & Kumar, P. (2025). Transparency in Diagnosis: Unveiling the Power of Deep Learning and Explainable AI for Medical Image Interpretation. *Arabian Journal for Science and Engineering*, *50*(19), 15751–15767. Advance online publication. DOI: 10.1007/s13369-024-09896-5

Gartner. (2021). *Innovation insight for data fabric*. Gartner Research Report.

Gerantia, M. (2024). Artificial intelligence in psychiatry: A comprehensive literature review. *European Psychiatry : the Journal of the Association of European Psychiatrists*, *67*(S1), S61–S61. DOI: 10.1192/j.eurpsy.2024.173

Gerke, S., Minssen, T., & Cohen, I. G. (2020). Ethical and legal challenges of artificial intelligence-driven healthcare. In Cohen, I. G., Lynch, H. F., Vayena, E., & Gasser, U. (Eds.), *Biomedical Innovation and the Law* (pp. 295–336). Cambridge University Press., DOI: 10.1016/B978-0-12-818438-7.00012-5

Germack, H. D., Leung, L., Zhao, X., Zhang, H., & Martsolf, G. R. (2022). Association of team-based care and continuity of care with hospitalizations for veterans with comorbid mental and physical health conditions. *Journal of General Internal Medicine*, *37*(1), 40–48. DOI: 10.1007/s11606-021-06884-5 PMID: 34027614

Giron-Michel, J., Padelli, M., Oberlin, E., Guenou, H., & Duclos-Vallée, J.-C. (2025). State-of-the-Art Liver Cancer Organoids: Modeling Cancer Stem Cell Heterogeneity for Personalized Treatment. *BioDrugs*, *39*(2), 237–260. DOI: 10.1007/s40259-024-00702-0

Glikson, E., & Woolley, A. W. (2020). Human trust in artificial intelligence: Review of empirical research. *The Academy of Management Annals, 14*(2), 627–660. DOI: 10.5465/annals.2018.0057

Gobinath, A., Rajeswari, P., Kumar, S. N., & Anandan, M. (2025). Quantum Robotics in Health Care: Innovations and Applications. In The Quantum Evolution (pp. 211-225). CRC Press.

Goktas, P., & Grzybowski, A. (2025). Shaping the future of healthcare: Ethical clinical challenges and pathways to trustworthy AI. *Journal of Clinical Medicine, 14*(5), 1605. Advance online publication. DOI: 10.3390/jcm14051605 PMID: 40095575

Goldfarb, A., & Teodoridis, F. (2022). Why is AI adoption in health care lagging? *Brookings Papers on Economic Activity, 2022*(1), 1–83.

Gomes, D., & Saifuddin Saif, A. F. M. (2021). Robust Underwater Fish Detection Using an Enhanced Convolutional Neural Network. *International Journal of Image. Graphics and Signal Processing, 13*(3), 44–54. DOI: 10.5815/ijigsp.2021.03.04

Goodfellow, I., Pouget-Abadie, J., Mirza, M., Xu, B., & Warde-Farley, D. (2014). Generative adversarial Nets. *Advances in Neural Information Processing Systems, 27*, 2672–2680.

Gorelik, A. J., Li, M., Hahne, J., Wang, J., Ren, Y., Yang, L., Zhang, X., Liu, X., Wang, X., Bogdan, R., & Carpenter, B. D. (2025). Ethics of AI in healthcare: A scoping review demonstrating applicability of a foundational framework. *Frontiers in Digital Health, 7*, 1662642. DOI: 10.3389/fdgth.2025.1662642 PMID: 41000336

Goswami, S. A., Dave, S., Patel, K. C., & Raval, M. N. (2025). Application of quantum artificial intelligence in healthcare. In *Quantum Computing for Healthcare Data* (pp. 119–138). Academic Press. DOI: 10.1016/B978-0-443-29297-2.00007-1

Gottesman, O., Kuivaniemi, H., Tromp, G., Faucett, W. A., Li, R., Manolio, T. A., Sanderson, S. C., Kannry, J., Zinberg, R., Basford, M. A., Brilliant, M., Carey, D. J., Chisholm, R. L., Chute, C. G., Connolly, J. J., Crosslin, D., Denny, J. C., Gallego, C. J., Haines, J. L., & Williams, M. S. (2013). The Electronic Medical Records and Genomics (eMERGE) Network: Past, present, and future. *Genetics in Medicine, 15*(10), 761–771. DOI: 10.1038/gim.2013.72 PMID: 23743551

Graham, S., Depp, C., Lee, E. E., Nebeker, C., Tu, X., Kim, H.-C., & Jeste, D. V. (2019). Artificial intelligence for mental health and mental illnesses: An overview. *Current Psychiatry Reports, 21*(11), 116. DOI: 10.1007/s11920-019-1094-0 PMID: 31701320

Grand View Research. (2023). *AI in healthcare market size, share & trends analysis report.* https://www.grandviewresearch.com/industry-analysis/artificial-intelligence-ai-healthcare-market

Grannis, S. J., Xu, H., Vest, J. R., Kasthurirathne, S., Bo, N., Moscovitch, B., Torkzadeh, N., & Rising, J. (2019). Evaluating the effect of data standardization and validation on patient matching accuracy. *Journal of the American Medical Informatics Association : JAMIA, 26*(5), 447–456. DOI: 10.1093/jamia/ocy191 PMID: 30848796

Grant, M. J., & Booth, A. (2009). A typology of reviews: An analysis of 14 review types and associated methodologies. *Health Information and Libraries Journal, 26*(2), 91–108. DOI: 10.1111/j.1471-1842.2009.00848.x PMID: 19490148

Gray, R., Campbell, L., Goharian, A., & Iredale, H. (2022). Health informatics: Engaging modern healthcare units: A brief overview. *Frontiers in Digital Health, 4*, 814775. DOI: 10.3389/fdgth.2022.814775

Greenhalgh, T., Wherton, J., Papoutsi, C., Lynch, J., Hughes, G., Hinder, S., & Shaw, S. (2017). Beyond adoption: A new framework for theorizing and evaluating nonadoption, abandonment, and challenges to the scale-up, spread, and sustainability of health and care technologies. *Journal of Medical Internet Research, 19*(11), e8775. DOI: 10.2196/jmir.8775 PMID: 29092808

Guerreiro, R., & Bras, J. (2015). The age factor in Alzheimer's disease. *Molecular Neurobiology, 51*(1), 1–7. PMID: 24733588

Gulshan, V., Peng, L., Coram, M., Stumpe, M. C., Wu, D., Narayanaswamy, A., Venugopalan, S., Widner, K., Madams, T., Cuadros, J., Kim, R., Raman, R., Nelson, P. C., Mega, J. L., & Webster, D. R. (2016). Development and validation of a deep learning algorithm for the detection of diabetic retinopathy in retinal fundus photographs. *Journal of the American Medical Association, 316*(22), 2402–2410. DOI: 10.1001/jama.2016.17216 PMID: 27898976

Gupta, A. D. (2022). Adoption of Digital Healthcare with the Concept of the Patient as an Organisation. https://doi.org/DOI: 10.21203/rs.3.rs-1712476/v1

Gupta, R. S.. (2025). A systematic review of quantum machine learning for digital health and clinical decision support. *npj* [REMOVED HYPERLINK FIELD]. *Digital Medicine.*

Hair, J. F., Risher, J. J., Sarstedt, M., & Ringle, C. M. (2019). When to use and how to report the results of PLS-SEM. *European Business Review, 31*(1), 2–24. DOI: 10.1108/EBR-11-2018-0203

Hampel, H., Toschi, N., Babiloni, C., Baldacci, F., & Lista, S. (2021). Biomarker-guided diagnosis and treatment of Alzheimer's disease. *Nature Reviews. Neurology, 17*(3), 127–143. PMID: 33452494

Haque, M. A., Kumar, V., Khan, S. N., & Kim, J. J. (2025). Quantum intelligence in drug discovery: Advancing insights with quantum machine learning. *Drug Discovery Today, 30*(10), 104463. DOI: 10.1016/j.drudis.2025.104463 PMID: 40907599

Harry, A. (2023). The future of medicine: Harnessing the power of AI for revolutionizing healthcare. *International Journal of Multidisciplinary Sciences and Arts, 2*(1), 36–47. DOI: 10.47709/ijmdsa.v2i1.2395

Hasan, D. Md. M., Alam, M. S., Hossain, S., & Gomes, D. (2024). Fair Use Policies of Digital Contents: Some Observations and Recommendations. *Proceedings of the 3rd International Conference on Computing Advancements*, 192–199. DOI: 10.1145/3723178.3723204

Hasan, M. R., Li, Q., Saha, U., & Li, J. (2024). Decentralized and secure collaborative framework for personalized diabetes prediction. *Biomedicines, 12*(8), 1916. DOI: 10.3390/biomedicines12081916 PMID: 39200380

Hasei, J., Nakahara, R., Otsuka, Y., Nakamura, Y., Hironari, T., Kahara, N., Miwa, S., Ohshika, S., Nishimura, S., Ikuta, K., Osaki, S., Yoshida, A., Fujiwara, T., Nakata, E., Kunisada, T., & Ozaki, T. (2024). High-quality expert annotations enhance artificial intelligence model accuracy for osteosarcoma X-ray diagnosis. *Cancer Science, 115*(11), 3695–3704. DOI: 10.1111/cas.16330 PMID: 39223070

Hashim, F., Shuaib, K., & Sallabi, F. (2021). MedShard: Electronic health record sharing using blockchain sharding. *Sustainability (Basel), 13*(11), 5889. DOI: 10.3390/su13115889

Hashimov, E. (2015). Qualitative Data Analysis: A Methods Sourcebook and The Coding Manual for Qualitative Researchers: Matthew B. Miles, A. Michael Huberman, and Johnny Saldaña. Thousand Oaks, CA: SAGE, 2014. 381 pp. Johnny Saldaña. Thousand Oaks, CA: SAGE, 2013. 303 pp.https://doi.org/DOI: 10.1080/10572252.2015.975966

He, K., Zhang, X., Ren, S., & Sun, J. (2016). Deep residual learning for image recognition. *Proceedings of the IEEE Conference on Computer Vision and Pattern Recognition*, 770–778.

Higgins, O., Short, B. L., Chalup, S. K., & Wilson, R. L. (2023). Artificial intelligence (AI) and machine learning (ML) based decision support systems in mental health: An integrative review. *International Journal of Mental Health Nursing*, *32*(4), 966–978. DOI: 10.1111/inm.13114 PMID: 36744684

Hogan, A., Blomqvist, E., Cochez, M., d'Amato, C., de Melo, G., Gutierrez, C., & Zimmermann, A. (2021). Knowledge graphs. *ACM Computing Surveys*, *54*(4), 1–37. DOI: 10.1145/3447772

Holden, R. J., & Karsh, B. T. (2010). The technology acceptance model: Its past and its future in health care. *Journal of Biomedical Informatics*, *43*(1), 159–172. DOI: 10.1016/j.jbi.2009.07.002 PMID: 19615467

Holeman, I., & Kane, D. (2020). Human-centered design for global health equity. *Information Technology for Development*, *26*(3), 477–505. DOI: 10.1080/02681102.2019.1667289 PMID: 32982007

Holzinger, A., et al. (2022). Guideline for software life cycle in health informatics. Methods of Information in Medicine, 61(5-06), 193-204. DOI: 10.1055/s-0042-1758476

Hoque, M. R., & Bao, Y. (2015). Cultural influence on adoption and use of e-Health: Evidence in Bangladesh. *Telemedicine Journal and e-Health*, *21*(10), 845–851. DOI: 10.1089/tmj.2014.0128 PMID: 26348844

Hosain, M. N., Kwak, Y.-S., Lee, J., Choi, H., Park, J., & Kim, J. (2024). IoT-enabled biosensors for real-time monitoring and early detection of chronic diseases. *Physical Activity and Nutrition*, *28*(4), 60–69. DOI: 10.20463/pan.2024.0033

Hoseini, M. (2023). Patient experiences with AI in healthcare settings. *AI and Tech in Behavioral and Social Sciences*, *1*(3), 12–18. DOI: 10.61838/kman.aitech.1.3.3

Hripcsak, G., Duke, J. D., Shah, N. H., Reich, C. G., Huser, V., Schuemie, M. J., & Ryan, P. B. (2015). Observational Health Data Sciences and Informatics (OHDSI): Opportunities for observational researchers. *Studies in Health Technology and Informatics*, *216*, 574–578. DOI: 10.3233/978-1-61499-564-7-574 PMID: 26262116

Huang, Y., Cao, R., & Rahmani, A. (2022). *Reinforcement learning for sepsis treatment: A continuous action space solution*. In Proceedings of the Machine Learning for Healthcare Conference. https://proceedings.mlr.press/v182/huang22a/huang22a.pdf

Huang, L., Shea, A. L., Qian, H., Masurkar, A., Deng, H., & Liu, D. (2019). Patient clustering improves efficiency of federated machine learning to predict mortality and hospital stay time using distributed electronic medical records. *Journal of Biomedical Informatics*, *99*(103291), 103291. DOI: 10.1016/j.jbi.2019.103291 PMID: 31560949

Hu, D., Guo, Y., Zhou, Y., Flores, L., & Zheng, K. (2025). A systematic review of early evidence on generative AI for drafting responses to patient messages. *Npj Health Systems*, *2*(1), 27. DOI: 10.1038/s44401-025-00032-5

Hussain, S. A., Bresnahan, M., & Zhuang, J. (2025). The bias algorithm: How AI in healthcare exacerbates ethnic and racial disparities – a scoping review. *Ethnicity & Health*, *30*(2), 197–214. DOI: 10.1080/13557858.2024.2422848

Islam, Md. R., Mahmud, M. A. A., Tanvir, K., Das Joy, S., Rahman, M., Dey, N., & Gomes, D. (2025). IoMT Architecture for Healthcare: Integration, Security, and Real-Time Decision Support. In S. N. S. Al-Humairi, P. Naronglerdrit, N. Chantarapanich, & S. Wanchat (Eds.), *Robotics and IoT Synergy in Next-Generation Healthcare* (pp. 305–340). IGI Global Scientific Publishing. DOI: 10.4018/979-8-3373-5447-7.ch010

Issa, W. B., Shorbagi, A., Al-Sharman, A., Rababa, M., Al-Majeed, K., Radwan, H., Refaat Ahmed, F., Al-Yateem, N., Mottershead, R., Abdelrahim, D. N., Hijazi, H., Khasawneh, W., Ali, I., Abbas, N., & Fakhry, R. (2024). Shaping the future: Perspectives on the Integration of Artificial Intelligence in health profession education: a multi-country survey. *BMC Medical Education*, *24*(1), 1166. DOI: 10.1186/s12909-024-06076-9

Iturria-Medina, Y., Sotero, R. C., Toussaint, P. J., & Evans, A. C. (2017). Early role of vascular dysregulation on late-onset Alzheimer's disease. *Nature Communications*, *7*(1), 11934. DOI: 10.1038/ncomms11934 PMID: 27327500

Jabarulla, M. Y., & Lee, H.-N. (2021). A blockchain and artificial intelligence-based, patient-centric healthcare system for combating the COVID-19 pandemic: Opportunities and applications. *Healthcare (Basel)*, *9*(8), 1019. DOI: 10.3390/healthcare9081019 PMID: 34442156

Jack, C. R.Jr, Bennett, D. A., Blennow, K., Carrillo, M. C., Dunn, B., Haeberlein, S. B., Holtzman, D. M., Jagust, W., Jessen, F., Karlawish, J., Liu, E., Molinuevo, J. L., Montine, T., Phelps, C., Rankin, K. P., Rowe, C. C., Scheltens, P., Siemers, E., Snyder, H. M., & Silverberg, N. (2018). NIA-AA Research Framework: Toward a biological definition of Alzheimer's disease. *Alzheimer's & Dementia*, *14*(4), 535–562. DOI: 10.1016/j.jalz.2018.02.018 PMID: 29653606

Jafleh, E. A., Alnaqbi, F. A., Almaeeni, H. A., Faqeeh, S., Alzaabi, M. A., & Al Zaman, K. (2024). The Role of Wearable Devices in Chronic Disease Monitoring and Patient Care: A Comprehensive Review. *Cureus*. Advance online publication. DOI: 10.7759/cureus.68921

Jathissa, P., Rohatsch, L., Sauermann, S., & Hussein, R. (2024). OMOP-on-FHIR: A FHIR server development to facilitate data interaction with the OMOP-CDM and FHIR for PGHD. *Studies in Health Technology and Informatics*, *316*, 157–158. DOI: 10.3233/SHTI240367 PMID: 39176696

Jessica, H., Britney, R., Sarira, E.-D., Parisa, A., Joe, Z., & Betty, B. (2025). Applications of artificial intelligence in current pharmacy practice: A scoping review. *Research in Social & Administrative Pharmacy*, *21*(3), 134–141. DOI: 10.1016/j.sapharm.2024.12.007

Jiang, F., Jiang, Y., Zhi, H., Dong, Y., Li, H., Ma, S., Wang, Y., Dong, Q., Shen, H., & Wang, Y. (2017). Artificial intelligence in healthcare: Past, present and future. *Stroke and Vascular Neurology*, *2*(4), 230–243. Advance online publication. DOI: 10.1136/svn-2017-000101 PMID: 29507784

JMIR Medical Informatics Editorial Board. (2024). Health informatics research trends and methodologies. *JMIR Medical Informatics*, *12*(1), e45127. DOI: 10.2196/45127

Kahn, M. G., Callahan, T. J., Barnard, J., Bauck, A. E., Brown, J., Davidson, B. N., Estiri, H., Goerg, C., Holve, E., Johnson, S. G., Liaw, S.-T., Hamilton-Lopez, M., Meeker, D., Ong, T. C., Ryan, P., Shang, N., Weiskopf, N. G., Weng, C., Zozus, M. N., & Schilling, L. M. (2016). A harmonized data quality assessment terminology and framework for the secondary use of electronic health record data. *EGEMS (Washington, DC)*, *4*(1), 1244. DOI: 10.13063/2327-9214.1244 PMID: 27713905

Kanwar, V., Chaudhary, S., & Sharma, A. K. (2023). Challenges in implementing digital health services in rural India. *The International Society for Telemedicine and eHealth, 11*(1), 1-5. https://hdl.handle.net/10520/ejc-jisfteh_v11_n1_a3

Kasralikar, P., Polu, O. R., Chamarthi, B., Veer Samara Sihman Bharattej Rupavath, R., Patel, S., & Tumati, R. (2025). Blockchain for securing AI-driven healthcare systems: A systematic review and future research perspectives. *Cureus*, *17*(4), e83136. DOI: 10.7759/cureus.83136 PMID: 40438823

Kasyapa, M. S. B., & Vanmathi, C. (2024). Blockchain integration in healthcare: A comprehensive investigation of use cases, performance issues, and mitigation strategies. *Frontiers in Digital Health*, *6*, 1359858. DOI: 10.3389/fdgth.2024.1359858

Kayarian, F., Patel, D., O'Brien, J. R., Schraft, E. K., & Gottlieb, M. (2024). Artificial intelligence and point-of-care ultrasound: Benefits, limitations, and implications for the future. *The American Journal of Emergency Medicine*, *80*, 119–122. DOI: 10.1016/j.ajem.2024.03.023 PMID: 38555712

Keerthana, R., Savitha, S., Logeswaran, K., Rajivkannan, A., & Namasivayam, M. (2025). AI Technologies for Predicting Susceptibility and Outcomes of Immunological Disorders. In AI-Assisted Computational Approaches for Immunological Disorders (pp. 107-142). IGI Global Scientific Publishing. DOI: 10.4018/979-8-3693-9725-1.ch004

Kerketta, A., & Balasundaram, S. (2024). Leveraging AI Tools to Bridge the Healthcare Gap in Rural Areas in India. medRxiv, 2024-07. **doi:** https://doi.org/ DOI: 10.1101/2024.07.30.24311228

Kernberg, A., Gold, J. A., & Mohan, V. (2024). Using ChatGPT-4 to Create Structured Medical Notes From Audio Recordings of Physician-Patient Encounters: Comparative Study. *Journal of Medical Internet Research*, *26*, e54419. DOI: 10.2196/54419

Khalid, N., Qayyum, A., Bilal, M., Al-Fuqaha, A., & Qadir, J. (2023). Privacy-preserving artificial intelligence in healthcare: Techniques and applications. *Computers in Biology and Medicine*, *158*, 106848. DOI: 10.1016/j.compbiomed.2023.106848

Khan, A. A., Laghari, A. A., Almansour, H., Jamel, L., Hajjej, F., Estrela, V. V., Mohamed, M. A., & Ullah, S. (2025). Quantum computing empowering blockchain technology with post quantum resistant cryptography for multimedia data privacy preservation in cloud-enabled public auditing platforms. *Journal of Cloud Computing (Heidelberg, Germany)*, *14*(1), 43. DOI: 10.1186/s13677-025-00771-8

Khan, F., & Driessen, J. (2018). Bridging the telemedicine infrastructure gap: Implications for long-term care in rural America. *The Public Policy and Aging Report*, *28*(3), 80–84. DOI: 10.1093/ppar/pry027

Khosravi, M., Zare, Z., Mojtabaeian, S. M., & Izadi, R. (2024). Artificial Intelligence and Decision-Making in Healthcare: A Thematic Analysis of a Systematic Review of Reviews. *Health Services Research and Managerial Epidemiology*, *11*, 23333928241234863. DOI: 10.1177/23333928241234863

Khurana, A., Subramonyam, H., & Chilana, P. K. (2024). Why and when llm-based assistants can go wrong: Investigating the effectiveness of prompt-based interactions for software help-seeking. *arXiv.org*. Retrieved from /arxiv.2402.08030DOI: 10.1145/3640543.3645200

Killi, K., Mettu, T. R., Srirambhatla, J., Maddali, S., & Kuna, A. (2025). Quantum approaches and technologies to transform cancer care: Opportunities and challenges in the Indian healthcare landscape. *Medical Journal, Armed Forces India*. Advance online publication. DOI: 10.1016/j.mjafi.2025.09.003

Kolding, S., Lundin, R. M., Hansen, L., & Østergaard, S. D. (2024). Use of generative artificial intelligence (AI) in psychiatry and mental health care: A systematic review. *Acta Neuropsychiatrica, 37*, e37. DOI: 10.1017/neu.2024.50 PMID: 39523628

Kraft, S. A., Cho, M. K., Gillespie, K., Halley, M., Varsava, N., Ormond, K. E., & Wilfond, B. S. (2018). Beyond consent: Building trusting relationships with diverse populations in precision medicine research. *The American Journal of Bioethics, 18*(4), 3–20. DOI: 10.1080/15265161.2018.1431322 PMID: 29621457

Kraus, S., Feuerriegel, S., & Oztekin, A. (2023). Artificial intelligence in healthcare: Past, present, and future. *California Management Review, 65*(2), 5–27.

Kreimeyer, K., Foster, M., Pandey, A., Arya, N., Halford, G., Jones, S. F., Forshee, R., Walderhaug, M., & Botsis, T. (2017). Natural language processing systems for capturing and standardizing unstructured clinical information: A systematic review. *Journal of Biomedical Informatics, 73*, 14–29. DOI: 10.1016/j.jbi.2017.07.012 PMID: 28729030

Krittanawong, C., Zhang, H., Wang, Z., Aydar, M., & Kitai, T. (2017). Artificial intelligence in precision cardiovascular medicine. *Journal of the American College of Cardiology, 69*(21), 2657–2664. DOI: 10.1016/j.jacc.2017.03.571 PMID: 28545640

Kruse, C. S., Argueta, D. A., Lopez, L., & Nair, A. (2015). Patient and provider attitudes toward the use of patient portals for the management of chronic disease: A systematic review. *Journal of Medical Internet Research, 17*(2), e40. DOI: 10.2196/jmir.3703 PMID: 25707035

Kubanek, M., & Szymoniak, S. (2022). *ETHICAL CHALLENGES IN AI INTEGRATION: A COMPREHENSIVE REVIEW OF BIAS, PRIVACY, AND ACCOUNTABILITY ISSUES.*

Kumar, H. (2025). AI-powered Mental Health diagnostics using Multimodal Data: A Deep Learning-based approach. *International Scientific Journal of Engineering and Management, 04*(06), 1–9. DOI: 10.55041/ISJEM04560

Kuo, T.-T., & Zhang, P. (2023). Editorial: Blockchain and distributed ledger technology—enabled architectures for improving healthcare. *Frontiers in Blockchain, 6*(1275474), 1275474. Advance online publication. DOI: 10.3389/fbloc.2023.1275474

LaBoone, P. A., & Marques, O. (2024). Overview of the future impact of wearables and artificial intelligence in healthcare workflows and technology. *International Journal of Information Management Data Insights, 4*(2), 100294. DOI: 10.1016/j.jjimei.2024.100294

Lang, M., Ghandour, S., Rikard, B., Balasalle, E. K., Rouhezamin, M. R., Zhang, H., & Uppot, R. N. (2024). Medical Extended Reality for Radiology Education and Training. *Journal of the American College of Radiology*, *21*(10), 1583–1594. DOI: 10.1016/j.jacr.2024.05.006

Leemans, J. (2024). Setting up Oracle Database 23ai with AI Vector Search. Medium. Retrieved from https://jan-leemans.medium.com/setting-up-oracle-database-23ai-with-ai-vector-search-3b61725d7f51

Lee, P., & Kesselheim, A. S. (2018). Trust in artificial intelligence requires trust in the humans behind it. *JMIR Medical Internet Research*, *20*(6), e10428. DOI: 10.2196/10428

Leslie, D. (2020). *Understanding artificial intelligence ethics and safety*. The Alan-Turing Institute. https://www.turing.ac.uk/sites/default/files/2019-06/understanding_artificial_intelligence_ethics_and_safety.pdf

Leslie, D., Mazumder, A., Peppin, A., Wolters, M. K., & Hagerty, A. (2021). Does "AI" stand for augmenting inequality in the era of COVID-19 healthcare? *BMJ (Clinical Research Ed.)*, *372*(304), n304. Advance online publication. DOI: 10.1136/bmj.n304 PMID: 33722847

Liang, H., & Xue, Y. (2009). Avoidance of information technology threats: A theoretical perspective. *Management Information Systems Quarterly*, *33*(1), 71–90. DOI: 10.2307/20650279

Li, C., Wang, J., Wang, S., & Zhang, Y. (2024). A review of IoT applications in healthcare. *Neurocomputing*, *565*, 127017. DOI: 10.1016/j.neucom.2023.127017

Li, G., Shen, D., & Yap, P. T. (2022). Deep learning in Alzheimer's disease: Progress and challenges. *NeuroImage*, *248*, 118830.

Li, J., Dada, A., Puladi, B., Kleesiek, J., & Egger, J. (2024). ChatGPT in healthcare: A taxonomy and systematic review. *Computer Methods and Programs in Biomedicine*, *245*, 108013. DOI: 10.1016/j.cmpb.2024.108013

Li, T., Li, J., Jiang, H., & Skiles, D. B. (2025). Deep Learning Prediction of Drug-Induced Liver Toxicity by Manifold Embedding of Quantum Information of Drug Molecules. *Pharmaceutical Research*, *42*(1), 109–122. DOI: 10.1007/s11095-024-03800-4 PMID: 39663331

Li, T., Sahu, A. K., Talwalkar, A., & Smith, V. (2020). Federated learning: Challenges, methods, and future directions. *IEEE Signal Processing Magazine*, *37*(3), 50–60. DOI: 10.1109/MSP.2020.2975749

Liu, J. C., Goetz, J., Sen, S., & Tewari, A. (2021). Learning from others without sacrificing privacy: Simulation comparing centralized and federated machine learning on mobile health data. *JMIR mHealth and uHealth*, *9*(3), e23728. DOI: 10.2196/23728 PMID: 33783362

Liu, S., La, H., Willms, A., & Rhodes, R. E. (2022). A "no-code" app design platform for mobile health research: Development and usability study. *JMIR Formative Research*, *6*(8), e37737. DOI: 10.2196/38737 PMID: 35980740

Livingston, G., Huntley, J., Sommerlad, A., Ames, D., & Mukadam, N. (2020). Dementia prevention, intervention, and care: 2020 report of the Lancet Commission. *Lancet*, *396*(10248), 413–446. DOI: 10.1016/S0140-6736(20)30367-6 PMID: 32738937

Luz, S., Haider, F., & de la Fuente, S. (2021). Alzheimer's Dementia Recognition through Spontaneous Speech: A Multilingual Approach. *Computer Speech & Language*, *68*, 101199.

M, T., & Annamalai, A. (2020a). Telepsychiatry and the role of artificial intelligence in mental health in post-COVID-19 India: A scoping review on opportunities. Indian Journal of Psychological Medicine, 42(5), 428–434. DOI: 10.1177/0253717620952160

Ma, T. (2025). Integration of blockchain and Artificial Intelligence in healthcare: Enhancing data security and operational efficiency. ITM Web of Conferences, 73, 03007. DOI: 10.1051/itmconf/20257303007

Mahapatra, P., Sahoo, K. C., Jitendriya, P., Samal, M., & Pati, S. (2021). Qualitative research methods in psychiatry in India: Landscaping the terrain. *Indian Journal of Psychiatry*, *63*(1), 5–14. DOI: 10.4103/psychiatry.IndianJPsychiatry_665_20 PMID: 34083815

Maleki Varnosfaderani, S., & Forouzanfar, M. (2024). The Role of AI in Hospitals and Clinics: Transforming Healthcare in the 21st Century. *Bioengineering (Basel, Switzerland)*, *11*(4), 337. DOI: 10.3390/bioengineering11040337

Manik, M. M. T. G., Mohonta, S. C., Karim, F., Miah, M. A., Islam, M. S., Chy, M. A. R., Adnan, M., & Saimon, A. S. M. (2025). AI-driven precision medicine leveraging machine learning and big data analytics for genomics-based drug discovery. *Journal of Posthumanism*, *5*(5), 4895–4915. DOI: 10.63332/joph.v5i5.1993

Marcus, D. S., Fotenos, A. F., Csernansky, J. G., Morris, J. C., & Buckner, R. L. (2010). Open Access Series of Imaging Studies (OASIS). *Journal of Cognitive Neuroscience*, *22*(2), 2677–2684. DOI: 10.1162/jocn.2009.21407 PMID: 19929323

Marengo, A., & Santamato, V. (2025). Quantum algorithms and complexity in healthcare applications: A systematic review with machine learning-optimized analysis. *Frontiers of Computer Science*, *7*, 1584114. DOI: 10.3389/fcomp.2025.1584114

Martin, C. P., & Lamb, J. (2025). Generative AI in healthcare: Current trends and future outlook. McKinsey & Company. Retrieved from https://www.mckinsey.com/industries/healthcare/our-insights/generative-ai-in-healthcare-current-trends-and-future-outlook

Mason, A. J. C., Bhavsar, V., Botelle, R., Chandran, D., Li, L., Mascio, A., Sanyal, J., Kadra-Scalzo, G., Roberts, A., Williams, M., & Stewart, R. (2024). Applying neural network algorithms to ascertain reported experiences of violence in routine mental healthcare records and distributions of reports by diagnosis. *Frontiers in Psychiatry*, *15*, 1181739. DOI: 10.3389/fpsyt.2024.1181739 PMID: 39319350

Mathkor, D. M., Mathkor, N., Bassfar, Z., Bantun, F., Slama, P., Ahmad, F., & Haque, S. (2024). Multirole of the internet of medical things (IoMT) in biomedical systems for managing smart healthcare systems: An overview of current and future innovative trends. *Journal of Infection and Public Health*, *17*(4), 559–572. DOI: 10.1016/j.jiph.2024.01.013

Mayer, A. H., da Costa, C. A., & Righi, R. da R. (2020). Electronic health records in a Blockchain: A systematic review. *Health Informatics Journal*, *26*(2), 1273–1288. DOI: 10.1177/1460458219866350 PMID: 31566472

McArdle, S., Endo, S., Aspuru-Guzik, A., Benjamin, S. C., & Yuan, X. (2020). Quantum computational chemistry. *Reviews of Modern Physics*, *92*(1), 015003. DOI: 10.1103/RevModPhys.92.015003

McCradden, M., Hui, K., & Buchman, D. Z. (2023). Evidence, ethics and the promise of artificial intelligence in psychiatry. *Journal of Medical Ethics*, *49*(8), 573–579. DOI: 10.1136/jme-2022-108447 PMID: 36581457

McGreevey, J. D.III, Mallozzi, C. P., Perkins, R. M., Shelov, E., & Schreiber, R. (2020). Reducing alert burden in electronic health records: State of the art recommendations from four health systems. *Applied Clinical Informatics*, *11*(1), 1–12. DOI: 10.1055/s-0039-3402715 PMID: 31893559

McKhann, G. M., Knopman, D. S., Chertkow, H., & Hyman, B. T. (2021). The new diagnostic criteria for Alzheimer's disease: Updating the NIA-AA guidelines. *Neurology*, *96*(2), 59–67. PMID: 33310876

McKinney, S. M., Sieniek, M., Godbole, V., Godwin, J., Antropova, N., Ashrafian, H., Back, T., Chesus, M., Corrado, G. S., Darzi, A., Etemadi, M., Garcia-Vicente, F., Gilbert, F. J., Halling-Brown, M., Hassabis, D., Jansen, S., Karthikesalingam, A., Kelly, C. J., King, D., & Shetty, S. (2020). International evaluation of an AI system for breast cancer screening. *Nature*, *577*(7788), 89–94. DOI: 10.1038/s41586-019-1799-6 PMID: 31894144

McMahan, B., Moore, E., Ramage, D., Hampson, S., & Arcas, B. A. (2017). Communication-efficient learning of deep networks from decentralized data. *Proceedings of the 20th International Conference on Artificial Intelligence and Statistics*, 54, 1273-1282.

Mehrabi, N., Morstatter, F., Saxena, N., Lerman, K., & Galstyan, A. (2021). A survey on bias and fairness in machine learning. *ACM Computing Surveys*, *54*(6), 1–35. DOI: 10.1145/3457607

Mehraeen, M., & Mahmoudi, L. (2024). Tracing the Blockchain Challenges in Healthcare: A Topic Modeling and Bibliometric Analysis. *Blockchain in Healthcare Today*, *7*(3). Advance online publication. DOI: 10.30953/bhty.v7.335

Mehta, N., & Devarakonda, M. V. (2018). Machine learning, natural language programming, and electronic health records: The next step in the artificial intelligence journey? *The Journal of Allergy and Clinical Immunology*, *141*(6), 2019–2021.e1. DOI: 10.1016/j.jaci.2018.02.025 PMID: 29518424

Mei, P., & Zhang, F. (2024). A framework for processing large-scale health data in medical higher-order correlation mining by quantum computing in smart healthcare. [REMOVED HYPERLINK FIELD]. *Frontiers in Digital Health*, *6*, 1502745. DOI: 10.3389/fdgth.2024.1502745 PMID: 39633967

Merchán-Cruz, E. A., Gabelaia, I., Savrasovs, M., Hansen, M. F., Soe, S., Rodriguez-Cañizo, R. G., & Aragón-Camarasa, G. (2025). Trust by Design: An Ethical Framework for Collaborative Intelligence Systems in Industry 5.0. *Electronics (Basel)*, *14*(10), 1952. DOI: 10.3390/electronics14101952

Mesinovic, M., Watkinson, P., & Zhu, T. (2025). Explainability in the age of large language models for healthcare. *Communications Engineering*, *4*(1), 128. Advance online publication. DOI: 10.1038/s44172-025-00453-y

Meskó, B., Hetényi, G., & Győrffy, Z. (2018). Will artificial intelligence solve the human resource crisis in healthcare? *BMC Health Services Research*, *18*(1), 545. DOI: 10.1186/s12913-018-3359-4 PMID: 30001717

Meurers, T., Halilovic, M., Otte, K., Despraz, J., Kaabachi, B., Kulynych, B., Raisaro, J. L., & Prasser, F. (2025). Phantom Anonymization: Adversarial testing for membership inference risks in anonymized health data. *Computers in Biology and Medicine*, *196*, 110738. DOI: 10.1016/j.compbiomed.2025.110738

Miner, A. S., Shah, N., Bullock, K. D., Arnow, B. A., Bailenson, J., & Hancock, J. (2019). Key considerations for incorporating conversational AI in psychotherapy. *Frontiers in Psychiatry*, *10*, 746. DOI: 10.3389/fpsyt.2019.00746 PMID: 31681047

Mirbabaie, M., Hofeditz, L., Frick, N. R. J., & Stieglitz, S. (2022). Artificial intelligence in hospitals: Providing a status quo of ethical considerations in academia to guide future research. *AI & Society*, *37*(4), 1361–1382. DOI: 10.1007/s00146-021-01239-4

Mittelstadt, B. (2019). Principles alone cannot guarantee ethical AI. *Nature Machine Intelligence*, *1*(11), 501–507. DOI: 10.1038/s42256-019-0114-4

Modi, N. D., Menz, B. D., Awaty, A. A., Alex, C. A., Logan, J. M., McKinnon, R. A., Rowland, A., Bacchi, S., Gradon, K., Sorich, M. J., & Hopkins, A. M. (2025). Assessing the System-Instruction Vulnerabilities of Large Language Models to Malicious Conversion Into Health Disinformation Chatbots. *Annals of Internal Medicine*, *178*(8), 1172–1180. Advance online publication. DOI: 10.7326/ANNALS-24-03933

Mohsin Khan, M., Shah, N., Shaikh, N., Thabet, A., alrabayah, T., & Belkhair, S. (2025). Towards secure and trusted AI in healthcare: A systematic review of emerging innovations and ethical challenges. *International Journal of Medical Informatics*, *195*, 105780. DOI: 10.1016/j.ijmedinf.2024.105780

Morley, J., Machado, C. C., Burr, C., Cowls, J., Joshi, I., Taddeo, M., & Floridi, L. (2020). The ethics of AI in health care: A mapping review. *Social Science & Medicine*, *260*, 113172. DOI: 10.1016/j.socscimed.2020.113172 PMID: 32702587

Morley, J., Murphy, L., Mishra, A., Joshi, I., & Karpathakis, K. (2022). Governing Data and Artificial Intelligence for Health Care: Developing an International Understanding. *JMIR Formative Research*, *6*(1), e31623. DOI: 10.2196/31623

Muhunzi, D., Kitambala, L., & Mashauri, H. L. (2024). Big data analytics in the healthcare sector: Opportunities and challenges in developing countries. A literature review. *Health Informatics Journal*, *30*(4), 14604582241294217. DOI: 10.1177/14604582241294217

Munia, A. A., Abdar, M., Hasan, M., Jalali, M. S., Banerjee, B., Khosravi, A., Hossain, I., Fu, H., & Frangi, A. F. (2025). Attention-guided hierarchical fusion U-Net for uncertainty-driven medical image segmentation. *Information Fusion*, *115*, 102719. DOI: 10.1016/j.inffus.2024.102719

Murala, D. K., Panda, S. K., & Dash, S. P. (2023). MedMetaverse: Medical Care of Chronic Disease Patients and Managing Data Using Artificial Intelligence, Blockchain, and Wearable Devices State-of-the-Art Methodology. *IEEE Access : Practical Innovations, Open Solutions*, *11*, 138954–138985. DOI: 10.1109/ACCESS.2023.3340791

Murdoch, B. (2021). Privacy and artificial intelligence: Challenges for protecting health information in a new era. *BMC Medical Ethics*, *22*(1), 122. DOI: 10.1186/s12910-021-00687-3 PMID: 34525993

Mustapha, A. Y., Ikhalea, N., Chianumba, E. C., & Forkuo, A. Y. (2022). Developing an AI-powered predictive model for mental health disorder diagnosis using electronic health records. *International Journal of Multidisciplinary Research and Growth Evaluation*, *3*(1), 914–931. DOI: 10.54660/.IJMRGE.2022.3.1.914-931

Nałęcz-Charkiewicz, K., Charkiewicz, K., & Nowak, R. M. (2024). Quantum computing in bioinformatics: A systematic review. *Briefings in Bioinformatics*, *25*(5), bbae391. DOI: 10.1093/bib/bbae391 PMID: 39140856

Narayan, S. M., Kohli, N., & Martin, M. M. (2025). Addressing contemporary threats in anonymised healthcare data using privacy engineering. *NPJ Digital Medicine*, *8*(1), 145. DOI: 10.1038/s41746-025-01520-6

Nassir, N., Hashmi, M. A., Raji, K. G., Jamalalail, B., Maksymowsky, A., Scherer, S. W., Alsheikh-Ali, A., & Uddin, M. (2025). Quantum computing and the implementation of precision medicine. npj. *Genomic Medicine*, *10*(1), 80. DOI: 10.1038/s41525-025-00537-w PMID: 41330918

National Family Health Survey-5 (NFHS-5). (2021). Ministry of Health and Family Welfare. https://rchiips.org/nfhs/

Navarro, D. F., Lewis, M., Shah, R., Delacroix, S., & Lehman, R. (2025). Generative AI and the changing dynamics of clinical consultations. *BMJ (Clinical Research Ed.)*, *391*, e085325. Advance online publication. DOI: 10.1136/bmj-2025-085325

Navath, S. (2023). Transforming healthcare: The impact and future of Artificial Intelligence in healthcare. *Journal of Artificial Intelligence and Machine Learning*, *1*(1), 16–21. DOI: 10.55124/jaim.v1i1.234

Nordmann, K., Redlich, M. C., Schaller, M., Sauter, S., & Fischer, F. (2025). Toward a conceptual framework for digitally supported communication, coordination, cooperation, and collaboration in interprofessional health care: Scoping review. *Journal of Medical Internet Research*, *27*(1), e69276. Advance online publication. DOI: 10.2196/69276 PMID: 40418789

Obermeyer, Z., & Emanuel, E. J. (2016). Predicting the future—Big data, machine learning, and clinical medicine. *The New England Journal of Medicine*, *375*(13), 1216–1219. DOI: 10.1056/NEJMp1606181 PMID: 27682033

Obermeyer, Z., Powers, B., Vogeli, C., & Mullainathan, S. (2019). Dissecting racial bias in an algorithm used to manage the health of populations. *Science*, *366*(6464), 447–453. DOI: 10.1126/science.aax2342

Odat, M, R., Marsool Marsool, M. D., Nguyen, D., Idrees, M., Hussein, A. M., Ghabally, M., A Yasin, J., Hanifa, H., Sabet, C. J., Dinh, N. H., Harky, A., Jain, J., & Jain, H. (2024). Presurgery and postsurgery: Advancements in artificial intelligence and machine learning models for enhancing patient management in infective endocarditis. *International Journal of Surgery (London, England)*, *110*(11), 7202–7214. DOI: 10.1097/JS9.0000000000002003 PMID: 39051669

Odhus, C. O., Kapanga, R. R., & Oele, E. (2024). Barriers to and enablers of quality improvement in primary health care in low-and middle-income countries: A systematic review. *PLOS Global Public Health*, *4*(1), e0002756. DOI: 10.1371/journal.pgph.0002756 PMID: 38236832

Okoro, Y. O., Ayo-Farai, O., Maduka, C. P., Okongwu, C. C., & Sodamade, O. T. (2023). EMERGING TECHNOLOGIES IN PUBLIC HEALTH CAMPAIGNS: ARTIFICIAL IN LIGENCE AND BIG DATA. *Acta Informatica Malaysia, 8*(1), 05–10. DOI: 10.26480/aim.01.2024.05.10

Okpete, U. E., & Byeon, H. (2024). Challenges and prospects in bridging precision medicine and artificial intelligence in genomic psychiatric treatment. *World Journal of Psychiatry*, *14*(8), 1148–1164. DOI: 10.5498/wjp.v14.i8.1148 PMID: 39165556

Olawade, D. B., David-Olawade, A. C., Wada, O. Z., Asaolu, A. J., Adereni, T., & Ling, J. (2024). Artificial intelligence in healthcare delivery: Prospects and pitfalls. *Journal of Medicine, Surgery, and Public Health*, *3*, 100108. DOI: 10.1016/j.glmedi.2024.100108

Olorunsogo, T., Adenyi, A. O., Okolo, C. A., & Babawarun, O. (2024). Ethical considerations in AI-enhanced medical decision support systems: A review. *World Journal of Advanced Engineering Technology and Sciences*, *11*(1), 329–336. DOI: 10.30574/wjaets.2024.11.1.0061

Oracle Corporation. (2024). Oracle APEX 24.2 release notes: AI-enhanced capabilities and vector search integration. Oracle APEX Documentation. Retrieved from https://apex.oracle.com/en/learn/documentation/release-notes/

Organization, W. H. (2024). *Ethics and governance of artificial intelligence for health: large multi-modal models. WHO guidance*. World Health Organization.

Osorio, C., Fuster, N., Chen, W., Men, Y., & Juan, A. A. (2024). Enhancing accessibility to analytics courses in higher education through AI, simulation, and e-collaborative tools. *Information (Basel)*, *15*(8), 430. DOI: 10.3390/info15080430

Pagar, S., & Dr D Y Patil Institute of Engineering Akurdi Pune, M. and R. (2024). Revolutionizing healthcare: AI-driven advances in EMR management. INTERANTIONAL JOURNAL OF SCIENTIFIC RESEARCH IN ENGINEERING AND MANAGEMENT, 08(05), 1–5. DOI: 10.55041/IJSREM34631

Pai, F. Y., & Huang, K. I. (2011). Applying the technology acceptance model to the introduction of healthcare information systems. *Technological Forecasting and Social Change*, *78*(4), 650–660. DOI: 10.1016/j.techfore.2010.11.007

Pallumeera, M., Giang, J. C., Singh, R., Pracha, N. S., & Makary, M. S. (2025). Evolving and novel applications of artificial intelligence in cancer imaging. *Cancers (Basel)*, *17*(9), 1510. Advance online publication. DOI: 10.3390/cancers17091510 PMID: 40361437

Panigrahi, S. (2025). *Carbon Quantum Dots Prepared by Hydrothermal Method for Drug Delivery*. Photocatalysis, and Bioimaging Applications.

Pan, Y., Liu, J., He, Y., Xie, X., & Shen, D. (2022). Multimodal learning for Alzheimer's disease diagnosis: A review. *Medical Image Analysis*, *78*, 102419.

Park, S. Y., et al. (2019). Identifying challenges and opportunities in human-AI collaboration in healthcare. Conference Companion Publication of the 2019 on Computer Supported Cooperative Work and Social Computing, 506-510.

Park, S. Y., Kuo, P. Y., Barbarin, A., Kaziunas, E., Chow, A., Singh, K., . . . Lasecki, W. S. (2019, November). Identifying challenges and opportunities in human-AI collaboration in healthcare. In *Companion Publication of the 2019 Conference on Computer Supported Cooperative Work and Social Computing* (pp. 506-510). https://doi.org/DOI: 10.1145/3311957.3359433

Patel, R., Wee, S. N., Ramaswamy, R., Thadani, S., Guruswamy, G., Garg, R., Calvanese, N., Valko, M., Rush, A., Rentería, M., Sarkar, J., & Kollins, S. (2022). NeuroBlu: A natural language processing (NLP) electronic health record (EHR) data analytic tool to generate real-world evidence in mental healthcare. *European Psychiatry : the Journal of the Association of European Psychiatrists*, *65*(S1), S99–S100. DOI: 10.1192/j.eurpsy.2022.286

Pattanaik, P., Himanshu, U., Bhushan, B., Thakur, M., & Pani, A. K. (2024). A study of the adoption behaviour of an electronic health information exchange system for a green economy. *International Journal of Logistics*, *27*(4), 512–537. DOI: 10.1080/13675567.2021.2008336

Pencina, M. J., Silcox, C., Economou-Zavlanos, N., & McClellan, M. (2025). Bridging the Gap Between Developers and Implementers in Health AI. *JAMA Health Forum*, *6*(6), e251692. DOI: 10.1001/jamahealthforum.2025.1692

Peoples, K. (2021). *How to write a phenomenological dissertation: A step-by-step guide* (Vol. 56). SAGE.

Pereira, T., Morgado, J., Silva, F., Pelter, M. M., Dias, V. R., Barros, R., Freitas, C., Negrão, E., Flor de Lima, B., Correia da Silva, M., Madureira, A. J., Ramos, I., Hespanhol, V., Costa, J. L., Cunha, A., & Oliveira, H. P. (2021). Sharing biomedical data: Strengthening AI development in healthcare. *Healthcare (Basel)*, *9*(7), 827. DOI: 10.3390/healthcare9070827 PMID: 34208830

Pesqueira, A., Barr, N. M., & Almeida, D. (2025). Leveraging AI and Blockchain for privacy and security in smart medical systems. In *AI and Blockchain Applications for Privacy and Security in Smart Medical Systems* (pp. 279–308). IGI Global., DOI: 10.4018/979-8-3373-0593-6.ch011

Pfitzner, B., Steckhan, N., & Arnrich, B. (2021). Federated learning in a medical context: A systematic literature review. *ACM Transactions on Internet Technology*, *21*(2), 1–31. DOI: 10.1145/3412357

Pham, K. T., Nabizadeh, A., & Selek, S. (2022). Artificial intelligence and chatbots in psychiatry. *The Psychiatric Quarterly*, *93*(1), 249–253. DOI: 10.1007/s11126-022-09973-8 PMID: 35212940

Prates, L., & Pereira, R. (2025). DevSecOps practices and tools. *International Journal of Information Security*, *24*(1), 11. Advance online publication. DOI: 10.1007/s10207-024-00914-z

Prathibha, S., Narayanamoorthy, S., Kishore, M. A., & Sandhiya, A. (2025, February). Quantum AI-Enhanced Health Care Diagnostic Pod: A Leap Towards Accurate and Accessible Diagnostics. In International Conference on Computational Intelligence in Data Science (pp. 122-137). Cham: Springer Nature Switzerland.

Prégent, J., Chung, V.-H.-A., El Adib, I., Désilets, M., & Hudon, A. (2025a). Applications of artificial intelligence in psychiatry and psychology education: Scoping review. *JMIR Medical Education*, *11*, e75238. DOI: 10.2196/75238 PMID: 40720804

Price, W. N.II, Gerke, S., & Cohen, I. G. (2019). Potential liability for physicians using artificial intelligence. *Journal of the American Medical Association*, *322*(18), 1765–1766. DOI: 10.1001/jama.2019.15064 PMID: 31584609

Prince, E. W., Hankinson, T. C., & Görg, C. (2025). A visual analytics framework for assessing interactive AI for clinical decision support. Pacific Symposium on Biocomputing. *Pacific Symposium on Biocomputing*, *30*, 40–53. DOI: 10.1142/9789819807024_0004 PMID: 39670360

Punia, A., Bhakuni, P., & Sharma, N. (2025). Development of AI- and NLP-driven chatbots and virtual assistants for mental health support. In Advances in Psychology, Mental Health, and Behavioral Studies (pp. 229–262). IGI Global. DOI: 10.4018/979-8-3693-9341-3.ch010

Putica, A., Khanna, R., Bosl, W., Saraf, S., & Edgcomb, J. (2025). Ethical decision-making for AI in mental health: The Integrated Ethical Approach for Computational Psychiatry (IEACP) framework. *Psychological Medicine*, *55*(e213), e213. DOI: 10.1017/S0033291725101311 PMID: 40702980

Qaddumi, B., Ayaad, O., Al-Ma'aitah, M. A., Akhu-Zaheya, L., & Alloubani, A. (2021). The factors affecting team effectiveness in hospitals: The mediating role of using electronic collaborative tools. *Journal of Interprofessional Education & Practice*, *24*, 100449. Advance online publication. DOI: 10.1016/j.xjep.2021.100449

Qi, K. (2025). Advancing hospital healthcare: Achieving IoT-based secure health monitoring through multilayer machine learning. *Journal of Big Data*, *12*(1), 1. DOI: 10.1186/s40537-024-01038-w

Quazi, F., Mohammed Abdul Sajid, P., & Gorrepati, N. (2024). Transforming treatment and diagnosis in healthcare through AI. International Journal of Global Innovations and Solutions (IJGIS). DOI: 10.21428/e90189c8.072ffbe8

Rahman, A., Hossain, M., Muhammad, G., Kundu, D., Debnath, T., Rahman, M., Khan, M. S. I., Tiwari, P., & Band, S. S. (2023). Federated learning-based AI approaches in smart healthcare: Concepts, taxonomies, challenges and open issues. *Cluster Computing*, *26*(4), 2271–2311. DOI: 10.1007/s10586-022-03658-4

Rajkomar, A., Dean, J., & Kohane, I. (2019). Machine Learning in Medicine. *The New England Journal of Medicine*, *380*(14), 1347–1358. DOI: 10.1056/NEJMra1814259

Rajkomar, A., Hardt, M., Howell, M. D., Corrado, G., & Chin, M. H. (2019). Ensuring fairness in machine learning to advance health equity. *The New England Journal of Medicine*, *380*(26), 2498–2500. DOI: 10.1056/NEJMp1814149 PMID: 31242381

Rajpurkar, P., Chen, E., Banerjee, O., & Topol, E. (2022). AI in health care: The surprising performance of foundation models. *The Lancet. Digital Health*, *4*(8), e538–e545. 100.1038/s41591-021-01614-0

Rane, N., Patil, D., & Rane, J. (2025). Artificial Intelligence-Enabled Drug Development: Deep Learning and Computational Chemistry for Accelerating Therapeutics. *Available at SSRN* 5521819. DOI: 10.2139/ssrn.5521819

Rani, S., Jining, D., Shah, D., Xaba, S., & Singh, P. R. (2023). The potential application of Artificial Intelligence in healthcare and hospitals. ITM Web of Conferences, 53, 01005. DOI: 10.1051/itmconf/20235301005

Rao, A., & Aalami, O. (2023). Towards improving the visual explainability of artificial intelligence in the clinical setting. *BMC Digital Health*, *1*(1), 23. DOI: 10.1186/s44247-023-00022-3

Rasool, M., Ahmad, H. F., Ahmed, M., & Khan, S. (2023). Quantum-assisted drug discovery and molecular simulation for personalized medicine. *Journal of Molecular Modeling*, *29*(8), 215. DOI: 10.1007/s00894-023-05512-9

Rathinavel, P., Ravikumar, R. N., Aarthi, S., Habib, M., Salaeva, N., & Pardaev, J. (2025). Augmenting human capabilities. In *Advances in Computational Intelligence and Robotics* (pp. 1–30). IGI Global Scientific Publishing., DOI: 10.4018/979-8-3373-2372-5.ch001

Raveesh, B. N., & Munoli, R. N. (2020). Ethical and legal aspects of telepsychiatry. *Indian Journal of Psychological Medicine*, *42*(5, Suppl), 63S–69S. DOI: 10.1177/0253717620962033 PMID: 33354067

Ravikumar, R. S., Manujakshi, Aarthi, S., Urazbaeva, Y., & Tamilselvi, S. (2025). Navigating data privacy, security, and regulatory challenges in healthcare AI ensuring fairness, bias mitigation, interpretability, and trust. In Transformative Role of Transformer Models in Healthcare (pp. 25–54). IGI Global Scientific Publishing. DOI: 10.4018/979-8-3373-2038-0.ch002

Ravikumar, R. N., Aarthi, S., Dilshodbek, A., Satheesh Kumar, A., Eshkaraev, S., & Shanmugam, K. B. (2025). Integrating blockchain, smart contracts, and AI for decentralized healthcare in the metaverse. In *Blockchain-Based Healthcare Management in the Metaverse* (pp. 261–294). IGI Global Scientific Publishing., DOI: 10.4018/979-8-3373-1225-5.ch010

Rawat, K. S., & Yadav, M. (2025). Analyzing Quantum Computing Applications Across Key Scientific Domains Using Trends and Visual Analytics: K. Rawat, M. Yadav. *Archives of Computational Methods in Engineering*, •••, 1–32.

Rector, A. L., Nowlan, W. A., & Kay, S. (1991). Foundations for an electronic medical record. *Methods of Information in Medicine*, *30*(3), 179–186. DOI: 10.1055/s-0038-1634836 PMID: 1943789

Reddy, S., Fox, J., & Purohit, M. P. (2019). Artificial intelligence-enabled healthcare delivery. *Journal of the Royal Society of Medicine*, *112*(1), 22–28. DOI: 10.1177/0141076818815510 PMID: 30507284

Rieke, N., Hancox, J., Li, W., Milletari, F., & Roth, H. R. (2020). The future of digital health with federated learning. npj. *Digital Medicine*, *3*(1), 119. PMID: 33015372

Rigas, E. S., Lagakis, P., Karadimas, M., Logaras, E., Latsou, D., Hatzikou, M., Poulakidas, A., Billis, A., & Bamidis, P. D. (2024). Semantic interoperability for an AI-based applications platform for smart hospitals using HL7 FHIR. *Journal of Systems and Software*, *215*, 112093. Advance online publication. DOI: 10.1016/j.jss.2024.112093

Risvas, C., & Spanoudaki, K. (2025). *Quantum computing in medicine: From molecular simulation to global health systems*. Springer Nature., DOI: 10.1007/978-3-031-56789-2

Rodriguez, R., ... (2025). AI in healthcare: What to expect in 2025. Chief Healthcare Executive. Retrieved from https://www.chiefhealthcareexecutive.com/view/ai-in-healthcare-what-to-expect-in-2025

Rogers, E. M. (2003). *Diffusion of innovations* (5th ed.). Free Press.

Rojas, J. C.. (2025). Adoption of artificial intelligence in healthcare: Survey of health system priorities, successes, and challenges. *Journal of the American Medical Informatics Association : JAMIA*, *32*(5), ocaf065. Advance online publication. DOI: 10.1093/jamia/ocaf065 PMID: 40323320

Rony, M. K. K., Das, D. C., Khatun, M. T., Ferdousi, S., Akter, M. R., Khatun, M. A., Begum, M. H., Khalil, M. I., Parvin, M. R., Alrazeeni, D. M., & Akter, F. (2025). Artificial intelligence in psychiatry: A systematic review and meta-analysis of diagnostic and therapeutic efficacy. *Digital Health*, *11*, 20552076251330530. DOI: 10.1177/20552076251330528 PMID: 40162166

Roosan, D., Nirzhor, S., Khan, R., & Hai, F. (2025). Quantum Gradient Optimized Drug Repurposing Prototype for Omics Data. arXiv preprint arXiv:2506.19097. DOI: 10.5220/0013524900003967

Rossi, M., & Rehman, S. (2025). Integrating artificial intelligence into telemedicine: Evidence, challenges, and future directions. *Cureus*, *17*(8), e90829. DOI: 10.7759/cureus.90829 PMID: 40988810

Ross, M. K., Wei, W., & Ohno-Machado, L. (2014). "Big data" and the electronic health record. *Yearbook of Medical Informatics*, *9*(1), 97–104. DOI: 10.15265/IY-2014-0003 PMID: 25123728

Sabrina, F., Sohail, S., & Tariq, U. U. (2024). A Review of Post-Quantum Privacy Preservation for IoMT Using Blockchain. *Electronics (Basel)*, *13*(15), 2962. DOI: 10.3390/electronics13152962

Saeed, U.. (2023). Algorithms in low-code-no-code for research applications: A practical review. *Algorithms*, *16*(2), 108. DOI: 10.3390/a16020108

Saeidnia, H. R., & Nilashi, M. (2025). From MYCIN to MedGemma: A Historical and Comparative Analysis of Healthcare AI Evolution. *InfoScience Trends*, *2*(6), 18–28. DOI: 10.61186/ist.202502.06.02

Saenz, A. D., Zhang, Z., Shah, A., Brawarsky, P., Omar, M., Rajkomar, A., & Zai, A. H. (2024). Establishing responsible use of AI guidelines: A comprehensive case study for healthcare institutions. *npj. NPJ Digital Medicine*, *348*(7), 348. Advance online publication. DOI: 10.1038/s41746-024-01300-8

Sarker, D., Sadi, M. T. H., Gomes, D., & Hasan, Md. M. (2025). Securing Patient Privacy and Data Protection by Federated Learning in AI-Driven Healthcare: In N. K. Mun, C.-S. Shieh, D. Ather, A. Panwar, & V. Jain (Eds.), *Advances in Computational Intelligence and Robotics* (pp. 317–352). IGI Global Scientific Publishing. DOI: 10.4018/979-8-3373-3306-9.ch012

Sarraf, S., & Tofighi, G. (2017). DeepAD: Alzheimer's disease classification via deep convolutional neural networks. *Proceedings of the International Conference on Image Processing Theory, Tools and Applications*, 1–6.

Savitha, S., Keerthana, R., Logeswaran, K., Vennila, V., Manjuladevi, R., & Sangeetha, M. (2025). Sustainable AI-Powered Systems and Cybersecurity for Health Diagnostics: Addressing Bias and Fairness in AI for Early Disease Detection. In AI-Driven Healthcare Cybersecurity and Privacy (pp. 205-244). IGI Global Scientific Publishing.

Savitha, S., Kannan, A. R., & Logeswaran, K. (2025). Augmenting Cardiovascular Disease Prediction Through CWCF Integration Leveraging Harris Hawks Search in Deep Belief Networks. *Cognitive Computation*, *17*(1), 52. DOI: 10.1007/s12559-025-10406-4

Scarfone, K., Souppaya, M., & Dodson, D. (2022). Secure Software Development Framework (SSDF) Version 1.1: Recommendations for Mitigating the Risk of Software Vulnerabilities. *NIST Special Publication*, *800*(218), 800–218. DOI: 10.6028/NIST.SP.800-218

Secinaro, S., Calandra, D., Secinaro, A., Muthurangu, V., & Biancone, P. (2021). The role of artificial intelligence in healthcare: A structured literature review. *BMC Medical Informatics and Decision Making*, *21*(1), 125. DOI: 10.1186/s12911-021-01488-9

Senn, H. M., & Thiel, W. (2009). QM/MM methods for biomolecular systems. *Angewandte Chemie International Edition*, *48*(7), 1198–1229. DOI: 10.1002/anie.200802019 PMID: 19173328

Seyyed-Kalantari, L., Zhang, H., McDermott, M. B. A., Chen, I. Y., & Ghassemi, M. (2021). Underdiagnosis bias of artificial intelligence algorithms applied to chest X-rays. *Nature Medicine*, *27*(12), 2176–2182. DOI: 10.1038/s41591-021-01595-0 PMID: 34893776

Shah, K., Kanani, S., Patel, S., Devani, M., Tanwar, S., Verma, A., & Sharma, R. (2023). Blockchain-based object detection scheme using federated learning. *Security and Privacy*, *6*(1), e276. Advance online publication. DOI: 10.1002/spy2.276

Shah, N. H., Milstein, A., & Bagley, S. C. (2019). Making machine learning models clinically useful. *Journal of the American Medical Association*, *322*(14), 1351–1352. DOI: 10.1001/jama.2019.10306 PMID: 31393527

Shahriar, S., Allana, S., Hazratifard, S. M., & Dara, R. (2023). A Survey of Privacy Risks and Mitigation Strategies in the Artificial Intelligence Life Cycle. *IEEE Access : Practical Innovations, Open Solutions*, *11*, 61829–61854. DOI: 10.1109/ACCESS.2023.3287195

Shah, W. S., Elkhwesky, Z., Jasim, K. M., Elkhwesky, E. F. Y., & Elkhwesky, F. F. Y. (2024). Artificial intelligence in healthcare services: Past, present and future research directions. *Review of Managerial Science*, *18*(3), 941–963. DOI: 10.1007/s11846-023-00699-w

Shanafelt, T. D., Dyrbye, L. N., Sinsky, C., Hasan, O., Satele, D., Sloan, J., & West, C. P. (2016). Relationship between clerical burden and characteristics of the electronic environment with physician burnout and professional satisfaction. *Mayo Clinic Proceedings*, *91*(7), 836–848. DOI: 10.1016/j.mayocp.2016.05.007 PMID: 27313121

Shanmuga, S. M., Jupally, S. H., & Vempalli, N. R. (2025). Models and Frameworks for Digital Preservation of Indigenous Knowledge Systems. In Revaluation and Preservation of Indigenous Knowledge Systems in Modern Society (pp. 511-534). IGI Global Scientific Publishing DOI: 10.4018/979-8-3693-7964-6.ch025

Shickel, B., Tighe, P. J., Bihorac, A., & Rashidi, P. (2018). Deep EHR: A survey of recent advances in deep learning techniques for electronic health record (EHR) analysis. *IEEE Journal of Biomedical and Health Informatics*, *22*(5), 1589–1604. DOI: 10.1109/JBHI.2017.2767063 PMID: 29989977

Shneiderman, B. (2020). Human-centered artificial intelligence: Reliable, safe & trustworthy. *International Journal of Human-Computer Interaction*, *36*(6), 495–504. DOI: 10.1080/10447318.2020.1741118

Shuaib, A. (2024). Transforming healthcare with AI: Promises, pitfalls, and pathways forward. *International Journal of General Medicine*, *17*, 1765–1771. DOI: 10.2147/IJGM.S449598 PMID: 38706749

Si, J. (2025). Exploring AI literacy, attitudes toward AI, and intentions to use AI in clinical contexts among healthcare students in Korea: A cross-sectional study. *BMC Medical Education*, *25*(1), 1233. DOI: 10.1186/s12909-025-07766-8

Sindakis, S., & Showkat, G. (2024). The digital revolution in India: Bridging the gap in rural technology adoption. *Journal of Innovation and Entrepreneurship*, *13*(1), 29. DOI: 10.1186/s13731-024-00380-w

Singh, S., ... (2025). An overview of 2025 AI trends in healthcare. HealthTech Magazine. Retrieved from https://healthtechmagazine.net/article/2025/01/overview-2025-ai-trends-healthcare

Singh, A. (2025). Chemical space exploration with quantum computing. *Nature Methods*, *22*(3), 452–452. DOI: 10.1038/s41592-025-02638-x PMID: 40074964

Singhal, K., Azizi, S., Tu, T., Mahdavi, S. S., Wei, J., Chung, H. W., Scales, N., Tanwani, A., Cole-Lewis, H., Pfohl, S., Payne, P., Seneviratne, M., Gamble, P., Kelly, C., Babiker, A., Schärli, N., Chowdhery, A., Mansfield, P., Demner-Fushman, D., & Natarajan, V. (2023). Large language models encode clinical knowledge. *Nature*, *620*(7972), 172–180. DOI: 10.1038/s41586-023-06291-2 PMID: 37438534

Singh, R. P., Hom, G. L., Abramoff, M. D., Campbell, J. P., & Chiang, M. F. (2020). Current challenges and barriers to real-world artificial intelligence adoption for the healthcare system, provider, and the patient. *Translational Vision Science & Technology*, *9*(2), 45. DOI: 10.1167/tvst.9.2.45 PMID: 32879755

SNOMED International. (2021). *SNOMED CT starter guide*. https://confluence.ihtsdotools.org/display/DOCSTART

Solanki, P., Grundy, J., & Hussain, W. (2023). Operationalising ethics in artificial intelligence for healthcare: A framework for AI developers. *AI and Ethics*, *3*(1), 223–240. DOI: 10.1007/s43681-022-00195-z

Solenov, D., Brieler, J., & Scherrer, J. F. (2018). The potential of quantum computing and machine learning to advance clinical research and change the practice of medicine. [REMOVED HYPERLINK FIELD]. *Mie Medical Journal*, *115*(5), 463–467. PMID: 30385997

Squires, M., Tao, X., Elangovan, S., Gururajan, R., Zhou, X., Acharya, U. R., & Li, Y. (2023). Deep learning and machine learning in psychiatry: A survey of current progress in depression detection, diagnosis and treatment. *Brain Informatics*, *10*(1), 10. DOI: 10.1186/s40708-023-00188-6 PMID: 37093301

Sreenu, N. (2019). Healthcare infrastructure development in rural India: A critical analysis of its status and future challenges. *British Journal of Health Care Management*, *25*(12), 1–9. DOI: 10.12968/bjhc.2018.0072

Srinivasan, S., Patel, T., Amer, S., & Rojas, J. C. (2024). How are US hospitals adopting artificial intelligence? Early evidence from 2022. *Health Affairs Scholar*, *2*(10), qxae123. Advance online publication. DOI: 10.1093/haschl/qxae123 PMID: 39403132

Srinivasulu, A., Agrawal, A., & Vedaiyan, R. (2025). Overcoming diagnostic and data privacy challenges in viral disease detection: An integrated approach using generative AI, vision transformers, explainable AI, and federated learning. *Frontiers in Virology*, *5*(1625855), 1625855. Advance online publication. DOI: 10.3389/fviro.2025.1625855

Steyvers, M., & Kumar, A. (2024). Three challenges for AI-assisted decision-making. Perspectives on Psychological Science: A Journal of the Association for Psychological Science, 19(5), 722–734. DOI: 10.1177/17456916231181102

Strika, Z., Petkovic, K., Likic, R., & Batenburg, R. (2025). Bridging healthcare gaps: A scoping review on AI in medical deserts. *Postgraduate Medical Journal*, *101*(1191), 4–16. DOI: 10.1093/postmj/qgae122 PMID: 39323384

Sufian, M. A., Alsadder, L., Hamzi, W., Zaman, S., Sagar, A. S. M. S., & Hamzi, B. (2024). Mitigating Algorithmic Bias in AI-Driven Cardiovascular Imaging for Fairer Diagnostics. *Diagnostics (Basel)*, *14*(23), 2675. DOI: 10.3390/diagnostics14232675

Sun, K., Liu, D., & Wang, J. (2022). Deep learning for neurodegenerative diseases. *Pattern Recognition Letters*, *157*, 69–76.

Sunki, K., Reddy, C. K. K., Reddy, D. M. K., & Doss, S. (2025). The role of quantum artificial intelligence in healthcare advancements. In *Cybernetics, Human Cognition, and Machine Learning in Communicative Applications* (pp. 137–158). Springer Nature Singapore. DOI: 10.1007/978-981-97-8533-9_10

Suvvari, T. K., Pradeep, K. V. S. B., Muppavarapu, R. S., & Nithya, A. (2025). The Potential Role of Quantum Computing in Biomedicine and Healthcare: The Next Frontier Beyond Artificial Intelligence. *Cureus*, *17*(4). Advance online publication. DOI: 10.7759/cureus.82759 PMID: 40406784

Taherdoost, H. (2023). Blockchain and healthcare: A critical analysis of progress and challenges in the last five years. *Blockchains*, *1*(2), 73–89. DOI: 10.3390/blockchains1020006

Taimoor, N., & Rehman, S. (2022). Reliable and Resilient AI and IoT-Based Personalised Healthcare Services: A Survey. *IEEE Access : Practical Innovations, Open Solutions*, *10*, 535–563. DOI: 10.1109/ACCESS.2021.3137364

Terra, M., Baklola, M., Ali, S., & El-Bastawisy, K. (2023). Opportunities, applications, challenges and ethical implications of artificial intelligence in psychiatry: A narrative review. *The Egyptian Journal of Neurology, Psychiatry and Neurosurgery*, *59*(1), 80. Advance online publication. DOI: 10.1186/s41983-023-00681-z

Thirunavukarasu, A. J., Ting, D. S. J., Elangovan, K., Gutierrez, L., Tan, T. F., & Ting, D. S. W. (2023). Large language models in medicine. *Nature Medicine*, *29*(8), 1930–1940. DOI: 10.1038/s41591-023-02448-8 PMID: 37460753

Thomas, V., Jenkins, J., & George, J. (2024). A systematic review and qualitative evidence synthesis of factors affecting mHealth adoption in India. *Oxford Open Digital Health*, *2*, oqae046. Advance online publication. DOI: 10.1093/oodh/oqae046 PMID: 40237014

Tirado-Domínguez, P., Perdomo-Ortiz, A., & Orús, R. (2025). Quantum approximate optimization algorithms for large-scale scheduling and healthcare logistics. *arXiv*. https://arxiv.org/abs/2501.04567

Tiwari, A., Mishra, S., & Kuo, T.-R. (2025). Current AI technologies in cancer diagnostics and treatment. *Molecular Cancer*, *24*(1), 159. DOI: 10.1186/s12943-025-02369-9

Tjhin, Y., Kewlani, B., Singh, H. K. S. I., & Pawa, N. (2024). Artificial intelligence in colorectal multidisciplinary team meetings. What are the medicolegal implications? *Colorectal Disease*, *26*(9), 1749–1752. DOI: 10.1111/codi.17091

Toni, E., Toni, E., Fereidooni, M., & Ayatollahi, H. (2024). Acceptance and use of extended reality in surgical training: An umbrella review. *Systematic Reviews*, *13*(1), 299. DOI: 10.1186/s13643-024-02723-w

Topol, E. (2019). *Deep Medicine: How Artificial Intelligence Can Make Healthcare Human Again*. Basic Books.

Topol, E. J. (2019). High-performance medicine: The convergence of human and artificial intelligence. *Nature Medicine*, *25*(1), 44–56. DOI: 10.1038/s41591-018-0300-7 PMID: 30617339

Torab-Miandoab, A., Samad-Soltani, T., Jodati, A., & Rezaei-Hachesu, P. (2023). Interoperability of heterogeneous health information systems: A systematic literature review. *BMC Medical Informatics and Decision Making*, *23*(1), 18. DOI: 10.1186/s12911-023-02115-5

Tun, H. M., Rahman, H. A., Naing, L., & Malik, O. A. (2025). Trust in Artificial Intelligence–Based Clinical Decision Support Systems Among Health Care Workers: Systematic Review. *Journal of Medical Internet Research*, *27*(1), e69678. DOI: 10.2196/69678

Ueda, D., Kakinuma, T., Fujita, S., Kamagata, K., Fushimi, Y., Ito, R., Matsui, Y., Nozaki, T., Nakaura, T., Fujima, N., Tatsugami, F., Yanagawa, M., Hirata, K., Yamada, A., Tsuboyama, T., Kawamura, M., Fujioka, T., & Naganawa, S. (2024). Fairness of artificial intelligence in healthcare: Review and recommendations. *Japanese Journal of Radiology*, *42*(1), 3–15. DOI: 10.1007/s11604-023-01474-3

Uganda, F. of M. K. I. U., & Mukamurera P., N. (2025). Telepresence in Healthcare: Engineering Remote Consultations. IDOSR JOURNAL OF BIOCHEMISTRY, BIOTECHNOLOGY AND ALLIED FIELDS, 10(1), 21–27. DOI: 10.59298/IDOSR/JBBAF/2025/1012127

Ullah, F.. (2022). What about the usability in low-code platforms? A systematic literature review. *Computer Standards & Interfaces*, *84*, 103698. DOI: 10.1016/j.csi.2022.103698

Union, E. (2024). *Regulation (EU) 2024/1689 of the European Parliament and of the Council laying down harmonised rules on artificial intelligence (Artificial Intelligence Act)*. Official Journal of the European Union.

Upreti, D., Yang, E., Kim, H., & Seo, C. (2024). A comprehensive survey on federated learning in the healthcare area: Concept and applications. Computer Modeling in Engineering & Sciences. *Computer Modeling in Engineering & Sciences*, *140*(3), 2239–2274. DOI: 10.32604/cmes.2024.048932

Uymaz, A. O., Uymaz, P., & Akgül, Y. (2024a). The shift from disease-centric to patient-centric healthcare: Assessing physicians' intention to use AI doctors. *Environment and Social Psychology*, *9*(4). Advance online publication. DOI: 10.54517/esp.v9i4.2308

Uymaz, P., Uymaz, A. O., & Akgül, Y. (2024). Assessing the behavioral intention of individuals to use an AI doctor at the primary, secondary, and tertiary care levels. *International Journal of Human-Computer Interaction*, *40*(18), 5229–5246. DOI: 10.1080/10447318.2023.2233126

Uzuner, Ö., South, B. R., Shen, S., & DuVall, S. L. (2011). 2010 i2b2/VA challenge on concepts, assertions, and relations in clinical text. *Journal of the American Medical Informatics Association : JAMIA*, *18*(5), 552–556. DOI: 10.1136/amiajnl-2011-000203 PMID: 21685143

Vale, M. D. (2024). Moral entrepreneurship and the ethics of artificial intelligence in digital psychiatry. *Socius: Sociological Research for a Dynamic World*, *10*, 23780231241259641. Advance online publication. DOI: 10.1177/23780231241259641 van der Laan, A. L., Boenink, M., Broerse, J. E., & Spreeuwenberg, P. (2022). Systematic review of barriers to and facilitators of artificial intelligence adoption in healthcare organizations. *Journal of Healthcare Management, 67*(5), 359–374.

Van Veen, D., Van Uden, C., Blankemeier, L., Delbrouck, J. B., Aali, A., Bluethgen, C., & Langlotz, C. P. (2024). Adapted large language models can outperform medical experts in clinical text annotation. *Nature Medicine, 30*(4), 1088–1097. DOI: 10.1038/s41591-024-02855-5 PMID: 38413730

Veinot, T. C., Mitchell, H., & Ancker, J. S. (2018). Good intentions are not enough: How informatics interventions can worsen inequality. *Journal of the American Medical Informatics Association : JAMIA, 25*(8), 1080–1088. DOI: 10.1093/jamia/ocy052 PMID: 29788380

Venkatesh, V., & Bala, H. (2008). Technology acceptance model 3 and a research agenda on interventions. *Decision sciences, 39*(2), 273-315. Venkatesh, V., & Davis, F. D. (2000). A theoretical extension of the technology acceptance model: Four longitudinal field studies. *Management Science, 46*(2), 186–204. DOI: 10.1287/mnsc.46.2.186.11926

Venkatesh, V., Morris, M. G., Davis, G. B., & Davis, F. D. (2003). User acceptance of information technology: Toward a unified view. *Management Information Systems Quarterly, 27*(3), 425–478. DOI: 10.2307/30036540

Venkatesh, V., Thong, J. Y., & Xu, X. (2012). Consumer acceptance and use of information technology: Extending the unified theory of acceptance and use of technology. *Management Information Systems Quarterly, 36*(1), 157–178. DOI: 10.2307/41410412

Verghese, A., Shah, N. H., & Harrington, R. A. (2018). What this computer needs is a physician: Humanism and artificial intelligence. *Journal of the American Medical Association, 319*(1), 19–20. DOI: 10.1001/jama.2017.19198 PMID: 29261830

Vokinger, K. N., Feuerriegel, S., & Kesselheim, A. S. (2021). Mitigating bias in machine learning for medicine. *Communications Medicine, 1*(1), 25. https://www.nature.com/articles/s43856-021-00028-w. DOI: 10.1038/s43856-021-00028-w PMID: 34522916

Voss, E. A., Makadia, R., Matcho, A., Ma, Q., Knoll, C., Schuemie, M., DeFalco, F. J., Londhe, A., Zhu, V., & Ryan, P. B. (2015). Feasibility and utility of applications of the common data model to multiple, disparate observational health databases. *Journal of the American Medical Informatics Association : JAMIA, 22*(3), 553–564. DOI: 10.1093/jamia/ocu023 PMID: 25670757

Wadden, J. J. (2022). Defining the undefinable: The black box problem in healthcare artificial intelligence. *Journal of Medical Ethics*, *48*(10), 764–768. DOI: 10.1136/medethics-2021-107529 PMID: 34290113

Wagner, G., Ringeval, M., Raymond, L., & Paré, G. (2025). Digital health competences and AI beliefs as conditions for the practice of evidence-based medicine: A study of prospective physicians in Canada. *Medical Education Online*, *30*(1), 2459910. Advance online publication. DOI: 10.1080/10872981.2025.2459910 PMID: 39890587

Wakili, A., & Bakkali, S. (2024). Internet of Things in healthcare: An adaptive ethical framework for IoT in digital health. *Clinical eHealth, 7*, 92–105. DOI: 10.1016/j.ceh.2024.07.001

Wang, D., & Qin, Q. (2024). Artificial intelligence technology on layered water injection in oilfield development process. *International Journal of e-Collaboration*, *20*(1), 1–15. DOI: 10.4018/IJeC.352596

Wang, Y., Wang, L., Rastegar-Mojarad, M., Moon, S., Shen, F., Afzal, N., Liu, S., Zeng, Y., Mehrabi, S., Sohn, S., & Liu, H. (2020). Clinical information extraction applications: A literature review. *Journal of Biomedical Informatics*, *77*, 34–49. DOI: 10.1016/j.jbi.2017.11.011 PMID: 29162496

Wang, Z., Cao, L., Jin, Q., Chan, J., Wan, N., Afzali, B., Cho, H.-J., Choi, C.-I., Emamverdi, M., Gill, M. K., Kim, S.-H., Li, Y., Liu, Y., Luo, Y., Ong, H., Rousseau, J. F., Sheikh, I., Wei, J. J., Xu, Z., & Sun, J. (2025). A foundation model for human-AI collaboration in medical literature mining. *Nature Communications*, *16*(1), 8361. DOI: 10.1038/s41467-025-62058-5

Warnat-Herresthal, S., Schultze, H., Shastry, K. L., Manamohan, S., Mukherjee, S., Garg, V., & Schultze, J. L. (2024). Swarm learning for decentralized and confidential clinical machine learning. *Nature*, *625*(7995), 545–550. DOI: 10.1038/s41586-023-06851-5 PMID: 34040261

Weiner, M. W., Veitch, D. P., Aisen, P. S., Beckett, L. A., Cairns, N. J., & Cedarbaum, J. (2020). The Alzheimer's Disease Neuroimaging Initiative: A review of papers published since its inception. *Alzheimer's & Dementia*, *16*(12), 1551–1581.

Weng, L., Ren, H., Xu, R., Xu, J., Lin, J., Shen, J. W., & Zheng, Y. (2025). Translocation mechanism of anticancer drugs through membrane with the assistance of graphene quantum dot. *Colloids and Surfaces. B, Biointerfaces*, *245*, 114340. DOI: 10.1016/j.colsurfb.2024.114340 PMID: 39476655

Whitelaw, A., Mamas, M. A., Topol, E., & Van Spall, H. G. C. (2020). Applications of digital health in the COVID-19 pandemic: Policy implications and lessons. *Journal of the American College of Cardiology*, *76*(23), 2980–2995. DOI: 10.1016/S2589-7500(20)30142-4 PMID: 32835201

Wilson, H. J., & Daugherty, P. R. (2018). Collaborative intelligence: Humans and AI are joining forces. *Harvard Business Review*, *96*(4), 114–123.

Wong, Z. S.-Y., Gong, Y., & Ushiro, S. (2025). A pathway from fragmentation to interoperability through standards-based enterprise architecture to enhance patient safety. *NPJ Digital Medicine*, *8*(1), 41. DOI: 10.1038/s41746-025-01442-3

World Economic Forum. (2023). *Quantum computing applications in healthcare and life sciences*. World Economic Forum.

World Economic Forum. (2025). 6 ways AI is transforming healthcare. Retrieved from https://www.weforum.org/stories/2025/03/ai-transforming-global-health/

World Health Organization. (2021). Ethics and governance of artificial intelligence for health. World Health Organization. https://apps.who.int/iris/handle/10665/341996

World Health Organization. (2023). Dementia: Key facts. https://www.who.int/news-room/fact-sheets/detail/dementia

Xie, Y., Wang, X., Yang, H., Zhang, J., Wang, H., Yan, Z., Yang, J., Yan, Z., Hao, Z., Liu, P., Kuang, Y., & Ye, Z. (2025). Swarm learning network for privacy-preserving and collaborative deep learning assisted diagnosis of fracture: A multi-center diagnostic study. *Frontiers in Medicine*, *12*, 1534117. DOI: 10.3389/fmed.2025.1534117 PMID: 40678137

Xu, J., Glicksberg, B. S., Su, C., Walker, P., & Johnson, K. (2021). Federated learning for healthcare: Systematic review and roadmap. *Journal of the American Medical Informatics Association : JAMIA*, *28*(9), 1980–1993.

Xu, R., & Wang, Z. (2024). Generative artificial intelligence in healthcare from the perspective of digital media: Applications, opportunities and challenges. *Heliyon*, *10*(12), e32364. DOI: 10.1016/j.heliyon.2024.e32364

Yadav, N. (2025). AI for mental health: The use of chatbots and NLP to support therapy and early detection. *International Scientific Journal of Engineering and Management*, *04*(05), 1–7. DOI: 10.55041/ISJEM03402

Yang, Q., Liu, Y., Chen, T., & Tong, Y. (2019). Federated machine learning: Concept and applications. *ACM Transactions on Intelligent Systems and Technology*, *10*(2), 12. Advance online publication. DOI: 10.1145/3298981

Yang, Y. (2024). Application of wearable devices based on artificial intelligence sensors in sports human health monitoring. *Measurement. Sensors*, *33*, 101086. DOI: 10.1016/j.measen.2024.101086

Yazici, C.. (2022). Experimental evidence of effective human–AI collaboration in medical decision-making. *Scientific Reports*, *12*(1), 14952. DOI: 10.1038/s41598-022-18751-2 PMID: 36056152

Ye, J., Woods, D., Jordan, N., & Starren, J. (2024). The role of artificial intelligence for the application of integrating electronic health records and patient-generated data in clinical decision support. *AMIA Joint Summits on Translational Science Proceedings AMIA Summit on Translational Science*, *2024*, 459–467. PMID: 38827061

Yuan, K. (2024). Research on music teaching systems assisted by artificial intelligence. *International Journal of e-Collaboration*, *20*(1), 1–17. DOI: 10.4018/IJeC.349746

Zhang, X., Ma, L., Sun, D., Yi, M., & Wang, Z. (2024). Artificial Intelligence in Telemedicine: A Global Perspective Visualization Analysis. *Telemedicine Journal and e-Health*, *30*(7), e1909–e1922. DOI: 10.1089/tmj.2023.0704

Zhang, Y., Li, X., & Chen, Z. (2025). Quantum signal processing for high-dimensional medical imaging. *IEEE Transactions on Medical Imaging*, *44*(2), 456–469. DOI: 10.1109/TMI.2024.3398765

Zhou, J., Liu, J., & Ye, J. (2020). Graph neural networks in Alzheimer's disease analysis. *Frontiers in Neuroscience*, *14*, 143.

Zhu, X., Suk, H. I., & Shen, D. (2016). A novel matrix-similarity based loss function for Alzheimer's disease diagnosis. *Medical Image Analysis*, *33*, 159–177.

Zhu, Y. (2025). Decentralized altruism: How Solo-Founder AI-driven nonprofit mode (SFADNM) with anarchist principles is reshaping nonprofits in the digital age. *Proceedings of the World Conference on Social Sciences and Humanities*, 2(1), 15–34. DOI: 10.33422/shconf.v2i1.1020

Zhu, Y., Matsuyama, Y., Ohashi, Y., & Setoguchi, S. (2017). When to conduct probabilistic linkage vs. deterministic linkage? A simulation study. *Journal of Biomedical Informatics*, *27*, 96–105. PMID: 26004791

Zirikly, A., Desmet, B., Newman-Griffis, D., Marfeo, E. E., McDonough, C., Goldman, H., & Chan, L. (2022). Information extraction framework for disability determination using a mental functioning use-case. *JMIR Medical Informatics*, *10*(3), e32245. DOI: 10.2196/32245 PMID: 35302510

Zondag, A. G. M., Rozestraten, R., Grimmelikhuijsen, S. G., Jongsma, K. R., Van Solinge, W. W., Bots, M. L., Vernooij, R. W. M., & Haitjema, S. (2024). The Effect of Artificial Intelligence on Patient-Physician Trust: Cross-Sectional Vignette Study. *Journal of Medical Internet Research*, *26*, e50853. DOI: 10.2196/50853

Zreikat, A. I., AlArnaout, Z., Abadleh, A., Elbasi, E., & Mostafa, N. (2025). The Integration of the Internet of Things (IoT) Applications into 5G Networks: A Review and Analysis. *Computers*, *14*(7), 250. DOI: 10.3390/computers14070250

Zukaib, U., Cui, X., Hassan, M., Harris, S., Hadi, H. J., & Zheng, C. (2023). Blockchain and machine learning in EHR security: A systematic review. *IEEE Access : Practical Innovations, Open Solutions*, *11*, 130230–130256. DOI: 10.1109/ACCESS.2023.3333229

About the Contributors

Jingyuan Zhao obtained her PhD in Management Science and Engineering from University of Science and Technology of China. She completed four postdoctoral programs respectively in Mathematical and Computational Science with University of Toronto Mississauga, in Innovation and Governance with University of Toronto, in Management of Technology with Université du Québec à Montréal, and in Technological Economics with Harbin Institute of Technology. Dr. Zhao's research expertise includes management of technology innovation, innovation and entrepreneurship, behaviour and information technology, human-computer interaction, and science and technology policy. She has teaching experience of 15 years at the graduate and undergraduate level. Research portfolio includes peer-reviewed articles in highly regarded journals, authored books, multiple book chapters, and conference presentations. Dr. Zhao also has extensive industry experience and provides consulting services to major corporations, such as China Mobile. She serves as editor-in-chief of International Journal of e-Collaboration (IJeC).

***

Sharmila A is an Assistant Professor with a background in dentistry, hospital administration, and academic research. She earned her Bachelor of Dental Surgery (BDS) from Saveetha University and subsequently completed a Fellowship in Medical Cosmetology (FMC) from ILAMED. She also holds a Postgraduate Diploma in Medico Legal Systems from Symbiosis University and an MBA in Hospital Management from Saveetha School of Management. Currently, she is pursuing her PhD in Hospital Management, further deepening her expertise in healthcare systems and operations. Her career spans over a decade with 4 years of clinical experience, 3 years in hospital administration, 1 year in human resources, and 3 years in academia. Dr. Sharmila brings a well-rounded perspective to healthcare, combining medical knowledge, legal understanding, and managerial skills to drive quality care and organizational efficiency.

Frank Billingsley has had a diverse and extensive career spanning multiple domains, including education, social services, and administration. He has had extensive international experience, and qualifications in higher education administration and teaching are prominent, with notable roles as a program director, head of department, and faculty member at various institutions. He has contributed to academic publications and presented at conferences on topics related to higher education and gender studies. Beyond academia, the candidate has a social work and counseling background, demonstrating a versatile skill set. His precise community service and involvement in various organizations further underscore their commitment to positively impacting.

Rahul Biswas is a computer science engineer from Bangladesh who has had an exciting journey in the field of technology. He earned his bachelor's degree in computer science and engineering, specializing in Information Security, from the esteemed Vellore Institute of Technology (VIT) in Vellore, India, in 2021. He then completed his Master's degree at the renowned Indian Institute of Technology Ropar in 2023. During his academic pursuit, he was part of a significant government project known as iHub-AWaDH (Agriculture and Water Technology Development Hub) at IIT Ropar. Under the expert guidance of the Domain Coordinator, he embarked on a research endeavor that resulted in the creation of an Intelligent Chatbot Assistant in the Agriculture Domain. This project showcased his proficiency in Natural Language Processing (NLP) and Agriculture Data Collection and emphasized the potential of technology in agriculture. He gained practical experience through an internship at CTG IT Service Limited, where he took on roles as a web developer and software tester. Furthermore, he extended his reach beyond national borders by actively participating in international conferences as a volunteer. His research interests encompass a wide range of areas, including Agriculture Technology Development, Natural Language Processing (NLP), Applied Machine Learning, and Agriculture Data Analysis..

G.S. Gigi is an Associate Professor at Saveetha School of Management, SIMATS, Chennai, brings 16 years of academic experience with a strong focus on research in human resource management, particularly employee engagement in the IT sector. She is currently guiding three Ph.D. research scholars and serves as a Research Advisory Committee (RAC) member for ten others across various universities. Her scholarly work includes numerous presentations and publications at national and international conferences and in reputed journals. Her research is driven by a commitment to addressing real-world HR challenges, blending academic rigor with practical insight to advance the field meaningfully.

C. Daniel Nesa Kumar MCA., M.Phil, Ph.D., is having 15+ years of teaching experience and currently working as Assistant Professor in the Department of Computer Applications(BCA) at Sri Ramakrishna College of Arts and Science, Coimbatore. He has completed his B.Sc Computer Science at CSI Bishop Appasamy College of Arts and Science, Coimbatore. His Masters in Computer Applications at Bishop Heber College, Trichy, M.Phil and Ph.D in Computer Science at Hindusthan College of Arts and Science – Bharathiar University, Coimbatore. His area of specialization is Networking, His research interest includes Digital Image Processing, Cloud Computing, Machine Learning etc. He has published several research papers in the field of Networking, Machine Learning, Image Processing in many reputed International Journals. Also presented his research work at various International and National conferences.

K. C. Raja Shree is a biomedical engineer with a doctorate in Healthcare Management and eight years of academic experience. She is known for her energy, enthusiasm, and multitasking abilities in academics and beyond. Her expertise lies in hospital quality management, supported by a proficiency certification as Quality Coordinator in Hospitals. She has published in Web of Science, Scopus, and UGC-listed journals and actively participates in conferences, workshops, and MOOCs to stay updated. Recipient of the Young Academician Award and Young Teacher Award, she is recognized for her dedication to teaching, research, and student development. Her professional interests also extend to organizing academic and cultural programs, contributing to a holistic learning environment

Noboranjan Dey currently serving as a Lecturer in the Computer Science department under the faculty of science and technology at American International University Bangladesh. He was granted an ICCR scholarship for his Master's degree. He pursued M.Tech in Computer Science and Engineering from National Institute of Technology Warangal, India, and Bachelor's degree from AIUB. His current research interests include Deep Learning, Neural Networks, Computer Vision, Image Processing, Medical Imaging, Biometrics.

Rameshkumar J is a Ph.D. Degree Candidate in the Department of Electronics and Communication Engineering, K.S.R. College of Engineering, Tamil Nadu, India. His research interests include signal and image processing. He has 15 years of academic experience and is also an active professional member of IETE and ISTE.

Hanh Le is a passionate researcher and accomplished Full Stack Software Developer with deep expertise in software development, data analytics, data science, and cloud computing. She holds a Ph.D. in Information Technology and a Master's in Computer Science, bringing both academic rigor and a solution-driven mindset to her work. With extensive experience in front-end and back-end development, she specializes in scalable, database-driven applications that support evidence-based decision-making. Dr. Le has led transformative tech initiatives across healthcare, law enforcement, and retail, translating complex needs into high-performing systems. She values interdisciplinary collaboration, believing that impactful innovation often arises at the intersection of fields. Her blend of technical skill, research excellence, and collaborative spirit continues to drive progress in academia and industry alike.

P. Praveen Kumar holds an MCom, MBA, and PhD in Finance from Pondicherry University. He secured the University 1st Rank in his Under Graduation. His teaching interests include Financial Accounting, Financial Management, Mergers & Acquisitions, Security Analysis & Portfolio Management, and other finance-related courses. His research interests extend to interdisciplinary areas.

Nehal Padalkar is an aspiring computer science professional specializing in Artificial Intelligence, with a strong focus on natural language processing, generative AI, and user-centered application design. She is currently pursuing a Bachelor of Technology in Computer Science and Engineering (Artificial Intelligence) at Jain (Deemed-to-be University), Bengaluru, where she maintains a strong academic record. Nehal has gained hands-on experience through internships at Rural Handmade (London, remote) and NexGen Architects (Bengaluru, hybrid), contributing to AI-driven solutions and collaborative product development. Her project portfolio includes real-time AI body-language detection using MediaPipe and OpenCV, a university policy conversational question-answering system using LangChain and Gemini API, and an AI smart PDF summarizer leveraging large language models for multi-format document processing. His technical expertise spans Python, MySQL, computer vision, NLP, RAG systems, LangChain, LangGraph, TensorFlow, OpenCV, and vector databases, along with experience in Figma-based interface design. She holds multiple certifications, including Harvard's CS50P in Python and advanced courses in cloud computing, neural networks, and agentic AI engineering. Known for strong problem-solving ability, leadership, and communication skills, Nehal is building a career at the intersection of AI engineering, human–computer interaction, and intelligent automation, with active contributions on GitHub and LinkedIn and a growing portfolio of practical AI applications.

Amitabh Patnaik is a seasoned academician and management scholar with a Ph.D. in Organizational Management. He holds an MBA with specializations in Marketing and Human Resource Management, along with a B.Tech in Agriculture, reflecting his strong interdisciplinary foundation. With over ten years and nine months of teaching experience, Dr. Patnaik has been contributing to higher education as a Professor at Dr. D. Y. Patil Institute of Management Studies since August 2008. His core areas of expertise include Organizational Management and Economics. He is proficient in SPSS and applies quantitative analytical techniques in both research and teaching. Dr. Patnaik's research interests encompass Agri-tourism, Servant Leadership, Behavioral Finance, Fintech, Leader–Member Exchange (LMX), Employee Engagement, and Organizational Behavior. His work reflects a commitment to integrating traditional sectors such as agriculture with contemporary management practices and emerging financial technologies. A dedicated educator and researcher, Dr. Patnaik actively engages in academic research, scholarly publications, and thought leadership, contributing meaningfully to the advancement of management education and organizational studies.

R. Keerthana is an Assistant Professor in the Department of Computer Science and Engineering at K.S.R. College of Engineering, Tiruchengode, Namakkal. She obtained her B.E. degree in Computer Science and Engineering from Vivekanandha Institute of Engineering and Technology for Women, affiliated with Anna University, Chennai. In 2018, she secured the 25th rank from Anna University and received the Best Outgoing Student Award from Vivekanandha College of Technology for Women. She has four years of teaching experience and one year of industrial experience. Ms. Keerthana also serves as a Placement Trainer at K.S.R. College of Engineering and has been recognized as a Wipro Certified Faculty by Wipro Limited. She has attended and presented papers at five international and national conferences and seminars, participated in various Faculty Development Programmes, and published two research articles in reputed journals. Additionally, she has delivered guest lectures at several institutions.

Manju Priya R, currently an Associate Professor at the School of Commerce, JAIN (Deemed-to-be) University in Bangalore, holds a M.Com., M.Phil, MBA, PGDCA, and Ph.D. She is a distinguished educator known for her ability to inspire, engage and guide students towards high academic achievement. With 20 years of teaching experience and 10 years of research expertise, she excels in maintaining students' interest and fostering a dynamic learning environment. She has guided numerous undergraduate, postgraduate and M.Phil students and is presently mentoring Ph.D candidates. Her academic interests are focused on Marketing and Human Resources(HR). She has served as a resource person for various colleges, sharing her insights with both students and faculty members. She has actively participated in over 50 National and International seminars and conferences, and has published more than 45 research papers in UGC care listed journals, Scopus, WOS, ABDC. Furthermore, she has authored 3 books and she has also contributed 10 book chapters to various academic publications.

Ravikumar R. N. is currently a Postdoctoral researcher at Universiti Malaysia Perlis, Malaysia. Also, working as an Associate Professor in the department of Computer Engineering at Marwadi University, Rajkot, Gujarat. He has 12+ years of national and international teaching experience. He completed his PhD at Amity University, Rajasthan, M.E at VMRF Deemed University, B.E at Anna University, Chennai. He is the co-founder of the Research Activities Club at Marwadi University and trains students on research activities, which leads to the publication of 7 Scopus/SCI journals, 20 Book chapters, 25 Conference papers, and 10 patents. His specialization is ML, DL, Federated Learning, Recommendation Systems, and Optimization Techniques.

Mahfujur Rahman is an Assistant Professor in the Department of Computer Science at American International University-Bangladesh (AIUB). He received his B.Sc. in Computer Science and M.Sc. in Computer Science with a specialization in Intelligent Systems from AIUB. He began his academic career at AIUB as a Teaching Assistant and later served as an Instructor and Lecturer before being promoted to Assistant Professor in 2023. In addition to his academic experience, he has industry exposure as a Web Application Developer at RF Builder Ltd., where he was involved in web application development and maintenance. He has over five years of experience supervising undergraduate thesis projects and actively contributes to research and academic activities. His research interests include Intelligent Systems, Natural Language Processing, Machine Learning, Data Science, Medical Image Processing, Internet of Things (IoT), and Big Data Analytics. He also serves as a reviewer for several local and international peer-reviewed journals and conferences.

Mrinmoy Roy is an interdisciplinary researcher and educator specializing in AI-driven healthcare, public policy, and behavioral science. He is Associate Professor and Research Lead at NSB Academy, Bengaluru, where he leads multidisciplinary projects in healthcare analytics, patient experience design, and digital health innovation. He earned his PhD in Management (Operations) from the Mittal School of Business, Lovely Professional University, with doctoral research focused on the adoption of AI-based diagnostic interventions for diabetes care in India. His scholarly work bridges behavioral science, digital health governance, and quantitative modeling, employing structural equation modeling, rare-event simulation, and agent-based policy modeling. His publications appear in reputed outlets including Hospital Topics (Taylor & Francis) and the Journal of Public Health (Springer), along with contributions to IntechOpen volumes, ICSSR monographs, and practitioner-oriented books on health IT. Dr. Roy has filed multiple patents, reflecting his emphasis on translational research and innovation. With prior leadership experience in AstraZeneca, Glenmark, Lupin, and Cipla, he integrates academic rigor with practical perspectives on healthcare operations and digital transformation. He has presented his research at leading forums such as IIM Bangalore, University Putra Malaysia, Goa Institute of Management, Universitas Andalas, and the Bengaluru Tech Summit. His current research interests include behavioral decision-making in healthcare policy, equity in digital health adoption, data governance in AI-enabled care, and sustainable healthcare operations. He serves as a peer reviewer for international journals and actively mentors students and professionals in digital health and applied analytics. Recipient of honors including "Pride of Indian Education: Most Profound Researcher & Educationist of the Year" and "Most Distinguished Professor of Business Management," Prof. Roy has over 40 publications and more than two decades of combined industry and academic experience.

Aarthi S is a dedicated Assistant Professor in Computer Science with over six years of teaching experience. She is currently pursuing her Ph.D. at Marwadi University, Gujarat, and holds an M.Phil. and MCA from Bharathiar University, Tamil Nadu. Throughout her academic career, Aarthi has specialized in programming languages such as C++, Java, and C, and contributed to research in recommender systems and AI-related data privacy. She has published journal articles, contributed to book chapters, and actively participated in technical workshops. Known for her student mentorship and engagement in academic events, Aarthi remains committed to fostering innovation and excellence in computer science education.

S.Hemalatha,M.E., working as an Assistant Professor in the Department of Computer Science and Engineering at K.S.R. College of Engineering (Autonomous), Namakkal, Tamil Nadu. Her area of specialization includes Artificial Intelligence and Machine Learning, Networking and Cybersecurity. She has obtained her Bachelor of Engineering degree in Computer Science and Engineering from Hindusthan College of Engineering and Technology and Master of Engineering degree in Computer Science and Engineering from Hindusthan College of Engineering and Technology. She is very innovative and active in exploring new technologies. She has published number of research papers in reputed International Conferences and Scopus Index.

S. Savitha is an Assistant Professor in the Department of Computer Science and Engineering, K.S.R. College of Engineering (Autonomous), India. She received her Master of Engineering degree in Computer Science and Engineering in 2012 from Anna University, Chennai, India. She completed her Ph.D. degree in Faculty of Information in Communication Engineering in 2024 from Anna University, Chennai, India. She has published more than 40 papers in referred journals and conference proceedings. Her research interest includes Data Mining, Big Data, Cloud computing, Databases,Artificial Intelligence and Machine Learning. She is a professional member of ISTE. She has published 2 patents and granted 4 design patents.

N Sathyanarayana has over 15 years of teaching experience at both undergraduate and postgraduate levels. He holds a Master of Business Administration degree from VTU and a Master of Commerce degree from Periyar University. He has completed his Ph.D. in Banking and Finance from Dayananda Sagar University. Currently, he serves as an Assistant Professor in the School of Commerce at Jain (Deemed-to-be University), Bangalore. He has published 24 research papers in international journals, including three indexed in Scopus, and seven papers in national journals. Additionally, he has presented 14 research papers at international conferences and 11 at national conferences. He has co-authored two books at the national level and contributed 21 Scopus-indexed book chapters.

Kazi Tanvir is a Bangladeshi computer-science lecturer and early-career researcher whose work joins machine learning, explainable AI and bioinformatics. He currently teaches in the Department of Computer Science at American International University-Bangladesh (AIUB). Kazi Tanvir has an MSc in Data Science at Vellore Institute of Technology (VIT), Vellore, Tamil Nadu, India. He has completed his BSc in Computer Science and Engineering majoring in Computational Theory from American International University-Bangladesh (AIUB). He has passed his Secondary and Higher Secondary from Birshrestha Noor Mohammad Public College, Dhaka. He aims to become a successful researcher in his domain. His fields of interest are Data Science, Image Processing, and Biostatistics. He has taken part in various international conferences and also have published some papers, data, book chapters and patents.

SathyaU. is an Assistant Professor in the Department of Computer Science and Engineering at Vivekanandha College of Technology for Women, Tiruchengode, Namakkal. She obtained her B.E. degree in Computer Science and Engineering from Vivekanandha Institute of Engineering and Technology for Women, affiliated with Anna University, Chennai. In 2016. She has 2.5 years of teaching experience . She has attended and presented papers at five international and national conferences and seminars, participated in various Faculty Development Programmes and workshops, and published two research articles in reputed journals.

Savdeep Vasudeva is an academic and researcher in the field of Business Administration with over 24 years of experience spanning teaching, research, and academic leadership. He is currently serving as Associate Professor at Amity Business School, Amity University Rajasthan, Jaipur. He holds a PhD in Business Administration (Management) from I. K. Gujral Punjab Technical University, completed in 2017, with his doctoral research focused on Customer Perception Towards Mobile Banking in Punjab – A Study of Personal Banking. His research expertise includes artificial intelligence, healthcare, technology adoption, e-services, and mobile commerce. Dr. Vasudeva has a strong publication record, including research papers indexed in Scopus, Web of Science, ABDC listed journals, and other reputed outlets. Throughout his career, Dr. Vasudeva has been engaged in guiding students, contributing to curriculum development, and advancing research in emerging areas at the intersection of technology and management. His academic qualifications include a B.Sc., MBA (IT), and PhD, and his work continues to focus on artificial intelligence applications in management, technology-enabled banking, and digital service adoption in emerging markets. He is currently based at Amity Business School, Amity University Rajasthan, India.

Index

F

H

I

L

M

N

O

www.ingramcontent.com/pod-product-compliance
Lightning Source LLC
LaVergne TN
LVHW081318300926
849161LV00008B/1797